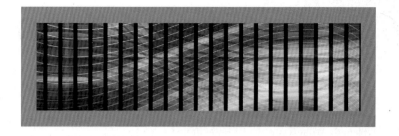

STUTTERING

An Integrated Approach to Its Nature and Treatment

FOURTH EDITION

BARRY GUITAR, PH.D.

Professor Department of Communication Sciences
the University of Vermont
Burlington, Vermont

Wolters Kluwer | Lippincott Williams & Wilkins
Health

Philadelphia · Baltimore · New York · London
Buenos Aires · Hong Kong · Sydney · Tokyo

Acquisitions Editor: Michael Nobel
Product Manager: Staci Wolfson
Marketing Manager: Shauna Kelley
Designer: Joan Wendt
Artist: Bot Roda
Compositor: SPi Global

4th Edition
Copyright © 2014 Lippincott Williams & Wilkins, a Wolters Kluwer business.

351 West Camden Street   **Two Commerce Square**
Baltimore, MD 21201   **2001 Market Street**
                                 Philadelphia, PA 19103

Printed in China

Library of Congress Cataloging-in-Publication Data
Guitar, Barry.
    Stuttering : an integrated approach to its nature and treatment / Barry Guitar. — 4th ed.
       p. ; cm.
    Includes bibliographical references and index.
    ISBN 978-1-60831-004-3 (pbk.)
  I. Title.
    [DNLM: 1. Stuttering—diagnosis. 2. Stuttering—etiology. 3. Stuttering—therapy. WM 475.7]
    616.85'54—dc23

                                         2012034909

DISCLAIMER
Care has been taken to confirm the accuracy of the information present and to describe generally accepted practices. However, the authors, editors, and publisher are not responsible for errors or omissions or for any consequences from application of the information in this book and make no warranty, expressed or implied, with respect to the currency, completeness, or accuracy of the contents of the publication. Application of this information in a particular situation remains the professional responsibility of the practitioner; the clinical treatments described and recommended may not be considered absolute and universal recommendations.

To purchase additional copies of this book, call our customer service department at (800) 638-3030 or fax orders to (301) 223-2320. International customers should call (301) 223-2300.

Visit Lippincott Williams & Wilkins on the Internet: http://www.lww.com. Lippincott Williams & Wilkins customer service representatives are available from 8:30 am to 6:00 pm, EST.

9 8 7 6 5 4 3

CONTENTS

PREFACE

This 4th edition of *Stuttering: An Integrated Approach to Its Nature and Treatment* contains some major renovations. As before, I've included new research that has been published since the previous edition. Most of the new studies have been in the areas of (1) constitutional factors and (2) developmental, environmental, and learning factors. To make this dense material more digestible, I've divided each of these areas into a chapter that gives a broad overview of the research and a chapter that gives the fine details.

The chapters on assessment and treatment have been updated as new material has become available and as I've gained a better understanding of how to assess and treat clients. I think the chapters on treating school-age children and on treating adolescents and adults are most different from those in the previous edition. My clinical experiences in these intervening seven years have given me a better sense of how to sequence treatment and what are crucial experiences for clients.

Finally, I have provided some video clips online at LWW's *thePoint* to illustrate our work with a variety of clients. These, along with new test material and PowerPoint slides, will make this a more complete text from which to teach.

Comments on the last edition—from students, clinicians, and instructors—have made this edition better. I look forward to hearing how it works for you.

— *Barry Guitar*

ACKNOWLEDGMENTS

Many people have made this book a pleasure to write, especially the individuals who stutter and the students who have worked with me over the span of 40-something years.

I would also like to thank my publisher, Lippincott Williams & Wilkins, who took a big chance on me and this text more than 20 years ago. One of their fine staff members, Staci Wolfson, has managed this project from beginning to end, with encouragement, direction, gentle prodding, and tact. I am most grateful to her. In addition, I appreciate the support from Mike Nobel, acquisitions editor; Shauna Kelley, marketing manager; Jen Clements, art director; and Bot Roda, the artist whose fine work you see throughout the book.

As with earlier editions, Rebecca McCauley and Charles Barasch have contributed immensely to this text in many ways, from editing my chaotic writing to suggesting drawings and ancillary material to providing organizational ideas. I am indeed obliged to them.

Finally, I wish to thank my wife, Carroll, who has listened patiently to my endless talk of stuttering and who has also carefully edited every page and chased down every reference, in addition to giving great help with the video clips.

This edition is dedicated to Cully Gage and the memory of Charles Van Riper.

1

Nature of Stuttering

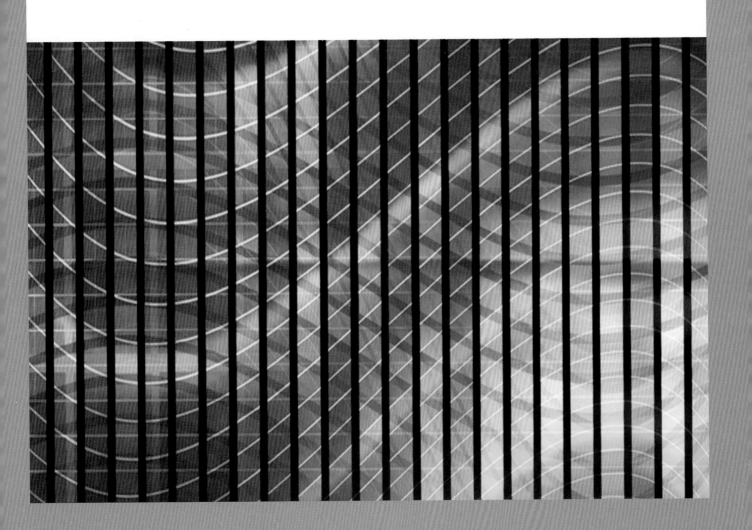

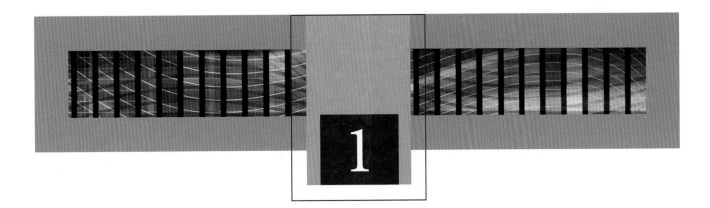

Introduction to Stuttering

CHAPTER OBJECTIVES

After studying this chapter, readers should be able to:

- Explain why it is good practice to use the term "person who stutters" rather than "stutterer"
- Describe factors that may (a) predispose a child to stutter, (b) precipitate stuttering, and (c) make stuttering persistent
- Name and describe the *core* behaviors of stuttering
- Name and describe the two major categories of *secondary* stuttering behaviors
- Name and describe different feelings and attitudes that can accompany stuttering
- Describe the elements of the new International Classification of Functioning, Disability, and Health (ICF) system that are most relevant to stuttering
- Discuss the age range of stuttering onset and the types of onset, and explain why the onset of stuttering is often difficult to pinpoint
- Describe the meanings of the terms "prevalence" and "incidence," and give current best estimates of each
- Give an estimate of the number of children who recover without treatment, and describe factors that predict this recovery
- Give an estimate of the sex ratio in stuttering at onset and in the school-age population
- Explain what is meant by "anticipation," "consistency," and "adaptation" in stuttering
- Explain some relationships between stuttering and language, and suggest what they mean about the nature of the disorder
- Describe several conditions under which stuttering is usually reduced or absent, and suggest why this may be so

KEY TERMS

Disfluency: An interruption of speech—such as a repetition, hesitancy, or prolongation of sound—that may occur in both typically developing individuals and those who stutter

Normal disfluency: An interruption of speech in a typically developing individual

Fluency: The effortless flow of speech

Repetition: A sound, syllable, or single-syllable word that is repeated several times. The speaker is apparently "stuck" on that sound and continues repeating it until the following sound can be produced

Prolongation: A stutter in which sound or air flow continues but movement of the articulators is stopped

Block: A stutter that is an inappropriate stoppage of the flow of air or voice and often the movement of articulators as well

Core behavior: The basic speech behavior of stuttering—repetition, prolongation, and block

Secondary behavior: A speaker's reactions to his or her repetitions, prolongations, and blocks in an attempt to end them quickly or avoid them altogether. Such reactions may begin as random struggle but soon turn into well-learned patterns. Secondary behaviors can be divided into two broad classes: escape and avoidance behaviors

Escape behavior: A speaker's attempts to terminate a stutter and finish the word. This occurs when the speaker is already in a moment of stuttering

Avoidance behavior: A speaker's attempt to prevent stuttering when he or she anticipates stuttering on a word or in a situation. Word-based avoidances are commonly interjections of extra sounds, like "uh," said before the word on which stuttering is expected

Attitude: A feeling that has become a pervasive part of a person's beliefs

Heterogeneity: Differences among various types of a disorder

Developmental stuttering: A term used to denote the most common form of stuttering that develops during childhood (in contrast to stuttering that develops in response to a neurological event or trauma or emotional stress)

Prevalence: A term used to indicate how widespread a disorder is

Incidence: An index of how many people have stuttered at some time in their lives

Anticipation: An individual's ability to predict on which words or sounds he or she will stutter

Consistency: The tendency for speakers to stutter on the same words when reading a passage several times

Adaptation: The tendency for speakers to stutter less and less (up to a point) when repeatedly reading a passage

PERSPECTIVE

No one is sure what causes stuttering, but it is an age-old problem that may have its origins in the way our brains evolved to produce speech and language. Its sudden appearance in some children is triggered when they try to talk using their just-emerging speech and language skills. Its many variations and manifestations are determined by individual learning patterns, personality, and temperament. It also provides lessons about human nature: the variety of responses that stuttering provokes in cultures around the world is a reflection of the many ways in which humans deal with individual differences.

This description of stuttering makes it seem like a very complicated problem—one that will take a long time to learn about. It's true that you could spend a lifetime and still not know everything there is to know about stuttering. But you don't need to understand everything in order to help people who stutter. If you read this book critically and carefully, you will get a basic understanding of stuttering and a foundation for evaluating and treating people who stutter and their families. And once you start working with people who stutter, your understanding and ability can expand exponentially.

If you continue to work with stuttering, you will soon outgrow this book and begin to make your own discoveries. You will experience the satisfaction of helping children, adolescents, and adults regain an ability to communicate easily. Someday you may even write about your therapy procedures and your assessment of their effectiveness. Those of us who have spent many years engaged in stuttering research and treatment all began where you are right now, at the threshold of an exciting and rewarding profession.

The Words We Use

In any field—whether it's law, medicine, or speech-language pathology—words may be used in specific ways. Definitions of many of the specialized terms used in our field are provided in the glossary at the back of this book. But some words and phrases deserve to be discussed at the beginning.

People Who Stutter

Until recently, it was common practice to refer to people who stutter as "stutterers." In fact, some of us who stutter refer to ourselves as *stutterers* and feel some pride in this term. However, many people prefer not to be labeled "a stutterer" and want to be called "people who stutter." They feel, and rightly so, that stuttering is only a small part of who they are.

Adults who stutter often say that changing the way they think of themselves—as people who happen to stutter but with many more important attributes—was one of the most significant things they did to break free of the bonds of stuttering. Such reports remind us that clients are far more than people who stutter. They are people, each with a galaxy of characteristics, one of which happens to be that they stutter. This way of thinking enables us to help not only our clients but also their families. Families learn to listen beyond the sounds of stuttering to the thoughts and feelings that their children are communicating. It helps everyone view disfluencies in perspective as only a small part of the whole child.

Some authors abbreviate "people who stutter" as "PWS." Personally, I feel that substituting an acronym that highlights stuttering is not really different from using "stutterer," so I won't employ that as a euphemism. However, I know that the language in this book would grow stale and cumbersome if I were to use "person who stutters" over and over. So I often refer to the "adult," "child," or "adolescent you are working with," and may sometimes use "stutterer." That, too, I feel is acceptable when used occasionally. After all, a stutterer may be someone who is proud that he sometimes stutters but doesn't let it get in the way of his life.

Disfluency

In our literature, "**disfluency**" is used to denote interruptions of speech that may be either normal or abnormal. That is, it can apply to pauses, repetitions, and other hesitancies that occur in the speech of persons with normal speech. It can also apply to moments of stuttering and is a handy term to use when describing the speech of young children whose diagnosis is unclear.

I'll use "disfluency" interchangeably with "stutter" to make the writing more varied. When someone's speech hesitancies are unequivocally *not* stuttering, I'll use the term "**normal disfluency**." I won't use the older term for abnormal hesitations, "dysfluency" with a "y," because it can easily be mistaken for "disfluency" when you see it on the page and because the two are indistinguishable when spoken.

OVERVIEW OF THE DISORDER

This section previews the next few chapters on the nature of stuttering and gives me a chance to reveal my own slant on the disorder. I think this may be helpful for anyone, but especially for those readers who have not had a course in stuttering and who may, therefore, know few details of its nature.

Do All Cultures Have Stuttering?

Stuttering is found in all parts of the world and in all cultures and races. It is indiscriminate of occupation, intelligence, and income; it affects both sexes and people of all ages, from toddlers to the elderly. It is an old curse, and there is evidence that it was present in Chinese, Egyptian, and Mesopotamian cultures more than 40 centuries ago. Moses was said to have stuttered (Garfinkel, 1995) and to have used a trick typical of many of us who stutter—getting his brother to speak for him. I did something similar when I was asked to read a prayer aloud in Sunday school.

What Causes People to Stutter?

The cause of stuttering is still something of a mystery. Scientists have yet to discover what causes stuttering, but they have many clues. First, there is strong evidence that stuttering often has a *genetic* basis—that is, something is inherited that makes it more likely a child will stutter. This genetic "something" has to do with the way a child's brain develops its neural pathways for speech and language. For example, the neural pathways for talking may have bottlenecks, dead ends, or other obstacles to the rapid flow of information. The pathways may also be vulnerable to disruption by other brain activity, such as emotions. Another clue about the nature of stuttering is that most stuttering begins in children between ages 2 and 5. Thus, the onset of stuttering occurs about the same time that many typical stresses of early childhood are occurring. One child may begin to stutter during a dramatic growth in vocabulary and syntax. Another's stuttering may first appear when the family moves to a new home. Still another child may start soon after a baby brother or sister is born. Many different factors, acting singly or in combination, may *precipitate* the onset of stuttering in a child who has a neurophysiological *predisposition*, or inborn tendency, for stuttering.

Once stuttering starts, it may disappear within a few months, or it may get gradually worse. When it gets worse, learned reactions may be an important factor in its severity. Playmates at school or thoughtless adults may cause a child to become highly self-conscious about his stuttering. The child will quickly learn that by pushing hard, he can get traction on a word that has been stuck. He may find that an eye blink or an "um" said quickly before trying to say a hard word may short-circuit stuttering temporarily. By the time a child is a teenager, learned reactions influence many of the symptoms. He has learned to anticipate stuttering and may thrash around in a panic when he speaks, trying to escape or avoid it. By adulthood, his fear of stuttering and desire to avoid it can permeate his lifestyle. An adult who stutters often copes with it by limiting his work, friends, and fun to those situations and people that put few demands on speech. Figure 1.1 provides an overview of many of the contributing factors in the evolution of stuttering. In this and the subsequent four chapters, I'll describe in detail our current understanding of these influences.

Can Stuttering Be Cured?

As implied above, it often cures itself. Some young children who begin to stutter recover without treatment. For others, early intervention may be needed to help the child develop normal fluency and prevent the development of a chronic problem. Once stuttering has become firmly established, however and the child has developed many learned reactions, a concerted treatment effort is needed. Good treatment of mild and moderate stuttering in preschool and early elementary school children may leave them with little trace of stuttering, except perhaps when they are stressed, fatigued, or ill. Most of those who stutter severely for a long time or who are not treated until after puberty make only a

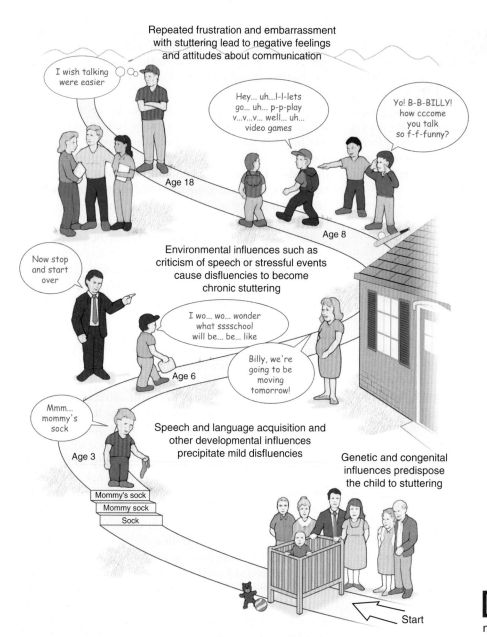

Figure 1.1 Factors contributing to the development of stuttering.

partial recovery. They often learn to speak more slowly or stutter more easily and learn to be less bothered by it. Some, however, will not improve, despite our best efforts.

DEFINITIONS

Fluency

By beginning with a definition of **fluency** rather than stuttering, I am pointing out how many elements must be maintained in the flow of speech if a speaker is to be considered fluent. It is an impressive balancing act; little wonder that everyone slips and stumbles from time to time when they talk.

Fluency is hard to define. In fact, most researchers have focused on its opposite, *dis*fluency. (I use the term disfluency to apply both to stuttering and to normal hesitations, making it easier to refer to hesitations that could be either normal or abnormal.) One of the early fluency researchers, Freida Goldman-Eisler, showed that normal speech is filled with hesitations (Goldman-Eisler, 1968). Other researchers have acknowledged this and expanded the study of fluent speech by contrasting it with disfluent speech. Dalton and Hardcastle (1977), for example, distinguished fluent from disfluent speech by differences in the variables listed in Table 1.1. Inclusion of intonation and stress in this list may seem unusual. It could be said that speakers who reduce stuttering by using a monotone are not really fluent. We would

Table 1.1	Variables Suggested by Dalton and Hardcastle (1977) as Useful in Distinguishing between Fluent and Disfluent Speech

1. Presence of extra sounds, such as repetitions, prolongations, interjections, and revisions
   - If a speaker says "I-I-I nnnnneed to have uh my uh, well, I-I-I should get mmmmmy car fixed," he sounds disfluent.
2. Location and frequency of pauses
   - If a speaker says, "Whenever I remember to bring my umbrella (pause), it never rains," he sounds fluent. But if he says, "Whenever (pause) I remember to bring (pause) my (pause) umbrella, it never (pause) rains," he sounds disfluent.
3. Rhythmical patterning in speech
   - English is typically spoken with stressed syllables at relatively equal intervals; in general, stressed syllables are followed by several unstressed syllables. When marked deviations from this pattern occur, as when a speaker with cerebellar disease stresses all syllables equally, the speaker sounds disfluent.
4. Intonation and stress
   - If a speaker does not vary intonation and stress and is therefore monotonous, he may be considered disfluent. Abnormal intonation and stress patterns may also be considered disfluent.
5. Overall rate
   - If a speaker has a very slow rate of speech or has bursts of fast rates interspersed with slower rates, he may be considered disfluent.

argue that it is not their fluency but the "naturalness" of their speech that is affected. Nonetheless, both will be of interest to the clinician who works to help clients with all aspects of their communication.

Starkweather (1980, 1987) suggested that many of the variables that determine fluency reflect temporal aspects of speech production. These include such variables as pauses, rhythm, intonation, stress, and rate that are controlled by when and how fast we move our speech structures. So, our temporal control of the movements of these structures determines our fluency. Starkweather also noted that the rate of information flow, not just sound flow, is an important aspect of fluency. Thus, a speaker who speaks without hesitations but has difficulty conveying information in a timely and orderly fashion might not be considered a fluent speaker.

In his description of fluency, Starkweather (1987) also included the effort with which a speaker speaks. By effort, he means both the mental and physical work a speaker exerts when speaking. This is difficult to measure, but it may turn out that listeners can make such judgments reliably. Moreover, mental and physical effort may reflect important components of what it feels like to be a person who stutters.

In essence, fluency can be thought of simply as the effortless flow of speech. Thus, a speaker who is judged to be "fluent" appears to use little effort when speaking. However, the components of such apparently effortless speech flow are hard to pin down. As researchers analyze fluency more carefully, they may find that the appearance of excess effort may give rise to judgments that a person is stuttering. However, other elements, such as unusual rhythm or slow rate of information flow, may result in judgments that a person is not a fluent speaker, but is not a stutterer either. I will discuss aspects of fluency again when I relate some of the elements of fluency, such as rate and naturalness, to various therapy approaches.

Stuttering

General Description

Stuttering appears at first to be complex and mysterious, but much of it is based on human nature and can be easily understood if you think about your own experiences. In some ways, it is like a problem you might have with your car.

Imagine you had a car that would suddenly stop when you were driving in traffic (Fig. 1.2). Sometimes it would sputter and jerk when you pulled away from a stop sign. Other times, it would drop into neutral, and the engine would race, but the wheels wouldn't turn. Still other times, the brakes would jam by themselves and wouldn't release until you stomped repeatedly on the pedal.

Compare this with what the "core" of stuttering behavior is: Stuttering is characterized by an abnormally high frequency and/or duration of stoppages in the forward flow of speech. These stoppages usually take the form of (a) **repetitions** of sounds, syllables, or one-syllable words, (b) **prolongations** of sounds, or (c) "blockages" or "**blocks**" of airflow or voicing in speech.

Returning to the car analogy: *After you'd repeatedly had problems with your car, you would probably develop some coping strategies to get it going again. You might, if it sputtered and jerked, push harder on the gas pedal to try to make it speed up.*

Similarly, speakers who are stuttering usually react to their repetitions, prolongations, or blocks by trying to force words out or by using extra sounds, words, or movements in their efforts to become "unstuck" or to avoid getting stuck.

If your car's problem persisted for several days or longer, you would probably develop some bad feelings about it. The first time it happened, you would be surprised. Then, as it happened more and more, surprise would give way to frustration. If your car frequently quit in the middle of traffic and other

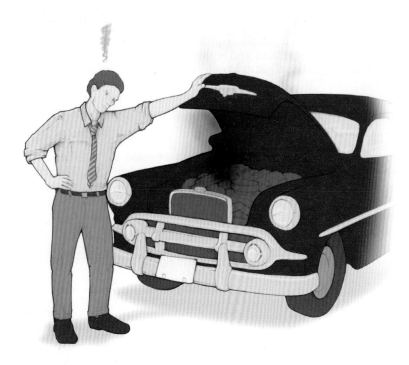

 Stuttering can be like having an old car that often breaks down.

drivers nearly hit you and started honking, you would begin to anticipate problems and become afraid they would happen whenever you drove the car.

The child who begins to stutter goes through many of the same feelings—surprise, frustration, embarrassment, and fear. These feelings—in combination with the difficulty the child has in speaking—may cause the stutterer to limit himself in school, social situations, and at work. This might be similar to your responses to a troublesome car. After your car quit on you in traffic many times, you'd probably leave it in the garage and walk, or you'd just stay home.

Another aspect of any description of stuttering involves specifying what it is not. For example, an important distinction must be made between the stuttering behaviors just described and normal hesitations. Children whose speech and language are developing normally often display repetitions, revisions, and pauses—which are not stuttering. Neither are the brief repetitions, revisions, and pauses in the speech of most nonstuttering adults when they are in a hurry or uncertain. Chapter 7 describes the differences between normal disfluency and stuttering in more detail to prepare you for the task of differential diagnosis of stuttering in children.

A distinction should also be made between stuttering and certain other fluency disorders. Disfluency resulting from cerebral damage or disease or psychological trauma differ from stuttering that begins in childhood. In addition, stuttering differs from cluttering, which is another fluency disorder involving rapid, garbled speech that I will talk about in Chapter 15. These disorders may be treated somewhat

differently, although some of the techniques that clinicians use with stuttering are also useful with other fluency disorders. These disorders are discussed in Chapter 15.

Core Behaviors

I have adopted the term "**core behaviors**" from Van Riper (1971, 1982), who used it to describe the basic speech behaviors of stuttering: repetitions, prolongations, and blocks. These behaviors seem involuntary to the person who stutters, as if they are out of her control. They differ from the "**secondary behaviors**" that a stutterer acquires as learned reactions to the basic core behaviors.

Repetitions are the core behaviors observed most frequently among children who are just beginning to stutter and are simply a sound, syllable, or single-syllable word that is repeated several times. The speaker is apparently "stuck" on that sound and continues repeating it until the following sound can be produced. In children who have not been stuttering for long, single-syllable word repetitions and part-word repetitions are much more common than multisyllable word repetitions. Moreover, children who stutter will frequently repeat a word or syllable more than twice per instance, li-li-li-li-like this (Yairi, 1983; Yairi & Lewis, 1984).

Prolongations of voiced or voiceless sounds also appear in the speech of children beginning to stutter. They usually appear somewhat later than repetitions (Van Riper, 1982), although both Johnson and associates (1959) and Yairi (1997a) reported that prolongations—as well as repetitions—may be present at onset. I use the term *prolongation* to denote those stutters in which sound or air flow continues but movement of the articulators is stopped. Prolongations as short as half a second may be perceived as abnormal, but in rare cases they may last as long as several minutes (Van Riper, 1982). In contrast to my use of the term, older writers include stutters with no sound or airflow as well as stopped movement of the articulators in their definitions of prolongations (e.g., Van Riper, 1982; Wingate, 1964).

Repetitions and sound prolongations are usually part of the core behaviors of more advanced stutterers, as well as of children just beginning to stutter. Sheehan (1974) found that repetitive stutters occurred in every speech sample of 20 adults who stuttered. Indeed, 66 percent of their stutters were repetitions. Although many of their stutters were also prolongations, as defined above, how many is not clear, because Sheehan's definition of prolongations seems to differ from mine.

Blocks are typically the last core behavior to appear. However, as with prolongations, some investigators (Johnson and associates, 1959; Yairi, 1997a) have observed blocks in children's speech at or close to stuttering onset. Blocks occur when a person inappropriately stops the flow of air or voice and often the movement of her articulators as well. Blocks may involve any level of the speech production mechanism—respiratory, laryngeal, or articulatory. There is some evidence and much theorizing that inappropriate muscle activity at the laryngeal level characterizes most blocks (Conture, McCall, & Brewer, 1977; Freeman & Ushijima, 1978; Kenyon, 1942; Schwartz, 1974). Others disagree (Smith, Denny, Shaffer, Kelly, & Hirano, 1996).

As stuttering persists, blocks often grow longer and more tense, and tremors may become evident. These rapid oscillations, most easily observable in the lips or jaw, occur when someone has blocked on a word or sound. The individual closes off the airway, increases air pressure behind the closure, and squeezes her muscles particularly hard (Van Riper, 1982). You can duplicate these tremors by trying to say the word "by" while squeezing your lips together hard and building up air pressure behind the block. Imagine this happening to you unexpectedly when you were trying to talk.

People who stutter differ from one another in how frequently they stutter and how long their individual core behaviors last. Research indicates that a person who stutters does so on average on about 10 percent of the words while reading aloud, although individuals vary greatly (Bloodstein, 1944; Bloodstein & Ratner, 2008). Many people who stutter mildly do so on fewer than 5 percent of the words they speak or read aloud, and a few with severe stuttering stutter on more than 50 percent of the words. The durations of core behaviors vary much less, averaging around one second, and are rarely longer than five seconds (Bloodstein, 1944; Bloodstein & Ratner, 2008).

Secondary Behaviors

People who stutter don't enjoy stuttering. They react to their repetitions, prolongations, and blocks by trying to end them quickly if they can't avoid them altogether. Such reactions may begin as a random struggle but soon turn into well-learned patterns. I divide secondary behaviors into two broad classes: **escape behaviors** and **avoidance behaviors**. I make this division, rather than follow the traditional approach of dealing with secondary behaviors as "starters" or "postponements," for example, because my treatment procedures focus on the principles by which secondary behaviors are learned.

The terms "escape" and "avoidance" are borrowed from behavioral learning literature. Briefly, escape behaviors occur when a speaker is stuttering and attempts to terminate the stutter and finish the word. Common examples of escape behaviors are eye blinks, head nods, and interjections of extra sounds, such as "uh," which are often followed by the termination of a stutter and are therefore reinforced. Avoidance behaviors, on the other hand, are learned when a speaker anticipates stuttering and recalls negative experiences he has had when stuttering. To avoid stuttering and the negative experience that it entails, he often resorts to behaviors he has used previously to escape from moments of stuttering—eye blinks or "uhs," for example. Or, he may try something different, such as changing the word he was planning to say.

In many cases, especially at first, avoidance behaviors may prevent the stutter from occurring and provide highly rewarding emotional relief from the increasing fear that a stutter will occur. Soon these avoidance behaviors become strong habits that are resistant to change. The many subcategories of avoidances (e.g., postponements, starters, substitutions, and timing devices such as hand movements timed to saying the word) are described in Chapter 7.

When trying to decide if a secondary behavior is an escape or an avoidance, just remember that an escape behavior occurs only after a moment of stuttering has begun, and an avoidance behavior occurs before the moment of stuttering begins.

Feelings and Attitudes

A person's feelings can be as much a part of the disorder of stuttering as his speech behaviors. Feelings may precipitate stutters, just as stutters may create feelings. In the beginning, a child's positive feelings of excitement or negative feelings of fear may result in repetitive stutters that he hardly notices. Then, as he stutters more frequently, he may become frustrated or ashamed because he can't say what he wants to say—even his own name—as smoothly and quickly as others. These feelings make speaking harder as frustration and shame increase effort and tension and impede fluent speech. Feelings that result from stuttering may include not only frustration and shame but also fear of stuttering again, guilt about not being able to help oneself, and hostility toward listeners as well.

Attitudes are feelings that have become a pervasive part of a person's beliefs. As a person who stutters experiences more and more stuttering, for example, he begins to believe that he is a person who generally has trouble speaking, just as you might believe that your car is a lemon if you continue to have trouble with it. Adolescents and adults who stutter usually have many negative attitudes about themselves that are derived from years of stuttering experiences (Blood, Blood, Tellis, & Gabel, 2001; Gildston, 1967; Rahman, 1956; Wallen, 1960). A person who stutters often projects his attitudes on listeners, believing that they think he is stupid or nervous. Sometimes, however, listeners may contribute directly to the person's attitudes. Research has shown that most people, even classroom teachers and speech-language pathologists, stereotype people who stutter as tense, insecure, and fearful (e.g., Turnbaugh, Guitar, & Hoffman, 1979; Woods & Williams, 1976). Such listener stereotypes can affect the way individuals who stutter see themselves, and changing a client's negative attitudes about himself can be a major focus of treatment.

The three components of stuttering—core behaviors, secondary behaviors, and feelings and attitudes—are depicted in Figure 1.3. The core behavior is the individual's block on the "N" in "New York." The secondary behaviors

consist of postponement devices such as "uh," "well," and "you know" and substitution of "the Big Apple" for "New York." Feelings and attitudes are depicted as the individual's thoughts that he won't succeed in saying the word fluently and the individual's belief that listeners will think he is dumb because he stutters.

Functioning, Disability, and Health

Some time ago, the World Health Organization (WHO) adopted the International Classification of Impairment, Disabilities, and Handicaps (WHO, 1980) to describe the consequences of various diseases and disorders. A number of authors have applied this framework to stuttering (Curlee, 1993; McClean, 1990; Prins, 1991, 1999; Yaruss, 1998, 1999). A decade ago, WHO changed their taxonomy to the International Classification of Functioning, Disability, and Health (ICF) (WHO, 2001). In the following paragraphs, I will suggest ways in which this system may be applied to stuttering.

The taxonomy begins with "Functioning and Disability," wherein body structures and body functions are considered. Structures that are dysfunctional in stuttering, as brain

Core Behavior

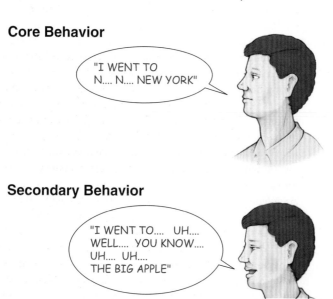

Secondary Behavior

Feelings and Attitudes

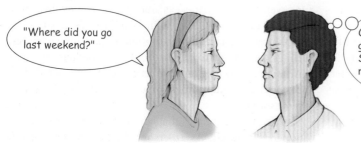

Figure 1.3 Components of stuttering: core behaviors, secondary behaviors, and feelings and attitudes.

imaging studies have shown, are cortical and subcortical structures, such as white matter tracts that may be critical for coordinating planning, execution, and sensory feedback for speech. Functions that differ in stuttering are the interruptions of speech flow that characterize the disorder. The ICF system becomes more useful when "Activity and Participation" are considered. Individuals who stutter may be affected to a greater or lesser extent in two of the ICF areas, "Speaking" and "Conversation." These are domains in which stuttering is noticeable. A third area, "Interpersonal Interactions," may also be affected if speaking and conversation are restricted by the stuttering to the extent that the person who stutters refrains from fully engaging with others.

A new and important section of the latest ICF system is titled "Contextual Factors." One component of this section is "The Environment." This is particularly relevant to individuals who stutter because people in the environment may range from unsupportive (e.g., a home with great stress or classmates who tease a child) to highly supportive (e.g., a family that is accepting of the child and encouraging of her participation). Also under "Contextual Factors" is the category of "Personal Factors." These are the attributes of a person who stutters—her character and personality.

Consider the influence of environmental and personal factors on two individuals who stutter. The first is the successful former CEO of General Electric, Jack Welch, who authored *Jack: Straight from the Gut*. His assertive temperament and early acceptance of his stuttering by his family were no doubt important in helping him succeed in the high-pressure world of corporate boardrooms. From an early age, Welch refused to let stuttering stand in the way of his goals (Welch & Byrne, 2001). In contrast, actor James Earl Jones initially reacted to his stuttering in a vastly different way. When he was 6 years old, he was so traumatized by his stuttering, he pretended that he was mute so that he wouldn't have to speak. Only later, with the support of someone in his environment—a high school English teacher—did he begin to learn that he could overcome his stuttering by facing difficult situations and practicing reading aloud in front of an audience (Jones & Niven, 1993).

Another two examples come to mind—men who had stuttered severely since childhood but obtained excellent college educations, were highly successful in business, and used their wealth to help others. One is Malcolm Fraser, who was a cofounder of the National Auto Parts Association and created the Stuttering Foundation of America. The other is Walter Annenberg, who established a media empire and later the Annenberg Foundation, a large philanthropic organization.

In all four cases, their functioning may have been impaired, but environmental and personal factors enabled them to overcome potential limitations in the domains of speaking and interpersonal interactions. You can see in this classification system why clinicians play a vital role in the lives of children and adults who stutter. They can influence environmental factors by helping families, teachers, and entire schools become supportive of the individuals who stutter and facilitative of increased fluency. And they can build the personal attributes of each client through counseling, insightful listening, educating, and caring.

THE HUMAN FACE OF STUTTERING

Before I delve deeper into the basic facts about stuttering, I'd like to touch briefly on the personal side of the problem. Some of you may never have had a friend who stutters or may never have worked with a stutterer in treatment, so I will present several examples of what stuttering can be like. Even if you are familiar with stuttering, these brief sketches, which portray four individuals who differ in age and in their accommodations to stuttering, may expand your sense of what stuttering is like for the person who experiences it. These case studies begin on page 12. You may also visit *thePoint* to watch video clips of these different levels of stuttering.

BASIC FACTS ABOUT STUTTERING AND THEIR IMPLICATIONS FOR THE NATURE OF STUTTERING

This section relates some of the best-known "facts" about stuttering. These are replicated research findings that pertain to the occurrence and variability of stuttering in the population and in individuals. As we discuss these findings, we will note what they suggest about the nature of stuttering. Thus, as you read the rest of this chapter, you will become increasingly aware of my perspective on the nature and treatment of stuttering.

Much has been made of the "**heterogeneity**" of stuttering; a number of authors have suggested that stuttering is not one disorder, but many. Researchers have proposed various divisions of the disorder, such as Van Riper's (1982) four "tracks" of stuttering development and St. Onge's (1963) triad of speech-phobic, psychogenic, and organic stutterers. My approach is to focus on the majority of people who stutter—those whose stuttering begins during childhood without an apparent link to psychological or organic trauma. This most common type of stuttering has been called "**developmental stuttering**," because symptoms usually emerge gradually as a child develops, especially during the period of intense speech and language acquisition. I simply call it "stuttering." In denoting similar fluency problems that are associated with psychological problems, brain damage, cognitive impairment, and cluttering, I refer to their assumed etiology, such as "disfluencies associated with brain damage."

Note, however, that even within the group of individuals whose stuttering begins in early childhood during rapid speech and language development, there is a great deal of variability in the behaviors we call stuttering and in how these behaviors change (or don't) as the child progresses toward persistence or recovery.

Case Examples

A Young Preschool Child: Borderline Stuttering

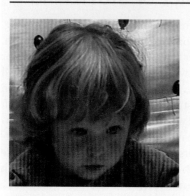

Ashley was a happy, outgoing child who was advanced in her language development; she spoke in well-formed sentences when she was 18 months old. Then suddenly, when she was 21 months old, she began to stutter. Her stuttering took the form of multiple repetitions, most often at the beginnings of sentences. For example she would say "I-I-I-I want some water" or "Ca-ca-ca-ca-can you lift me up?" Despite the fact that she would sometimes repeat a syllable 10 or more times before getting the word out, she didn't show obvious signs of frustration when she stuttered. She continued to develop language rapidly, talk copiously, and socialize easily.

About six months after she started stuttering, her parents contacted a speech-language pathologist who evaluated Ashley. The evaluation indicated that Ashley's language development was advanced for her age, that her phonological development was also advanced, and that she stuttered on 4 percent of the syllables she spoke. (This means that when a few minutes of her speech were analyzed and the number of syllables she spoke was counted, Ashley stuttered on 4 percent of those syllables.)

Ashley's parents told the clinician that they had no idea why Ashley started stuttering. She was happy, secure, and talkative; no big event occurred around the time of stuttering onset; and she didn't have any relatives who stuttered.

For a description of Ashley's treatment and its outcome, turn to Chapter 11.

Discussion

The two segments in this video show Ashley talking about a picture (a cat named Cookie knocking a plant off a shelf) that the clinician has previously described to her. In the first segment, the clinician elicits Ashley's response by asking "What happened to Cookie, again?" Ashley's response

is "*Cat….nn…de-de-de …. Coo-Coo-(approximately 15 repetitions of this syllable)-Cookie knocked the plant down.*" In the second segment, the clinician says "Let's take another one. Tell me. Remember?" Ashley replies "*Then Coo-Coo-Coo-Coo-Cookie knocked the plant down.*"

These segments are a pretty good illustration of what stuttering can be like when it first starts in a preschool child. What are the primary core behaviors that Ashley shows? Repetitions? Prolongations? Blocks?

When we are trying to determine whether a child needs immediate and direct treatment for stuttering, it is often helpful to assess the child's emotional reaction to her stuttering. Can you tell from the video whether Ashley is frustrated or embarrassed by her stuttering? What do you see in the video that gives you clues about this?

An Older Preschool Child: Beginning Stuttering

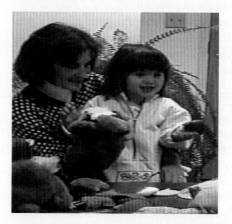

Katherine developed speech and language normally, speaking her first word at about 1 year and beginning to combine words at 15 months with complete fluency. When she was 3, after a particularly hectic Christmas holiday, she began to stutter. Her first disfluencies were easy part- and whole-word repetitions, but she soon began to tense her articulators, momentarily blocking the flow of speech until the word "popped out." Sometimes, when she was completely stuck for several seconds, she responded by hitting her parents or crying out. She also showed much less interest in talking and using new words and phrases.

Her parents soon brought her to a speech and language clinic for an evaluation. Katherine was found to be stuttering on 21 percent of the syllables she spoke—a very high percentage for any child. Her overall severity was assessed with the *Stuttering Severity Instrument*, which rated it as severe. Her receptive language was found to be far above average for her age. Her expressive language was found to be typical for her age, but it was likely that she was inhibited in expressing herself because of her stuttering. Her phonological development was found to be appropriate for her age.

For a description of Katherine's treatment, see Chapter 12.

Discussion

In Segment 1, Katherine responds to a question from her mother by saying "O-O-O-O…an…an…an…OK now…I think he is still hungry…[unintelligible]…a leaf." This may be an example of a child getting stuck on an attempt to say a word ("OK") and then, finding herself in a block, changing the word she tries to say (from "OK" to "and"). Then she is able to say the original word and go on.

In Segment 2, still with her mother, she is stuck on the first sound of the word "OK," then she seems to be able to move on to the "kay" but gets stuck there too, and so she doubles back to the "o" and finally finishes the word by pushing out of the stutter on "o" and then having a slight stutter on the first sound of "kay." Whew! You can see how much work this 3-year-old must do just to get a few words out. No wonder she doesn't seem as expressive as she did before her stuttering started.

In Segment 3, Katherine is playing with the clinician and says "uh…nnnnn…ne…ne…nnnn…na…now, what is this?" The "uh" might be Katherine's way of getting ready for the stutter she anticipates on "now."

In Segment 4, Katherine is playing with both of her parents and says "Lo-look what I made. Oh…uh…bbbbb…buh…bbbbb…buh…" The first stutter is a part-word repetition ("lo-look") that is so mild it might be considered a normal disfluency in another context. But the second stutter (on a word beginning with "b") is quite a long stutter in which Katherine struggles heroically to produce the word but is interrupted by the door opening before she can finish. How would you describe this last stutter? Repetition? Prolongation? Block? What emotions do you think she's feeling? Why do you think so?

A School-Age Child: Intermediate Stuttering

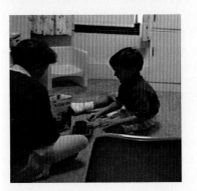

David was the second of three children in a family with no history of speech or language disorders. His speech was developing normally until age 4, when he began to show excessive part-word and whole-word repetitions. After several months, when David's stuttering had not decreased, his mother took him to his pediatrician who assured her it would resolve on its own.

When David was almost 6, his stuttering was growing steadily more severe, and he was avoiding talking in many situations. His mother then decided to consult a speech-language pathologist at a university clinic, who evaluated David. In the evaluation, David was stuttering on 8 percent of his syllables spoken; many stutters were tightly squeezed blocks with evident struggle behavior.

David's subsequent treatment and his current status as a 20-something-year-old are described in Chapter 13.

Discussion

In this video, you can see how stuttering may be more complicated as children grow older and become more self-conscious. In the video for the first child, Ashley's moments of stuttering seemed to pop up out of the blue and surprise her. In the video for the second child, Katherine's stuttering was a little more predictable to her, but it was mostly confined to those few words on which she got blocked. Now we will see that David's stuttering affects more of his entire speech pattern and is characterized by much avoidance and struggle.

In Segment 1, showing David talking with his mother, David's style of speaking is hesitant, with many stops, "ums," false starts, and changes in direction. He says something like "and then…it like that…and then…then put…um the same a-mount of…of…of…of …um… [then some unintelligible words, after which he seems to give up on the sentence and begins counting]." As you can imagine, it's hard to assess what percentage of syllables are stuttered when David avoids saying the words on which he expects to stutter.

Segment 2 shows a block on the word "whoever," preceded by several words that seem to postpone David's attempt on this word. He says "and then …uh …whoever gets um …um the four, four… an, an … um … um these [unintelligible word]." Do you think he expects to stutter on "whoever?" What are the cues that tell you so? What escape behaviors does David use as he struggles with this block?

In Segment 3, David has another block with a few avoidance behaviors before and escape behaviors during the stutter. He says "He … [unintelligible word] … he goes home automatically because … um … because he-he has done the shortcut an-an he goes all the way home." Can you describe the avoidance and escape behaviors David shows in this clip?

(Continued)

An Adult: Advanced Stuttering

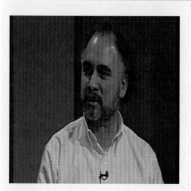

Sergio is a 44-year-old musician who has stuttered since he was 3 years old. Eight of his maternal aunts and uncles stuttered, suggesting a genetic origin to his problem. His stuttering began as multiple repetitions of one-syllable words and parts of words. Much of his speech was fluent, but whenever he was excited or hurried, Sergio's stuttering flared up, sending his parents into a state of alarm and concern for his future. At first, his father's solution for Sergio's stuttering was hitting him on the head with his knuckles when he blocked. When this failed and Sergio developed physically tense prolongations and blocks that occurred regularly in his speech, his parents took him to various therapists, including a hypnotist and a psychotherapist who prescribed tranquilizers. None of these seemed to have more than a temporary effect, and Sergio's stuttering grew steadily worse. During his elementary and junior high school years, he was frequently ridiculed for his stuttering, even by teachers, and Sergio found himself an outcast among his peers.

This changed, however, soon after "Beatlemania" swept through America. Sergio bought a guitar and taught himself to sing "I Want to Hold Your Hand" and other Beatles songs. As a result, his popularity with schoolmates shot up, even though his stuttering continued to worsen. He had so much difficulty speaking in class, and his teachers were so unsympathetic, he finally dropped out of school and pursued a vagabond lifestyle as a singer and songwriter.

As he traveled, working various jobs by day and singing at night, Sergio continued to stutter severely, with one happy exception. When he was performing with his band, not only did he sing fluently, but he also spoke to the audience easily, announcing each number and making casual, funny comments between songs. As a result of his constant battle with stuttering, Sergio developed a wide variety of avoidances. He dodged making phone calls, and whenever he received calls, he used elaborate facial grimaces and starter sounds to fight his way through stutters.

Discussion

The telephone is a difficult situation for most people who stutter, and Sergio is no exception. Segment 1 shows Sergio talking about his experiences on the phone when he had long silent blocks in the past, and Segment 2 is a phone call Sergio made more recently. On both clips you'll see a mix of avoidance and escape behaviors that are now well entrenched in Sergio's speech pattern after years of stuttering. There are also some straightforward stutters without escape and avoidance behaviors that are witness to Sergio's attempts to stutter in a simpler way. See if you can identify the types of stutters that Sergio has on both segments, as well as his particular escape and avoidance behaviors, more of which are seen in Segment 2.

Onset

Imagine yourself in your doctor's office with an annoying cold that just won't go away—runny nose, sore throat, and cough. She asks you to describe when the first signs of your illness appeared and what they were like at onset. It is quite likely you won't remember exactly when your symptoms first occurred and exactly what they were like, especially if they came and went over the course of a week or two before they became persistent. This is the problem with determining the onset of stuttering. Parents are asked to recall exactly when the child's stuttering started and what it was like when they first noticed it; thus some of our information on onset—especially from older studies—may be inaccurate. The description of stuttering onset given here is relatively brief. More details are given in Chapter 7 when I describe the

differences between normal disfluency and the beginning stages of stuttering.

Let's first consider the question of how old children are, on average, when they begin to stutter. In the earliest studies (e.g., Milisen & Johnson, 1936), researchers asked parents a year or more after the onset of stuttering had occurred, to recall the age of stuttering onset in their children. The average age of onset, taken from nine pre-1990 studies summarized in Bloodstein and Ratner (2008), is roughly 4 years. After 1990, led by Ehud Yairi and his colleagues at the University of Illinois, researchers were careful to interview parents of children who began to stutter within 12 months of the parent interview. Bloodstein and Ratner (2008) list six studies conducted after 1990 in which parents were interviewed closer to onset than earlier studies. The average age of onset of these newer studies is about 2.8 years. Thus, either the newer studies are getting a more accurate picture of the age of onset, the age of onset is getting younger, or both.[1] The current consensus is that the onset of stuttering typically occurs just before age 3, and most onsets occur between ages 2 and 3.5 years (Yairi & Ambrose, 2005). Some older children—up to about age 12—may begin to stutter, but these are much rarer cases. Stuttering onset in adolescents and adults is likely to be a different form of disfluency—psychogenic or neurogenic—which I will discuss in Chapter 15.

Next, let's look at the first signs of stuttering, as reported by parents. Most early reports of stuttering onset (e.g., Bluemel, 1932) indicated that simple, relaxed repetitions of syllables and words were the typical first signs of stuttering. However, some early studies (e.g., Taylor, 1937) and the carefully conducted interviews by Yairi (1983) found that, in many cases, parents described prolongations and blocks, along with signs of struggle, as the first stutters shown by their child. Summarizing their own and others' research, Yairi & Ambrose (2005) suggest that even when only repetitions are the first signs of stuttering, the percentage of spoken syllables that are repeated and the number of iterations in each repetition are markedly higher in children who stutter than in their normal peers.

Lastly, there is the question of whether onset is sudden, intermediate, or gradual. In other words, do parents conclude their child is stuttering because of marked disfluencies seen in the course of a day or two, does it take a week or two for them to make that determination, or does it take longer, many weeks? Remember our example of getting a cold and trying to remember the onset? No doubt some colds come on suddenly, with sore throat and running nose appearing overnight and getting worse quickly. Other colds tiptoe into your life, with a sore throat that comes and goes and later turns into a runny nose and cough.

In contrast to the earliest reports on stuttering always having a gradual onset, Yairi and Ambrose (2005) found in their sample of 163 children many cases (41 percent) in which onset was reported to be sudden, with another group (32 percent) reported as intermediate, and a third group (27 percent) as gradual. These figures may be influenced by

how attentive to their child's speech these parents were; no doubt, parents who had relatives who stuttered would have been more likely to recognize stuttering sooner.

Prevalence

The term "**prevalence**" is used to indicate how widespread a disorder is. Information about the prevalence of stuttering tells us how many people currently stutter. Accurate, up-to-date information on the prevalence of stuttering is difficult to obtain. The research literature contains studies having many methodological differences, which can result in wide differences in estimates of prevalence. For example, the prevalence of stuttering probably varies considerably with age, and not all studies measure stuttering in the same age groups. Moreover, definitions of stuttering may vary from study to study. Some studies may include relatively normally disfluent individuals in their count; others may exclude them.

Beitchman, Nair, Clegg, and Patel (1986) assessed the prevalence of speech and language disorders in kindergarten children, using a representative sample. They retested children who failed the initial screening as well as a random sample of children who passed. The prevalence of stuttering in this sample of kindergarten children was 2.4 percent. Although this is only one study's finding, the care with which the data were collected increases its credibility.

Bloodstein and Ratner (2008) reviewed and summarized the results of 44 studies of school-age children in the United States, Europe, Africa, Australia, and the West Indies. These studies showed that the prevalence of stuttering throughout the school years is about 1 percent. Andrews, Hoddinott, Craig, Howie, Feyer, and Neilson (1983) came to the same conclusion—about 1 percent of the schoolchildren worldwide are likely to be stutterers at any given time. If the 2.4 percent prevalence among kindergartners noted above is valid, a considerable number of recoveries must take place between kindergarten and the upper grades.

There appear to be no reliable prevalence data for stuttering in adults. However, both Andrews and colleagues (1983) and Bloodstein and Ratner (2008) suggest that the prevalence of stuttering is lower after puberty. If so, the prevalence for adults would be less than 1 percent.

Incidence

The **incidence** of stuttering is an index of how many people have stuttered at some time in their lives. Like the data on prevalence, incidence figures are not clear-cut because different researchers have used different definitions of stuttering and methods for obtaining their data. Some researchers only report stuttering that lasted six months or more, not wanting to include shorter episodes of disfluency. Others report any speech behaviors that informants or parents considered to be stuttering. Estimates of incidence, when reports of

---

[1]Yairi and Ambrose (2005) ask whether the age of stuttering onset is getting younger and whether this reflects a general trend of earlier language acquisition. In this regard, Nan Ratner (*personal communication*, July, 2009) has surveyed a number of language acquisition experts through the Childes discussion group, and their consensus seems to be that there is no clear evidence that the age of language acquisition (i.e., ages at which major language milestones are achieved) has changed over the last few decades. She points out, however, that there is some evidence from differing results achieved by older versus more recent studies of phonological development that children may be acquiring articulatory targets earlier. Whether this would affect the age of stuttering onset is not known.

informants and parents are considered, are as high as 15 percent, a figure that includes those children who stuttered for only a brief period (Bloodstein & Ratner, 2008). When only the cases of stuttering that lasted longer than six months are included, incidence appears to be about 5 percent (Andrews et al., 1983). We think the latter estimate may more accurately reflect the chronic disorder we call stuttering, but the former illustrates how close perceptions of normal disfluency and early stuttering may be.

A report by Mansson (2000) of all children born on the Danish island of Bornholm supports the suggested incidence of 5 percent. This population is homogeneous and stable, making a careful, longitudinal study quite possible. Of the 1,042 children born on the island in 1990 and 1991, 98 percent were screened for speech and language problems at age 3. The children were followed for nine years, and it was then found that 5.19 percent went through some period of stuttering.

Incidence figures tell us something else about the nature of stuttering. The difference between incidence (5 percent) and prevalence (1 percent in school-age children and less in adults) suggests that most people who stutter at some time in their lives recover from it, and we know that prevalence declines after puberty. Thus, unless treatment alone is responsible for such remissions, some aspect of growth or maturation allows many individuals to recover from stuttering.

Recovery without Treatment

Recovery from stuttering without treatment, also referred to as "spontaneous" or "natural" recovery, has long been a puzzling issue. Putting aside the important question about *why* children recover without treatment, there is debate about what percentage of children who start to stutter recover in this way.

Reviews of early research report findings that range from 20 percent to 80 percent natural recovery (Bloodstein & Ratner, 2008; Andrews et al., 1983). This wide range may be from different methodologies used by different studies. Some asked large numbers of adults if they ever stuttered when they were children. This method, which is called "retrospective" may be affected by faulty memories, poor definitions of stuttering, and the inclusion of individuals who may have stuttered for only brief periods.

Recent research has proceeded more carefully by first identifying a group of children close to the onset of their stuttering and then following them for several years without offering treatment and assessing how many recover and how many persist. Those who persist are then referred for therapy. Several studies using this methodology have been published. Yairi and Ambrose (1999) followed a group of 84 children for a minimum of four years after the onset of their stuttering and determined that over this span of time, 74 percent had recovered without treatment. Kloth, Kraaimaat, Janssen, and Brutten (1999) followed 23 children for six years and

discovered that 70 percent had recovered. Mansson (2000) identified 51 children between the ages of 3 and 5 who started to stutter and found that 71 percent recovered within two years. When the follow-up continued for another few years until the children were 8 or 9 years old, recoveries were up to 85 percent. However, this latter figure may be affected by speech therapy given to some after the two-year follow-up.

Several studies have compared children who recover and those who persist to determine what might characterize children who recover. Research at the University of Illinois (Yairi & Ambrose, 2005) over the past 20 years indicates that there are several factors that are useful for indicating the likelihood that a child's stuttering will persist rather than disappear naturally. You may wish to follow up on this brief overview by reading the reference, given above, that describes these findings in detail. The following factors appear to be among the most important predictors:

Family history: When a child's family includes stutterers whose stuttering persisted, there is increased risk of persistence.

Gender: Boys have a greater risk of persistence. However, girls typically recover more quickly; therefore, a girl who has been stuttering for a year is at more risk than a boy who has been stuttering for a year.

Age at onset: Children who begin to stutter "later" have a greater risk of persistence. Onsets occur most frequently between ages 2 and 3.5 years, so children with onset after 3.5 years are more at risk.

Trend of stuttering frequency and severity: Children whose stuttering (defined as part-word repetitions and single-syllable word repetitions, prolongations, and blocks) frequency and severity is not decreasing over a period of a year after onset are at more risk of persistence.

Duration since onset: The longer the child continues to stutter beyond a year after onset, the greater the risk of persistence, especially for girls.

Duration of stuttering moments: Continued presence of more than one repetition unit, especially more than three (li-li-li-li-like this) is a sign of increased risk. Also, continued rapid repetitions are a sign of increased risk. Children who recover tend to have fewer repetition units (li-like this) and slower repetitions (li.......like this).

Continued presence of sound prolongations and blocks: The percentage of prolongations and blocks at onset doesn't predict persistence, but if prolongations and blocks do not decrease as stuttering goes on, the child is more likely to persist.

Phonological skills: Children whose phonological skills are below the norms have a greater risk for continued stuttering.

Two other studies examined factors associated with recovery. A longitudinal study by Brosch, Haege, Kalehne, and Johannsen (1999) followed a group of 79 stuttering children for several years. The group that persisted in stuttering had a significantly larger proportion of left-handed children. Because this is a preliminary report from an ongoing study, caution should be exercised in considering this factor as critical to recovery. Nonetheless, the factor of laterality may be one of the additional genetic factors that influence recovery; replication of this work is critical.

In the study by Kloth et al. (1999) described earlier, results indicated that children who recovered had a more mature (less variable) speech motor system, a slower speaking rate, and a mother whose interaction style was nondirective and whose language was less complex. Rommel, Hage, Kalehne, and Johannsen (2000) followed 71 children identified as stuttering soon after onset and followed them for three years. The mothers of those who recovered naturally compared to the mothers of those who persisted had less complex syntax and a smaller number of different words used when talking to their children.

In summary, early studies of recovery reported wide variations in results. Their findings depend on many factors—among them, the accuracy with which stuttering is differentiated from normal disfluency, whether the study is retrospective or longitudinal, and the size of the group studied. The most careful studies are longitudinal assessments of children who are identified soon after the onset of stuttering and are followed for several years. In these studies, about 75 percent of the children who begin to stutter recover without formal treatment. Many factors have been suggested as associated with recovery. These include having relatives who recovered from stuttering or no relatives who stuttered; having an early onset; showing a decrease in frequency and severity of stuttering in the year after onset; having a slower speech rate; having a more stable speech-motor system; having a mother who has a nondirective interaction style and uses less complex language when speaking to the child; being right-handed; having less severe stuttering (although some studies dispute this); having good phonological, language, and nonverbal skills; and being female. We now consider the latter variable, the sex factor, in more detail.

Sex Ratio

Studies of the sex ratio in stuttering were first published in the 1890s and have been published every decade since. With this steady stream of information, we ought to have reliable data on this phenomenon. In fact, we do. The results from studies of people who stutter at many ages and in many cultures put the ratio at about three male stutterers to every one female stutterer. There is strong evidence, however, that the ratio may increase as children get older. For example, Yairi (1983) reported that of 22 children who were 2 and 3 years

of age and whose parents believed they were stuttering, 11 were boys, and 11 were girls. In a larger study of 87 children between 20 and 69 months, Yairi and Ambrose (1992b) found a male:female ratio of 2.1:1 overall, although the 20 youngest subjects, those under 27 months, showed a 1.2:1 ratio.

Bloodstein and Ratner's (2008) review indicated that the male-to-female sex ratio is about 3:1 in the first grade and 5:1 in the fifth grade, confirming the hypothesis that the sex ratio increases as children get older. Evidence of the increasing male-to-female ratio was provided by two recent studies. Kloth and colleagues (1999) found a male:female ratio of 1.1:1 ratio near onset, which rose to 2.5:1 six years later. Mansson (2000) found a male:female ratio of 1.65:1 at the initial screening (age 3), which rose to a ratio of 2.8:1 two years later. The nearly even sex ratio among very young children who stutter and the gradually increasing proportion of boys who stutter may be a consequence of several factors. West (1931) presented data indicating that the change in sex ratio was the result of an increasing proportion of boys beginning to stutter in the late preschool and early school-age years. However, recent data indicate that girls begin to stutter a little earlier than boys (Yairi, 1983; Yairi & Ambrose, 1992b) and recover earlier and more frequently (Andrews et al., 1983; Yairi & Ambrose, 1992b; Yairi & Ambrose, 1999; Yairi, Ambrose, & Cox, 1996).

Females who stutter and don't recover by adulthood may be an interesting subpopulation to study. They may have inherited a stronger predisposition to stutter, have been subjected to strong environmental pressures on their speech, or both (Andrews et al., 1983). Alternately, they may lack the "recovery factor" that most young female stutterers appear to have, or they may have inherited additional factors that interact with stuttering to inhibit recovery.

Variability and Predictability of Stuttering

Another important piece of background information about stuttering is how it varies yet is surprisingly predictable in its occurrence despite the fact that it seems so inconsistent and so idiosyncratic. This predictability is an important clue to its nature. As we trace the research on stuttering's variability, we will see how this information reflects changing theoretical perspectives on the disorder.

Before the 1930s, stuttering had been commonly regarded as a medical disorder. Lee Edward Travis, the first person trained as a Ph.D. to work with speech and hearing disorders, set up a laboratory at the University of Iowa in 1924 to study stuttering from a neurophysiological perspective. He hypothesized that stuttering was the result of an anomalous or inefficient organization of the brain's two cerebral hemispheres. To Travis and his fellow researchers, the variability of stuttering behaviors was seen as part of an organic disorder, and an unimportant part at that. Far more relevant to their research were stutterers' brain waves, heart rates, and breathing patterns. But in the 1930s, psychologists at Iowa and elsewhere began taking a keen interest in behavioral approaches to the study of human disorders, which spilled over into research on stuttering. Scientists who had been trying to understand the neurophysiology of stuttering gradually began trying to examine the social, psychological, and linguistic factors that govern its occurrence and variability (Bloodstein & Ratner, 2008).

Anticipation, Consistency, and Adaptation

Before describing these interesting findings, I'll briefly explain these terms that are best understood in the context of someone who stutters reading a passage several times. "**Anticipation**" refers to an individual's ability to predict what words or sounds he or she will stutter on (Johnson & Solomon, 1937; Knott, Johnson, & Webster, 1937; Milisen, 1938; Van Riper, 1936). "**Consistency**" is the tendency for people to stutter on the same words when they read a passage more than once (Johnson & Inness, 1939; Johnson & Knott, 1937). "**Adaptation**" is the finding that when speakers read a passage several times, they gradually stutter less and less over the course of five or six readings (Johnson & Knott, 1937; Van Riper & Hull, 1955).

These studies were usually carried out by giving the stutterer a passage and asking him to read it aloud. If the experimenter were studying consistency, for example, he would have his own copy of the passage on which he would mark every word on which the speaker stuttered. Then he would ask the speaker to read it again, and the experimenter would again mark the words stuttered in the second reading. From this he could calculate the percentage of words stuttered in two (or more) readings. These findings, called anticipation, consistency, and adaptation, respectively, changed some assumptions about the disorder. Stuttering, it seemed, was not simply a neurophysiological disorder. It showed characteristics of learned behavior, as well.

These studies not only changed existing views of stuttering, they also opened the door to new treatment possibilities. If much of stuttering is learned, it may be unlearned. The challenge was to determine how much is learned and how to help people who stutter develop new responses. Many of the treatment approaches we discuss later in the book use principles of learning to help clients acquire new, fluent responses and reduce the tension and avoidance of their old stuttering responses.

Language Factors

One of the Iowa researchers, Spencer Brown, pushed investigations of the predictability of stuttering into the realm of language. In seven studies completed over a stretch of 10 years, Brown found correlations between stuttering and seven grammatical factors during reading aloud. These findings were reported in a remarkable series of papers Brown published from 1935 to 1945 (Brown, 1937, 1938a, 1938b, 1938c, 1943, 1945; Brown & Moren, 1942; Johnson & Brown,

1935). Brown showed that most adults who stutter do so more frequently

- On consonants
- On sounds in word-initial position
- In contextual speech (vs. isolated words)
- On nouns, verbs, adjectives, and adverbs (vs. articles, prepositions, pronouns, and conjunctions)
- On longer words
- On words at the beginnings of sentences
- On stressed syllables

These findings strongly suggest that stuttering is highly influenced by these linguistic factors.

Later investigators applied Brown's hypotheses to the speech of children who stutter. An advantage in studying language factors in children's stuttering is that the loci (places where it occurs in speech) and frequency of stuttering might be less influenced by responses learned from years of stuttering and more by innate language processing difficulties. Indeed, researchers discovered that although stuttering in elementary school children follows the same linguistic patterns as adult stuttering, the loci and frequency of stuttering in *preschool* children are different. Stuttering in these very young children occurs most frequently on pronouns and conjunctions, not on nouns, verbs, adjectives, and adverbs. It occurs *not* as repetitions, prolongations, or blocks of sounds in word-initial positions, but as repetitions of parts of words and single-syllable words in sentence-initial positions (Bloodstein & Gantwerk, 1967; Bloodstein & Ratner, 2008). This led researchers to hypothesize that in its incipient stage, stuttering is located at the beginning of syntactic units (sentences, clauses, and phrases), as if the task of linguistic planning and preparation was a key ingredient in the recipe for disfluency (Bernstein Ratner, 1997; Bloodstein, 2001, 2002; Bloodstein & Ratner, 2008).

Conture (2001) and others (e.g., Byrd, Wolk, & Davis, 2007) have focused particular attention on the phoneme or sound selection component of linguistic planning in individuals who stutter. Findings that recovery from stuttering may be associated with good phonological skills, a slower speech production rate, and a stable speech-motor system suggest that some individuals who stutter may overcome a linguistic planning delay by relying on strengths in related language areas or by slowing their rates of speech production to compensate for such deficits. We will revisit these modes of compensation when we discuss treatment approaches.

In summary, there are strong links between language and stuttering. As mentioned in the section describing onset, stuttering usually first appears when children are going through the most intense period of language acquisition (Bloodstein & Ratner, 2008). It is also clear that deficits in language (including phonology) often accompany stuttering and may predict its persistence (Yairi & Ambrose,

1999, 2005). Future studies may also confirm what several researchers have suggested, that even stutterers who show no clinically significant language disorders may have subtle language or phonological deficits that contribute to their stuttering (e.g., Byrd, Wolk, & Davis, 2007).

Fluency-Inducing Conditions

One of the researchers at the University of Iowa, Oliver Bloodstein, wrote his Ph.D. dissertation on "Conditions under Which Stuttering Is Reduced or Absent" (Bloodstein, 1948, 1950). In studying the speech of stutterers in 115 conditions, Bloodstein found that stuttering is markedly decreased in many of these conditions. Some of these conditions are speaking when alone, when relaxed, in unison with another speaker, to an animal or an infant, in time to a rhythmic stimulus or when singing, in a different dialect, while simultaneously writing, and when swearing. In later studies, reviewed in Andrews, Howie, Dosza, and Guitar (1982), additional conditions were found to reduce stuttering. These conditions included speaking in a slow prolonged manner, speaking under loud masking noise, speaking while listening to delayed auditory feedback, shadowing another speaker (repeating what they say immediately afterward), and speaking when reinforced for fluent speech.

Various explanations have been proposed to account for the impact of these conditions. Most are compatible with the idea that stuttering has a substantial learned component and is affected by such external stimuli as communicative pressure. Recent brain imaging studies—reviewed in Chapters 2 and 3—indicate that left-hemisphere speech and language structures and functions are impaired in people who stutter. This may make it difficult for a speaker to orchestrate rapid and coordinated production of phonological and lexical items, syntax, intonation, and other subcomponents of spoken language. Thus, many conditions may induce fluency by providing timing cues, reducing rate, lowering stress on vulnerable pathways, or marshaling attentional resources to overcome the limitations of an impaired neurological system.

An Integration

Modern research on stuttering has taken a long and complex journey from Travis's laboratory in Iowa in 1924. Yet, in many ways, those early findings are not entirely irrelevant. Travis's theory of stuttering as a problem of coordinating the two sides of the brain for speech has reemerged as a view of stuttering as a problem of coordinating multiple brain networks for speech with those for language, cognition, and emotion. This juggling act breaks down in all speakers when the resources needed to process language, cognition, or emotion momentarily drain available central nervous system capacities, leaving too little capacity for the intricacies of rapid, smooth speech production. The result is normal disfluency. Those individuals who stutter appear

to have trouble allocating resources to speech production under conditions of high demand. They have inherited or acquired a more vulnerable speech production system— one that is less able to deal with the norm of rapid, smooth speech under a wide variety of conditions, perhaps because the neural pathways used to produce speech are not as efficient as they need to be.

This vulnerable speech production system may heal itself and become more resistant to disruption in children who recover naturally from stuttering. Because of that great neural plasticity characteristic of the very young, some of these children's brains spontaneously develop new, more efficient pathways for speech and become entirely fluent. Others may recover because they learn to compensate by speaking more slowly or finding other ways to marshal their resources to resist disruption. The children who don't recover appear to fall into a cycle of reacting to their disfluencies by tensing muscles, struggling to escape, and even avoiding difficult words and situations. These highly learned reactions—which are influenced by an individual's personality and the people around him—become part of an individual's stuttering patterns and influence the way he thinks and feels about speaking.

This updated view is essentially the model of stuttering presented in this book. To state it more formally, stuttering is an inherited or congenital disorder that first appears when a child is learning the complex and rapid coordinations of speech and language production. Children who do not recover but persist in stuttering are those who may have more extensive deficits in the neural networks of the brain. As stuttering persists, they learn maladaptive responses to their disfluencies. This learning is influenced by their biological temperament, developing social and cognitive awareness, and the response of the environment to their speech.

The next few chapters expand on this theme and prepare you to use this information in diagnosis and treatment.

SUMMARY

- Stuttering appears in all cultures and has been a problem for humankind for at least 40 centuries.
- It is characterized by a high frequency or severity of disruptions that impede the forward flow of speech.
- It begins in childhood and usually becomes more severe as the child grows to adulthood unless he recovers with or without formal treatment.
- Core behaviors of stuttering are repetitions, prolongations, and blocks. Secondary behaviors are the result of attempts to escape or avoid core behaviors and include physical concomitants of stuttering, such as eye blinks or verbal concomitants, such as word substitutions.
- Feelings and attitudes can also be important components of stuttering that reflect the stutterer's emotional reactions

to the experience of being unable to speak fluently and to listener responses to her stuttering. Feelings are immediate emotional reactions and include fear, shame, and embarrassment. Attitudes crystallize more slowly from repeated negative experiences associated with stuttering. An example is a stutterer's belief that listeners think she is stupid when they hear her stuttering.

- Stuttering begins between 18 months of age and puberty, but most often between ages 2 and 5 years, with a peak just before age 3. Its first appearance may be either a gradual increase in easy repetitions of words and sounds or a sudden onset of multiple repetitions, sometimes with prolongations or blocks as well.
- Prevalence of stuttering is about 1 percent. Incidence is about 5 percent. Recovery rate without professional treatment is about 75 percent of children who ever stuttered. The male-to-female ratio in schoolchildren and adults is about 3:1 but may be lower, close to 1:1, in very young children who start to stutter. More girls recover during early childhood, increasing the proportion of males with the disorder after the preschool years.
- Many persons who stutter are able to predict the words in a reading passage they will stutter on before reading it aloud (anticipation), and most tend to stutter on many of the same words each time in repeated readings of a passage (consistency). Stuttering frequency decreases for most stutterers when they read a passage many times (adaptation).
- Stuttering occurs more frequently in certain grammatical contexts. The nature of these grammatical contexts differs somewhat for adults and children.
- A variety of conditions reduces the frequency of stuttering. Their effects may be attributable to changes in speech pattern, reductions in communicative pressure, or both. Research on these fluency-inducing conditions suggests that stuttering may be decreased by conditions that reduce the demands on speech motor control and language formulation functions.

STUDY QUESTIONS

1. What might make some children's core behaviors change from repetitions to prolongations to blocks?
2. What are the differences between core and secondary behaviors in stuttering?
3. When stuttering is defined, from what other kinds of hesitation must it be distinguished?
4. What are some feelings and attitudes people who stutter might have, and what is their origin? Do nonstutterers ever have these feelings?
5. What is the age range for the onset of stuttering (the youngest and oldest ages at which onset is commonly reported)? Why might it occur at that time?
6. What is the difference between "incidence" and "prevalence?"
7. What problems do researchers encounter when they try to determine how many stutterers recover without treatment?
8. Why might the ratio of male-to-female stutterers change with age?
9. In what ways is stuttering predictable? In what ways does it vary?
10. Why is it difficult to answer the question, "What is *the* cause of stuttering?"
11. The International Classification of Functioning, Disability, and Health (ICF) indicates that with some conditions, interpersonal interactions may be affected. How might stuttering affect these interactions?
12. How can stuttering treatment help change factors affecting the individual in the ICF area called "Contextual Factors?"
13. How would you describe the etiology of stuttering to a parent who has had limited education and is not used to discussing abstract concepts?

SUGGESTED PROJECTS

1. Enlist the help of an adult who stutters, and have him teach you to stutter. Then ask him to go with you while you use some voluntary stuttering in public. Write a brief report of what feelings you experienced and how people reacted to you.
2. Use an Internet search engine like Google to find an online discussion group of people who stutter and clinicians. Join the group and observe what issues they discuss.
3. Attend a support group for people who stutter.
4. Listen to some *preschool* children talking and note their normal disfluencies. Then listen to *elementary* school children talking, and compare their disfluencies to those of the preschool children.
5. If you are a fluent speaker, record your own speech and observe the types of disfluencies you hear. Do they differ from stuttering? In what ways?
6. Conduct a search on the Internet for resources that guide you to critically evaluate Web sites (for example, http://www.library.ucla.edu/libraries/college/help/critical). Using that format, critically evaluate a Web site you find when searching for "stuttering" sites with your search engine.

SUGGESTED VIEWING

The King's Speech. This film depicts King George VI of England who stuttered severely, but found a great deal of help with his Australian speech therapist, Lionel Logue. The movie provides an excellent depiction of the emotions surrounding stuttering.

SUGGESTED READINGS

Bloodstein, O. (1993). *Stuttering: The search for a cause and cure.* Boston: Allyn and Bacon.

This book is part history and part analysis, written with charm and clarity. Bloodstein covers early treatments for stuttering, the burgeoning of research in the 1930s, 1940s, and 1950s, and more recent findings in the realm of neurophysiology. His own orientation on the learning-environmental basis of stuttering comes through, but he gives good coverage of other possible factors as well. Bloodstein is particularly good at conveying the excitement that accompanies research.

Bobrick, B. (1995). *Knotted tongues—Stuttering in history and the quest for a cure.* New York: Simon and Schuster.

A highly readable account of various treatments for stuttering throughout the ages and of famous people who stutter.

Carlisle, J. (1985). *Tangled tongue: Living with a stutter.* Toronto: University of Toronto Press.

An eloquent autobiography by a man with a severe stutter and a great sense of humor.

Helliesen, G. (2002). *Forty years after therapy: One man's story.* Newport News, VA: Apollo Press.

An autobiography of someone who stuttered severely and was treated by Charles Van Riper, the world-renowned stuttering clinician. This book presents a unique view of stuttering therapy from the client's viewpoint.

Jezer, M. (1997). *Stuttering: A life bound up in words.* New York: Basic Books.

A compelling, sensitive book about the frustrating and sometimes funny things that happen to someone growing up with a severe stuttering problem and learning to cope with it.

Murray, F.P. (undated). *A stutterer's story.* Memphis: Stuttering Foundation of America. (www.stutteringhelp.org).

An autobiography depicting the long struggle of someone who stuttered severely and spent his life searching for answers. The author describes his acquaintance with many of the pioneers of stuttering therapy.

Shields, D. (1989). *Dead languages.* New York: Knopf.

This is a novel about a young boy who stutters. It conveys the feelings associated with being a stutterer in a world that prizes spoken language. It is recommended for students who would like to understand a child who stutters.

St. Louis, K. (Ed.) (2001). *Living with stuttering—Stories, basics, resources, and hope.* Morgantown, WV: Populore Publishing Company.

The life stories of 25 people who stutter and how they have coped with their stuttering.

Constitutional Factors in Stuttering

CHAPTER OBJECTIVES

After studying this chapter, readers should be able to:

- Describe the evidence supporting genetic inheritance of stuttering from (a) family studies, (b) twin studies, and (c) adoption studies

- Explain how genetic studies are done and what has been found about how chromosomes and genes are associated with stuttering
- Explain why congenital and early childhood factors are thought to contribute to a predisposition to develop stuttering and what some of these factors may be
- Describe the ways in which brain structures in stuttering individuals differ from those of nonstuttering individuals
- Describe the ways in which brain functions in stuttering individuals differ from those of nonstuttering individuals
- Describe changes in the brain that are associated with improvements in fluency as the result of treatment
- Describe differences in these areas found between groups of individuals who stutter and groups of individuals who don't: (a) sensory processing, (b) central auditory processing, (c) dichotic listening, (d) auditory feedback, (e) sensory-motor control, (f) reaction time, (g) fluent speech, and (h) nonspeech motor control
- Suggest why differences in each of the above areas could contribute to stuttering
- Describe how language development and performance in individuals who stutter have been found to differ from individuals who don't
- Describe the ways in which stuttering and emotion may be related.

KEY TERMS

Anomaly: A difference from the normal structure or function

Family studies: Examination of family trees of individuals who stutter to determine the frequency and pattern of the occurrence of stuttering in relatives. These studies can answer questions such as whether males or females are more likely to have children who stutter and whether persistent stuttering (as opposed to natural recovery) is a trait that is inherited

Twin studies: Research on the co-occurrence of stuttering of both members of a twin pair if one twin stutters; questions such as whether identical twins show more concordance than fraternal twins can be answered, shedding light on the extent of a genetic basis of stuttering

Adoption studies: Investigations of stuttering in siblings who were adopted soon after birth and placed with different families. A higher incidence of stuttering among biological relatives than adoptive family members also provides evidence of a genetic basis of stuttering rather than an environmental basis

Persistent stuttering: Stuttering that persists for several years after onset, beyond the time at which natural recovery is likely to occur

Natural recovery (from stuttering): Stuttering that disappears within a year or two after onset from natural causes rather than from treatment

Concordance (in twins): If one twin has a condition, such as stuttering, the other twin also has the condition

Gene: A segment of DNA that determines an individual's traits, such as height and weight

DNA: A double-stranded molecule passed on from a mother and a father to a child containing the "instruction book" for passing on traits

Congenital factor: A physical or psychological trauma that occurred at or near birth that may predispose an individual to develop stuttering

Predisposition: A susceptibility to developing a condition

Sensory processing: Activity of the brain as it interprets information coming from the senses, such as sounds arriving via the ears and auditory nerves

Sensory-motor control: The way all movement is carried out with sensory information used before, during, and after to improve the precision of movement

Temperament: Aspects of an individual's personality, such as sensitive versus thick skinned, that are thought to be innate rather than learned

I have written this chapter to be a readable summary of perspectives and research on constitutional factors in stuttering. Details of important studies are provided in Chapter 3. Figure 2.1 illustrates the major areas covered in this chapter and how the topics are related.

Taking it from the top, you will learn that heredity and congenital and/or early childhood trauma are background factors that can contribute to stuttering. They influence how brain structure and function develop. You will also learn how the brains of those of us who stutter may be different from those of typical speakers and how that may influence what I believe is the major direct link to stuttering—sensory-motor control. You will also learn about two other factors that appear to be influences on stuttering onset and development via their influences on sensory-motor control of speech: language factors and emotional factors. Both of these

are to some extent products of brain structure and function. Language and emotional factors are also influenced by the environment, a major determinant of stuttering that will be covered in Chapters 4 and 5.

BIOLOGICAL BACKGROUND

Hereditary Factors

Two individuals contributed a vast amount to our understanding of the mechanisms of heredity. One was the Austrian monk, Gregor Mendel, whose experiments in breeding varieties of peas gave rise to his insights about genetic inheritance. He established the principle that each parent in a breeding pair contributes equally to the genetic makeup of the offspring, and he developed the understanding of dominant and recessive traits. The other major contributor to the science of genetics was Charles Darwin, who, interestingly, is thought to have inherited stuttering from his grandfather, Erasmus (Thomson, 2009). Darwin's theory of evolution suggested that while specific characteristics (such as height, weight, and skin color) could be inherited by one generation from another, variations in how those characteristics expressed themselves produced slight differences in members of a species. These differences favored some individuals more than others, depending on the environment; the most favorable traits for the current environment of the species would be increased because individuals possessing them would thrive and reproduce most frequently.

Stuttering often runs in families, a fact long recognized by researchers (e.g., Andrews et al., 1983; Bloodstein & Ratner, 2008). For many years, researchers debated about what this meant. Some suggested that the appearance of stuttering in several generations of a family must mean that it is caused by an inherited neurological difference or **anomaly**. Others disagreed, countering that political beliefs often run in families too, but aren't inherited. Some researchers argued that stuttering develops in response to a critical attitude toward normal disfluency that has been handed down from one generation to the next (Johnson & associates, 1959). A child whose parents were critical of her normal disfluencies would grow afraid and would "hesitate to hesitate." This would start a spiral of more hesitations leading to greater fear and so on.

For many years, researchers aligned themselves with one side of this argument or the other. Currently, however, there is broad agreement that stuttering can be inherited (Bloodstein & Ratner, 2008; Yairi & Ambrose, 2005). In other words, for many people who stutter, one or both of their parents had some predisposition to stuttering that was transmitted in their genes. Current thinking may be due to strong newer evidence about heredity in stuttering but is probably also due to the rise of less deterministic views of heredity. Research has shown, for a number of inherited disorders, that genes do not work alone. Stuttering, asthma, migraine headaches,

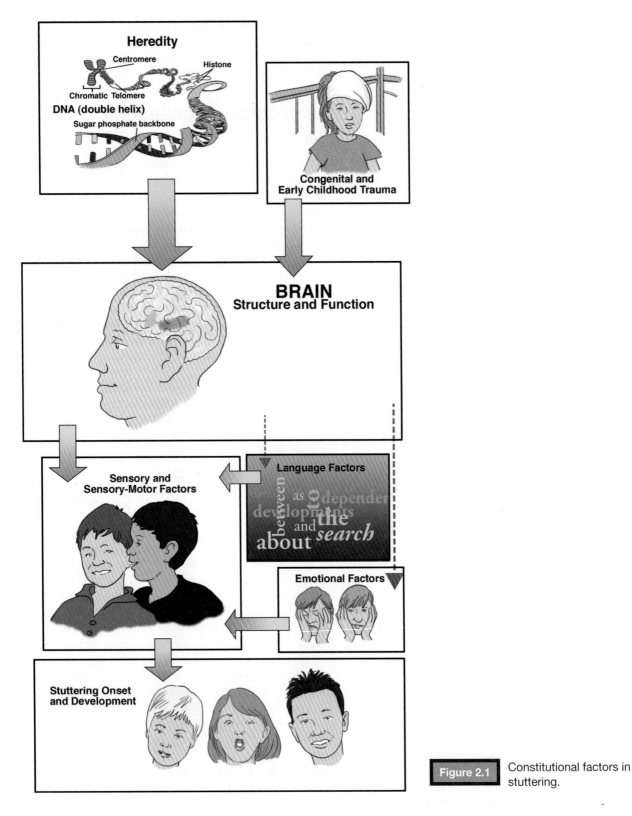

Figure 2.1 Constitutional factors in stuttering.

and certain other disorders are seen as the result of heredity *and* environment acting together with elements of chance thrown in (Kidd, 1984). The interaction between heredity and environment is something we commonly encounter. For example, this year I grew all my tomato plants from the same seed packet, giving them an identical heredity. But I planted some near Burlington, in a relatively warm environment (for Vermont), and I planted others in the Northeast Kingdom of Vermont, a colder, cloudier summer environment. As you might guess, by mid-August the tomatoes near warmer, sunnier Burlington were plump and red, while those in the Northeast Kingdom were shriveled and sickly green, showing that environment had a strong differential effect on heredity. And so it is with stuttering.

Going back to the topic at hand, a child in one family may inherit genes predisposing him to stutter, but his home environment may be so low key that stuttering never develops. A different child, inheriting similar genes, may grow up in a demanding, hectic, fast-talking home and begin to stutter at age 3. And lest this comment appear to hearken back to a period when parents were blamed, it may often be the case that which aspects of the environment play a role for any given child will remain a mystery.

In this chapter, I will review three approaches to the study of heredity and stuttering: **family studies**, **twin studies**, and **adoption studies**. These different ways of gathering evidence all suggest that for many individuals, stuttering is partly attributable to heredity. The insights we gain from these studies are vital to us in counseling individuals and families about the nature of stuttering.

Family Studies

In family studies, researchers gather evidence of the inheritance of stuttering by studying family trees. They begin with a group of individuals who stutter, for example, a group of 100. They then make up a group of 100 individuals who don't stutter, matched with the first group by age and gender. The researchers interview all the relatives in each group member's family to determine the average number of stuttering relatives each person has. Then they compare the findings in each group to answer the question: Do individuals who stutter have more relatives who stutter than individuals who don't stutter?

As scientists study family trees of stutterers, they also search for patterns of occurrence of stuttering. Geneticists know that certain inherited traits occur in specific patterns in families, and they ask whether stuttering follows a known pattern of inheritance. For example, some traits appear only if both the mother and father have the trait; other traits are more common in children when the mother has the trait than when the father has the trait. Therefore, when scientists find these known patterns of family occurrence in a disorder like stuttering, it provides more evidence to support the idea that the disorder is inherited rather than simply the result of imitation, critical family attitudes about disfluency, or some other aspect of their shared environment.

To summarize the research, despite the small number of studies and their limitations, family studies have provided strong evidence for a genetic predisposition in many individuals who stutter. Males tend to be at more risk to develop persistent stuttering, while females seem to have some natural resistance to persistent stuttering and tend to recover from stuttering more easily. Some evidence also suggests that there may be more than one genetic mechanism involved in **persistent stuttering**; one or more genes may carry the predisposition for the speech breakdown evident in children who

begin to stutter, while an additional genetic predisposition may prevent or facilitate **natural recovery** from stuttering.

Twin Studies

The genetic transmission of stuttering can also be investigated by comparing the incidence of stuttering in fraternal and identical twins. Identical twins (also called monozygotic twins) have completely identical genes. In fraternal twins (dizygotic), only 25 percent of their genes are identical, like any other two siblings. Greater similarities in the traits of identical twins compared with those of fraternal twins are generally attributed to inheritance.

The many studies of stuttering in twins reveal two major findings. One is that compared to fraternal, same-sex twins, identical twins show more **concordance** (if one twin stutters, the other also does). The second is that even though there is much concordance among identical twins, there are still many identical twin pairs in which one twin stutters and the other doesn't (discordance). These two findings suggest that genes don't work alone; the environment must interact with genes to produce the behavior in question, and even in twins, their environments (both before they are born and after) may not be as similar as they might superficially seem.

Adoption Studies

One of the most powerful methods to examine the relative contributions of genes and the environment to stuttering is to look at the families of stutterers who were adopted soon after birth. Higher incidence of stuttering among the *biological* relatives of adopted stutterers would support a greater role of genetics in causing stuttering, whereas higher incidence among *adoptive* relatives would support a greater role of the environment. The few studies that have been done had mixed results, but one study that investigated both biological and adoptive families found that although both heredity and environment play a role in the occurrence of stuttering, heredity plays a slightly stronger role (Felsenfeld, 1997).

Genes

Humans have between 25,000 and 35,000 different genes. These **genes** are segments of DNA that determine various individual traits. **DNA** contains the "instruction book" that tells the body how to make various chemicals that determine such characteristics as a person's height, weight, eye color, emotional vulnerability, athletic ability, and everything else that is influenced by heredity. Very long strings of DNA (containing many genes) are wrapped into the little worm-like structures called chromosomes (see Fig. 2.2).

Almost every cell in the body contains 23 pairs of chromosomes—one member of each pair from the individual's mother and one from the father. Some traits may be determined more by the mother's genes and others more by the father's. Some traits are determined by one gene, others by multiple genes acting together. The hunt for genes related to stuttering is conducted by looking at the chromosomes in

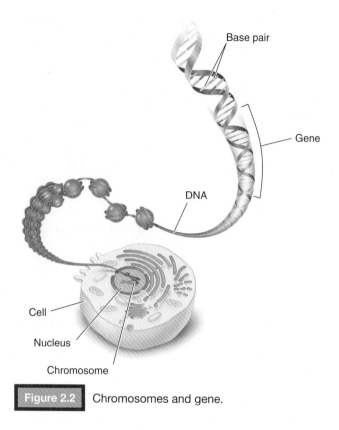

Figure 2.2   Chromosomes and gene.

many related individuals, some of whom stutter and some of whom don't. Thus, many chromosomes in related individuals will all be the same, but if genetics is a factor in stuttering, the subgroup of related people who stutter will have one or more chromosomes that will be different from the subgroup of related people who don't stutter.

Researchers looking at families and communities with large concentrations of individuals who stutter have identified seven different chromosomes that appear to be associated with stuttering. One of these chromosomes has been shown to carry three genetic mutations, one of which is associated with motor control and emotional regulation (Kang, Riazuddin, Mundorff, Krasnewich, & Friedman et al., 2010). The many different chromosomes and genes found to be associated with stuttering in the studies described in Chapter 3 testify to how varied and complex the origins of stuttering may be. Many different factors may contribute to stuttering, and these factors interact with others to create a neurological substrate for stuttering. For example, neurophysiological deficits may give rise to problems and delays in speech motor control, sensory processing, language planning and execution, and/or emotional vulnerability. Combinations of these problems may result in the repetitions, prolongations, and blocks that appear in children as they develop speech and language in "one great blooming, buzzing confusion" (James, 1890) that is the child's normal environment in the typical family.

When talking with parents about the genetics of stuttering, be aware that parents may have mixed feelings about

the possibility that their child inherited a predisposition to stutter. On the one hand, it may help them realize that their parenting style didn't cause the stuttering; on the other, parents may feel guilty for passing on genes that may have resulted in stuttering. However, it is important for them to know that genetic variations are neither all good nor all bad. Remember the genius of Charles Darwin: Genes that predispose a child to stuttering may also pass on very beneficial or even extraordinary talents (Table 2.1).

Congenital and Early Childhood Factors

It has been estimated that 30 to 60 percent of individuals who stutter have family histories of stuttering (Yairi, Ambrose, & Cox, 1996). Therefore, 40 to 70 percent of individuals who stutter have *no* family history and may have developed the disorder by mechanisms other than inheritance of a predisposition that has caused stuttering in relatives. However, we do not know how many of these individuals inherited a factor or several factors that predisposed them to stuttering but did not produce stuttering in other family members. On the other hand, some individuals who stutter may not have inherited any factor, which predisposed them to stutter. Instead, they may have experienced a physical or psychological trauma that predisposed them to stuttering or even precipitated its onset. Such traumas may have occurred at or near birth and would be viewed as **congenital factors**. Some events or factors may also have occurred during early childhood rather than at or near birth, but for simplicity's sake, I will refer to them all in the remainder of this section as congenital.

Unfortunately, there is relatively little research on congenital factors related to stuttering. The research that has been done can be divided into studies which examined stutterers who had no family history of stuttering and studies that examined large groups of individuals who sustained brain injuries at birth or in childhood to determine if there were more cases of stuttering in populations with early brain injuries than in the general population.

In summary, studies of individuals who stuttered but had no family history of stuttering found that this group had more history of infectious diseases, anoxia at birth, childhood surgery, head injury, mild cerebral palsy, mild retardation, and intense fear prior to the onset of stuttering. Studies of young adults who had brain injuries found a greater incidence of stuttering, especially if the individuals had been unconscious for a time following the injury. Finally, although the results are not uniform in this, studies of stutterers with family histories of stuttering found that these individuals had more prolongations and silent blocks in stuttering and a slower rate and more variability in fluent speech, compared with stutterers without a family history of stuttering.

As we've just seen, the **predisposition** for stuttering may come not only from genetic inheritance but may also come from congenital factors. Thus, it may be most appropriate to use the term "constitutional predisposition" (Table 2.2).

Table 2.1	Summary of Hereditary Factors in Stuttering	
Area of Interest	**Important Findings**	**Major Clinical Implications**
Family Studies	Stuttering appears to be inherited in many cases. There may be a single gene for transitory stuttering and that gene combines with others for persistent stuttering. Sex ratio at onset is fairly equal—less than 2:1, males to females. Females are more likely to recover within two years, making the ratio 3:1 in early school years. Factors that predict recovery include (a) being female, (b) no family members who stuttered or only transitory stuttering, (c) early onset of stuttering (prior to age 3), and (d) good language, phonological, and nonverbal abilities.	Parents should be told that stuttering is often inherited rather than the result of their parenting. Prognosis improves as more of the four recovery factors are true for the child.
Twin Studies	Greater concordance among identical compared to fraternal twins. At least two-thirds of the influence on the occurrence of stuttering appears to be related to genes, one-third or less to environmental factors.	Both genetic and environmental factors are important, so the child's home environment might be an influence in occurrence of stuttering and recovery.
Adoption Studies	More than chance occurrence of biological and adopted relatives who stuttered among adopted children. These studies provide evidence for the importance of both genetic and environmental factors.	Presence of relatives who stutter does not make it certain that a child will stutter.
Genes	Genes associated with stuttering have been found on chromosomes 1, 7, 9, 12, 13, 15, 16, and 18. Both persistent and recovered stuttering are associated with chromosome 9, but persistent stuttering by itself is associated with chromosome 15. Studies in very different cultural groups have identified chromosome 12 as significantly related to stuttering. Mutations of three different genes on this chromosome have been identified as being associated with stuttering.	Research is underway to identify genes associated with stuttering. This may lead to earlier identification and preventative treatment. For parents, these studies may provide support for understanding that they did not cause their child's stuttering by anything they did. Parents concerned that they may have passed on genes that predisposed their child to stuttering should know that they may also have passed on traits that are highly desirable.

Brain Structure and Function

Whether an individual's stuttering results from an inherited predisposition or from an early brain injury or other trauma, it seems likely that structures and functions in the central nervous system would be different or "anomalous" in those who stutter. Brain structures and functions would be, in effect, the bridge between the etiology of the disorder and the behavior. In other words, a genetic predisposition,

Table 2.2	Summary of Congenital and Early Childhood Factors	
Area of Interest	**Important Findings**	**Major Clinical Implications**
Congenital and Early Childhood Factors	Of stutterers, 40–70 percent have no family history of stuttering. Onset of stuttering, especially in cases without family history, has been associated with such factors as brain injury before or soon after birth, premature birth, surgery, head injury, retardation, and intense fear. Evidence shows that individuals with family histories that include stuttering exhibit more evidence of neuromotor instability.	Heredity shouldn't be assumed to be the only cause of stuttering. Clinician should ask family about child's experiences and events near the time of stuttering onset. Clinician should be mindful that a purpose of exploring etiology is to relieve guilt of parents. Statements about cause should be made tentatively and without blaming family.

injury, trauma, or some unknown cause might result in brain structures and/or functions that delay or disrupt normal neural processing for speech and language. This delay or disruption might, in turn, result in the repetitions, prolongations, and/or blocks that characterize the disorder.

The search for how these brain structures or functions are different in people who stutter has been underway at least since the experiments of Lee Edward Travis at the University of Iowa in the 1930s, described in Chapter 1. In the following sections, I will review studies of brain structure and brain function in separate sections, even though they obviously influence each other. I will follow the discussion of structures and functions by talking about how stuttering may have changed brain structure and how treatment may have changed brain function. I am indebted to the chapter by Neumann and Euler (2010) for some of the recent brain imaging information. As you read about specific anatomical areas, consult Figure 2.3 to orient yourself to landmarks related to speech and language production in both stutterers and nonstutterers.

Brain Structure Differences in People Who Stutter

Compared to the search for anomalous function in the brains of people who stutter, research on actual structural differences in their brains has begun relatively recently. Several studies between 2000 and 2007 (see Chapter 3) examined the brain anatomy of adults who stuttered by measuring the shape, size, and density of speech and language areas. The findings suggest that sensory, planning, and motor areas in the left hemisphere of these individuals developed differently from those in matched nonstuttering individuals. For example, white matter tracts, which convey information from sensory centers that may store phonological representations of sounds to motor execution areas of the left hemisphere, have been shown to be less dense than those in normal speakers, whereas the same tracts were found to be *denser* in the *right* hemisphere of those who stuttered. It is as if the right hemisphere had taken over some typically left hemisphere functions.

By 2008, neuroimaging researchers had developed techniques that were safe enough to use with children. In that year, two groups of investigators published studies of school-age

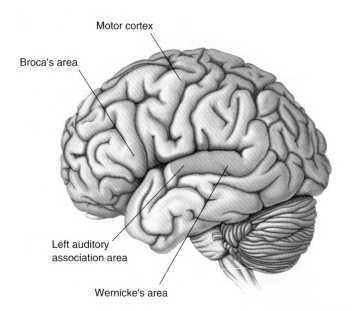

Motor cortex

Broca's area

Left auditory association area

Wernicke's area

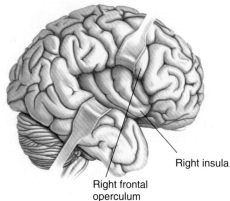

Right insula

Right frontal operculum

Figure 2.3 Areas in the left and right sides of the brain that may be involved in speech and language processing in stutterers and nonstutterers.

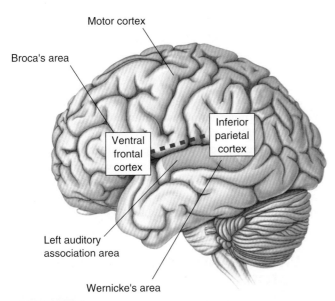

Motor cortex

Broca's area

Ventral frontal cortex

Inferior parietal cortex

Left auditory association area

Wernicke's area

Figure 2.4 The superior longitudinal fasciculus III is a bi-direction pathway between the inferior parietal cortex (sensory integration) and the ventral frontal cortex (motor planning).

children who had stuttered in their preschool years. One study of children who recovered from stuttering compared to those who hadn't (and a control group) showed that both recovered and persistent stutterers had reduced volumes of gray matter around Broca's area, as well as in bilateral temporal lobe areas that may be related to auditory perception of speech (Chang, Erickson, Ambrose, Hasegawa-Johnson, & Ludlow, 2008). The subgroup that persisted in stuttering also showed less dense white matter tracts connecting phonological representations of sounds to speech motor execution areas, the same deficit as discovered in adult stutterers, described earlier. This finding was reported again in a second study of slightly older children in that same year, suggesting that this structural abnormality in the left hemisphere may be a major factor in stuttering (Watkins, Smith, Davis, & Howell, 2008).

The 2008 findings of the two groups cited above were replicated by Cykowski, Fox, Ingham, Ingham, and Robin (2010), using more extensive brain imaging technology. They suggested that the most robust difference between stutterers and nonstutterers is in left-hemisphere fiber tracts that communicate between the inferior parietal cortex (sensory integration) with the ventral frontal cortex (motor planning) (see Fig. 2.4). As in earlier studies, the authors found that in individuals who stutter compared to nonstutterers, certain nerve fibers aren't structured as effectively to conduct impulses along the directional flow of the nerve bundle. Thus, conduction is not as fast as it might be. The fiber tract in question is the superior longitudinal fasciculus; its function is to provide sensory-motor integration for speech. See the next chapter for more details on these research findings.

Brain Function Differences in People Who Stutter

Research on functional differences has a long history beginning in the 1920s with what now seems like primitive technology. Interestingly, more recent studies using modern technology have validated many of those old findings.

In essence, both old and new studies have shown that individuals who stutter have a greater activity in their right hemispheres than in their left hemispheres, during both fluent and stuttered speech. This is the reverse of the pattern shown by fluent control subjects who show considerable left-hemisphere activity and little right-hemisphere activity during speech. Figure 2.5 shows this difference between stutterers and nonstutterers. The activity seen in the stutterers' right hemispheres was often in those very areas that are homologous (parallel) to the left-hemisphere areas most active in fluent speakers.

Neuroimaging studies have also revealed a great deal of underactivation of left-hemisphere structures typically active for speech, such as areas around the white matter tracts presumed to carry information from sensory and sound representation areas to motor execution areas (see Figs. 2.4 and 2.6).

Nonstuttering speakers

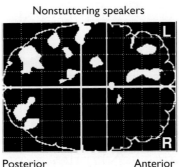

Posterior   Anterior

Stuttering speakers

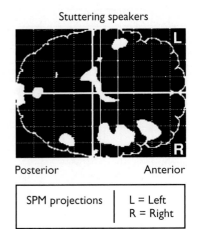

Posterior   Anterior

| SPM projections | L = Left |
| | R = Right |

Figure 2.5 PET scans of brains of nonstuttering (*left*) and stuttering (*right*) adults while reading aloud. SPM, statistical parametric mapping. (From De Nil, L., Kroll, R., Kapur, S., & Houle, S. (1995). *Silent and oral reading in stuttering and nonstuttering adults: A positron emission tomography study*. Paper presented at the Annual Convention of the American Speech-Language-Hearing Association, Orlando, Florida, December.)

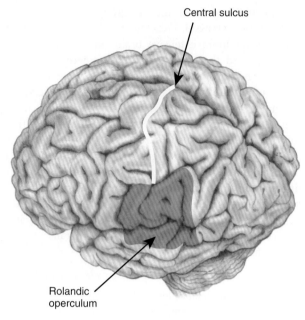

Central sulcus

Rolandic
operculum

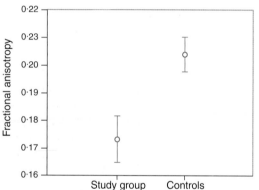

Figure 2.6 Density of white matter tracts between sensorimotor areas and speech planning areas in stutterers (study group) and nonstutterers (control group).

Studies of stutterers after treatment have generally revealed a reversal of right-hemisphere overactivation and left-hemisphere underactivation just described. Both short-term and long-term treatment outcome studies using brain imaging suggested that areas of the left-hemisphere that were previously underactivated were now reactivated, and right-hemisphere sites were now more normally underactivated.

Figure 2.7 depicts the differences in brain activity between stutterers before and after treatment. It is evident, particularly in the brain images of stutterers in Figure 2.7 (a) before treatment and (b) immediately after treatment, that activity levels shift from greater in the right hemisphere to greater in the left hemisphere (Table 2.3).

SENSORY AND SENSORY-MOTOR FACTORS

As you can see in Figure 2.1, sensory and motor factors that influence stuttering emerge from an individual's brain structure and function. They influence the onset and development of stuttering because they limit how well the individual can produce rapid and fluent speech. For example, earlier I described the findings that suggest that the fiber tracts integrating sensory, planning, and motor functions for speech appear to be significantly less dense in individuals who stutter. This may mean that sensory-motor tasks, such as saying "ah" after hearing a bell, will be slower in stutterers.

The findings summarized in the following sections compare stuttering and nonstuttering speakers' sensory and sensory-motor functions, using a variety of experiments. Keep in mind that the purpose of these comparisons is to learn more about deficits in those who stutter. When sensory and sensory-motor functions are poorer in stutterers, there is an assumption that it reflects a brain structure or function difference that may be causally related to stuttering.

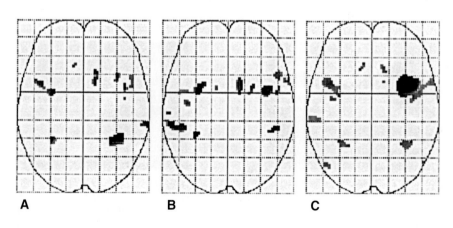

A   B   C

Figure 2.7 Overt reading: statistical parametrical maps of between-group comparisons (people who stutter versus people who do not stutter) **(A)** before therapy, **(B)** immediately after therapy, **(C)** two years after therapy (Neumann, Euler, Wolff von Gudenberg, Giraud, & Lanfermann et al., 2003).

Table 2.3	Summary of Brain Structure and Function in Stuttering	
Area of Interest	**Important Findings**	**Major Clinical Implications**
EEG Studies	Stutterers differ from nonstutterers in showing more activity on the right side of the brain in structures similar to those on left side active in nonstutterers. Stutterers show more left-hemisphere activity during speech after treatment.	Evidence that treatment is associated with greater activity in the left hemisphere during speaking. May have implications about the neurological changes that accompany improvement in fluency
Brain Imaging Studies Using MRI, PET, and Modern Techniques	Stutterers show the following differences from nonstutterers: • Overactivation of many areas of right hemisphere during speaking, especially when stuttering • Deactivation of left auditory cortex during stuttering • Anomalous symmetry in planum temporal (part of Wernicke's area) in stutterers • Less dense fibers in white matter tracts of left operculum, which are thought to connect sensory, planning, and motor areas After either transitory or long-term fluency is induced, right-hemisphere overactivity is reduced and left-hemisphere speech, language, and auditory areas are activated.	As above, evidence that improvement in fluency is associated with increase in left-hemisphere activity and decrease in right-hemisphere activity. Potential to refine treatments by increasing activities that involve left-hemisphere speech, language, and auditory areas. Treatments that encourage clients to carefully monitor their speech may engage the left hemisphere.

Some Caveats about Finding the Causes of Stuttering

As researchers have searched for the causes of stuttering, they have been hampered by the difficulty in demonstrating cause-and-effect relationships. In particular, the brain differences described in the preceding section could be the cause of the disorder or the result of how the brain has responded to years of stuttering (most likely, some of each is involved). Moreover, brain activity during stuttering may also be indirectly related to the behavior of stuttering; for example, some right hemisphere activity may be a manifestation of stutterers' fears and anxiety about stuttering. These fears might not cause the disorder in the first place, but they may make it worse.

In some speech disorders, which have a more clear-cut physical basis, cause and effect can be directly investigated. There may even be animal models of the disorder to work from. In a disorder that can occur in animals, factors thought to cause the disorder can be manipulated and their effects measured. For example, interfering with the genes or the embryonic development of dogs, cats, or rabbits can produce the clefting or spasticity that is respectively similar to cleft palate or cerebral palsy seen in humans. Thus, scientists can infer how inheritance, embryonic development, or brain trauma can cause these disorders. However, communication through spoken language does not occur in animals, which makes it less likely that animal models can be used to look for the cause of disorders like stuttering. And obviously, selective breeding

or surgery to create stuttering is not an option in humans. Therefore, researchers have turned to indirect approaches, or *descriptive* rather than *experimental* approaches. They compare groups of stutterers and nonstutterers on tasks they believe are related to speech fluency. If they find, again and again, that the two groups perform differently in certain tasks, they may have a clue about the disorder.

Such indirect research is complicated because the differences that are found might be a *result* of stuttering, not a cause of it. For example, reaction time studies of how quickly subjects can say a word that is flashed on a screen might show that subjects who stutter are slower than subjects who don't. This difference, however, might be the result of subjects who stutter saying words more slowly to keep from stuttering. Even if a difference is not the result of trying not to stutter, it is more likely to be only a correlated factor that has no causal relationship to stuttering. Even if groups of stutterers do respond more slowly, slower reaction times alone probably do not cause stuttering. If they did, people would start stuttering as they grew older or after they had imbibed a few beers. Finding something that co-occurs with something else but doesn't cause it is like finding that most basketball players have larger shoe sizes than most gymnasts. Shoe size itself doesn't determine who is better suited for each of these sports, but height may be a determining factor. Both shoe size and height are related to one's genetically determined bone size, so they end up being different in gymnasts and basketball players, but shoe size itself doesn't make one a better basketball player or gymnast.

Another problem with descriptive studies rather than experimental approaches to studying the nature of stuttering is that when comparing groups of people who do and do not stutter, there is often a great deal of overlap in the two groups' performances even though their averages might be statistically different. For example, some of the people who stutter will usually show coordination as good as the average person in the group of nonstutterers on a typical test of motor coordination, and some of the people who don't stutter will demonstrate the same level of coordination as an average person in the stuttering group. These overlaps remind us that we are usually not studying factors that are necessary or sufficient by themselves to cause stuttering. Such underlying differences between people who stutter and people who don't may provide us clues, however. And with those clues in hand, we may look more closely at certain abilities, brain functions, and neuroanatomical sites to see if there truly are things that distinguish all stutterers from all nonstutterers. Failing to find that, we will see if there are subgroups of stutterers, some of whom differ from nonstutterers in one way and others who differ in another way. This may then help us discover other paths leading to a better understanding of stuttering.

In the next section, I will review some of the literature on stutterer/nonstutterer performance differences. As you will see, when scientists try to repeat others' experiments to verify their results, inconsistent research findings are common. One study finds a difference; another study reports there isn't one. Differences in the findings of two studies may occur because different subjects were involved or because there were small differences in the way that the studies were done. For example, one study may use a 1,000-Hz tone as a stimulus, and another study may use a recording of the word "go." Despite the inconsistencies in many results, there are areas of agreement or trends that many studies find. As you read, try to determine for yourself which areas give us solid leads. In my summaries, I will share my own interpretation of these areas of overlap.

Sensory Processing

You might wonder why research has been conducted on the ability of individuals who stutter to process sensory information such as auditory, visual, and tactile signals. Stuttering, after all, appears to be a motor rather than a sensory problem. The answer is twofold. First, as patients with various injuries and diseases have taught us, normal speech depends on intact auditory as well as proprioceptive (feeling of position and movement) and tactile (feeling of touch) feedback. Researchers have been curious to see if stutterers' abnormal speech might be the result of some disturbance of feedback. Second, experiments, which have altered **sensory processing**, such as delayed auditory feedback (Black, 1951; Lee, 1951), have created repetitions, prolongations, and blocks in normal speakers, prompting scientists to ask whether this might be the cause of stuttering.

The findings that I'm about to review may be related to the results of the brain imaging studies discussed earlier. Remember that many studies found that areas of the auditory cortex are underactivated during stuttering (Beal, Gracco, Lafaille, & De Nil, 2007; Brown, Ingham, Ingham, Laird, & Fox, 2005), while others have found structural anomalies in the auditory cortex (Foundas, Bollich, Corey, Hurley, & Heilman, 2001). Still other research has discovered reduced density in stutterers' white matter fibers that support sensory-motor integration in speech production (Sommer, Koch, Paulus, Willer, & Bücher, 2002). It would not be surprising, then, if anomalies in these areas affect both the fluency of speech production and the accuracy of speech perception. For example, the superior temporal gyrus has been shown to contain systems that are important in the phonemic planning of utterances and the understanding of speech (Hickok, 2001). Moreover, efficient functioning of the auditory cortex is likely to be critical for fluent speech production because of the crucial role of auditory feedback in normal speaking and the deleterious effects on fluency of delaying auditory feedback.

Central Auditory Processing

A number of studies (see Chapter 3) have been conducted to assess how accurately and quickly individuals who stutter can identify or judge the duration of auditory signals, compared to nonstutterers. The major findings have been that stutterers are poorer at processing auditory signals. They are less accurate at identifying words and sentences in noisy conditions, and they are poorer at judging the durations of tones. Interestingly, researchers have also found that nonstutterers who are more disfluent perform more poorly at the tests than do nonstutterers who are more fluent. Remember the findings that individuals who stutter have deficits or anomalies in auditory processing areas of the brain? It seems likely that these deficits are responsible for the poorer scores on tests of central auditory processing.

Brain Electrical Potentials Reflecting Auditory Processing

Although there are conflicting findings when experimenters have looked at brain waves associated with listening to auditory stimuli, there appears to be a subgroup of stutterers who have anomalous responses. This subgroup showed longer delays between the stimuli and the brain wave responses, as well as smaller brain waves. This finding may reflect the findings in brain anatomy studies that identified a subgroup with anomalies in the auditory cortex that benefit more than others from delayed auditory feedback to promote fluency. These and other similar findings will be discussed further in Chapter 3.

Dichotic Listening Tests

In the early 1960s, a procedure was developed to assess hemispheric dominance for speech and language by testing which ear was more accurate at hearing speech sounds. Kimura

(1961), a Canadian psychologist, invented the "dichotic listening test," which simultaneously presented two different syllables (like "ba" and "da") dichotically—a different syllable to each ear. Listeners reported which syllable they heard. Auditory nerves connecting the ears to the cerebral hemispheres carry more information to the hemisphere on the opposite side than to the hemisphere on the same side. Results with normal speakers indicated that syllables presented to the right ear (opposite the left hemisphere, which is dominant for speech and language) were most frequently reported as heard, which was called a right ear advantage for speech.

This procedure has been used to assess laterality differences between stuttering and nonstuttering groups. Again there have been conflicting findings, but most of the dichotic tests that have used linguistic stimuli such as words and sentences have found that individuals who stutter have reversed hemispheric dominance for perception of speech. That is, nonstutterers tend to have left-hemisphere dominance, and stutterers have more right-hemisphere dominance. As with other studies of auditory processing, researchers are beginning to suspect that not all stutterers are alike in this respect; there may be a subgroup that has anomalous auditory processing.

Auditory Feedback

Ever since the ancient Greek stutterer Demosthenes improved his speech by orating above the roar of the Mediterranean Sea, it has been observed that changes in auditory feedback can affect fluency. Masking noise, delayed auditory feedback, frequency shifts, and other alterations in the properties of the auditory signal can create temporary fluency in persons who stutter (see Van Riper, 1982, for a review up to that date). On the other hand, delayed auditory feedback can create an artificial stutter in normal speakers (Black, 1951; Lee, 1951). A variety of explanations for the effects of altered feedback

on people who stutter have been offered, including that it (1) is a distraction, (2) causes stutterers to change how they talk (e.g., becoming louder), and (3) compensates for a defect in stutterers' auditory monitoring of their speech (Bloodstein, 1995; Garber & Martin, 1977).

Other Sensory Feedback

The findings reviewed in the last few sections are related to the auditory system, but other sensory systems are important for the control of speech—specifically, touch and movement. A number of studies have suggested that stutterers have poorer sensory feedback in several domains, but other studies don't find these differences. Perhaps that is why some of the sensory feedback enhancements used for treatment (e.g., SpeechEasy) are effective with some individuals who stutter but not others (Foundas, Bollich, Feldman, Corey, & Hurley et al., 2004; Pollard, Ellis, Finan, & Ramig, 2009) (Table 2.4).

Sensory-Motor Control

On the face of it, stuttering appears to be a disorder of speech motor control. Fluent speech depends on **sensory-motor control** of the muscles that move speech structures to produce airflow, voicing, and articulation in a coordinated fashion so that speech sounds are produced smoothly, in a specified sequence, and at a reasonable rate. Stuttered speech, then, must be the result of some disturbance in the smooth, sequenced muscle contractions necessary for coordinated structural movements. Van Riper described this as "a temporal disruption of the simultaneous and successive programming of muscular movements" (Van Riper, 1971, p. 404; 1982, p. 415).

The control of the smooth movements of speech depends in part on sensory input as well as motor output. In fact, part of the control of any complex movement uses sensory

Table 2.4	Summary of Sensory Processing and Stuttering	
Area of Interest	**Important Findings**	**Major Clinical Implications**
Sensory Processing	Stutterers show the following differences from nonstutterers: • Poorer central auditory processing, especially with regard to temporal information • Brain waves of stutterers may have longer latencies and lower amplitudes when listening to linguistically complex stimuli. • Some dichotic listening studies have found that stutterers have less right-ear/left-hemisphere advantage. More evident in more severe stutterers and more likely when stimuli are linguistically complex • A small number of studies suggest stutterers may be poorer at processing tactile and visual information. • Masking and other changes in the way that stutterers hear themselves speaking can decrease the frequency and severity of stuttering.	Dysfunction of auditory system implicated in stuttering. Temporary fluency can be obtained by masking or distorting auditory feedback.

information about where the structure is now and where it's going in order to produce just the right amount of contraction of all the muscles involved. When the brain plans the movements needed to produce sounds, it uses stored memories of past movements and their consequences in planning what must be moved as well as when and how to produce the desired acoustic and perceptual result—the sounds of speech. This section reviews several areas of research that have looked at stutterers' speech and nonspeech motor control. It's important to remember that even if it is not explicitly stated by researchers, investigations of motor skills are in fact investigations of sensory-motor skills.

Reaction Time

Figure 2.8 depicts an example of a reaction time experiment. The participant is told to watch the computer screen for a picture of an object and to say the name of the object the instant it appears. The time between the appearance of the object on the screen and the first sound or movement made by the participant is her reaction time. As indicated, reaction time involves sensory analysis, response planning,

and response execution. It is therefore a potentially useful measure in stuttering research if it is thought that the core deficit is a delay in some aspect of sensory processing, planning, or motor execution.

Beginning in 1976, experimenters have shown that individuals who stutter (including children) often have slower reaction times than individuals who don't (see Chapter 3 for detailed descriptions of these studies). This has been shown with both auditory and visual stimuli and with responses involving initiating and terminating a vowel sound, pressing lips together, and making respiratory movements. Differences were more frequently found when linguistically meaningful stimuli were used to test reaction time. These differences probably reflect the brain imaging evidence discussed earlier in this chapter that individuals who stutter have anomalies in brain areas related to sensory-motor integration.

Fluent Speech

Reaction time responses, such as lip pressing or saying "ahhh," are indirect measures of speech processing under normal conditions. Researchers have been able to make

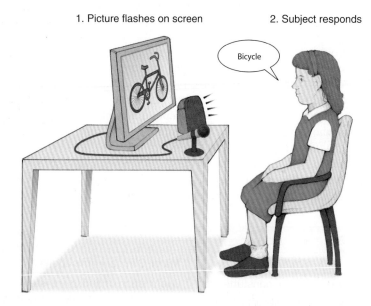

1. Picture flashes on screen   2. Subject responds

Bicycle

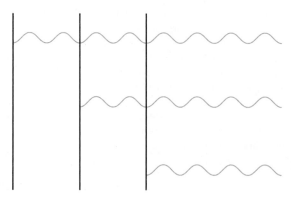

Sensory Analysis
Subject hears signal, sees image on screen, senses the position of speech structures and tension of muscles

Response Planning
Subject chooses word to say, selects phonemes and muscles to use

Response Execution
Subject activates muscles in proper sequence to say "bicycle"

Figure 2.8 Processing stages in a reaction time task.

more direct assessments by examining the speed and coordination of stutterers' speech movements when they are talking fluently and by analyzing the sound waves of their fluent speech. The findings generally show that people who stutter have slower speech movements and sometimes have abnormal sequencing in the movements of their articulators (see Chapter 3). There are different interpretations of these findings, including views that (a) stutterers have sensory-motor delays caused by abnormalities in brain pathways, (b) these findings only reflect strategies that stutterers use to be fluent, and (c) stutterers are slower in their speech production because, even in some of their apparently fluent speech, they abnormally tense speech muscles in a way that puts a drag on the movement of their articulators. I suspect that each of these three interpretations may be true for different subjects in different experiments.

Nonspeech Motor Control

Following in the wake of studies that showed individuals who stutter often have slower than normal reaction times and slower segments in their fluent speech, researchers began to examine complex motor coordination of *nonspeech* muscles and structures. One advantage of this approach is that it eliminates the effect of stuttering itself that may contaminate measures of speech movements. Second, complex motor coordination, such as sequential finger movements, appears to be planned and organized by areas of the brain, such as the supplementary motor area (SMA), which also appear to be involved in the sequential articulatory movements of speech (Goldberg, 1985). Interestingly, neurophysiological evidence that sequential finger movements are regulated by the same brain regions that control speech has been supported by arguments that spoken language in humans evolved from right-hand (and thus left-hemisphere) specialization for manipulating objects and hand gesturing in earlier hominids (Kent, 1997; MacNeilage, 1987).

A number of studies have shown that in various nonspeech tasks such as tapping with fingers in a prescribed sequence, stutterers are slower than nonstutterers. They may be significantly slower in *initiating* the sequence of taps, and more severe stutterers may be notably slower than mild stutterers or nonstutterers. Finger tapping experiments have also suggested that right-hemisphere activity may interfere with stutterers' dominant (right)-hand sequential finger tapping, which requires input from the left hemisphere. In fact, other experiments showed that both right-handed stutterers and left-handed non-stutterers are less able to focus on one hemisphere without interference by the other. Another interesting study of nonspeech motor control suggested that stutterers' optimal tapping rate was slower than that of nonstutterers; however, when instructed to tap at a fast rate, stutterers could tap very fast but became highly unstable (high degree of variability) when doing so (Subramanian & Yairi, 2006). This is in agreement with a study of children's hand clapping, which demonstrated that a subgroup of children who stuttered was highly variable compared to children who didn't stutter when clapping their hands at a specified rate (Olander, Smith, & Zeleznik, 2010). Researchers looking at adult stutterers' ability to follow auditory pitch changes using various motor outputs also found the stutterers to be slower and less accurate than nonstutterers.

These experiments suggest that stutterers are slower and/or more variable than nonstutterers at nonspeech motor tasks. Some of these tasks showed that stutterers are poorer at integrating sensory and motor information to produce a movement. Other tasks showed that when they were performing sensory-motor tasks, they lacked the left-hemisphere dominance shown by nonstutterers. The relationship of these findings to stuttering is that many, if not all, individuals who stutter have a basic deficit in sensory-motor control, whether for speech or for nonspeech motor activities (Table 2.5).

LANGUAGE FACTORS

Figure 2.1 depicts language factors as having their influence by affecting the primary deficit in stuttering, sensory-motor control of speech. The influence of language on stuttering is threefold—language development, language delays, and language complexity.

The first factor, language development, exerts its influence because of the stress that language development in a child puts on his speech production. The next chapter considers this factor in detail. But to put it in a nutshell here, the rapid language acquisition that occurs in all children between the ages of 2 and 5 places high demands on brain resources. Add this stress to a child's basic deficit in sensory-motor control of speech, and stuttering may emerge. As evidence for this hypothesis that children predisposed to stuttering are stressed by language development, researchers point to the fact that the stuttering usually begins at the very time when language growth is greatest (Bloodstein & Ratner, 2008). In fact, Yairi and Ambrose (2005) reported that in more than 50 percent of their sample of stuttering children, parents reported the onset of stuttering during a sudden increase in language development.

The second factor, language disorder or delay, may precipitate or worsen children's stuttering because these children essentially have two deficits to deal with—a speech motor control problem and a language problem. Again, this may cause children who stutter to divert resources or attention away from compensating for the speech motor control problem to deal with the language problem. Many studies have demonstrated language problems in some children who stutter, but the best recent compendium of these findings is a meta-analysis of 22 studies that compared language ability in samples of stuttering and nonstuttering children (Ntourou, Conture, & Lipsey, 2011). The authors found that four language measures showed significant differences between these two groups: overall

Table 2.5	Summary of Sensory-Motor Control and Stuttering	
Area of Interest	Important Findings	Major Clinical Implications
Sensory-Motor Control	Compared to nonstutterers, individuals who stutter appear to have these differences: • Stutterers' reaction times are slower, especially when linguistically meaningful stimuli are used. • Stutterers' fluent speech is slower; they have longer vowels, slower transitions, and delayed onset of voicing. • Stutterers are slower and make more errors on nonspeech tasks of sequencing. This may be truer for more severe stutterers. • Although stutterers are slower tapping at a comfortable rate, they are faster than controls during fast-tapping conditions but more variable. Close relatives of stutterers have slower tapping rates than stutterers and controls but less variability. Results of hand-tapping task experiment suggested that stutterers are not as able to focus on left-hemisphere motor control and may be vulnerable to interference from the right hemisphere or other areas of left hemisphere. Stutterers are poorer at auditory-motor tracking; they may not have left-hemisphere advantage for auditory-motor tracking, and they may be slower at developing a mental model of auditory-motor relationships.	There is a possibility that training in auditory speech motor control could improve fluency. Evidence that stutterers are slower at a variety of tasks suggests that slower speech rate may facilitate fluency. If stutterers try to speak at fast rates, they may be more likely to stutter because of unstable speech motor control. Possible that some close relatives of stutterers may be predisposed to stutter but may prevent stuttering by speaking more slowly. Modeling slow speech by parents of young children at risk may prevent stuttering by inducing a slower speech rate in children.

language, receptive vocabulary, expressive vocabulary, and mean length of utterance. They speculate that the effect of these language difficulties is that "…when planning/formulating sentences, [children who stutter] may experience subtle, but important difficulties in quickly and efficiently encoding and retrieving lexical items. The end product of such difficulties, it may be argued, is the disruption in the fluent initiation and/or continuation of speech-language, most typically characterized by production of speech disfluencies (e.g., revisions, hesitations)" (Ntourou, Conture, & Lipsey, 2011, pp. 174–175).

The third influence of language on stuttering, language complexity, appears to affect sensory-motor control of speech to trigger the occurrence of stuttering in a moment-to-moment fashion. Researchers have found that when individuals who stutter produce longer or more linguistically complex utterances, they are more likely to stutter, whether they are adults or children. Studies have also shown that certain grammatical word types (e.g., nouns and verbs), longer words, and words at the beginning of an utterance are more likely to be stuttered (see Chapter 1 for details). Again, it is as if the extra demand of processing language—in an individual perhaps with other factors such as a genetic predisposition for stuttering—impedes the individual's sensory-motor control of speech. As I will suggest in the next section, emotion is another brain activity that may disrupt speech production in these children with vulnerable systems. Details on some of these key studies are given in Chapter 3 (Table 2.6).

EMOTIONAL FACTORS

Because people who stutter are a heterogeneous group, the relationship between emotion and stuttering, like the relationship between language and stuttering, will vary among individuals. For some, emotion may be an important etiological factor that triggers the onset of stuttering and makes recovery difficult. For others, although emotion in strong doses may make stuttering change—sometimes for the worse, sometimes for the better—emotion may not be a major factor in its etiology. However, the experience of stuttering generates emotions such as frustration, fear, and anger in everyone who stutters. In other words, emotional arousal may cause stuttering, but stuttering may also cause emotional arousal.

I will begin the discussion of emotion and stuttering with a review of the link between stuttering and anxiety, and then I will describe the evidence suggesting that many people who stutter have more emotionally sensitive temperaments than fluent speakers.

Anxiety and Autonomic Arousal

The average listener may think that people stutter because they are nervous. Scientists, following up on this impression, have used such terms as "anxiety," "autonomic arousal," and "negative emotion" to specify the emotional states that may

Table 2.6	Summary of Language Factors in Stuttering	
Area of Interest	Important Findings	Major Clinical Implications
Language	Stuttering onset is often associated with language development.	In evaluating a child who has recently begun to stutter, it is important to determine if the child is/was in a period of intense language development when stuttering started.
	Children who stutter appear to have slightly less robust language processing abilities.	A complete evaluation of a child who stutters should include assessment of receptive and expressive language.
	More stuttering occurs in more complex sentences; stuttering is influenced by linguistic factors such as lexical class of word, length, and location in a sentence.	Decreasing linguistic load on children who are beginning to stutter may reduce their stuttering. In addition, the use of pauses and slower speech rate in older children and adults who stutter may increase fluency by decreasing linguistic demands on the speech production system.
	More linguistically complex stimuli result in poorer performances by stuttering on many performance tasks.	

cause or accompany stuttering. The broad term "anxiety" generally describes a state of alert concern about a future event. When the term "autonomic arousal" is used in a similar way, it denotes activation of the sympathetic nervous system, which prepares the body for action, such as in the fight-or-flight response. Research about anxiety and stuttering has been going on for more than 50 years. Recently, Bloodstein and Ratner (2008) reviewed more than a dozen studies comparing stutterers and nonstutterers on various measures of anxiety and found that more than half of the studies revealed no differences. However, a substantial number of them *did* find stutterers to be *more anxious* on some measures. It is possible that there is a subgroup of stutterers who are more anxious, and studies that happen to have more individuals from this subgroup in their study find the stuttering group to be more anxious. No doubt some of the studies of social anxiety may reflect the fact that years of stuttering can cause a person who stutters to be more anxious in social situations.

Several studies related to anxiety and stuttering are described in detail in Chapter 3. In summary, research has shown that high levels of anxiety produced by the threat of electric shock can produce stuttering-like behaviors in typical speakers. Moreover, there is evidence that changes in speech-related physiology occur in stutterers but not nonstutterers under conditions of anxiety. Finally, several studies using physiological measures of anxiety showed stutterers and nonstutterers to be equally anxious, but only stutterers showed the effects in their speech in terms of increased disfluencies.

Temperament

Many of us who work with children who stutter have often heard parents describe their children as particularly sensitive. Upon questioning, these parents frequently say that even before stuttering began, the child was more easily upset by changes in routine or was shyer with strangers than her siblings. These emotional and behavioral characteristics may be a part of the child's inherited physiology or **temperament**. Some children seem to be born with sensitive or inhibited temperaments and are more likely to react to new people and novel situations with increased muscle tension and physiological signs of stress (Kagan, Reznick, & Snidman, 1987).

An important early conceptualization of stuttering, temperament, and anxiety was presented in Brutten and Shoemaker's (1967) classic book *The Modification of Stuttering*. Rather than using the term "temperament," they referred to "individual differences in conditionability and autonomic reactivity." They suggested that some individuals have predispositions to stutter because they are constitutionally more likely to have an anxiety-based speech breakdown under stressful conditions. Moreover, these individuals are also thought to be more conditionable, making it more likely that initial breakdowns under stress will escalate into highly learned stuttering behaviors.

Following Brutten and Shoemaker, a number of authors have speculated about the possible importance of considering this kind of reactive temperament in gaining a better understanding of the nature of stuttering (e.g., Bloodstein, 1987, 1995; Bloodstein & Ratner, 2008; Conture, 1991; Guitar, 1997, 1998, 2000; Peters & Guitar, 1991; Walden, Frankel, Buhr, Johnston, Conture, & Karrass, 2012). A reactive temperament, for example, might trigger increased physical tension in a child when she is disfluent and thus create a learned cycle of disfluency begetting more severe disfluencies, leading to chronic stuttering. On the other hand, a placid temperament in an equally disfluent child might allow her to stay relaxed, ignore the disfluencies, and thereby outgrow early stuttering.

Data on the sensitivity of people who stutter are meager, but what is available is described in Chapter 3. Questionnaire studies have found indications that both adults and children who stutter are more sensitive than nonstutterers. This has been corroborated by at least one study of a physiological measure of sensitivity.

With evidence in hand that at least some individuals who stutter have more sensitive temperaments, we need to ask how this may shed light on the disruption of fluency by emotion. Psychologists who study temperament have looked carefully at the regulation and expression of emotion in persons with sensitive temperaments. There is good evidence from studies of both normal and brain-damaged patients that the regulation of emotion is a lateralized function (Kinsbourne, 1989; Kinsbourne & Bemporad, 1984). Emotions regulated by the left hemisphere appear to motivate such behaviors as approach, exploration, and action, whereas emotions regulated by the right hemisphere motivate behaviors such as avoidance, withdrawal, and the arrest of action. Studies of electrical activity in the brain indicate that individuals with sensitive temperaments are right hemisphere-dominant for emotionally based behaviors (Ahern & Schwartz, 1985; Calkins & Fox, 1994). This means that if stutterers are temperamentally reactive as a group, they may have an inborn proclivity toward behaviors motivated by right-hemisphere emotions—avoidance, withdrawal, and the arrest of action.

How this may affect speech is not yet clear, but Webster (1993b) speculates that when individuals who stutter are emotionally aroused, then right-hemisphere proclivities, such as avoidance and withdrawal, could affect their left-hemisphere SMAs, interfering with planning and initiation of speech. My own speculation about the relationship between emotion and stuttering is that one important aspect of right hemisphere–dominant, emotionally based behaviors is the arrest of ongoing behavior. This phenomenon is especially well described by Jeffrey Gray (1987), a psychologist who has studied the central nervous system's response to stress. He proposes that when an individual experiences fear or frustration, a behavioral inhibition system in the brain increases three distinct forms of behavior: (a) freezing, which involves widespread muscular contractions that produce tense and silent immobility; (b) flight; or (c) avoidance. It is possible that such behaviors may be manifested in speech by both core behaviors (repetitions, prolongations, and blocks) and secondary behaviors (escape and avoidance).

Indirect support for this possibility may be findings by Kagan, Reznick, and Snidman (1987) that more sensitive children manifest their reactivity by generating higher levels of physical tension, particularly in laryngeal muscles, when they are speaking in unfamiliar or threatening situations. I suspect that some children who are both sensitive and have vulnerable motor speech systems may respond to early repetitive disfluencies with increased tension, especially in the laryngeal region. This tightening may further interfere with speech, producing the abruptly terminated repetitions, prolongations, and blocks that develop in many children when stuttering persists. Other children who are highly sensitive and predisposed to have motor speech breakdowns may begin their disfluencies with tense prolongations and blocks in response to emotionally difficult situations. The heterogeneity of individuals who stutter and their

unique patterns of stuttering will be discussed further in upcoming chapter sections on developmental factors and learning.

Brain imaging studies have shown extensive activity during stuttering in an area called the right insula, shown in Figure 2.3 (Fox, 2003), and the anterior cingulate cortex (Braun, Varga, & Stager, 1997; Braun, Varga, Stager, Schulz, & Selbie et al., 1997; De Nil, Kroll, Kapur, & Houle, 2000). Both of these areas have strong connections with the amygdala (Allman, Hakeem, Erwin, Nimchinsky, & Hof, 2001; Habib, Daquin, Milandre, Royere, & Rey et al., 1995), which is a major structure in fear conditioning (LeDoux, 2002). It is possible that some of the right-hemisphere activity heightened during stuttering and reduced during induced fluency may reflect negative emotional arousal. My reasoning is that, first, many of the studies reviewed for this chapter suggest that stutterers' speech planning and production are localized in right-hemisphere regions homologous to Broca's, Wernicke's, and interconnecting areas. Second, emotions lateralized to the right hemisphere in the human brain are those associated with fear—avoidance, escape, and arrest of ongoing behavior (Kinsbourne, 1989). Third, because strong emotions tend to dominate the neural processes in surrounding areas (LeDoux, 2002), these emotions may disrupt ongoing speech processing in ways analogous to how they affect all behavior, including avoidance behaviors, escape behaviors, and blocks.

The section you have just read—on emotions and stuttering—suggests that emotions play a major role in the development of stuttering. In some cases, they may also play a role in the cause. All of this information needs to be pulled together into a unified description that explains more precisely how emotion influences stuttering (and vice versa), as well as how individuals may differ in this respect. Some aspects of a unified view of stuttering and emotions are suggested in a model proposed by Walden and colleagues (2012). Although their view ("dual diathesis-stressor model of stuttering") incorporates both emotional variables and speech-language variables, I will only describe what they hypothesize about emotions. They suggest that children who stutter may have constitutional predispositions (diatheses) that make them highly emotionally reactive to novel stimuli. This predisposition will be greater or lesser in different children. For the predisposition to be "activated," the child must encounter some environmental stress. Thus, the child may stutter more or less in any given situation, depending on the stress he experiences and the degree of predisposition he has. The stimulus the child is reacting to in this case is the experience of having some difficulty speaking (disfluencies or other speech disturbances). The child's emotional reaction to the difficulty will increase the difficulty in a cyclical fashion. Of course, any given child will have other predispositions, such as language or speech deficits that will interact with the emotional diathesis.

It is hoped that future research will provide evidence to support these hypotheses and other theoretical perspectives on stuttering. New theoretical frameworks need to include descriptions of how emotion may affect recovery from stuttering—via treatment or natural recovery—and suggest whether recovery can be

Table 2.7	Summary of Emotional Factors in Stuttering	
Area of Interest	Important Findings	Major Clinical Implications
Anxiety	Many studies find that stutterers are not more anxious than nonstutterers, but a few do indicate they are more anxious.	For many persistent stutterers, their treatment programs may benefit from components that facilitate the unlearning of fear-based stuttering behaviors.
Autonomic Arousal	Anxiety or autonomic arousal in stutterers is associated with stuttering. There is evidence that emotion caused by something like the threat of electric shock can cause disfluencies in even nonstutterers.	No clear clinical implications.
Temperament	There is some evidence that stutterers tend to have a more sensitive or inhibited temperament; there is speculation that this may be related to right-hemisphere activity associated with stuttering. Sensitivity may influence physical tension.	There may be a subgroup of particularly reactive/sensitive individuals who need more focus on emotions during treatment.

improved by treating emotions as well as stuttering behaviors. One example of new research that will help build models of the connection between stuttering and emotion is the research of Kang et al. (2010) on genes associated with stuttering, described earlier in this chapter. This work has identified one gene (GNPTG) that is associated with both motor control and emotional regulation. Exploration of how individuals with this gene respond to treatment and how treatment may be adjusted to modify the effect of this gene would be a vital step forward.

Complete theoretical models of stuttering must, of course, incorporate all of the constitutional factors described in this chapter—not only genetics and emotion (Table 2.7) but also brain structure and function, sensory processing, sensory-motor control, and language. In addition, developmental and environmental factors must be included as well.

A LAY DESCRIPTION OF CONSTITUTIONAL FACTORS

If you are talking with a person who stutters or a parent of a child who stutters, you may want to summarize current thinking about the causes of stuttering. I think it would be safe to say something like this:

"Recent scientific findings about stuttering suggest that individuals who stutter have a slightly different brain structure and function than fluent speakers. Because of heredity or possibly early injury, the brains of people who stutter seem to be a little less efficient at bringing together all the elements of spoken language—like what words to use and how to put those together into a sentence—at just the right time and speedily enough for rapid, fluent speech. This doesn't happen all the time, of course. But when a person is saying something complicated or is in a hurry or is really excited or upset, then being fluent is a little harder."

In this chapter, I have reviewed the evidence for a constitutional basis for stuttering, and in the next chapter, I've given more detail on the research findings that make up this evidence. In Chapter 4, I will discuss developmental and environmental factors, which may interact with the constitutional factors to produce the disorder. In the subsequent chapter, I will integrate these findings to provide a comprehensive view of how all of the factors may combine to precipitate stuttering in an individual.

SUMMARY

- Stuttering appears to have a genetic basis in many individuals. However, twin studies and adoption studies confirm that genes must interact with environmental factors for stuttering to appear.
- Recent research identifies some genes associated with stuttering in some individuals.
- Stuttering may have its etiology in congenital factors for some stutterers. These may include physical trauma at birth or in utero, cerebral palsy, retardation, and emotionally stressful situations.
- Slightly more boys begin to stutter than girls, but girls are more likely to recover, so by school age and beyond, there are many more boys who stutter than girls.
- Early childhood stuttering may be either *transitory*, in which the child recovers naturally within 18 months, with no or minimal treatment, or *persistent*, in which the child, if not treated, stutters three years or more.
- Persistent and transitory stuttering appear to be the result of a common genetic factor (either a single gene or several), but the persistent form of stuttering probably has additional genetic factors that impede recovery.

- Natural recovery from stuttering appears to be associated with the following factors: (a) good scores on tests of phonology, language, and nonverbal skills; (b) either no family history of stuttering or family members who had natural recovery from stuttering; (c) early age of onset of stuttering; and (d) being a girl.
- Brain imaging studies of adults who stutter have shown various anomalies during speaking and especially during stuttering. One anomaly is overactivation in right-brain areas homologous to left-hemisphere speech and language structures typically used by nonstutterers. Another anomaly is deactivation in the left auditory cortex.
- Neuroanatomical differences seen via brain imaging include (a) anomalies in the planum temporale (related to auditory processing) and in gyri (raised areas on brain's surface) in speech and language areas and (b) less dense fiber tracts connecting speech perception, planning, and execution areas.
- Inducement of short-term or long-term fluency in stutterers is accompanied by decreases in right-hemisphere activations and increases in activation of left-hemisphere speech, language, and auditory areas.
- On tasks of sensory processing, stutterers have less accurate and slower processing, particularly of auditory stimuli, and lack of left-hemisphere dominance for processing.
- Greatest performance deficits occur when linguistically complex stimuli are used.
- Masking and other changes in auditory feedback create temporary fluency, suggesting that distortions, deficits, or delays in auditory feedback may be associated with stuttering.
- On tasks of sensory-motor control, stutterers demonstrate slower reaction times, especially when stimuli are linguistically more complex. Stutterers are slower, less accurate, and less left hemisphere-dominant when performing sequential motor tasks and auditory-motor tasks.
- When there is a greater linguistic load, stutterers' speech motor systems are more variable; greater linguistic load is also associated with more stuttering.
- Stutterers do not appear to be more anxious than nonstutterers, but there is evidence that when their autonomic arousal levels are high, more stuttering is likely to occur.
- As a group, stuttering children and adults appear to have a more sensitive temperament. This sensitivity may be associated with more physical tension in speech musculature for some individuals.

STUDY QUESTIONS

1. How does each of the areas—family studies, twin studies, and adoption studies—provide evidence that stuttering is inherited?
2. A couple comes to you for advice. They tell you they are thinking of having children but are worried because each has a relative who stutters. What more information would you like to get from them? What would you tell them about the likelihood that they would have a child who stutters and whether they should be concerned?
3. How do studies provide evidence that stuttering is a product of both heredity and environment?
4. How would you summarize the brain imaging studies to someone who is not a professional in our field?
5. Why do almost all the brain imaging studies use right-handed males as participants?
6. Researchers have found many differences between groups of stutterers and nonstutterers. Why can't we say that these differences *cause* stuttering?
7. Explain how the deficits in sensory processing in people who stutter could be related to the actual behaviors of stuttering?
8. What are the differences between sensory processing and sensory-motor control?
9. Do you think difficulty with language processing may be a cause of stuttering for some individuals? Why or why not? How might language deficits be related to stuttering?
10. Describe the relationships between emotion and stuttering.
11. What research finding in this chapter do you think has the most relevance for the treatment of stuttering? Defend your answer.

SUGGESTED PROJECTS

1. Talk to someone who stutters and plot out his or her family tree, noting relatives who stutter and relatives who have other speech, language, or learning problems.
2. Make a family tree of your own relatives indicating which, if any, currently have or have had speech, language, hearing, or learning disabilities. Describe how you got the information and what the disabilities are.
3. On which side of the brain do you process speech and language? Find out how you could ascertain this information by asking speech-language pathology researchers or audiologists you know if they have tests you could take to find out. If this doesn't lead to a test for this kind of laterality, search the internet for self-administered tests, which tell you whether you are more "left-brained" or more "right-brained."
4. Use a digital stopwatch (how fast can you turn it on and off?) or similar instrument to determine your reaction time. Try this under many different conditions, such as at several times during the day and when sick or tired versus when feeling alert. Determine what variables affect your reaction times, and see if it is true for other people. Using this information, suggest why different studies of reaction times in stutterers get different outcomes.
5. Find a temperament test, such as those available online, and take it yourself. Do you think the results accurately describe you?

SUGGESTED READINGS

Bloodstein, O., & Ratner, N. (2008). *A handbook on stuttering* (6th ed.). Clifton Park, NY: Delmar Learning.

This is the most recent edition of a classic reference book on stuttering. It provides a thorough update of "the most important research in stuttering." Moreover, it is quite easy to read.

Maassen, B., Kent, R., Peters, H., van Lieshout, P., & Hulstijn, W. (Eds.) (2004). *Speech motor control in normal and disordered speech*. Oxford: Oxford University Press.

This book contains updated chapters by many scientists who presented their findings at a conference on speech motor control in 2001. Although not all of the contents are directly related to stuttering, there is much of great interest to clinicians and researchers interested in the neurophysiological bases of speech and stuttering.

Neumann, K., & Euler, H. (2010). Neuroimaging and stuttering. In B. Guitar & R. McCauley (Eds.), *Stuttering Treatment: Established and Emerging Approaches* (pp. 355–377). Baltimore: Lippincott Williams & Wilkins.

This chapter begins with a history of brain imaging and stuttering and then describes the most important findings in structural and functional brain imaging related to stuttering. This is followed by a section on neuroimaging findings before and after treatment, a specialty of the authors.

Van Riper, C. (1982). *The nature of stuttering* (2nd ed.). Englewood Cliffs, NJ: Prentice-Hall.

Although somewhat outdated, this book reviews an impressive amount of world literature on stuttering, from as long ago as the 20th century B.C. In a synthesis of the research, Van Riper presents his venerable hypothesis that stuttering is a disorder of timing.

Yairi, E. & Ambrose, N. G. (2005). *Early childhood stuttering*. Austin, TX: Pro-Ed.

The authors give an in-depth description of the results of 14 years of research on the development of stuttering conducted at the University of Illinois. Chapters are devoted to the onset and development of stuttering, characteristics of children's disfluency, genetics, and cognitive, psychosocial, and motor factors in stuttering. Elaine Paden and Ruth Watkins contributed chapters on phonological and language abilities of children who stutter, respectively. Like Wendell Johnson's magnum opus *The Onset of Stuttering*, this book reflects a monumental effort focused on childhood stuttering.

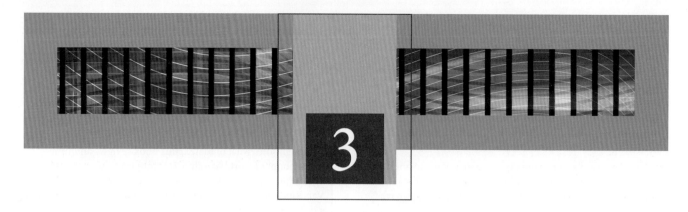

Research Findings about Constitutional Factors in Stuttering

CHAPTER OBJECTIVE

After studying this chapter, readers should be familiar with details of the research literature relevant to constitutional factors in stuttering.

In Chapter 2, I sketched the "big picture" of constitutional factors, summarizing the major themes so that you could see how an individual's neurological makeup could explain many of the behaviors of stuttering. In this chapter, I'll fill in the details from the multitude of scientific studies that have been carried out on stuttering for almost 100 years.

HEREDITARY FACTORS

Family Studies

The first "modern" reports on the genetics of stuttering were published by a group of researchers in Newcastle, England (Andrews & Harris, 1964; Kay, 1964). They investigated the family histories of 80 stuttering children and compared them with the families of nonstuttering children. These researchers found that (a) children who stuttered had far more stuttering relatives than did children who didn't stutter; (b) male children were at higher risk for developing stuttering than female children; and (c) female children who stuttered were more likely to have stuttering relatives than were male children who stuttered. Thus, a pattern of family occurrence emerged, providing evidence for a possible genetic explanation of stuttering. These results supported a model in which stuttering was transmitted by either a single gene or a combination of several genes contributing different factors. This early insight into the possibility of multiple genes is supported by more recent work. My own working hypothesis is that chronic or persistent stuttering is the result of genes affecting not only speech motor control but also language and temperament.

Ten years after the Newcastle studies, researchers at Yale University conducted further family studies of stuttering (Kidd, 1977; Kidd, Kidd, & Records, 1978; Kidd, Reich, & Kessler, 1973). Using the data from England (Kay, 1964) combined with new data they gathered themselves in the United States, the Yale researchers were able to develop statistical models, which predicted patterns of inheritance. They found, as in Kay's earlier study, that males were more likely to stutter than females and that females who stuttered were more likely to have relatives who stuttered. Kidd (1984) concluded that these patterns were best explained by an interaction between the environment and a combination of several genes.

The Newcastle and Yale family studies focused on children and adults, most of whom had been stuttering for several years. Researchers at the University of Illinois used a different approach. Ambrose, Yairi, and Cox (1993) studied the family histories of 69 very young children who had just been diagnosed with stuttering, including individuals who would recover from stuttering and those who would persist. The Illinois group found that two-thirds of these children had relatives who stuttered and that, as in earlier studies, more male relatives than female relatives stuttered. Unlike past studies, however, these researchers found that male and female children who stuttered had similar chances of having relatives who stuttered. This difference is likely to have come from the fact that females in the Kay and Kidd studies were older, with persistent rather than transient cases of the disorder. Kay and Kidd may have found that their females had more relatives who stuttered because they studied only those females whose stuttering persisted, and for a female (who is less likely to stutter than a male) to persist in stuttering, she can be assumed to have inherited more genetic material. Thus, she would naturally have more relatives who stuttered; her family would have a heavier "genetic loading." On the other hand, many of Ambrose, Yairi, and Cox (1993) very young female subjects recovered quickly from stuttering and thus may have had lower genetic loadings and fewer relatives who stuttered.

Kay's (1964) and Kidd's (1984) hypotheses that stuttering may be transmitted by several genes rather than a single gene received support from another study by the Illinois group that investigated differences between those young children who recover from stuttering without treatment and those who persist. Ambrose, Cox, and Yairi (1997) analyzed the family trees of 66 children who were identified soon after the onset of stuttering. The children were followed for several years and eventually grouped into those who persisted

in stuttering and those who recovered. The researchers found that the sex ratios of the two groups were quite different. The male: female ratio was 7:1 in the persistent group but about 2:1 in the recovered group, indicating a much higher percentage of boys in the persistent group. This provides more evidence that girls are more likely to recover than boys.

A second finding was that persistence tended to run in families. In other words, children who did not outgrow their stuttering were likely to come from families in which relatives who stuttered also persisted in their stuttering. Conversely, children who recovered were likely to come from families in which relatives who initially stuttered became fluent when they grew older. Further analysis of their data led the authors to propose that persistent and recovered stuttering are transmitted by the same major gene or genes, but that those individuals whose stuttering persists have additional genetic factors that hamper recovery. It is also possible that those who recovered have additional genetic factors that facilitate recovery. A contrasting view is given by Viswanath, Lee, and Chakraborty (2004), whose studies of persistent stutterers led them to hypothesize that persistent and recovered stuttering are two genetically different disorders.

The researchers in Illinois examined a number of genetic and nongenetic factors that might predict recovery or persistence and thereby might be useful in deciding which children are in immediate need of treatment. In an early study, Yairi, Ambrose, Paden, and Throneburg (1996) found that predictors of recovery include (a) good scores on tests of phonology, language, and nonverbal skills; (b) family members who had recovered from stuttering; and (c) early age of onset of stuttering. Some of the factors that impede recovery, such as problems in phonology or language, might be determined by other genes that may accompany a gene that is related to the initial onset of stuttering. In later studies (e.g., Yairi & Ambrose, 1999), the Illinois group refined this list of factors; this refined list, which includes eight factors, was presented in Chapter 1 in the section titled "Recovery without Treatment."

Before we leave the topic of family studies, it is worth mentioning several criticisms that have been made about genetic studies in reviews by Felsenfeld (1997) and Yairi, Ambrose, and Cox (1996). Many of the genetic studies used no matched control group, but instead relied on incidence figures from other studies. Other problems in past studies include the inadequacy of a definition of stuttering when searching for stuttering among relatives of children or adults who stutter and relying on testimony of others, rather than direct assessment to determine whether or not a relative stutters. These researchers suggest that future studies (a) look for subgroups of stutterers that may have different genetic etiologies; (b) examine family members who don't stutter to find factors that may resist stuttering; and (c) search for environmental factors that may interact with genetic factors to precipitate or maintain stuttering.

Twin Studies

Twin studies of stuttering have shown that the disorder occurs much more often in both members of identical twin pairs than in both members of fraternal, same-sex twin pairs (Andrews, Morris-Yates, Howie, & Martin, 1991; Felsenfeld, Kirk, Zhu, Statham, Neale, & Martin, 2000; Howie, 1981; Luchsinger, 1944; Seeman, 1937). To use the vocabulary of genetics, there is higher "concordance" of stuttering in identical than in fraternal twins. This supports the hypothesis that stuttering is inherited, but it doesn't reveal what exactly is inherited. How does a gene (or several genes) affect a child's speech so that stuttering results? No one is sure.

In addition to providing evidence of genetic factors in stuttering, twin studies demonstrate that heredity does not work alone. In one of the twin studies previously cited, although there was higher concordance for stuttering among identical twins, some pairs were discordant (Howie, 1981). Specifically, Howie found that in six of the 16 identical twin pairs, one twin stuttered, but the other didn't. This means that even though both members of the twin pair had the same genetic inheritance, only one of them stuttered, indicating that genes alone do not explain stuttering. However, this may not be surprising because genes must interact with the environment to produce their effects (LeDoux, 2002). A gene might not express itself in stuttering unless, for example, there is some kind of prenatal or postnatal stress on the child. In the case of stuttering, where there appears to be several genes working together to produce a chronic disorder, the situation is even more complex because several genetic tendencies may need to interact with different aspects of the child's internal and external environment to create stuttering. No wonder there were six discordant pairs in the Howie study!

An estimate of the relative proportions of genetic and environmental influences was suggested in a later study involving 3,810 unselected twin pairs (Andrews et al., 1991). They were deemed "unselected" because they were all part of the Australian Twin Registry rather than a population selected because of stuttering, thus making the sample less likely to be influenced by "ascertainment bias." This kind of bias might occur, for example, if subjects were found through newspaper ads; only individuals who read the ads in newspapers and were motivated to be in the study would participate in the study. Analyses of stuttering in these 3,810 unselected twin pairs estimated that 71 percent of the variance (the probability of whether or not one would stutter) is accounted for by genetic factors, and 29 percent is accounted for by the individual's environment (including factors influencing the fetus, as well as factors after birth). Felsenfeld and colleagues (2000) recently followed this study up by contacting a group of twins in the Australian Twin Registry different from those studied by Andrews and colleagues (1991). Felsenfeld and colleagues (2000) screened 1,567 pairs and 634 individuals, using questionnaires and telephone interviews. They found 17 monozygotic and eight dizygotic twin pairs

who were concordant for stuttering (both twins stuttered at some time in their lives) and 21 monozygotic and 45 dizygotic twins who were discordant for stuttering (only one of the twin pairs ever stuttered). Statistical analyses estimated that "additive genetic effects" (the effects of different genes working together) accounted for 70 percent of the variance and that an individual's unique environment (influences on one of the twins but not the other, such as illness) accounted for 30 percent of the variance. These proportions are essentially the same as those found by Andrews and colleagues (1991) and support current thinking that genes and environment interact to set the stage for stuttering.

In a study of 1,896 twin pairs in Japan, Ooki (2005) compared concordance in identical and fraternal twins. Using sophisticated statistical techniques, Ooki determined that the proportion of genetic influence on stuttering in males was 80 percent in males and 85 percent in females. In other words, for both males and females, genetic factors were strongly implicated—even more so than in the Andrews and team (1991) and Felsenfeld and team studies (2000). It is interesting that the females showed slightly more genetic influence than the males. Perhaps this echoes the evidence that females have some resistance to stuttering. For a female to develop stuttering, more genetic influence or "genetic loading" is needed.

A study by Dworzynski, Remington, Rijsdijk, Howell, and Plomin (2007) discovered interesting differences between a group of twins who recovered from stuttering ($n = 950$) and a group who persisted ($n = 150$). In the recovered group, concordance for stuttering was 40 percent for identical twins and 20 percent for fraternal twins. However, in the persistent stuttering group of twins, the concordance was 19 percent for identical twins and 0 percent for fraternal twins. This suggests that the genetics of persistent stuttering are complex. As we noted previously, the family studies of Ambrose, Cox, and Yairi (1997) indicated the possibility that while recovered and persistent stuttering are transmitted by the same major gene(s), persistent stuttering itself may have additional genetic factors that make recovery more difficult. The findings of Dworzynski and colleagues (2007) may support this supposition because there is so little concordance in the persistent fraternal twin group—meaning that to get concordance, the same array of multiple genes must be transmitted, far less likely in fraternal twins.

Van Beijsterveldt, Felsenfeld, and Boomsma (2010) conducted a study using a very large participant pool: 105,000 twin pairs at age 5. They bypassed the usual problem of parent identification of their children as stuttering by asking parents merely to estimate the frequency of repetitions, prolongations, and blocks they observed in their children's speech. Children were categorized by the experimenters as "probably stuttering" or "high nonfluency," or as having typical speech. Concordance for probable stuttering was higher in identical twins, supporting the genetic/heritability hypotheses. It was notable that high nonfluency also appeared to be genetically based.

In an interesting aside, Bloodstein and Ratner (2008) questioned the assumption that influence on stuttering that was not accounted for by genetic factors must be attributed to environmental factors. Research using animal models suggests that identical twins sometimes have discordance for certain traits not because of environmental influences but because of variations in the way two identical embryos develop. Some of these variations may be related to "epigenetics," non-DNA factors that are inherited and influence the expression of genes into specific behaviors or phenotypes. Two examples in humans are Angelman syndrome and Prader-Willi syndrome. These two syndromes appear very different but are the result of deletion of the same DNA sequence (gene) in the chromosome. The difference between the two syndromes is simply whether the chromosome is inherited from the mother or the father. In the two syndromes, the chromosome inherited from the mother has a different "tag" or expression controller than the chromosome inherited from the father. We describe this difference as an epigenetic factor because the genes are identical, but how they are triggered or expressed is different (Kempf & Weinberger, 2009). Readers wishing to understand recent developments in genetics, epigenetics, and other principles of gene variability may want to view "Ghost in Your Genes" a public broadcasting system NOVA program on genetics located at http://www.pbs.org/wgbh/nova/genes/.

Adoption Studies

Because the birth records of adopted children are difficult to obtain, studies of adopted stutterers are rare. Bloodstein (1961b) and Bloodstein and Ratner (2008) presented information obtained from 13 adopted stutterers whom Bloodstein interviewed about stuttering in their adoptive families (information on their biological families was not available). Four of the 13 stutterers reported having relatives who stuttered in their adoptive families, which is higher than would be expected by chance. This small sample, without data from biological families, supports the possibility that environmental factors may have an effect. If the relatives in the adoptive family were key figures, such as a parent or older sibling who was close to the child, this would be stronger evidence for the influence of the environment on stuttering. Unfortunately, this information is not available.

Felsenfeld (1997) reported some preliminary data on a small sample of adopted children who had speech disorders (primarily stuttering) and for whom data were available from *both* adoptive and biological families. These data indicated that a history of stuttering in the biological families was slightly more predictive of disorders in these children than was stuttering in the adoptive family.

Again, the evidence suggests that both genetic and environmental factors influence whether or not a child will stutter and that genetic inheritance appears to contribute more strongly.

Genes

A number of researchers are currently looking for genes that may predispose children to stuttering. Dennis Drayna (1997) at the National Institutes of Health has begun genetic linkage studies using large numbers of families to try to isolate genes for stuttering. Linkage analysis compares the chromosomes of family members who have a trait (the appearance of a trait in a person is called a "phenotype") with those of family members who do not. In this way, the chromosomal location of the stuttering gene or genes can be identified. Drayna has been studying families in which there is more than one individual who stutters. His work has brought him into contact with a family in Cameroon, Africa, in which 42 of 100 family members stutter. Preliminary results suggest genes on chromosome 18 may be related to stuttering, a set of genes that control intercellular communication (Shugart, Mundorff, Kilshaw, Doheny, & Doan et al., 2004).

Cox and Yairi (2000) have been studying individuals who stutter in a North Dakota community of Hutterites. This group is of interest because they do not marry outside the community, resulting in a homogeneous gene pool. These researchers have identified three chromosomes (numbers 1, 13, and 16), which may include the genes involved in stuttering. Riaz, Steinberg, Ahmad, Pluzhnikov, and Riazuddin et al. (2005) added another chromosome to the list of those that may contain a gene associated with stuttering. The researchers studied 46 Pakistani families who were highly inbred, increasing the probability that if a particular chromosome appears to be associated with stuttering, many stuttering individuals in different families would also have the same chromosome because they are all so highly interrelated. Their results suggest that chromosome 12 in these families is strongly linked to stuttering, and chromosome 1 is a little less strongly linked. The authors point out that their results and those of other groups suggest that all stuttering is not likely to be the result of the same chromosome location; there may be several different locations that can contribute to stuttering.

Not long after the Riaz team (2005) study, Suresh, Ambrose, Roe, Pluzhnikov, & Wittke-Thompson et al., (2006) published a genome linkage study of 100 families of European descent in the United States, Sweden, and Israel. Their research added some new ways of looking at genetic associations with stuttering. First, they compared chromosome locations associated with stuttering for individuals who had stuttered sometime in their lifetimes (some of whom had recovered, some of whom were still stuttering) versus a subgroup of these individuals who persisted in stuttering. Chromosome 9 appeared to be the location of a gene related to stuttering at sometime in one's lifetime; chromosome 15 was linked only to those whose stuttering was persistent. This is support for the idea that whether an individual naturally recovers from stuttering or not is determined, at least in part, by genetic makeup. It also supports the finding that one predictor of natural recovery is family history of recovery from stuttering (Yairi & Ambrose, 2005).

A second new twist in this study was comparing chromosome locations for stuttering that were specific to males compared to females. The researchers found that in males, stuttering was linked to a location on chromosome 7, and in females, it was linked to chromosome 15. They noted that chromosome 7 has also been associated with specific language impairment and autism. A secondary analysis of those families whose stuttering was associated with chromosome 7 found strong evidence of a linkage of stuttering to chromosome 12. This is of interest because of the evidence for chromosome 12 in the findings of Riaz and colleagues (2005), who examined a group of families in Pakistan who were culturally and geographically very different from those in the Suresh team (2006) study.

Recently, a follow-up study was conducted with those families in Pakistan that showed a link between stuttering and chromosome 12. Kang, Riazuddin, Mundorff, Krasnewich, Friedman, and colleagues (2010) studied the 123 Pakistanis who stuttered as well as 270 individuals in the United States and England who stuttered. They also used a control group of 372 individuals in these three countries who didn't stutter. Mutations of three genes (the genes were called GNPTAB, GNPTG, and NAGPA) on chromosome 12 were found to be associated with stuttering. Some individuals showed mutations of gene GNPTAB, others had mutations on GNPTG, and still others had mutations on NAGPA. The work of all three genes is related to controlling enzymes in a cell's lysosome structure, the part of a cell involved in recycling cell waste products. It is important to note that there are known genetic disorders (e.g., mucolipidoses) of this waste recycling process that affect joint, skeletal, and other body components. These disorders affect brain development, resulting in delays in movement coordination, and some forms of mucolipidoses are accompanied by speech problems (National Institute of Neurological Disorders and Stroke, 2011). Additionally important is the fact that one of the genes, GNPTG, is associated with motor control and emotional regulation by way of the gene's expression in the hippocampus and in the cerebellum.

CONGENITAL AND EARLY CHILDHOOD TRAUMA STUDIES

One of the first studies to look closely at stutterers who had no family history of stuttering, West, Nelson, and Berry (1939), examined a sample of 204 people who stuttered and found that 100 of them reported no family history of stuttering. Of these 100, 85 reported congenital factors that may have been related to the onset of stuttering. These factors included infectious diseases, diseases of the nervous system, and injuries—all reported to have occurred just prior to stuttering onset, although the exact proximity to onset was not reported. Thus, these congenital factors may have created a predisposition to develop stuttering.

A later study by Poulos and Webster (1991) found that 57 of the clients in a clinic sample of 169 adults and adolescents who stuttered reported no family history of stuttering. Of these without family histories, 37 percent reported congenital factors that may have been associated with the onset of stuttering, whereas only 2.4 percent of the clients having a positive family history of stuttering reported such factors. The factors reported included anoxia at birth, premature birth, childhood surgery, head injury, mild cerebral palsy, mild retardation, and experiencing intense fear.

A third study that began with a larger group of stutterers and then looked for possible etiological differences was reported by Alm and Risberg in 2007. At first they divided the group in half, using a scale that measured tendencies toward attention deficit hyperactivity disorder (ADHD). Looking closer at the two subgroups, they discovered that those with high ADHD tendencies had more neurological lesions prior to stuttering onset and also had less family history of stuttering. This again is support for the hypothesis of two different predispositions contributing to stuttering—genetic inheritance and brain injury.

There were two studies that looked at a brain-injured population and assessed whether there were more individuals who stuttered than in the general population. In the first, Böhme (1968) examined a sample of 313 individuals who had sustained brain damage at birth or in early childhood; 24 percent of those 313 developed stuttering (compared to 5 percent in the general population). Unfortunately, no information is given about family history of stuttering in those who developed it, but the implication is that congenital or early childhood brain injury can often result in stuttering. In a similar study, Segalowitz and Brown (1991) surveyed more than 600 high school students to ascertain how many had experienced head injury during their childhoods. Of the students, 92 reported head injury, and of those, nine (about 10 percent) reported having been diagnosed with stuttering. However, it was not clear that the stuttering appeared after the head injury. The authors found that there was a significant relationship between having a head injury and being diagnosed with stuttering, particularly for those children who were unconscious for a period of time after the head injury. Again, there is no information as to whether some of the children who stuttered and had head injuries also had family histories of stuttering.

The fact that neurological or psychological traumas may be associated with childhood stuttering in those without family histories of stuttering is not surprising. Adult onset of stuttering is often associated with head injury, neurological disease, stress, or psychological trauma as I will describe in Chapter 15. Thus, mechanisms similar to those precipitating adult onset may be involved in childhood stuttering in the absence of family history of stuttering, but this possibility raises as many questions as answers. Why would some children (and adults), but not others, begin to stutter as a result of intense fear or brain injury? Which brain structures and functions affected by head injury and neurological disease result in stuttering? How are they similar to and how do they differ from the effects of inheriting a predisposition to stutter?

In respect to the last question, a number of investigators have looked at whether stutterers who have family histories of stuttering showed any differences in their stuttering behavior, such as severity, compared to those without family histories. Andrews and Harris (1964) and Kidd, Heimbuch, Records, Oehlert, and Webster (1980) found no differences in the stuttering of those with and without family histories of stuttering. However, Janssen, Kraaimaat, and Brutten (1990) looked at a wider variety of speech and language-related variables in several different age groups. They found several significant differences (as well as similarities) between the group with family histories of stuttering and the group without such histories. In terms of similarities, the groups were not significantly different in responsiveness to treatment, reading ability, or speech-related anxiety. However, when stuttering behaviors were examined closely, those with family histories of stuttering showed more prolongations and blocks (silent prolongations) than those with no history of stuttering, although the frequency of repetitions was the same for both groups. Another difference between the groups was that those with positive family histories for stuttering showed significantly longer durations of voiced segments of speech and significantly greater variability in length of unvoiced segments during fluent speech than those with no family history of stuttering. The authors summarized this finding by suggesting that the stutterers with positive family histories were slower and more variable in their fluent speech.

It could be concluded from these studies that individuals with family histories of stuttering have inherited greater neuromotor instability than those without family histories of stuttering—an instability that produces more prolongations and blocks and that may require the individual to speak more slowly to maintain fluency. This is not to say that those without family history of stuttering did not inherit the predisposition to stutter. Their family histories may contain other speech-related deficits (e.g., articulation problems), and their underlying neuromotor anomalies may result in stuttering, but it is stuttering that is more characterized by repetitions than prolongations or blocks.

BRAIN STRUCTURE AND FUNCTION

Brain Structure Differences in People Who Stutter

In an early study of brain anatomy, researchers at Tulane University in New Orleans (Foundas, Bollich, Corey, Hurley, & Heilman, 2001) used magnetic resonance imaging (MRI) to assess the relative left-right size of the *planum temporale (PT)*, a part of Wernicke's area thought to be associated with higher-level auditory processing. Their results found that the

PT in nonstutterers was larger in the left hemisphere than in the right, but in stutterers, it was symmetrical in size in the two hemispheres or in some cases larger on the right. The researchers pointed out that a similar pattern has been found in individuals with dyslexia and specific language impairment. Additional anomalies found in participants who stutter were differences in various *gyri* (folds) in the speech and language areas of the brain. The authors of the study speculated that these differences in the brains of those who stutter may reflect deficits that interfere with information flow between Wernicke's area (auditory cortex) and Broca's (speech motor).

A follow-up study by Foundas, Bollich, Feldman, Corey, Hurley, and colleagues (2004) was launched to find evidence of behavior differences associated with the abnormal structure shown in the earlier study. These researchers found that matched groups of stutterers and controls had approximately the same PT asymmetry (64 percent had leftward asymmetry and 36 percent had rightward asymmetry in each group). However, the subgroup of stuttering participants who had *rightward* asymmetry of PT stuttered more severely and interestingly had a significantly greater response to the fluency-inducing condition of delayed auditory feedback. The authors attributed this finding to the fact that the PT is thought to be important in auditory processing of speech and language and perhaps in coordinating auditory feedback of speech with ongoing speech output. Delayed auditory feedback may have corrected an auditory feedback processing deficit causing stuttering in those with rightward PT asymmetry. It is not clear from the article whether the artificial delay in the feedback caused the stutterers to read more slowly than they would have otherwise. Slowing one's speech rate is a common response to delayed auditory feedback and may have been the means by which the stuttering subjects who had greater rightward asymmetry of PT improved their fluency. It is not clear, however, whether improved fluency was the result of (a) an improved synchrony between auditory feedback (arriving slightly later in the cortex) and speech production; (b) improved coordination of the subcomponents of speech-language production because coordination would seem to be enhanced if any motor behavior is slowed down; or (c) both.

Sommer, Koch, Paulus, Weiller, and Büchel (2002) conducted a third neuroanatomical study in Germany. Using a process called diffusion tensor imaging, these investigators examined the density of white matter fiber tracts in the area of the left operculum, fibers which are thought to connect sensory, planning, and motor areas of the brain. They chose this area of the brain to study because two years earlier, other researchers studying activity in the left operculum found asynchrony in the sequencing stages of speech processing in stutterers (Salmelin, Schnitzler, Schmitz, & Freund, 2000). Sommer and colleagues (2002) indeed found what they suspected; fibers in the left operculum in stuttering participants were less dense than those in fluent participants. These results suggested that this structural difference in stutterers' brains could be the basis for the dyssynchrony in processing found by Salmelin and colleagues (2000). These results complement the findings of Foundas and colleagues (2001) and Foundas and colleagues (2004), who also reported anomalies in this region of the brain. As we will see in more recent studies, the results of Sommers and colleagues (2002) are the harbinger of repeated findings of a deficit in pathways connecting speech planning areas with motor execution and sensory feedback areas that are critical in speech production.

Interesting structural anomalies—increased volumes of white matter—were found in right hemisphere structures in an MRI study of 10 adult stutterers and 10 controls (Jäncke, Hänggi, & Steinmetz, 2004). These larger volumes were found in the superior temporal gyrus, inferior frontal gyrus, and precentral gyrus in the right hemisphere. These researchers, as well as some others, have suggested that these enlarged structures may be compensatory in nature, representing a response to deficits in similar structures in the left hemisphere.

In a later brain imaging study using an updated version of the same methodology (voxel-based morphometry—that uses statistical techniques to measure size and density of very small areas of the brain), Beal, Gracco, Lafaille, and De Nil (2007) confirmed the Jäncke team (2004) findings and extended them. These authors provided evidence that auditory and speech production areas in both right *and* left hemisphere of stutterers had *increased* density compared to that of nonstutterers. Several specific brain areas were noted. First, the auditory cortex showed increased gray matter density in stutterers, supporting previously found differences in activation level apparent in the auditory cortical areas in stutterers. Second, there were areas of increased density of white matter in the *right* hemisphere (replicating Jäncke et al., 2004). Of particular interest is that these areas of increased density are in right-hemisphere locations homologous to the left-hemisphere locations found to show less dense white matter tracts by Sommer and colleagues (2002). In other words, it's as if either (a) the right-hemisphere white matter tracts originally developed in stutterers to have the functions of connecting sensory and motor functions that are typically seen in nonstutterers' left hemispheres or (b) these right-hemisphere white matter tracts grew denser as a result of the stutterers' inadequate left-hemisphere white matter tracts in a compensatory fashion.

Chang, Erickson, Ambrose, Hasegawa-Johnson, and Ludlow (2008) conducted an innovative neuroimaging study of recovered and persistent stuttering children (ages 9–12) who were all initially identified as stuttering in their preschool years. The findings were quite remarkable. Both recovered and persistent stuttering children were found to have deficits in areas related to speech production. These deficits were reduced gray matter volume in the left inferior frontal lobe area (including Broca's) and in bilateral temporal

lobe areas that may be related to auditory perception of speech and possibly storage of auditory-perceptual targets for speech production. On the other hand, only persistent stuttering children (not those who had recovered from stuttering) were found to have another deficit—reduced density in white matter tracts subserving speech motor control. Neumann and Euler (2010) suggest that these white matter fibers are essentially part of the arcuate fasciculus. This bundle of fibers is thought to send phonological representations of words, developed in Wernicke's area, to the motor planning and execution areas in Broca's area.

Using some of the same technology (diffusion tensor imaging, an approach that studies the density of fibers by measuring how water diffuses around them) with young stutterers (average age, 18 years) compared to nonstuttering controls, Watkins, Smith, Davis, and Howell (2008) also found reduced density of white matter tracts—pathways which they describe as serving "the integration of articulatory planning and sensory feedback, and via connections with primary motor cortex, a substrate for execution of articulatory movements" (p. 50). Findings of the same structural deficits in young stutterers by these two groups of researchers, along with the evidence of reduced gray matter volume in bilateral temporal lobe areas (Chang et al., 2008) provide neurophysiological evidence for long-standing hypotheses that stuttering is related to reduced capacity for sensory-motor processing (e.g., Neilson, 1980). Watkins and colleagues (2008) note that structural deficits in circumscribed areas of one hemisphere rarely lead to persistent speech or language disorders, so it is not surprising that their findings reflect reduced density of white matter tracts in several areas of both hemispheres. As we will see in the next section, these abnormalities in white matter tracts underlie functional abnormalities in neural processing related to speech and language production.

Researchers recently conducted a replication of the research described in the preceding paragraphs (Cykowski, Fox, Ingham, Ingham, & Robin, 2010). This group carried out diffusion tensor imaging of white matter tracts in sensorimotor integration and speech planning areas of the brain. They studied the directional properties of the axons in these pathways and found them less diffusive parallel to the axons and more diffusive perpendicular to the axons compared to nonstutterers. In other words, these nerve bundles appear to be less efficient at carrying information along the pathways.

Using more stringent statistical analysis techniques than earlier studies, Cykowski and colleagues (2010) found that the anomalies in stutterers were restricted to left-hemisphere white matter tracts similar to those originally identified by Sommer and colleagues (2002), rather than more widespread white matter tract anomalies seen in later studies. Cykowski and colleagues (2010) also found that the neural pathways affected were not the arcuate fasciculus, as some have suggested, but instead the third division of the superior longitudinal fasciculus (SLF III), which connects speech output planning areas of the ventral frontal cortex with sensorimotor integration areas of the inferior parietal lobe. They speculated that the etiology of the less efficient transport structure of the white matter tracts in individuals who stutter may be a result of delayed myelination of nerves in these pathways.

This explanation is essentially a reprise of Karlin's (1947) hypothesis that "the basic cause for stuttering is a delay in the myelination of the cortical areas in the brain concerned with speech" (p. 319). Karlin goes on to suggest that the myelin sheath surrounding nerves insulates them, and incomplete myelination results in slower transmission in nerves and in actions that are less precise and less coordinated. He further points out that myelination occurs earlier in girls than in boys (Flechsig, 1927), significant given the greater persistence of stuttering in boys.

It seems to me that an important effect of delayed myelination in these bidirectional nerve pathways may be that without adequate insulation provided by the myelin sheath, these pathways may be vulnerable to "cross talk" from high levels of activity in emotion and language processes (see Fig. 2.4 in Chapter 2). Vulnerability of poorly myelinated fibers in SLF III to interference by emotional activity seems possible given the evidence that the left frontal cortex is active for positive emotional arousal and the evidence reported by Johnson, Walden, Conture, and Karrass (2010) that stuttering may increase during positive emotional arousal. Furthermore, emotion-related disorders are reported to be associated with decreased myelination in the superior longitudinal fasciculus (Pavuluri & Passaroti, 2008).

In contrast to the effects of emotion (creating "noise" in the transmission lines), the effects of language processing may be more a phenomenon of overwhelming the transmission lines because so much information must be passed back and forth at such high speeds (e.g., longer sentences are spoken more quickly). Karlin (1947) points out that stuttering first appears when "sentence formation and flow of language has become more fully developed" (p. 319), implying that this increased demand of more developed language is too much for the pathways that are not fully myelinated, and thus stuttering results. Cykowski and colleagues (2010) also suggest that speech-language demands (such as when producing low-frequency or more complex words that require more careful monitoring) can put enough stress on the unmyelinated fiber tracts to provoke stuttering.

These findings indicate that stutterers' left-hemisphere structures for speech and language appear to have deficits or delays in development. This may prompt the use of homologous right-hemisphere structures, which themselves may not be as suited for rapid speech production as left-hemisphere structures (Geschwind & Galaburda, 1985). This results in stuttering, especially under the stress of increasing language demands as well as interference from nearby right hemisphere centers for emotion.

Brain Function Differences in People Who Stutter

Electroencephalographic Studies

Motivated by a theory that a lack of dominance of one cerebral hemisphere over the other caused stuttering (Orton, 1927; Orton & Travis, 1929; Travis, 1931), Travis and his students used electroencephalographs (EEGs) to measure brain waves in stuttering and nonstuttering subjects. Their hope was to find proof that the brains of stutterers didn't show the normal left-hemisphere dominance during speech and that this resulted in mistimed signals to muscles of the speech production system. EEG studies are carried out by pasting electrodes on the surface of the scalp to measure the electrical activity of brain. This procedure, like any assessment of the brain, was fraught with methodological quandaries (Bloodstein, 1995). How faithfully would electrical activity on the scalp plumb the activity of brain cells several centimeters below? How do we know that the electrical activity recorded isn't created by muscle contractions during speech or even the result of the subject blinking her eyes or wiggling her nose? How do we know which part of the brain is active when we see the squiggles on the chart paper that represent electrical impulses? These uncertainties make it likely that the EEG studies by different scientists in different laboratories will produce widely different findings due to different methodologies and different interpretations of the data.

Despite these problems, many EEG studies of stutterers and nonstutterers have been conducted, and some interesting findings have turned up. As with other experimental results, you should be cautious about accepting the results as final proof. Several EEG studies supported the notion that stutterers' brains functioned differently, although other studies did not. Studies by Travis and Knott (1937); Douglass (1943); Zimmermann and Knott (1974); Ponsford, Brown, Marsh, and Travis (1975); many by Moore and his colleagues (e.g., Moore & Haynes, 1980); and a study by Boberg, Yeudall, Schopflocher, and Bo-Lassen (1983) showed in different ways that individuals who stutter tended to have more activity on the right side of the brain during speech and especially during stuttering than did nonstutterers. This activity seemed to involve structures in the right hemisphere in a similar location as those in the left hemisphere that control speech and language (sometimes referred to as "homologous" areas). Although this was not exactly what Orton and Travis had predicted, it was close. Whereas the Orton-Travis theory hypothesized that stutterers lacked hemispheric dominance, findings from these EEG studies suggested that rather than lacking dominance, stutterers may be more likely to have a *right*-hemisphere dominance for speech and language (whereas nonstutterers generally have left hemisphere dominance).

Cerebral Blood Flow Studies

In the 1970s and 1980s, researchers developed new technology that was more precise than EEG in detecting where brain activity was occurring by measuring the amount of blood flowing to those areas. Cerebral blood flow (CBF) is usually detected by injecting a radioactive tracer into the bloodstream and taking the equivalent of x-ray pictures of the amount of radioactivity given off. The greater the amount of neural activity in an area, the greater the blood flow in that area and the greater the amount of radioactivity given off.

Interpretation of CBF and other brain imaging studies must take into account many different variables that can influence the results (Ingham, 2001). Two such variables are the spatial and temporal resolution of each technology. In other words, how accurately can CBF determine exactly *where* the activity is occurring and *when* it's occurring? Early studies could only observe areas of the brain in a relatively general way, but improved technologies have allowed researchers to differentiate the activity of different areas in more detail and reveal interactions among brain areas. Besides the problem of how good the resolution is, other variables that can influence outcomes of brain imaging studies are the gender of the participants, the severity of their stuttering, whether or not they've had speech therapy, what tasks the participants perform in the study, and techniques used to analyze the data (Lauter, 1995, 1997). Keep these factors in mind as you read about the research in this area.

Wood, Stump, McKeehan, Sheldon, and Proctor (1980) published the first study of CBF in stuttering, using only two participants. They found greater activity in the right-hemisphere region corresponding to Broca's area than in Broca's area (left hemisphere) itself during stuttering before treatment with the drug haloperidol. After two weeks of treatment with haloperidol, both participants showed that the greater activity had shifted from right- to left-hemisphere speech areas. The second CBF study of stuttering was not published until 11 years later. Pool, Devous, Freeman, Watson, and Finitzo (1991) studied the brains of 20 adult stutterers using single photon emission computed tomography, an improved technology that enabled scientists to view the brain from multiple angles and obtain better images of what was going on. The principal finding from this study was that the stuttering group showed less left-hemispheric dominance compared to controls in areas that are believed to be associated with language processing (middle temporal lobe), speech motor control (inferior frontal lobe), and motor initiation (anterior cingulate).

Positron Emission Tomography Studies and Beyond

Four years later, another CBF study took advantage of a new brain imaging tool, positron emission tomography, which allowed researchers to make more accurate inferences about where increased blood flow was occurring in the brain.

A large team of researchers studied the brains of four adults who stuttered and a matched group of control participants in two conditions: reading aloud alone and in unison with someone else called "choral reading" (Wu, Maguire, Riley, Fallon, & LaCasse et al., 1995). As you may remember from Chapter 1, when individuals who stutter read aloud along with someone else, they become fluent. These findings suggested that two important speech and language areas of the brain—Broca's area and Wernicke's area, both in the left hemisphere (see Fig. 2.3)—showed decreased activity (compared to their normal-speaking controls) when participants were stuttering, compared to when they were fluent during choral reading.

Broca's area is thought to be the major cortical area responsible for organizing and executing speech motor output. Wernicke's area, on the other hand, is vital for speech and language comprehension but may also be involved in speech output because it appears to be the storehouse for the sounds that form words—the phonological representations that are called upon before the motor commands are given.

In November 1995, four different research groups presented their findings at the annual convention of the American Speech-Language-Hearing Association in Orlando, Florida (De Nil, Kroll, Houle, Ludlow, Braun, & Ingham et al., 1995; Ingham & Fox, 1995; Wu, Maguire, Riley, Fallon, & LaCasse et al., 1995). As the presentations were given, the excitement in the room was palpable because so many of their findings were similar, although the groups were working entirely independently. Here at last was clear evidence that the brains of people who stutter worked differently than those of nonstutterers. Years of previous speculation and studies suggesting anomalous cerebral dominance, inadequate laterality, auditory processing problems, and language dysfunction in stuttering seemed to be confirmed. These findings and others are reviewed below, organized by the types of anomalies they suggest.

Brain Overactivation During Stuttering

Many studies have shown that certain areas of the brain show higher levels of activation in those who stutter than in controls. Sometimes this is present during stuttering, but it has also been shown to occur in stutterers' fluent speech. Researchers have suggested that some of the overactivations may be important etiological factors, while others may be compensatory.

Overactivation of Right-Hemisphere Cortical Areas During Stuttering

A common finding by several of the brain research teams in 1995 and afterward is that individuals who stutter demonstrate high levels of activity in the right hemisphere when they are speaking, especially when stuttering, as illustrated in Figure 2.5.

The focus of this activity is greatest in right-hemisphere structures that are homologous to those in the left hemisphere used by normal speakers (Braun, Varga, Stager, Schulz, Selbie, & Maisog et al., 1997; De Nil, Kroll, Kapur,

& Houle, 2000; Fox, Ingham, Ingham, Hirsch, & Downs et al., 1996; Fox, Ingham, Ingham, Zamarripa, Xiong, & Lancaster, 2000). One of those areas is called the *right frontal operculum* (see Fig. 2.3) and is in the same location in the right hemisphere that Broca's area is in the left hemisphere (Fox, 2003). Broca's area is thought to be active in planning the phonetic structure of an utterance to be spoken (Kent, 1997). Another area in the right hemisphere commonly found to be active during stuttering is the right *insula* (Fox, 2003). In the left hemisphere, the insula may function as a connection between Wernicke's area (which may be important for phonological representations of words and auditory monitoring of one's own speech) and Broca's area (Ingham, Ingham, Finn, & Fox, 2003).

A meta-analysis of many studies that compared stutterers and controls (Brown, Ingham, Ingham, Laird, & Fox, 2005) confirmed that a major difference between these groups was a general overactivation of right-sided areas that are homologous to left-sided areas active for speech production: the frontal operculum, Rolandic operculum, and anterior insula. It should be noted that these researchers also observed that a common finding was overactivation in left-hemisphere areas related to motor control of speech, perhaps as a result of the extra effort required to speak.

Researchers have considered two possible explanations for the overactivation of right-hemisphere structures during stuttering. One is that during embryonic development, the right side of the brain becomes "wired" to be the primary speech and language area (e.g., Geschwind & Galaburda, 1985). This may result in some difficulty speaking because right-hemisphere structures are not generally suited for the rapid processing of signals required for speech (such as the quick transitions in many consonant-vowel transitions). When a child with this right-hemisphere "wiring" for speech develops language beyond the single-word stage, stuttering may emerge as he tries to produce multiword utterances at the typically fast speech rates used for longer sentences (Kent, 1984). A second hypothesis is that the child who stutters initially tried to use left-hemisphere regions for speech and language, but the neural networks for speech and language failed to function adequately and resulted in stuttering. Only then did the child's brain begin to use right-hemisphere structures in a compensatory way to try to achieve more normal speech, similar to the way in which some individuals with aphasia use right-hemisphere structures to compensate for damaged areas in the left hemisphere (e.g., Sommer et al., 2002; Weiller, Isensee, Rijntjes, Huber, Müller et al., 1995).

Several researchers have provided evidence in favor of the second (compensation) hypothesis. Braun and colleagues (1997) found that activations of right-hemisphere sensory areas were negatively correlated with stuttering; that is, these regions became more active as speech became more fluent. Moreover, researchers in Germany (Neumann et al., 2003) found that right-hemisphere activations were greater in participants who stuttered moderately compared to those who stuttered severely, suggesting that right-hemisphere activity may indeed be a way in which individuals could partially overcome dysfunctions in the left-hemisphere areas. In other words, the moderate stutterers used more compensatory right-hemisphere activity to reduce the severity of their stuttering.

It is possible, of course, that both hypotheses are correct—that some individuals develop right-hemisphere processing for speech and language before they begin to stutter, and others develop right-hemisphere processing after they begin to stutter, as a compensatory response. Still others may in fact process speech and language in both hemispheres simultaneously. Each of these options is probably inefficient and may create the dyssynchrony in processing that results in stuttering.

Overactivation in Midbrain Areas

A number of researchers have reported unusually high levels of activity in midbrain structures that, via pathways to the cerebral cortex, may influence speech movements. Specifically, some structures of the basal ganglia have been shown to be overactive in those who stutter (e.g., substantia nigra, subthalamic nucleus, red nucleus, globus pallidus) (Fox et al., 1996; Watkins et al., 2008). This midbrain area is important in speech motor activity, via loops that send signals from the cortex to the basal ganglia, which then send "go" or "no go" signals to the supplementary motor area (SMA), which is responsible for initiating movement. Excess activity in the basal ganglia associated with stuttering could possibly result in inhibitory signals sent to SMA preventing the initiation of speech movements. Another perspective, given by Alm (2004), is that the excess *right*-hemisphere SMA activity during stuttering reported by Fox and colleagues (1996) may be the result of inadequate left-hemisphere SMA activity due to basal ganglia dysfunction in stutterers.

Underactive Brain Areas in Stuttering

Several areas of the brain, including both motor and sensory centers, have been found to be underactive in stuttering. Because speech motor control involves motor and sensory integration, it is not surprising that this is sometimes reported.

Underactivity in Speech Motor Areas

Watkins and colleagues (2008) found that during speech production, stutterers showed decreased activity compared to controls in areas related to using sensory and motor information and planning sequential movements: ventral premotor, Rolandic opercular, and sensorimotor cortex on both sides of the brain. This underactivity was in the same area of the brain as the structural differences found by Watkins and colleagues (2008)—less dense white matter tracts connecting articulatory planning and sensory feedback areas. Thus, structural differences seem to result in functional deficits that presumably interfere with the smooth flow of speech. The researchers point out that the fact that the decreased activity is present on both sides of the brain and is widespread may account for the fact that, unlike in cases of unilateral and limited brain lesions, these individuals' brains were unable to develop work-arounds to compensate for the problem.

Underactivity in Auditory Areas

Many brain imaging studies of stuttering have shown a lack of activity in the superior temporal lobe, including auditory association areas and Wernicke's area (Braun et al., 1997; De Nil, Kroll, Lafaille, & Houle, 2003; Fox et al., 1996; Fox et al., 2000). The meta-analysis by Brown and colleagues (2005) mentioned earlier indicated that a common finding among several of these studies was that auditory areas in both hemispheres were deactivated, suggesting that stutterers' mechanisms for guiding their speech by self-hearing were not functioning properly. More recently, Watkins et al. (2008) found in their study of adolescent and young adult stutterers that underactivity was notable in Heschl's gyrus, a part of the superior temporal lobe that is important for processing speech sounds. Another imaging study (Salmelin, Schnitzler, Schmitz, Jancke, Witte, & Freund, 1998) found that stutterers have a reversal of the normal pattern of activation of the left and right auditory cortices during stuttering. Evidence of auditory dysfunction during stuttering is especially pertinent in light of the many studies that have shown that stutterers may have difficulty performing auditory processing tasks (e.g., Barasch, Guitar, McCauley, & Absher, 2000; Molt, 1998) and that fluency can be induced by changing the way stutterers hear their own speech (e.g., Brayton & Conture, 1978; Howell, El-Yaniv, & Powell, 1987).

How does auditory self-monitoring affect fluency? It may provide a stimulus to synchronize or integrate the sequence of activities that run in parallel when a speaker decides what she will say, selects the linguistic elements for it, and executes the utterance. Thus, the asynchrony or timing disturbance that many researchers see as the basis of stuttering (e.g., Perkins, Kent, & Curlee, 1991; Van Riper, 1982) may be caused by a paucity of signals that synchronize the sequence for speech output. Therapies (e.g., Van Riper, 1973) that emphasize proprioception may be giving the client another feedback modality to use for timing; therapies that focus on the use of slow speech, gentle onsets, and light articulatory contacts may develop the client's auditory and proprioceptive monitoring of speech.

Other functions besides monitoring one's own speech may also reside in the deactivated regions of the superior temporal lobe. For example, Wernicke's area may be important for storing the phonological representations of words (Caplan, 1987; Paulesu, Frith, & Frackowiak, 1993). Activation of this region of the brain, therefore, may be a key stage in phonological planning for speech production. Lack of activation during stuttering may reflect a deficit in the sequence of phonological selection, phonetic planning, and motor execution.

SENSORY AND SENSORY-MOTOR STUDIES

Research has assessed how well individuals who stutter can process auditory signals in various parts of the brain. A number of studies have used the Synthetic Sentence Identification/ Ipsilateral Competing Message test (SSI-ICM) to compare stutterers and nonstutterers. This test requires participants to identify words in a nonsense phrase (such as "small boat with a picture has become") when competing noise is presented in the same ear (right on top of the nonsense phrase). Three studies using this test found that stutterers performed worse than normal participants (Hall & Jerger, 1978; Molt & Guilford, 1979; Toscher & Rupp, 1978). The same test was given to two groups of normal speakers—those who were judged to be more fluent and those who were judged to be less fluent. The more fluent normal speakers performed significantly better than the less fluent normal speakers (Wynne & Boehmler, 1982). This finding suggests that stuttering and normal disfluencies are not entirely different phenomena; both may be associated with some difficulty in central auditory processing. This difficulty may give rise to disfluencies in many children, only some of whom develop chronic stuttering. Some other factor in addition to an auditory processing difficulty may be necessary for high levels of normal disfluency to become stuttering.

In contrast to the above studies, Hannley and Dorman (1982) found no differences between stutterers and nonstutterers on the SSI-ICM, but the stutterers in their study had all recently completed a treatment program. This finding is intriguing in light of evidence from brain imaging studies that individuals who stutter who had demonstrated an absence of activity before treatment in the left auditory cortex showed normal levels of activity immediately after treatment (De Nil et al., 2003; Ingham, 2003; Neumann et al., 2003; Stager, Jeffries, & Braun, 2003).

Another tool for assessing central auditory processing is the Masking Level Difference (MLD) test, which requires listeners to detect the onset and offset of a tone in the presence of a masking noise. When masking noise is played in the same ear as the tone, there are fewer cues for listeners to use in "filtering" the tone from the masking noise. Listeners must use very subtle temporal cues to detect the tone; under these conditions, persons who stutter perform more poorly than groups of nonstutterers (Liebetrau & Daly, 1981; Kramer, Green, & Guitar, 1987). These results may be interpreted to support the outcome of the SSI studies because both tests require the participants to use temporal information—in one case (SSI), the information is in rapidly changing format frequencies (characteristic acoustic information) needed to identify words, and in the other case (MLD), the information is the onset and offset of a tone in masking.

Two other studies of central auditory processing tested the hypothesis that people who stutter have difficulty resolving temporal differences. Herndon (1966) found that stutterers were poorer than nonstutterers at distinguishing which of two brief tones was longer. Barasch and colleagues (2000) administered the Duration Pattern Sequence (DPS) test, which involves judging the relative lengths of three tones, and another measure in which subjects estimated the protensity (i.e., durations) of tones and silent intervals. These tests failed to distinguish between the stuttering and non-stuttering participants as groups, but they showed that less fluent participants in each group scored more poorly on the DPS than those who were more fluent. In addition, the more disfluent subjects in both groups judged temporal intervals to be longer than did less disfluent subjects. This finding is evidence that there may be a connection between normal disfluency and stuttering. The authors speculated that one of the possible connections between increased disfluency and longer protensity estimates is the effect of fear and anxiety on speaking. It has been suggested that fear and anxiety affect temporal processing (Fraisse, 1963) and that anomalies in temporal processing may be an underlying cause of both stuttering (Kent, 1984) and high levels of normal disfluency (Wynne & Boehmler, 1982). Given the evidence that stutterers are no more anxious than nonstutterers (Guitar, 1998), one might ask—why should stutterers' temporal processing for speech be any more susceptible to negative emotions than temporal processing in nonstutterers? The answer may be found in evidence that negative emotions such as fear and anxiety appear to be regulated by the right hemisphere along with evidence that stutterers process speech in widely distributed areas of the right hemisphere. Thus, the close proximity of areas regulating negative emotions and speech production may allow "cross talk" between these areas to interfere with speech, producing disfluency. It remains to be seen if highly normally disfluent speakers also use right-hemisphere structures for speech production.

As described in the earlier section on brain structure differences in stutterers, Foundas and colleagues (2004) looked for differences in auditory processing that might reflect the differences in the structure of a part of the auditory temporal cortex (PT). They did indeed find an auditory processing difference in a subgroup (36 percent) of stutterers who had an atypical rightward asymmetry in this part of the auditory cortex. As you may remember from the earlier discussion of this work, the difference was that stutterers with atypical auditory cortices became more fluent when speaking while listening to delayed auditory feedback. This suggests that for some stutterers, speech production timing and coordination difficulties may originate in dyssynchronies in central processing of auditory feedback.

Brain Electrical Potentials Reflecting Auditory Processing

Studies of electrical brain activity in response to auditory stimuli have provided further evidence that auditory

processing is abnormal in individuals who stutter. Studies by Hood (1987) and Dietrich, Barry, and Parker (1995) reflecting both subcortical and cortical activity have found group differences between stutterers and nonstutterers. However, the first study found stutterers' responses to be slower, and the second found them to be faster than those of nonstutterers. A study by Molt (1998) is more relevant to the question raised by brain imaging studies of whether persons who stutter have a deficit in the left auditory cortex. Molt found that stutterers had longer latencies and lower amplitudes of brain waves in the cortex when they were asked to make decisions about semantic incongruencies in sentences to which they listened when compared to nonstutterers.

In a study that combined behavioral and brain electrical activity measures related to auditory processing of non-linguistic material (tones), Hampton and Weber-Fox (2008) showed that while most of a group of 11 stutterers performed like a matched group of 11 nonstutterers, there was a sub-group of three stutterers who performed much more poorly than the nonstutterers on behavioral measures (accuracy and speed of identification of tones) and showed abnormalities in the brain electrical activity measures (early "P300" responses, positive-going peaks at a point 300 msec after the stimuli). This finding is reminiscent of the subgroup of stutterers described in the Foundas et al. (2004) study with an anomalous rightward asymmetry in the PT who showed a greater improvement in fluency while speaking under delayed auditory feedback than did those stutterers with more typical PT asymmetry. In other words, not all individuals who stutter may have auditory processing anomalies. A small group may have both structural and functional deviations from the norm, and this group may benefit from therapeutic approaches that help them compensate for these deviations.

Dichotic Listening Tests

More support for the notion that stutterers have abnormal auditory processing comes from speech perception studies. A number of experiments found that many persons who stutter do not show the typical right-ear advantage that non-stutterers do, evidence that people who stutter do not have left-hemisphere dominance for language (Blood, 1985; Curry & Gregory, 1969; Davenport, 1977; Liebetrau & Daly, 1981; Sommers, Brady, & Moore, 1975). Some dichotic studies, however, found no differences between stutterers and nonstutterers (Dorman & Porter, 1975; Pinsky & McAdam, 1980; Slorach & Noehr, 1973). Other studies found no significant group differences but found that fewer stutterers than nonstutterers showed the expected right-ear advantage (Brady & Berson, 1975; Quinn, 1972; Rosenfield & Goodglass, 1980; Strong, 1977) or found that the magnitude of difference between ears was greater for nonstutterers (Blood & Blood, 1989).

Looking over the myriad of studies that have been conducted, it appears that the more linguistically complex the stimulus (e.g., words versus syllables), the more likely that differences between stutterers and nonstutterers would be found. Thus, stutterers' differences appear to be related to their linguistic processing abilities; they appear more likely to process linguistically meaningful stimuli in their right hemispheres.

Like much research in this area, dichotic testing of stutterers also suggests there might be group differences or at least subgroups of stutterers who differ from nonstutterers on a critical dimension. Examples of such subgroups might be those with more severe stuttering (Davenport, 1977); those who show several abnormal signs on neuropsychological test batteries, suggesting an "organic" origin of stuttering; and those showing only a few abnormal signs, suggesting a "functional" origin (Liebetrau & Daly, 1981). Perhaps the best example, however, is the stuttering subgroup mentioned in the previous section—individuals who show structural and functional abnormalities in sensory—especially auditory—processing.

Auditory, Tactile, and Proprioceptive Feedback

A connection between stutterers' brain anomalies in auditory processing and speech performance was suggested by Stromsta (1957, 1972, 1986). His research on auditory feedback led him to suggest that stutterers' abnormal brain rhythms interfere with the smooth integration of auditory feedback from the speaker's own voice and his subsequent speech output. The result, he suggested, is a combination of a stoppage of phonation and an improper coarticulation of sounds (Stromsta, 1986). This proposal foreshadows the results of recent brain imaging studies reviewed earlier. For example, Stager, Jeffries, and Braun (2003) suggested that brain scans during conditions that promoted fluency showed increased activity in stutterers' central auditory cortex, reflecting "more effective coupling of auditory and motor systems" (p. 334) so that auditory feedback could facilitate the sequencing of speech motor output. And of course, the results of the studies by Foundas and colleagues (2004) showing atypical morphology in some stutterers' auditory temporal cortex also suggest that problems in processing auditory feedback may underlie stuttering.

The few studies that have been conducted of other feedback systems besides auditory also show some deficits, but the results are mixed. Baker (1967) found that people who stutter performed more poorly than nonstutterers on tests of oral sensation. However, this finding was not replicated by Jensen, Sheehan, Williams, and LaPointe (1975). On a test that required subjects to match spatially ordered visual patterns with temporally ordered auditory patterns, Cohen and Hanson (1975) found that individuals who stutter performed more poorly than those who didn't. Chuang, Fromm, Ewanowski, and Abbs (1980) evaluated stutterers' abilities to make the smallest movements possible with their

jaws and tongues. The stuttering group had significantly larger "difference limens" (smallest detectable difference) with or without the assistance of visual feedback for such movements. This means that they did not have the degree of fine sensory-motor control of the jaw and tongue that the nonstuttering group did. De Nil and Abbs (1991) followed up on this study and demonstrated that stutterers had less sensorimotor control for minimal movements with their jaws, lips, and tongues (but not finger movements) compared to nonstutterers, when using only kinesthetic feedback. There were no differences between the groups when using visual feedback.

Together with the findings about the auditory system, these studies may indicate that as a group, individuals who stutter have some difficulty using auditory, touch, and movement information to control speech. But Namasivayam, van Lieshout, McIlroy, and De Nil (2009) provided evidence that stutterers are as capable as nonstutterers in using sensory feedback to stabilize speech motor control in the face of experimental perturbations (masking noise and tendon vibration). If they are as good as nonstutterers at using sensory feedback to nullify the effects of external interference with speech movements, stutterers may be using sensory feedback to also nullify the effects of internal interference with speech (i.e., their innately poorer speech motor skills). In other words, when stutterers are fluent, as they naturally are some of the time, they may be achieving this fluency by making extra use of sensory feedback (van Lieshout, Hulstijn, & Peters, 2004). In summary, this literature is full of conflicting findings, and it is not clear whether all stutterers have deficits in sensory feedback or whether there is only a subgroup that shows these deficits.

| SENSORY-MOTOR CONTROL

The first experiments on people who stutter found that they were slower than nonstutterers in initiating and terminating a vowel in response to a buzzer (Adams & Hayden, 1976; Starkweather, Hirschman, & Tannenbaum, 1976). Later experiments showed that stutterers were slower than nonstutterers in reacting with respiratory (exhalation) and articulatory movements (lip closing) (McFarlane & Prins, 1978; Watson & Alfonso, 1987). They were also slower whether they were responding to auditory or visual signals (e.g., Cross & Cooke, 1979). Children who stutter were also found to have slower reaction times in studies by Cross and Luper (1979, 1983), Cullinan and Springer (1980), Maske-Cash and Curlee (1995), and Till, Reich, Dickey, and Sieber (1983).

Although not all studies showed group differences, De Nil (1995) pointed out that about 75 percent of the 44 voice reaction time studies that he reviewed found that people who stutter were significantly slower than people who don't stutter and that most of the other studies showed trends in that direction. He further noted that when investigators used linguistically meaningful stimuli to test reaction times (words or sentences, rather than isolated sounds), 80 percent of the studies found significant differences between stutterers and nonstutterers. These findings are likely to be related to the evidence from brain imaging studies indicating that individuals who stutter have anomalies in areas used for sensorimotor processing of speech and language. Not surprisingly, these anomalies may affect sensorimotor reaction times on nonspeech tasks, but are most evident in tasks requiring linguistic processing.

Fluent Speech

Acoustic studies have demonstrated that, on average, stutterers have longer vowel durations, slower transitions between consonants and vowels, and delayed onsets of voicing after voiceless consonants even when speaking fluently (Colcord & Adams, 1979; DiSimoni, 1974; Hillman & Gilbert, 1977; Starkweather & Myers, 1979). The findings of these acoustic studies have been supported by "kinematic" research, which has measured the movements of speakers' speech structures (e.g., Alfonso, Story, & Watson, 1987; Zimmermann, 1980). As a group, stutterers tend to move their lips and jaws more slowly, even during fluent speech, than do nonstutterers (e.g., Zimmermann, 1980). Kinematic research has also shown that some stutterers demonstrate abnormal sequencing of articulator movement onsets and velocities (Caruso, Abbs, & Gracco, 1988). Other kinematic studies, however, have not found group differences or have found them only in stutterers who had recently undergone therapy (e.g., McClean, Kroll, & Loftus, 1990), which may have taught them to speak more slowly.

So what does this mean? Why might many stutterers speak more slowly or use different sequences of articulatory movements than nonstuttering speakers even when they are fluent? Some researchers think that these findings reflect delays or other dysfunctions in processing incoming and outgoing signals. Stutterers may be unable to process neural signals fast enough to make the rapid, precise movements of normal conversational speech, especially when they are under the stress of planning a complex sentence or competing with other talkers. Their delays in voicing onset, slower transitions, and abnormal sequencing during fluent speech may just reflect a slower mechanism working at its normal rate. A different view, suggested by more skeptical researchers, is that such differences simply reflect the way stutterers have learned to talk to avoid stuttering, either on their own or as a result of therapy, and this way of speaking keeps them fluent even with an inefficient speech motor system.

Another interpretation of these slower movements is that they are the result of heightened tension in muscles having antagonistic functions for speech production (Starkweather, 1987). For example, increased tension in muscles that move a structure forward (agonists), as well as muscles that hold it

back (antagonists), would make movement of that structure considerably slower. Imagine two people pulling a rope in opposite directions. Even if one were stronger, that person would make slow progress in her direction because the other, weaker person would create a drag. The slowed movements of stutterers' speech structures would account for not only slower reaction times but also the longer movement durations in their fluent speech.

Findings from a number of studies support this view. They have shown that stutterers co-contract agonist and antagonist muscles of both the laryngeal (Freeman & Ushijima, 1975; Shapiro, 1980) and articulatory (Guitar, Guitar, Neilson, O'Dwyer, & Andrews, 1988) muscle groups during stuttering. These studies, like Starkweather's (1987) review, have noted that such co-contraction of agonist and antagonist muscles appears even in some of the apparently fluent speech of stutterers. This finding has led many researchers to posit that stuttering is not an "all-or-nothing" event (Adams & Runyan, 1981; Bloodstein, 1987). Sometimes, stutterers may speak freely, without a trace of excess tension. At other times, they may have excess tension that isn't heard by listeners as stuttering. At still other times, muscle tension may be so great that both listeners and the person who stutters are acutely aware of stuttering. This continuum of fluency reflects the subjective impression of many stutterers, including me.

Nonspeech Motor Control

In a study of both sequential finger movements and sequential counting aloud fluently, Borden (1983) found that severe stutterers, but not mild stutterers, were slower than nonstutterers in executing both finger movement and speech tasks. Thus, severe stutterers may have substantial deficits in certain sensory-motor tasks, but mild stutterers only slight deficits, and these may require special task conditions to be revealed.

Webster (1993a) developed a finger movement task 10 years later in which participants tapped four numbered keys in a predetermined sequence. To make the task somewhat like speech, participants were assigned a novel sequence of keys at the beginning of each trial (3-2-4-1 or 4-1-2-3, etc.). In both timed and untimed tests, stutterers made more errors sequencing and were slower initiating the task but were comparable to nonstutterers in execution time (once the movement was started). Unlike Borden's study, no effort was made to analyze the results by subjects' stuttering severity. Webster thought that these results suggested that stutterers may have difficulty in "response planning, organization, and initiation" (Webster, 1993b, p. 84) of novel sequences of movements.

To answer the question of why this difficulty may be present only intermittently in individuals who stutter (after all, they have a great deal of fluent speech), Webster (1993b) postulated what others (Cross, Sweet, & Bates, 1985; Curlee, 1993; Peters & Guitar, 1991) have also considered that at times, such as under stress, there is "cross talk" or interference between the hemispheres. Specifically, activity in the right hemisphere interferes with sequential movement control in the left hemisphere.

To test this, Webster used a task in which participants performed sequential finger tapping with the right hand while turning a knob with the left hand, in response to an auditory signal. If his hypothesis were true, the stuttering group's left hemisphere–controlled finger tapping would be vulnerable to interference by the right hemisphere–controlled knob turning. Indeed, the stuttering group's performance was significantly poorer than that of the nonstuttering group on both tasks.

Webster (1997) then wondered if interference of left-hemisphere sequential movement control mechanisms might be the result of stutterers' inability to focus attention on the left-hemisphere task and ignore interference from a competing source, whether from the right or left hemisphere. To test this, Webster used a procedure developed to investigate attention focus in right- and left-handed people. Participants were required to tap twice with one hand for every tap they made with the other hand. They were tested with the right-hand double tapping and the left single tapping, as well as vice versa. The nonstutterers were able to perform the task significantly better when they tapped twice with the right hand and once with the left; however, stutterers and nonstuttering left-handers performed the task equally well with either hand doing the double tapping. Webster interpreted this outcome as suggesting that stutterers and left-handed nonstutterers did not have the ability to focus predominantly on the left hemisphere, but had equal focus on both, making their left hemispheres vulnerable to interference from other activities. Webster's model of stuttering, derived from these experiments, postulates that individuals who stutter are unable to protect the integrity of speech production centers from interference or "cross talk" from emotions or other ongoing processes. It is not clear why then, all left-handers don't stutter. I would presume that this model proposes that stutterers have both a deficit in the sequencing of processing underlying speech production as well as an inability to focus on the left hemisphere.

Following up on Webster's studies, Subramanian and Yairi (2006) experimented with a version of the finger-tapping task, using not only stutterers and controls but a third group of "high-risk" participants. All participants were right-handed. The high-risk individuals were parents or siblings of the stutterers—of special interest because they were thought to be carriers of genetic material that could create stuttering except for the absence of some critical factor that would presumably cause them to stutter, too. All participants tapped in several conditions, including tapping at a comfortable rate and at a fast rate. Among the findings of this study was evidence that in the comfortable rate condition, the stuttering group and the high-risk group were slower than the control groups. However, in the fast rate condition, the stuttering group tapped faster than either of the other groups, both with their right hands and with their left hands. Along with their high rate, the stuttering group also had higher variability in tapping rate than either group.

Of great interest was the finding that in this fast rate condition, the high-risk group had slower tapping rates than either the stuttering group or the control group but had relatively low variability. The authors speculated that these findings may reflect that those in the stuttering and high-risk groups have motor systems that operate best at slow rates. When there is pressure to operate at a fast rate, the high-risk group is able to control their rate and maintain stability (low variability). But under this pressure, the stuttering group taps very rapidly, pushing their motor systems beyond their optimal operating speed, causing them to become unstable (high variability).

It is not too great a leap to imagine that individuals who stutter speak more rapidly than is optimal for their speech planning and execution systems, thus becoming disfluent. It is also possible that close relatives of individuals who stutter who may have inherited a predisposition for stuttering don't develop stuttering because they are able speak at slower speech rates, more appropriate for the limitations of the speech motor production system. It is interesting that this is the same conclusion drawn by Kloth, Janssen, Kraaimaat, and Brutten (1995, 1998) who found that in a high-risk-for-stuttering population of 93 children studied prior to onset, the 26 children who did develop stuttering spoke more rapidly than the 67 children who didn't. However, both groups' speech rates were within the normal range.

Subramanian and Yairi (2006) also found evidence that could support Webster's (1997) hypothesis that stutterers suffer from an inability to focus entirely on the left hemisphere when performing motor tasks and thus may activate both hemispheres for speech, as brain imaging studies have shown (e.g., Brown et al., 2005). Subramanian and Yairi's (2006) data showed that when participants were asked to tap simultaneously with both hands, but tap twice as fast with one hand than with the other, the stuttering and high-risk participants performed equally well with either the right or left hand tapping twice as fast. The control groups were better when they tapped twice as fast with their dominant (right) hands as with the left hands. This finding supports the speculation that the stuttering and high-risk groups did not suppress the right hemisphere and focus entirely on the left hemisphere. Another similarity to Webster's (1997) findings was that Subramanian and Yairi's (2006) stuttering group required more trials to learn to tap twice as fast with one hand than the other. Webster's similar finding that stuttering subjects took longer to initiate a pattern of tapping led him to speculate that it reflects stutterers' difficulty initiating speech movement at the beginning of an utterance, thus stuttering more at the beginnings of phrases.

Subramanian and Yairi's (2006) finding that adults who stutter manifest greater variability in a nonspeech motor task was recently discovered in children who stutter. Olander, Smith, and Zelaznik (2010) studied 17 children who stutter and controls, ages 4 to 6, using a task that required children to clap their hands in time to a metronome and then continue to clap at that rate after the metronome was turned off. Their results indicated that although 40 percent of the children performed like the control group, 60 percent showed variability outside the range of the controls. They speculate that nonspeech motor variability may be related to speech motor control deficits and that these deficits might be predictive of recovery or persistence of stuttering.

The last studies of nonspeech motor control I will review concern the use of auditory input to control motor output. A common paradigm in these studies is to have participants track or follow the changing frequency (pitch) of a target sound with a second sound, called a "cursor." A computer controls the pitch changes in the target's sound and participants follow these changes by using their hands or their jaws to move a lever that changes the pitch of the cursor. Using this paradigm, Sussman and MacNeilage (1975) found that normal speakers made fewer errors tracking the target sound when the cursor tone was presented to the right ear and the target tone to the left ear. Those who stuttered, on the other hand, made equal numbers of errors whether the cursor tone was in the right ear and the target tone in the left or vice versa, suggesting that they did not have a left-hemisphere advantage for integrating auditory information with motor output as the nonstutterers did.

Researchers in Australia replicated and extended this work on tracking (Neilson, 1980; Neilson & Neilson, 1987, 1988) using both visual and auditory targets and cursors. They demonstrated that participants who stuttered were significantly poorer using auditory targets and cursors than when using visual ones. They also showed that when both stuttering and nonstuttering participants practiced the tasks beforehand, the differences between the groups were even larger than when they had not practiced. The Neilsons proposed that stutterers were slow in developing a mental auditory-motor model of the relationship between their movement of the cursor control and the resulting sound change. They further hypothesized that the basic deficit in stuttering is difficulty in forming or accessing auditory-motor models of what speech movements are needed to produce the sounds they want to make. I suspect that the Neilsons would agree that stutterers can use their auditory-motor models better in situations where the demands on their neural resources are low but have more trouble when the demands are high.

As the Neilsons were working on their experiments in Australia, researchers at Baylor College of Medicine in Texas were also studying the auditory-motor tracking abilities of persons who stutter. In a series of publications (Nudelman, Herbrich, Hoyt, & Rosenfield, 1987; 1989; Nudelman, Herbrich, Hess, Hoyt, & Rosenfield, 1992), these researchers described experiments, which required participants to hum along with a tone that suddenly changed pitch. The pitch of the target tones was sometimes changed rapidly, sometimes slowly, while researchers measured how quickly participants could change their humming to match the changing pitch of the auditory target tone. The researchers found that stutterers were significantly slower than nonstutterers in detecting changes in the target's frequency, suggesting that stutterers need more time to process auditory signals. Once again, we find that research has produced evidence that, as a group, people who stutter have difficulty performing auditory processing tasks—perhaps more so when the auditory information is related to vocal output. Note that this limitation might be related to findings by Cykowski and colleagues (2010) and Sommer and colleagues (2002) that brain areas used for sensory integration are not efficiently connected to motor planning/motor execution areas.

LANGUAGE FACTORS

Studies of stutterer-nonstutterer differences on sensory and sensory-motor tasks, reviewed earlier in this chapter supported the notion that language factors are important in stuttering, affecting both speech and nonspeech tasks. For example, the results of dichotic listening studies and reaction time experiments indicate that there are greater stutterer-nonstutterer differences when the stimuli used are more linguistically complex and more meaningful (e.g., Curry & Gregory, 1969; De Nil, 1995). Moreover, Kleinow and Smith (2000) found that linguistic complexity affected the stability of speech motor control in stutterers. Using a measure called the spatiotemporal index that reflects the amount of variability in articulator movement when a sentence is said over and over, Kleinow and Smith demonstrated that longer and more syntactically complex sentences produced significantly more instability in stutterers' speech production than simpler and shorter sentences. The same was not true for nonstutterers. Kleinow and Smith interpreted these findings as suggesting that stutterers' speech production systems are more vulnerable to breakdown when language demands are high. Smith, Sadagopan, Walsh, and Weber-Fox (2010) also found increasing interarticulatory coordination breakdown as phonological complexity increased for adults who stutter but not controls.

Some researchers caution against the view that language factors are a primary causal influence in stuttering. De Nil, for example, suggests that the basic problem of stuttering may be in "sensorimotor processes involved in speech production" rather than in "cognitive language formulation processes" involved in speech production (De Nil, 2004, p. 123). He and his fellow researchers (De Nil, Kroll, & Houle, 2001) compared brain scans of stutterers and nonstutterers while they performed two tasks—one, reading single words aloud, and the other, generating verbs. While both tasks involved saying single words aloud, the verb-generation task engaged more language processing—specifically, semantic and phonological searching and encoding. To assess whether the two groups differed on the two tasks, the experimenters "subtracted" the scans of reading the words aloud from the scans of generating verbs. In other words, they wanted to see if the extra demand of generating verbs alone showed a big difference between the two groups, so they took out all activity in the verb-generating task that was also present just in reading words aloud. The subtraction indicated that there were minimal differences between the groups in the more linguistically involved task or generating verbs, although there were large differences between the groups in reading words aloud. This suggested that the added linguistic burden of having to think of verbs was not particularly more demanding on the stutterers than on the nonstutterers.

The two views (a) that language is not a primary factor in stuttering and (b) that language is a major influence in stuttering may be compatible if one assumes that the basic defect is in sensorimotor control of speech but that individuals who stutter achieve fluency by compensating for that sensorimotor defect by using additional neuronal resources, additional attention, or simplifying the task by slowing their speech rates. When language becomes more complex and/or sentences become longer, speech rate increases (Starkweather, 1981), and it would seem from evidence that there is more distributed brain activity when language is more complex that more neuronal resources and attention are devoted to the greater language demands. Thus, fewer extra resources are available to compensate for the sensorimotor defect and more stuttering results.

The notion that stutterers have a limitation on their neural resources during speech and language production is supported by the research program of Bosshardt (2006) that provides data to suggest that stutterers are poorer at tasks requiring linguistic processing while engaging in other cognitive activities. Bosshardt's interpretation of his results describes the connection between language and stuttering by hypothesizing that individuals who stutter have speech and language planning and production systems that are less protected from interference, either by heavy processing loads within the system or by other activities in the brain. One might extend that argument to suggest that when children are first learning to use new language constructions during childhood, the neuronal resource requirements for language planning are high. Thus, children with vulnerable speech and language systems will experience interference by language planning on the smooth production of speech. Even when these children have grown older and have learned adult language, their use of long, complex sentences at rapid rates while planning the next parts of a narrative can be disrupted.

EMOTIONAL FACTORS

Anxiety and Autonomic Arousal

A direct connection between a momentary experience of anxiety and stuttering-like behavior in *nonstutterers* was suggested by an early study by Harris Hill (1954). Subjects were trained to produce a sentence describing a picture when a red light came on. After several trials, they were then given an electric shock while speaking the sentence. Subsequently, no shock was given during sentence production, but the red light was assumed to be associated with electric shock. When speaking under the anticipation of shock, subjects produced "compulsive and preservative" repetitions, prolongations, and blocks. Electromyographic sensors detected increased muscle tension during these responses. Hill reported that many responses appeared to be "indistinguishable from what is generally termed stuttering. [Moreover, the responses of several subjects] would have been classed as severe in any speech clinic" (p. 8). Thus, it appears that even nonstutterers will show stuttering-like behaviors under threat of penalty, and some nonstutterers show severe instances of this. This study demonstrates that emotion (probably negative arousal, in this case) can cause disfluencies.

Using Bosshardt's (2006) model for the effect of increasingly complex linguistic tasks on fluency, we might suppose that if those who stutter have, as described above, speech and language planning and production systems that are less protected from interference by other brain activities, emotion can be one of those other brain activities that can interfere with the smooth flow of speech. Hill's finding that physical tension increases under threat of negative consequences (electric shock) would lead one to suspect that tension in stuttering also results from the threat of negative consequences. In the case of stuttering, however, those consequences may be the frustration, embarrassment, and shame that often arise when one can't perform the simple act of saying a word. It may be significant that in Hill's experiment, a subgroup of some subjects were much more severe than others. Perhaps this reflects individual differences in the vulnerability of the speech production system to interference. I will return to this point when I discuss temperament in the next section.

Another early study of anxiety and stuttering is of interest because of what it might tell us about emotion, speech physiology, and stuttering. Horovitz, Johnson, Pearlman, Schaffer, and Hedin (1978) looked at a phenomenon called the stapedial reflex, which had been previously shown to increase during anxiety in normal speakers. The stapedial reflex is muscle contraction in the middle ear, triggered by activation of the laryngeal nerve just prior to speaking, decreasing the loudness with which a speaker hears her own voice. The researchers found that stutterers demonstrated an increased stapedial reflex when they became more anxious (as measured by a physiological assessment of anxiety), compared to a no-anxiety condition. A group of matched nonstutterers showed no increase in stapedial reflex when their anxiety increased. Participants in both groups increased their anxiety by imagining themselves in stressful speaking situations. Although the results of this study are hard to interpret, it appears to show that an increase in anxiety in stutterers may result in changes in speech-related physiology even when only imagining some difficulty speaking. It may be relevant that the increase in stapedial reflex may have been brought about by an increase in laryngeal nerve activity. This connection between autonomic arousal and heightened laryngeal muscle activity may reflect a conditioned response that becomes part of the learning, which maintains stuttering in some individuals. I will revisit this connection between laryngeal tension and autonomic arousal when I discuss temperament and stuttering.

More recently, researchers have asked whether people who stutter are more anxious than people who don't. To answer this question, they have used various measures of physiological arousal, such as heart rate, skin conductance, and level of cortisol (a chemical secreted by the brain under conditions of stress) in saliva secretion. Four studies (Caruso, Chodzko-Zajko, Bidinger, & Sommers, 1994; Miller, 1993; Peters & Hulstijn, 1984; Weber & Smith, 1990) found that both stutterers and nonstutterers showed high levels of autonomic arousal when they had to speak or read aloud, indicating that people who stutter are not more anxious or more nervous than people who don't. However, several studies of autonomic arousal in individuals who stutter have reported that higher levels of arousal are associated with more stuttering (Caruso, Chodzko-Zajko, & McClowry, 1995; Miller, 1993; Weber & Smith, 1990). Although most speakers may show increased arousal when they have to speak, it may be that only the speech of those who stutter is vulnerable to breakdown (unless arousal is unusually high, as in the Hill's 1954 experiment).

Temperament

In a questionnaire study, Oyler (1992) found that adults who stutter were more emotionally sensitive than were adults who don't stutter; however, this hypersensitivity could be the result of many years of stuttering. Greater sensitivity in children who stutter has been reported by several studies. Fowlie and Cooper (1978) reported that mothers of children who stutter viewed them as more sensitive than did mothers describing children who do not stutter. Oyler and Ramig (1995) found that parents of children who stutter rated them as more sensitive than did control parents rating nonstuttering children.

Using the concept of "difficult" temperament, which includes some aspects of sensitivity as well as restlessness and impulsiveness, both Wakaba (1998) and Embrechts and Ebben (1999) found that parents of stuttering children rated their children as having this type of temperament to a greater degree than did parents of nonstuttering children.

LaSalle (1999) presented a paper indicating that, in contrast to parents of young children who don't stutter, parents of young children who do stutter rated their children as having high frustration reactions and lack of persistence. Both of these traits have been associated with sensitive temperament (Thomas & Chess, 1977). Anderson, Pellowski, Conture, and Kelly (2003), using the Behavioral Style Questionnaire (McDevitt & Carey, 1978) found that parents of children who stutter rated their children as slower to adapt novelty compared with how parents of nonstuttering children rated their children. They related this to Kagan's (1989, 1994) description of this personality trait as also being more shy and fearful when encountering unfamiliar events and people. More evidence of children who stutter having a more reactive temperament comes from an important study by Karrass, Walden, Conture, Graham, Arnold, and colleagues (2006). Their findings, using a scale of children's reactions to everyday stressful situations completed by parents, suggested that when compared to nonstuttering children, children who stutter are more emotionally reactive and are less able to regulate their emotional responses. The authors speculated that these traits may make it more likely that children who stutter will react emotionally to their disfluencies, producing more disfluencies in a cycle of reactivity and increasing stuttering, which the authors call "reverberant interaction." It should be remembered that emotional reactivity may increase laryngeal tension (e.g., Kagan, Reznick, & Snidman, 1987) and perhaps tension in other parts of the speech system, not only increasing stuttering, but making it more severe as well.

Some researchers (e.g., Kagan, 1994a, 1994b) have advocated for physiological or behavioral studies, rather than parent rating of children's temperament. In this spirit, using a physiological measure of sensitivity, Guitar (2003) found that the acoustic startle responses of adults who stutter were significantly greater than those of adults who do not. The startle paradigm, which measures the magnitude of the eye blink in response to a burst of white noise, is believed to differentiate individuals whose nervous systems have low thresholds of arousal from those whose nervous systems require larger stimuli to react (Vrana, Spence, & Lang, 1988). Moreover, it has demonstrated differences in children who have been categorized as temperamentally inhibited and temperamentally uninhibited (Snidman & Kagan, 1994). Guitar (2003) also found substantial correlations between startle responses and scores on the nervous subscale of the Taylor-Johnson Temperament Analysis (Taylor & Morrison, 1996).

It should be noted that two later studies, Alm and Risberg (2007) and Ellis, Finan, and Ramig (2008), failed to replicate Guitar's (2003) findings. This suggests that a sensitive temperament may not be a characteristic of all adults who stutter, and it is certainly not a trait limited to those who stutter. To the extent it is a component of stuttering for many individuals, it probably interacts with a basic predisposition for difficulty with speech motor control.

To close out this review of emotional temperament in stuttering, I would like to call attention to a recent theoretical paper that touches on this topic. Walden, Frankel, Buhr, Johnson, and Conture (2012) make a strong case for the relevance of emotional factors in at least some children who stutter. They argue that stuttering may emerge as the result of two possible predispositions (a) emotional vulnerability and/or (b) limitations on rapid speech-language processing. Stuttering's initial appearance and its day-to-day and moment-to-moment variability are a result of particular stressors or triggers for each of these predispositions. Triggers for the emotional predisposition involve environmental factors such as unexpected changes in the child's day-to-day life or events that cause strong positive or negative emotion. The researchers support their position with a wide array of studies, many of which they have carried out, that demonstrate the existence of both predispositions and the effect on a child's fluency of environmental stressors on each. Further evidence of the importance of environmental factors will be provided in Chapters 4 and 5.

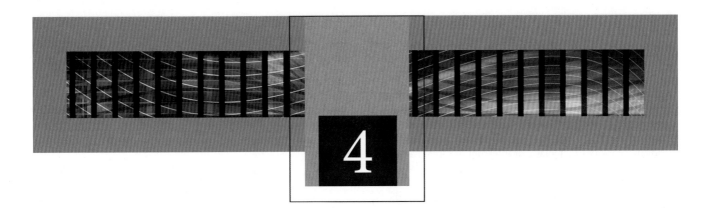

Developmental, Environmental, and Learning Factors in Stuttering

CHAPTER OBJECTIVES

After studying this chapter, readers should be able to:

- Describe the analogy made between a computer with limited resources and a child learning to speak fluently
- Explain how factors related to physical development can interfere with fluent speech
- Explain how factors related to speech and language development can interfere with fluent speech
- Explain how factors related to cognitive development can interfere with fluent speech
- Explain how factors related to social-emotional development can interfere with fluent speech
- Describe the evidence for the role of parents, the speech-language environment, and life events in the onset and development of stuttering
- Describe how classical, operant, and avoidance learning may play a role in the development of stuttering
- Describe the role of learning new behaviors and unlearning old ones in the treatment of stuttering

KEY TERMS

Competition for neural resources: The concept that the brain has a limited amount of resources that can be applied to tasks such as learning to speak and learning to walk. If some task requires a great deal of attention or uses a great deal of neural activity, other tasks performed at the same time will have fewer resources and may thus be less well performed

Speech and language environment: The communication style that characterizes people in a child's environment—usually his home. For example, some parents, siblings, and other relatives of a child may speak very rapidly, use advanced forms or language, or interrupt the child frequently. These aspects of the speech and language environment are thought to stress the child

Life events: Happenings in a child's life that may stress the child, such as parents' divorce or being hospitalized

Classical conditioning: Repeated pairing of a neutral stimulus (such as a person) with a stimulus (a humiliating long stutter) that elicits a response (such as fear), so that the neutral stimulus eventually elicits the response. This process explains the spread of stuttering to more and more situations and words. Stuttering treatment can break this link with procedures like "desensitization," which pairs the old behavior that elicited fear (e.g., a long stutter) with a different response (e.g., the clinician's positive interest in the client's long stutter)

Operant conditioning: Following a behavior with a reward or punishment so that the behavior becomes more frequent (if rewarded) or less frequent (if punished). Operant conditioning explains why stuttering behaviors become more and more abnormal as the child stutters more. But operant conditioning can be a powerful treatment tool as well

Avoidance conditioning: This type of learning occurs when a person uses a behavior to try to prevent an unpleasant occurrence by doing something; it is perpetuated by the successful prevention of the unpleasant experience, at least some of the time. In stuttering, avoidance conditioning may begin when a person first escapes from a stutter by saying an extra sound or word (like "uh"). Then he may make that sound even before saying the feared word, like "uh, can I have some pizza?"

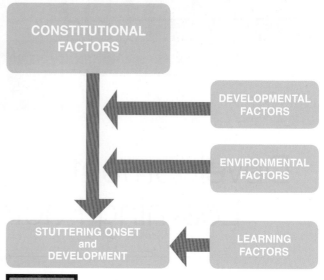

Figure 4.1   Predisposing constitutional factors interact with developmental, environmental, and learning factors to precipitate or worsen stuttering.

Many factors, both in children themselves and in their outside environments, create the conditions under which stuttering first emerges and then either disappears or grows worse. Some of these factors are part of the child's normal development, such as the explosive growth of speech and language skills during preschool years. Other factors may be common environmental situations that most children take in stride as they grow up, such as competing with siblings for attention and speaking time in a busy home. These developmental and environmental influences are not the cause of stuttering by themselves. Rather, they have their effects by interacting with the sensory-motor, language, and emotional factors discussed in Chapters 2 and 3 to precipitate stuttering sometime between the child's acquisition of short phrases and puberty. Figure 4.1 depicts the influence of developmental and environmental factors (as well as learning) on the onset and development of stuttering.

The interaction of sensory-motor, language, and emotional factors with a child's development and environment is ongoing, day by day. Such factors may have a gradual, cumulative

effect, just like the forces of weather have on the surface of the earth. For many children, there is not a sudden landslide of stuttering, but a more gradual erosion of fluency. For others, stuttering appears out of a clear blue sky, then diminishes and may or may not reappear. Conditions at the onset of stuttering are typically not dramatic; the child is usually not under great pressure, nor has he just experienced a traumatic event. In my experience, stuttering often starts during ordinary stress—one or both parents away on a trip, relatives visiting for a holiday, a new baby in the house, or even no stress at all. The ordinariness of situations when stuttering first appears is reflected in this observation by Van Riper (1973, p. 81):

> In the great majority of children we have carefully studied soon after onset, we were unable to state with any certainty … what precipitated the stuttering. In most instances there simply were no apparent conflicts, no illnesses, no opportunity to imitate, no shocks or frightening experiences. Stuttering seemed to begin under quite normal conditions of living and communicating.

Because children's lives are often so normal when stuttering first emerges, research to determine critical developmental and environmental factors affecting its onset and progression has not produced notable results. This is a domain of educated guesses and tentative conclusions. Evidence for developmental factors is inferred from the fact that almost all onsets of stuttering occur when children are developing most rapidly during their preschool years (Andrews et al., 1983; Wingate, 1983). Evidence of environmental influences comes in part from clinical reports of particular stresses sometimes associated with the onset of stuttering and its remission when these stresses are lessened (e.g., Van Riper, 1973,

1982). Environmental factors are also implicated by higher incidences of stuttering in those cultures that are more competitive, with high standards and less tolerance of differences (Bloodstein & Ratner, 2008). Finally, some sources of evidence for genetic factors in stuttering are also evidence for environmental factors. These studies show that genes alone cannot account for the occurrence of stuttering in all children but rather some other factors—probably environmental—must also be responsible (e.g., Andrews, Morris-Yates, Howie, & Martin, 1991). However, this research has not been able to identify which environmental factors might be involved. The paucity of objective data tying specific developmental and environmental factors to stuttering will make this chapter more speculative than the last. Wherever I can, however, I will try to support speculations with facts.

In addition to developmental and environmental factors that may precipitate stuttering, there are influences that act upon stuttering once it begins. These are various types of learning—classical, operant, and avoidance conditioning. Learning, of course, affects all of our behaviors throughout our lifetime, and it may cause a child who initially stuttered only when he was excited, tired, or stressed to eventually stutter in ordinary circumstances, day after day. Learning can escalate mild, repetitive stuttering to severe blocking with a complex pattern of extra sounds, substituted words, and avoidance of speaking situations. Understanding the principles of learning will help you understand what may have created the individual stuttering patterns of clients. More importantly, this knowledge will guide treatment procedures as you help your clients acquire more effective communication behaviors and skills.

In this chapter, I have divided developmental, environmental, and learning factors into separate sections, although they do not operate independently; their actions are influenced by each other and by sensory-motor, language, and emotional factors, such as those described in Chapters 2 and 3. A developmental variable, such as cognitive level, may determine at what age avoidance conditioning may occur. An environmental variable, such as the stress of moving to a new neighborhood, may have different effects on different children, depending on such factors as a child's sensitivity, physical development of speech production, and language maturation. It's also critical to keep in mind when evaluating and treating clients that every client is an individual whose stuttering has evolved from unique contributions of developmental, environmental, learning, and constitutional factors.

DEVELOPMENTAL FACTORS

Our view of how developmental factors affect children's fluency assumes that there is in the growing child a **competition for neural resources**; that is, the brain must share its resources in coping with many demands. Like a computer, the brain can work on several things at once, but the more tasks it performs simultaneously, the more slowly and less efficiently it does each one. Unlike a computer, if the tasks are dissimilar, such as driving a car and talking about the weather, there is less interference between them. On the other hand, if the tasks are similar, such as rubbing your stomach while patting your head, there is more interference between them (Kinsbourne & Hicks, 1978). The problem of shared resources is more acute in children because their immature nervous systems have less processing capacity to share (Hiscock & Kinsbourne, 1977, 1980). Some children are especially at risk for straining their developing resources. Their speech and language skills may be delayed, yet they have to compete in a highly verbal environment. Or, their language development may surge ahead of their speech motor control skills, giving them much to say, but limited capacity to say it at a rapid rate, as though they were trying to push a crowd of people through a small door in a hurry. Such children may become excessively disfluent as other developmental demands outpace their abilities to coordinate the complex movements of rapid, articulate speech.

Here is an example of this competition between burgeoning language and slower motor abilities. Several years ago, I evaluated a 4-year-old girl whose uncle and grandmother stuttered. Her parents were concerned because she had been repeating words and sounds excessively for a year and a half, sometimes up to 20 times per instance. However, her language development was well above average; she began to talk with single words at 9 months and to produce sentences intelligibly at 12 months. In contrast, her motor development was somewhat slower; she had not walked until 18 months. I think it is possible that her disfluencies emerged as a result of a high proportion of her cerebral resources being used to formulate and express language with less mature capacities for motor activities, including fluent speech. In other words, a disparity between language facility and motor speech ability may have been an important contributor to the emergence of stuttering.

To appreciate how many skills and abilities the child is developing at the same time, look carefully at Figure 4.2. This chart covers only social, motor, and language domains, but it is clear that children have to master many different abilities simultaneously. If a child's development is slower in one or more areas, her road to maturity may be steep and difficult at times. So, let us look at some of the domains of development and how they might contribute to the onset of stuttering.

Physical and Motor Skill Development

The mother of a 3-year-old child who recently began to stutter told me "Whenever he has a spurt of growth, his stuttering seems to increase." Why would this be? Between ages 1 and 6 years, children grow by leaps and bounds. Their bodies get bigger. Their nervous systems form new pathways and new connections. Their perceptual and motor

	SOCIAL	SELF-HELP	GROSS MOTOR	FINE MOTOR	LANGUAGE	
5-0 yr.	Shows leadership among children	Goes to the toilet without help	Swings on swing, pumping by self	Prints first name (four letters)	Tells meaning of familiar words	**5-0** yr.
4-6	Follows simple rules in board games or card games	Usually looks both ways before crossing street	Skips or makes running "broad jumps"	Draws a person showing at least three parts–head, eyes, nose, mouth, etc.	Reads a few letters (five+)	**4-6**
		Buttons one or more buttons	Hops around on one foot without support	Draws recognizable pictures	Follows a series of three simple instructions	
4-0 yr.	Protective toward younger children	Dresses and undresses without help, except for tying shoelaces			Understands concepts – size, number, shape	**4-0** yr.
3-6	Plays cooperatively, with minimum conflict and supervision	Washes face without help	Hops on one foot without support	Cuts across paper with small scissors	Counts five or more objects when asked "how many?"	**3-6**
				Draws or copies a complete circle	Identifies four colors correctly	
	Gives directions to other children	Toilet trained	Rides around on a tricycle, using pedals		Combines sentences with the words "and," "or," or "but"	
3-0 yr.	Plays a role in "pretend" games–mom, dad, teacher, space pilot	Dresses self with help	Walks up and down stairs–one foot per step	Cuts with small scissors	Understands four prepositions–in, on, under, beside	**3-0** yr.
2-6	Plays with other children –cars, dolls, building	Washes and dries hands	Stands on one foot without support	Draws or copies vertical lines	Talks clearly, is understandable most of the time	**2-6**
	"Helps" with simple household tasks	Opens door by turning knob	Climbs on play equipment–ladders, slides	Scribbles with circular motion	Talks in two- to three-word phrases or sentences	
2-0 yr.	Usually responds to correction–stops	Takes off open coat or shirt without help	Walks up and down stairs alone	Turns pages of picture books, one at a time	Follows two-part instructions	**2-0** yr.
	Shows sympathy to other children, tries to comfort them	Eats with spoon, spilling little	Runs well, seldom falls		Uses at least 10 words	
	Sometimes says "no" when interfered with	Eats with fork	Kicks a ball forward	Builds towers of four or more blocks	Follows simple instructions	
18 mo.	Greets people with "hi" or similar	Insists on doing things by self, such as feeding	Runs	Scribbles with crayon	Asks for food or drink with words	**18** mo.
	Gives kisses or hugs	Feeds self with spoon	Walks without help	Picks up two small toys in one hand	Talks in single words	
	Wants stuffed animal, doll, or blanket in bed	Lifts cup to mouth and drinks	Stands without support	Stacks two or more blocks	Uses one or two words as names of things or actions	
12 mo.	Plays patty-cake	Picks up a spoon by the handle	Walks around furniture or crib while holding on	Picks up small objects– precise thumb and finger grasp	Understands works like "no," "stop," or "all gone"	**12** mo.
	Plays social games, peek-a-boo, bye-bye		Crawls around on hands and knees		Word sounds–says "ma-ma" or "da-da"	
9 mo.	Pushes things away he/she doesn't want		Sits alone, steady, without support	Picks up object with thumb and finger grasp	Wide range of vocalizations (vowel sounds, consonant-vowel combinations)	**9** mo.
	Reaches for familiar persons	Feeds self cracker	Rolls over from back to stomach	Transfers toy from one hand to the other	Responds to name–turns and looks	
6 mo.	Distinguishes mother from others	Comforts self with thumb or pacifier	Turns around when lying on stomach	Picks up toy with one hand	Vocalizes spontaneously, social	**6** mo.
	Social smile	Reacts to sight of bottle or breast	Lifts head and chest when lying on stomach	Looks at and reaches for faces and toys	Reacts to voices; vocalizes, coos, chuckles	
Birth						Birth

Figure 4.2   Child development in the first five years. (Courtesy Harold Ireton, Ph.D.)

skills improve with maturation and practice. This intensive period of growth is a two-edged sword for children predisposed to stuttering. Neurological maturation may provide more "functional cerebral space" that supports fluency, but it also spurs development of other motor behaviors that may compete with fluency for available neuronal resources. An example of such competition is the common observation that children learn to walk first or talk first, but not both at the same time. For example, Netsell (1981, p. 25) said of this trade-off, "The practice of walking *or* talking seems sufficient to 'tie up' all the available sensorimotor circuitry because the toddler seldom, if ever, undertakes both activities at once." Likewise, Berk in his text on child development (1991, p. 194) suggested that "when infants forge ahead in spoken language, they seem to temporarily postpone mastery of new motor skills or vice versa." Studies are needed to explore the specific effects on speech and language of mastering other skills. In Chapter 6, on theoretical perspectives on stuttering, I will introduce the "capacities and demands" view of stuttering, which may be a useful framework for understanding the competition for resources that I have been discussing.

The learning of motor control of speech by itself, even without acquisition of other motor skills at the same time, puts enormous demands on the child's brain. Think about how difficult it must be to learn how to move the tongue, lips, and jaw to produce a desired sound when the relative size of these articulators is changing every day. Think about how the use of speech must draw on language resources as well. As Kent and Vorperian (2007, p. 73) remind us, "Speech development in children draws on a number of anatomical, motor, sensory, and cognitive resources. Ultimately, these various factors need to be integrated to account for a child's progress toward the faculty of speech." The integration of these factors may be a particular challenge for some children. Details about this process and evidence that individuals who stutter may be at a disadvantage are presented Chapter 5.

Before leaving the topic of motor skill learning, I would like to mention that another challenge to some children who stutter may be a delay in motor development. A review of studies of motor coordination in people who stutter can be found in Bloodstein and Ratner (2008). They cite several studies that have found children who stutter to be somewhat delayed as a group compared to nonstuttering children, but suggest it is not a clear-cut issue. I suspect that a significant delay in development of fine motor speech skills in a child with a strong urge to communicate and rapidly developing language abilities may set the stage for more serious disfluency. Such a delay may account for reduced speech intelligibility in some children, disfluency in others, and both problems in still other children. Given the evidence that boys are slower than girls in neuromotor development (Smith & Zelaznik, 2004), I suspect that boys are more at risk for the combination of reduced intelligibility and stuttering.

Speech and Language Development

The Onset of Stuttering

Although I discussed the interaction of speech-language development and the onset of stuttering in Chapters 2 and 3, it's worth revisiting this topic in the context of overall development. Most stuttering begins between ages 2 and 4, a time when children acquire new sounds and learn new words almost by the hour (Bloodstein & Ratner, 2008). Yairi and Ambrose (2005) point out that many authors suggest that when stuttering begins before age 3, its onset coincides with "qualitative and quantitative advancements in the child's articulation, phonology, morphology, and syntax" (p. 47). As with other developmental factors, we don't believe that the demands of speech and language development *cause* stuttering, but that for many children, these demands may be a precipitating factor.

What is happening to precipitate stuttering during this speech and language growth spurt? You will remember from Chapters 2 and 3 that brain imaging studies of adults who stutter have shown some unexpected patterns of activity during speech. For example, there are abnormally high levels of activity in some regions of the right hemisphere and abnormally low levels in some areas of the left. In addition, recent findings with children who stutter suggest that areas of the brain used for integration of articulator planning, sensory feedback, and motor execution are compromised (e.g., Chang, Erickson, Ambrose, Hasegawa-Johnson, & Ludlow, 2008). Thus, planning and production of speech and language may use atypical neural pathways that may be slow or inefficient. But the demands grow ever greater as a child produces longer, faster, and more complex sentences. Tasks using different neural networks for segment selection, grammatical formulation, and prosodic planning must be orchestrated precisely so that each element is in place at the proper time as utterances are produced. If some components are ready but others are delayed, initial sounds or syllables may be repeated, prolonged, or even blocked, waiting for the whole sentence to be put together in the brain. A child's reaction to this speech traffic jam may determine whether maladaptive learning occurs, or instead such moments soon disappear as the child develops compensatory strategies to pave the way to normal speech. We'll look more at these reactions later.

Delayed and Deviant Speech and Language Development

Because it is thought that stuttering arises from constitutional differences (e.g., inheritance or congenital injury) in some children, it is natural to wonder if other speech and language abilities besides fluency are affected. It is also important to understand how delays in speech and language development might be related to the appearance of stuttering or disfluency. In general, research has found that speech and language delays or difficulties are more common among children who stutter than those who don't, but the findings are neither simple nor clear-cut, and their implications are unclear.

More evidence of a possible relationship between language delays and stuttering is given in Chapter 5. Briefly, there are several possible relationships that can be hypothesized. One suggestion is that delays in language development may be related to stuttering because children with delayed language may become frustrated at their difficulty speaking, develop fears related to speaking, and thus learn to stutter as an anticipatory avoidance response (Bloodstein & Ratner, 2008). An example would be a child who has a gap between vocabulary development and growth of syntactic skills. This child may have the language form ready but unable to fill it with verbal content, making repetitions and even blocks possible as he tries to go ahead with speaking but is unable to. This may also happen to children who are not delayed, but advanced in one language component and typically developing in another.

Cognitive Development

I use the phrase "cognitive development" to refer to the growth of perception, attention, working memory, and executive functions that play roles in spoken language but are separate from it.

There may be two ways in which cognitive development affects stuttering. First, spurts in cognitive development may accompany the onset of stuttering as well as sudden increases in stuttering. Second, as a child who stutters develops more advanced cognitive abilities, he is more likely to become aware and even self-conscious of his stuttering.

Cognitive Development and the Onset and Fluctuation of Stuttering

Parents frequently report that the onset of their child's stuttering occurred under the most normal of circumstances—no extra stresses in the household and no apparent increases in the child's anxiety. The same "normal circumstances" are also frequently true for sudden changes in the ongoing stuttering of a preschool child—suddenly his stuttering is worse, and just as suddenly, it's better. One factor that may not be obvious to the parent but nonetheless may be an influence on stuttering is the child's cognitive growth. Earlier in this chapter, I suggested that aspects of physical development may affect stuttering; for example, learning to walk may make great demands on sensory-motor abilities, making fewer resources available for fluency. Now I am proposing that learning to think may make great demands on cognitive-linguistic abilities, leaving fewer resources available for rapid production of fluently spoken language.

This argument has been made before. Lindsay (1989) pointed out that during Jean Piaget's "preoperational period" of childhood development from 2 to 6 years, a child goes through a series of transitions in which new cognitive learning must be assimilated and consolidated with current knowledge. These transitions are times when a child's linguistic and cognitive systems are temporarily unstable before new concepts are mastered. As a consequence, children's speech and language production during this period of adjustment may be vulnerable to disfluencies.

A number of authors have made other arguments that support a connection between cognition and stuttering, including the high frequency of disfluencies in children with developmental delays and traumatic brain injuries. These studies are summarized in Chapter 5.

Cognitive Development and Reactions to Stuttering

In the preceding section, I have suggested that children's cognitive development may influence the onset of stuttering through competition for resources in the child's brain. Now, I would like to argue that the role of cognitive development is also important in explaining how and when a child begins to form negative attitudes and beliefs about herself and her speech. Between ages 3 and 4, children's cognitions mature enough so that they internalize the standards of behavior of those around them, including peers (Fagan, 2000). It is only at this point, according to Lewis (2000), that all children can evaluate how they are performing in comparison to others and will experience the "self-conscious" emotions of embarrassment, pride, shame, and guilt.

In regard to stuttering, once children who stutter compare their speech with others, they are likely to conclude that they are doing something wrong. Because some of the conclusions that children who stutter draw about their speech may come from other children's reactions to their speech, a study by Ezrati-Vanacour, Platzky, and Yairi (2001) is of importance. These researchers looked at awareness of stuttering in typically developing children and found that some children were aware of stuttering in puppets at age 3, but most were not aware until age 5. Notably, most children at age 4 showed a preference for fluent speech, suggesting a negative evaluation of disfluent speech. Thus, peers of children who stutter may respond negatively to the speech of stuttering children at this age.

Emotions such as embarrassment and shame that arise from the increasing cognitive maturity of children who stutter and their peers may play an important role in the discomfort children feel when they stutter, and thus, it may affect the persistence of the stuttering. The embarrassment and shame some children feel about their stuttering are probably the most important cognitive-emotional factors that give rise to increases in tension, escape, and avoidance responses that make stuttering a self-sustaining disorder and increasingly difficult to overcome. In my experience, most children who recover completely from stuttering with treatment are younger than 5, perhaps a significant age, given the evidence cited above about peer awareness of stuttering.

Social and Emotional Development

Interference With Speech by Emotion

At some time in your life, you have probably experienced the effects of strong emotion on your speech. If you've been nervous when talking in front of an audience, your voice may have quavered or you may have been talking faster than you meant to but couldn't help it. When you get really worked up, like when you have to make a phone call in an emergency, rapid breathing and tension in your larynx can make it difficult to talk. The same sort of interference by emotion may be even more prevalent in early childhood, because a child's speech and language neural networks and structures are immature, not fully myelinated, and may not be buffered from "cross talk," or interference by the limbic (emotional) system structures and pathways involved in the regulation and expression of emotion. Such interference may be even more likely among many children predisposed to stutter. Their slower maturing speech and language functions may not be optimally localized or adequately insulated from interference and may be closer to centers of emotion in the right hemisphere, a hypothesis I discussed in Chapter 2. Thus, when such children are emotionally aroused, fluency may suffer because neural signals for properly timed and sequenced muscle contractions may be interrupted in some way. I see evidence of this when I ask parents when their child first began to stutter. They frequently tell me that they noticed stuttering for the first time when their child was highly excited about something.

Excitement is commonly mentioned in the literature as a stimulus that elicits disfluency. Starkweather (1987) noted that "all children speak more disfluently during periods of excitement." Dorothy Davis (1940), who conducted one of the first studies of normal disfluency, reported that of the 10 situations in which children showed repetitions in their speech, "excitement over own activity" was when they most frequently repeated sounds and words. In a later study, Johnson and associates (1959) asked parents of children identified as stutterers to describe the situation in which they first observed their child's stuttering. They most often reported that the first appearance of stuttering occurred when the child was in a hurry to tell something or was in an excited state. Thus, both stuttering and normal disfluency seem to occur most often or noticeably during states of transitory emotional arousal.

Stages of Social and Emotional Development

Some stages of development may provide more social and emotional stress than others. For example, the processes of separation and individuation are known to be periods of stress. After a child passes his second birthday, he strives harder for autonomy, creating the conflicts of the "terrible twos." Most parents gradually relinquish control, while at the same time helping their child learn the limits of his freedom. In some cases, however, the transition from a dependent infant to an independent preschooler may occur too rapidly for a parent or a child. If the child is pushed toward independence faster than he wants, he may feel frustrated and insecure because his mother seems less nurturing. A mother may become alarmed if she isn't ready for her child's quest for independence and may try to restrain her child. A child may conform to these restraints but feel angry and frustrated. Yet, the child cannot easily express these feelings to someone he depends on so much, and disfluency may result in those interactions in which such emotional ambivalence and conflict affect motor control of speech (Lidz, 1968).

Emotional Security

As a young child grows older, other members of the family besides the mother play a role in social and emotional changes. Although a child's father and siblings comprise a wider support system, a child's resentment at having to share his mother's attention may elicit feelings of anger, aggression, and guilt. It seems possible that if such feelings are punished or ignored, transient disfluency or more severe stuttering may result in some children.

One of the more common provocations for feeling resentment is the birth of a sibling. I discuss the effect of a sibling's birth on fluency later in the section on environmental factors, but it warrants mentioning here too because a child's strong emotions may often reflect his developmental level as well as the environmental event that triggered the emotions. Theodore Lidz (1968, p. 246), a developmental psychiatrist with interests in speech and language, provided this example:

> Psychoanalytically oriented play therapy with children also indicates that many of their forbidden wishes and ideas have relatively simple access to consciousness. A 6-year-old boy who started to stammer severely after a baby sister was born was watched playing with a family of dolls. He placed a baby doll in a crib next to the parent dolls' bed and then had a boy doll come and throw the baby to the floor, beat it, and throw it into a corner. He then put the boy doll into the crib. In a subsequent session, he had the father doll pummel the mother doll's abdomen, saying, "No, no!" At this point of childhood, even though certain unacceptable ideas cannot be talked about, they are still not definitely repressed.

Although we feel, as does Lidz, that stuttering may be triggered by the birth of a sibling, our belief about the underlying cause is not so Freudian. Many threats to feelings of security can create emotional stress that may disrupt the speech of children who are predisposed to stutter. As we will see in the section on treatment, we have found that therapy strategies that increase a child's sense of security and help him learn to speak more fluently will suffice for many children who begin stuttering under these emotional stresses.

Self-Consciousness and Sensitivity

As we noted earlier in the section on cognitive development, the emergence of self-consciousness, which begins during the child's second year, may be another source of social and emotional stress. This reflects the child's growing awareness of how he is performing relative to adult expectations. Although this process is not thoroughly understood, Jerome Kagan presents an interesting description of it in his book, *The Second Year* (1981). In a relevant example, Kagan proposes that the self-corrections a child makes in his speech are evidence of this self-awareness. Taking this further, we can surmise that increasing self-awareness in a child who is excessively disfluent might lead to self-corrections and stoppages that only worsen the problem.

In Chapter 2, we briefly discussed the hypothesis that people who stutter, as a group, may have unusually sensitive temperaments. Research on temperament in nonstuttering children, especially the longitudinal studies of Calkins and Fox (1994) and Kagan and Snidman (1991), indicates that the social-emotional traits of fearfulness and withdrawal that accompany more sensitive temperaments can change over the course of a child's preschool years. Some children become better able to modulate their temperamental tendencies, but others remain hostages to their temperaments. Such individual adaptations may be crucial in determining which children who begin to stutter will continue to do so and which will stop.

Recent reports on sensitive temperament have included the positive as well as negative aspects of this personality type. In an overview article, Ellis and Boyce (2008) suggest that a reactive temperament in a child may produce very different outcomes, depending on whether a child encounters a stressful environment or a nurturing one. For example, Boyce, Chesney, Alkon-Leonard, Tschann, Adams, and colleagues (1995) found that, compared to relatively unreactive children, sensitive children in stressful environments had more respiratory illnesses than typical children, whereas sensitive children in nurturing environments had fewer. In other words, a sensitive temperament can give a child protection against illness if the environment is favorable. What are the implications for stuttering? Future research may show that sensitive children with family histories of stuttering who experience stressful childhoods develop persistent stuttering. But those with the same background who grow up in highly supportive environments recover from any stuttering they have in early preschool years. And those with family histories of stuttering but an unreactive temperament may have a mix of persistence and recovery. This view of children who stutter who also have sensitive temperaments suggests that treatments may be most effective if they can help parents create maximally supportive, nurturing environments.

Before leaving this section, I want to comment on stutterers' psychological adjustments in general. Many people who have little exposure to stuttering believe that stutterers are essentially nervous people or that stuttering is a sign of neurosis. If this were true, we should have found evidence of psychological maladjustment or excessive anxiety in people who stutter, particularly when stuttering first begins in childhood. However, research on the personalities and adjustments of people who stutter has found no convincing evidence that they differ from nonstutterers in these ways (Bloch & Goodstein, 1971; Bloodstein & Ratner, 2008; Van Riper, 1982). A few findings suggest that adults who stutter may not be as socially well adjusted as those who do not, but this may reflect the influence of stuttering on social experiences (Bloodstein, 1987; Bloodstein & Ratner, 2008).

Summarizing the effect of social and emotional development on fluency, I have suggested that many of the normal social and emotional stresses that children experience may result in disfluent speech, although the evidence is mostly anecdotal. Moreover, we suspect that children who are neurophysiologically vulnerable to stuttering may be especially prone to difficulty when social conflicts and emotions create extra "noise" in their neural circuitry for speech. This would be particularly true for those children who are both predisposed to stuttering and who have emotionally reactive temperaments. In general, however, children who stutter appear to be as psychologically well adjusted as those who do not stutter, despite the extreme emotional stress that stuttering itself can impose.

ENVIRONMENTAL FACTORS

Some children who have predispositions for stuttering may show initial signs of stuttering in response to developmental pressures alone, but most who become stutterers are probably affected by environmental pressures as well. Such pressures typically result from attitudes, behaviors, or events that occur in their homes. One example is a family's anxiety about the child's speech, which may be readily apparent in the facial expressions of parents and siblings when the child is disfluent. Another pressure may be the conversational style in the child's home that is distinguished by lots of interruptions as well as rapid, complex speech that is beyond the child's level. There are many things in a child's environment—some subtle and some not so subtle—that can add enough stress to a child with a predisposition to stutter to trigger the onset and promote the growth of stuttering.

When I described the effects of developmental factors on a child's speech, I used the analogy of a computer that is overloaded by too many simultaneous tasks. The computer analogy is also appropriate to depict environmental factors, but now you need to imagine that a computer being used for programs that exceed its capacities is also being subjected to periodic power surges or external commands that its programs cannot process. It is easy to imagine that similar circumstances would likely create fluency breakdowns in a vulnerable child. These kinds of environmental pressures can also worsen the symptoms of stuttering, as I describe in Chapter 5. I will begin this discussion of environmental factors by reviewing research on the most important factor in family environments, the parents.

Parents

Much of the early research on parents of children who stutter was done in the 1950s at the University of Iowa. These studies suggested that parents of children who stutter are more critical and perfectionistic. This perspective shaped the public's view of stuttering for many generations and still has some influence. For example, parents of the children I work with sometimes tell me in our first meeting that they think they may have caused their child's stuttering by being too demanding of him when he first started to speak.

Valid criticisms of this early research point out that these studies didn't use control groups of parents of children with other disorders; thus, we can't dismiss the possibility that rather than causing stuttering, these differences in parenting may be the result of stuttering. This possibility is all the more likely given that these parents were interviewed more than a year after the onset of their child's stuttering. Perhaps any parent of a child with a disorder would appear to have high standards for him. Another objection to the claim that parents of children who stutter caused the stuttering by their perfectionism is that their brothers and sisters would have stuttered also, but this appears not to have been the case.

More recent studies of parents of stutterers and parents of nonstutterers—reviewed in Chapter 5—produced mixed results. Some indicate that parents of stutterers are more anxious or more rejecting, while others find no differences. On balance, it seems likely that some children who stutter grew up with parents who were a little more demanding or anxious than average, and this may have made a difference. Assuming they already had a constitutional predisposition to stutter, their early speech may have been peppered with disfluencies, which would have alarmed their parents. The children then, picking up their parents' dismay, may have become self-conscious about their minor disfluencies and thus have unwittingly added tension and struggle, which blossomed into more noticeable stuttering.

It is interesting to speculate that in some cases a child's hypersensitivity to parents' concern and their increased tension as a response to their disfluencies is a component of an overall vulnerable temperament found in some children who stutter (Anderson, Pellowski, Conture, & Kelly, 2003; Karrass et al., 2006; Oyler & Ramig, 1995), which may be inherited. Their parents, the genetic source of these temperaments, may be the anxious, overprotective mothers or fathers that have been described in the literature on parents of stutterers. Such children are, therefore, in double jeopardy for persistent stuttering because of their own temperaments and because one or both parents are overly concerned about their children's stuttering because of *their* own temperaments. On the other hand, some parents may have an ameliorating effect on a child's vulnerable temperament, making it possible for a child who begins to stutter and who is emotionally reactive to recover from stuttering. In a discussion of environmental influences on biological predispositions of children who do not stutter, Calkins and Fox (1994, p. 209) said that "the child's interactions with a parent provide the context for learning skills and strategies for managing emotional reactivity."

Once again we see that influences on stuttering are numerous and complex, coming from both the child and the environment. Some of these influences may precipitate stuttering, others may interact to make remission difficult, and still others may provide the kinds of support that make remission possible.

Speech and Language Environment

Because every preschool-age child is tuned into the speech and language around him, especially that of his parents, the communication style surrounding him may be an important influence on the child who stutters. Writers have hypothesized that as a child tries to emulate adult models of speech and language, to use longer words and longer sentences, to try less familiar words, and to pack more meaning into his utterances, he will be more likely to stutter. Van Riper (1973) expressed it this way: "Stuttering usually begins at the very time that great advances in sentence construction occur, and it seems tenable that, when the speech models provided by the parents or siblings of the child are too difficult for him to follow, some faltering will ensue" (p. 381). Later, in the same volume, Van Riper goes on to cite nine references in which clinicians point to parental speech models as a major source of stress on a child's fluency (pp. 380–383). This stress includes not only the parents' speech and language but also the conditions under which the child tries to speak.

Following in Van Riper's footsteps, many other clinicians have speculated that speech and language environments are a potential source of stress for children who stutter (e.g., Gottwald, 2010; Richels & Conture, 2007; Shapiro, 1999; Starkweather, Gottwald, & Halfond, 1990; Zebrowski & Kelly, 2002). Table 4.1 lists a variety of sources of possible communicative stress.

Table 4.1	Possible Speech and Language Stresses
Stressful Adult Speech Models	
Rapid speech rate	Complex syntax
Polysyllabic vocabulary	Use of two languages in home
Stressful Speaking Situations for Children	
Competition for speaking	Hurried when speaking
Frequent interruptions	Frequent questions
Demand for display speech	Excited when speaking
Loss of listener attention	Many things to say

Two writers have moved beyond clinical speculation to develop informal theories about the influence of adult models on a child's fluency. Crystal (1987) proposed an "interactive" view of many speech and language disorders, which suggested that demands at one level of language production (e.g., syntax) may deplete resources for other levels (e.g., prosody or phonology) and result in breakdown. His supporting data nicely illustrate how stuttering may be exacerbated by a child's use of advanced language. He presented evidence that the more complex the syntax and semantics that a child used, the more he stuttered. Starkweather (1987), describing a demands-and-capacities view of stuttering, commented that "the production of speech and the formulation of language place a simultaneous demand on the young person. If the demands in either of these two dimensions are excessive, performance in the other dimension may be reduced." These two views imply that stuttering may increase when an individual uses longer words, less frequently occurring words, more information-bearing words, and longer sentences. Stuttering may also increase when the individual is uttering a more linguistically complex sentence. By implication, the child's **speech and language environment**—usually conversation by adults talking to the child—may be responsible for influencing a child to use more advanced language.

What do we know about the speech and language of parents of children who stutter? Research on this topic is summarized in the appendix, and all citations are given there. It is important to note that not all of the conclusions given below are supported by every study, but there are some generalizations we can make about four aspects of parents' speech that are thought to increase stuttering: speech rate, frequency of interruptions, frequency of questions, and complexity of language. Specifically, (1) speech rates of parents of children who stutter may be faster, and this may be more reliably so for parents of children who are severe stutterers. (2) Mothers of stutterers and even mothers of nonstutterers who interacted with children who stuttered interrupted the stuttering children more frequently when these children were stuttering than when they were fluent; additionally, the durations of the mothers' interruptions may be related to the severity of the child's stuttering. (3) Parents of children who stutter may ask about the same number of questions as parents of nonstuttering children, but when children give longer answers to questions, they stutter more. (4) For children who began to stutter, the more complex the mothers' language, the less likely the children are to recover naturally.

What are the clinical implications of this view? Even the most cautious researchers examining the parent-child interactions of stuttering children are hopeful about the possible therapeutic value of changing some parents' verbal behaviors. They advocate clinical research on the therapeutic effects of reducing parents' speech rates (Nippold & Rudzinski, 1995), changing their language patterns (Miles & Ratner, 2001), or

even combining these approaches with direct treatment of children's fluency.

Life Events

Certain **life events** can deliver a blow to a child's stability and security. When this happens, stuttering may suddenly appear out of nowhere, or previously easy repetitions may be transformed into hard, struggled blocks. To have someone close to you die, to be hospitalized for an operation, or to have parents divorce is difficult for any of us, but it is especially difficult for children. Obviously, many children go through such events and adapt to them without apparent major problems. But children who are predisposed to stuttering often show the effects of such events in their speech. Kagan (1994a) noted that some children who begin life with relaxed temperaments may even become shy and fearful under the onslaught of stressful events. This may well set the stage for stuttering if other constitutional factors predispose the child for it. You may wonder what the mechanism is by which stress can precipitate or worsen stuttering. I don't know the answer, but it seems likely that if a child's brain pathways for speech and language are slightly compromised, extra resources are needed to maintain fluency. When stress increases negative emotions such as anxiety, it seems possible that the negative emotions would consume the extra resources. However, it still leaves us with an incomplete picture. How exactly do extra resources compensate for deficits? How does anxiety consume extra resources?

There is little research on the relationship between stressful life events and stuttering, but many authors have observed the connection. Starkweather (1987), for example, wrote, "All children speak more disfluently during periods of tension—when moving or changing schools, when their parents divorce, or after the death of a family member" (pp. 146–147). These increases in disfluency could easily result in the onset of stuttering or in increased stuttering in children who are vulnerable to such stresses. Johnson and associates (1959) noted that the following events were among the 16 situations in which parents first noticed their child's stuttering: (a) child's physical environment changed (e.g., moving to new house); (b) child became ill; (c) child realized his mother was pregnant; (d) a new baby arrived. In discussing the onset of stuttering, Van Riper (1982) acknowledged that various studies have found no differences in the amount of emotional conflict in the homes of children who developed stuttering versus those who didn't. However, he went on to note, "Nevertheless, we have studied individual cases in which stuttering did seem [to be] triggered by such conflicts, and it is difficult for us to ignore these experiences" (p. 79).

My own clinical experience is similar. In the past several years, for example, during which I've evaluated dozens of children who stutter, I've encountered four children in four different families who began to stutter when their parents were in the early stages of divorce. However, this turmoil was not the only factor in their stuttering. Three of the children had relatives who stuttered, and the father of the fourth child was a stutterer. Moreover, all four were preschoolers and were probably experiencing various growth and development pressures. But for all of them, their parents' divorce appeared to be a factor that pushed them from normal speech to stuttering.

In another case of a life event–precipitating stuttering, I evaluated a 9-year-old girl who began to stutter when her classroom teacher had an emotional breakdown that was apparent in the classroom. The teacher's outbursts of anger and crying, interspersed with high demands for rapid performance on frequent examinations, were apparently extremely stressful for this student. Under this stress she developed tight blocks, with physical tension at the level of the larynx and abdomen. Even though I was convinced through extensive interviews with the family that the child had no prior stuttering, I noted several predisposing factors for stuttering. First, her younger sister had significant learning disabilities, including auditory processing problems. Second, her mother described herself and her daughter who stuttered as shy and emotionally reactive. These two factors—a family history of learning disability and a vulnerable temperament—may have provided a fertile matrix for the sudden germination of stuttering when a stressful life event occurred. Happily, after a year of treatment, this child became fluent.

In a few cases, traumatic life events appear to precipitate stuttering in children as well as in adults who appear to have no predisposition to stuttering. These unusual onsets are discussed in Chapter 15 when we explore "psychogenic stuttering." Such individuals often stutter in unusual ways, which differ from the "garden variety" stuttering of those who begin stuttering when a stressful life event interacts with various predisposing conditions. Table 4.2 lists some of the life events that we have found to be stressful to children's fluency.

Table 4.2	Stressful Life Events That May Increase a Child's Disfluency
1. The child's family moves to a new house, a new neighborhood, or a new city.
2. The child's parents separate or divorce.
3. A family member dies.
4. A family member is hospitalized.
5. The child is hospitalized.
6. A parent loses his or her job.
7. A baby is born, or a child is adopted.
8. An additional person comes to live in the house.
9. One or both parents go away frequently or for a long period of time.
10. Holidays or visits occur, which cause a change in routine, excitement, or anxiety.
11. A discipline problem involving the child.

LEARNING FACTORS

When I was in high school, I stuttered severely. If I had to make a phone call, I dreaded it for hours beforehand. When I finally got up the courage to pick up the phone and dial, an invisible hand seemed to tighten around my throat. When someone answered, all I could get out was a series of "ums" punctuated by the listener's repeated "Hello? Hello? Hello?" Finally I could say "Is Mmmmmm" and there I was, stuck fast, until with a huge head jerk I would blurt out, "Is Molly there?" And the listener would say, typically, "What?"

I had gone downhill a long way since my stuttering began at age 3 with simple repetitions of words like "I-I-I-I..." So, how did this change take place? The answer is learning—the change that takes place in a person or animal as a result of their experiences in the environment (Lefton, 1997). Learning created my more severe stuttering symptoms as I went through elementary school, junior high, and high school. Learning also helped me—with the guidance of a good stuttering therapist—to reduce those symptoms to the mild form of stuttering that I have today. In this section, you will learn more about how learning works, so that you will understand your client's stuttering behaviors and then can help him change them. The different components of my stuttering were created by different types of learning. Specific types of learning are often referred to as different kinds of conditioning. These include **classical conditioning**, **operant conditioning**, and **avoidance conditioning**.

Classical Conditioning

Classical conditioning was first scientifically described by the Russian physiologist, Ivan Pavlov. As with many discoveries, it was serendipitous. Pavlov was actually studying how dogs digested their food, which he did by measuring their saliva when they were fed. One morning he happened to notice that the dogs were salivating even before they were fed, seemingly in response to just seeing him walk in the door of his laboratory. This observation led him to abandon his study of dogs' digestion and begin a series of studies of how the anticipatory salivation worked. Would any sight or sound occurring just before the dogs were fed elicit salivating? First, he rang a bell just before the dogs were fed; then, he rang the bell without food. At first the bell alone didn't elicit anticipatory salivation. But then, like a good scientist, he persisted. His intuition about his earlier observation led him to carry out many pairings of the bell and subsequent feeding. At last he saw results; after many pairings (conditioning), the bell elicited salivation even though the food was nowhere in sight.

Pavlov's observation provided the first scientific understanding of classical conditioning. Since then, classical conditioning has been studied extensively, and scientists have

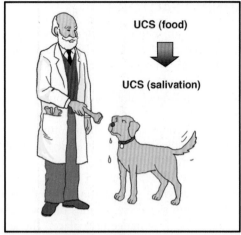

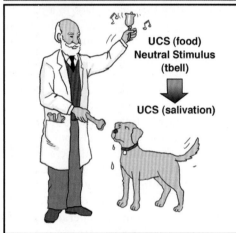

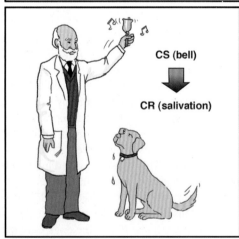

Figure 4.3 Classical conditioning paradigm. Dog salivates naturally when given food. Food is paired frequently with sound of bell. Bell without food then elicits salivation.

- A stimulus that reliably elicits a response must be present. This stimulus is called the unconditioned stimulus (UCS), and the response it elicits—often a reflexive or hardwired response—is called an unconditioned response (UCR).
- Then a neutral stimulus that doesn't elicit any particular response must be paired with the UCS. The neutral stimulus is called the conditioned stimulus (CS) because it will be *conditioned* to elicit a response.
- After repeated pairing of the CS with the UCS (which reliably elicits the UCR), the CS is then presented without the UCS, and *voila!* The CS elicits the UCR.

Classical Conditioning and Stuttering

Remember my description of my stuttering in high school? The feelings of dread I had before making a phone call and the tightening of my throat were the result of classical conditioning. The neutral stimulus (CS) was the phone or the thought of making a phone call. Because I had had lots of experience with stuttering at that time and it was all unpleasant, embarrassing, and shameful, the expectation of stuttering (UCS) elicited strong negative emotions for me (UCR). Those emotions, like many people's fear of public speaking, resulted in considerable tension in my larynx and other muscles related to speech. Repeated experiences that paired the phone with the experiences of stuttering conditioned me to experience fear when contemplating making a phone call. The fear elicited muscle tension that undoubtedly worsened my stuttering every time I made a phone call. I think my experiences are typical of how classical conditioning can make stuttering worse for many people who stutter.

An excellent theoretical account of classical conditioning and stuttering was provided by Eugene Brutten, a speech-language pathologist, and Donald Shoemaker, a psychologist, who worked together at the University of Southern Illinois (Brutten & Shoemaker, 1967). They hypothesized that the earliest stuttering symptoms (often repetitions) result from the cognitive and motor disorganization that occurs when a child's anxiety is conditioned to speech.

Although the description of classical conditioning and stuttering I am giving here owes much to Brutten and Shoemaker's (1967) pioneering work, I believe classical conditioning is seldom responsible for the earliest signs of stuttering. Instead, I believe, along with Starkweather (1987, p. 372), that "it seems likely that [neuro]physiological sources play more of a role in stuttering onset, whereas conditioning processes play more of a role in stuttering development." I also agree with a similar assessment by Van Riper (1982) that "the real contribution of classical conditioning theory as it is applied to stuttering lies in its ability to explain the development of the disorder."

Illustration of Classical Conditioning and Stuttering

Let me give you a description of how classical conditioning might actually work in the development of childhood stuttering. For ease of explanation, I will refer to hypothesized increases in muscle tension (and perhaps speech rate) during

been able to describe how it takes place. Figure 4.3 depicts the "paradigm" (a model or diagram of how a process takes place) for classical conditioning.

For classical conditioning to take place, several things must occur:

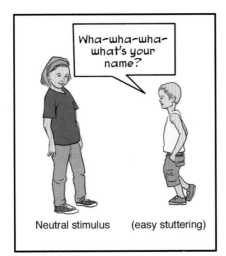

Neutral stimulus   (easy stuttering)

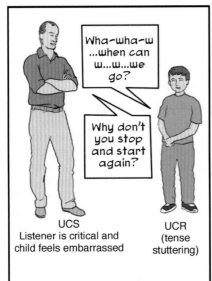

UCS
Listener is critical and
child feels embarrassed

UCR
(tense
stuttering)

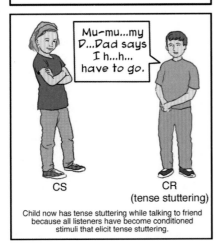

CS

CR
(tense stuttering)

Child now has tense stuttering while talking to friend
because all listeners have become conditioned
stimuli that elicit tense stuttering.

Figure 4.4   Example of classical conditioning of tension in a beginning stutterer. The repeated pairing of easy stuttering with a critical listener or internal frustration, which elicits tension, makes the easy stuttering a conditioned stimulus for tension. Consequently, tense stuttering occurs in more and more situations.

disfluencies under conditions of negative emotion as "the tension response." The paradigm to illustrate this conditioning is shown in Figure 4.4.

To illustrate how this paradigm applies to an individual child who stutters, I will use a hypothetical 4-year-old I'll call Richard.

In this example, Richard's stuttering up to this point has been relaxed, slow part-word repetitions. This will be the CS, but it hasn't been conditioned yet, so it's still neutral. When he experiences this easy stuttering, Richard doesn't respond to it in any particular way. It doesn't bother him, and he doesn't react to it. As I describe this process, I will sometimes refer to the CS as "easy stuttering" or as "disfluency." The point I'm trying to make here is that a child's early stuttering may often go unnoticed and does not include tension or hurry. But with conditioning, it becomes tense and hurried.

Now we observe Richard as he goes along in his daily life, growing up and becoming more aware of how he is performing compared to other kids. Different things may happen to pair the neutral stimulus (Richard's easy stuttering) with a UCS (something that causes Richard to react to his stuttering in a way he didn't previously). This pairing will turn the neutral stimulus into a CS. For example, Richard may notice that as he is stuttering, he is not getting his words out as fast as he'd like compared to his peers or his own internal expectations. This may cause an emotional response, such as frustration. With frustration comes an increase in his body tension, especially in speech muscles (see the section on temperament in Chapter 6 for a full description of this). This is Richard's UCR. Other things may also occur—for example, Richard's stuttering may elicit negative responses from his parents or playmates, causing him to feel embarrassed or ashamed. His father may frown and suggest impatiently that he stop speaking and start again. Richard's emotional response to this may also trigger a tension response—tightening speech muscles and repeating sounds a little faster. The important thing to understand is that this repeated pairing of the previously neutral stimulus (stuttering) with the UCR (tension response) will turn the first moments of stuttering and even the anticipation of stuttering into a CS that elicits the UCR.

Other factors influencing Richard's UCR may be in his external environment. For example, Richard may have a new baby brother or his family may have just moved to a new town. These factors may increase a child's anxiety (autonomic arousal), particularly in a sensitive child, and may thus make the UCR (tension response) more likely and stronger and also make the learning more powerful. This will be described at greater length in the later section on individual differences.

Now, the experience of stuttering or the anticipation of stuttering elicits the tension response, even in the absence of any threatening stimuli. Previously, Richard used to stutter with only easy disfluencies in friendly situations like talking with his mother or playing with a peer; now he stutters with tension and hurry in those situations because his stuttering

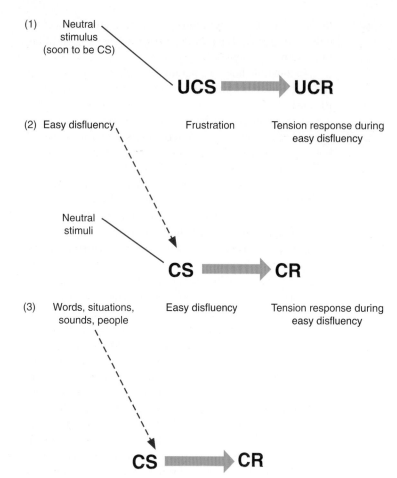

(1)   Neutral
       stimulus
       (soon to be CS)

UCS ➡ **UCR**

(2) Easy disfluency   Frustration   Tension response during
                                                   easy disfluency

    Neutral
    stimuli

CS ➡ **CR**

(3) Words, situations,   Easy disfluency   Tension response during
     sounds, people   easy disfluency

CS ➡ **CR**

Words, situations,   Tension response at
sounds, people   onset of utterance

Figure 4.5 Spread of conditioning. (*1*) Easy disfluency repeatedly elicits the tension response, producing tense stuttering. (*2*) Easy disfluency, which occurs with various words, situations, sounds, and people, is then a conditioned stimulus that elicits the tension response and tense stuttering. (*3*) Words, situations, sounds, and people become the conditioned stimuli, which elicit the tension response at the onset of an utterance, producing fixed articulatory postures (or blocks) when the child begins an utterance.

(CS) or anticipation of it triggers the tension response. This conditioning process also involves generalization of Richard's stuttering to more and more situations, involving a process that we will describe in the following section.

Spread of Conditioning

Conditioning is an active and continuing process. When a child is disfluent (CS) and experiences the tension response (CR) (a CS elicits a conditioned response), a host of other stimuli are present, incidentally. When the child stutters, he is talking to someone, uttering a particular word or sound, speaking in a particular room, and talking about a particular topic. Because of the power of classical conditioning, the pairing of these other stimuli with the CS (disfluency) gives them the potency to elicit the CR. The particular sound on which he stutters, for example, may become conditioned to elicit the CR, so in the future he is more likely to stutter on that sound with tension and hurry. Thus, as conditioning takes place again and again, the stimulus becomes a complex of many things, including words and sounds, listeners, and physical surroundings or situations. This chaining of stimuli is called

"higher-order conditioning" or "second-order conditioning." Figure 4.5 illustrates the process.

It is important to note that to maintain the effects of the CS, a UCS must occur periodically. Stuttering must occasionally provoke frustration or another negative emotion for it to continue to elicit the tension response.

The spread of conditioning to other conditioned stimuli results in changes in stuttering as well. Initially, a child might emit several repetitive disfluencies or a long prolongation before the tension response occurs. Soon, however, muscle tension occurs earlier and earlier in the stutters. When other conditioned stimuli, such as words, elicit the tension response, the easy repetitive disfluencies may not occur at all. Instead, a child will increase muscle tension on the very first sound he tries to utter, resulting in the "fixed articulatory postures" that are a sign of advancing stuttering.

As a child's stuttering frequency increases as a result of the spread of conditioning to more and more stimuli, the duration of the child's stuttering may also increase. This may be explained by the fact that the tension response soon becomes a stimulus that elicits more tension. After all, the tension response makes it harder to utter a word, and the experience of "squeezing hard" without being able to speak for a second or two elicits frustration, leading to another tension response.

Individual Differences in Conditioning

Before we leave our discussion of classical conditioning, I would like to touch on the topic of individual differences and conditioning. The rapid learning and widespread generalization that is apparent in stuttering may parallel the "prepared classical conditioning" of some animals that are rapidly and deeply conditioned to such naturally dangerous objects as snakes (Mineka, 1985). In humans, rapid conditioning can occur in those with temperaments that are more alert to threatening stimuli. For example, individuals with an anxious temperament are more prone to acquire fears and phobias (Biederman, Rosenbaum, Chaloff, & Kagan, 1995), and animals, which have been exposed to stressful situations, are more easily classically conditioned (Shors, Weiss, & Thompson, 1992). Thus, it seems likely that children who stutter and who are especially sensitive may rapidly condition to such threatening stimuli as a critical parent or a peer who makes fun of the child's stuttering.

Undoing the Classical Conditioning

How can you use the principles of classical conditioning to help someone who stutters talk more fluently? Treatment of the conditioned tension response in young children can involve behavioral therapy that gives the child enough experience with fluent speech that the old conditioned response is finally extinguished. For this to occur, fluency-facilitating conditions are set up on a daily basis. This may involve a one-on-one relaxed conversation with a parent, starting with simple language so that the child repeatedly has conditioned stimuli (parent, anticipation of speaking) followed by the absence of the conditioned tension response. Instead, the conditioned stimuli are associated with fluent speech. This repeated pairing is first done with one parent and then with other members of the family, as well as situations outside the home so that gradually, fluency is generalized to many situations. Operant or instrumental conditioning is an important component of this process and will be described in an upcoming section.

When the conditioned tension response has been deeply learned, as is often the case with older children, adolescents, and adults, considerable unlearning must take place. The clinician has a number of options, but one of several tools I use frequently is desensitization. Remember that when I described the original conditioning, I suggested that there is an emotional reaction, such as frustration, that triggers a UCR of tensing and speeding up. Desensitization aims to reduce the emotional response by helping the client go ahead and stutter but feel emotionally accepting of it and relaxed about it. This is achieved by rewarding the client for staying in the stutter and staying calm while in it, decreasing the emotional response. Once the client can do this in many situations, the client is helped to stutter in a new way that sounds like the typical speech of an average speaker. A full description of this aspect of treatment will be given in the chapters on treating school-age children (Chapter 13) and adults (Chapter 14).

Because the CS has been associated with many different people, situations, and words, undoing the conditioning must involve pairing many different conditioned stimuli (people, situations, words) with the new responses.

Operant Conditioning

When I stuttered severely in high school, I would often end stutters by jerking my head just as I made a big push that finally got the word out. Operant conditioning was responsible for my learning this behavior and for the fact that it remained part of my stuttering pattern for many years. In this type of learning, the frequency at which a behavior occurs is related to the consequences that follow. If a behavior is followed by a reward, it increases; if it is followed by an aversive consequence, it decreases. Like many operant behaviors, my head nod had begun as random struggles when I was jammed on a word. Several times the word I was stuck on popped out of my mouth just as I jerked my head up. The relief I felt in freeing myself of the stutter and being able to finish the word caused my head jerking to increase whenever I stuttered. The escape behaviors described in Chapter 1, such as eye blinks, are learned through operant conditioning. They begin as part of random struggle efforts to escape from a stutter, and they are rewarded by the release of the word.

A common type of operant conditioning is called *positive reinforcement*. The next time you're in a public building with an elevator, watch what happens when people are waiting for the elevator to arrive and it's delayed. One person will usually keep pressing the elevator button several times even though the button is illuminated and the elevator is on its way. Like everyone else, this person has been reinforced many times by the prompt arrival of the elevator after pushing the button just once. At some later time, however, he must have encountered a delayed elevator, and after pressing the button repeatedly, he was rewarded by the eventual arrival of the elevator. Thus, positive reinforcement conditioned him to repeat this behavior even though he had to have known that it wasn't necessary. The same is true if you have a "lucky shirt" to wear to an exam. If you do well, you will probably be more likely to wear the same shirt—even if it is in need of a wash—to your next exam in spite of intellectually knowing that it doesn't actually affect the outcome.

Another kind of operant conditioning is *punishment*. It has probably shaped your behavior if you've ever gotten a ticket for speeding. The punishing effect of an expensive fine makes you drive more cautiously when you are on the same section of road. You can appreciate the disadvantage of punishment, however, if you can remember referring to the police officer as a "weasel" when you described the incident to your friends and family. Unless it is mild and delivered with good humor, punishment usually is not beneficial to clinical relationships.

A third kind of operant conditioning, *negative reinforcement*, is the mechanism behind the escape behaviors, like eye blinks and head nods, that are part of many stuttering patterns. The head jerks that were part of my own stuttering pattern were the result of just this type of conditioning. Negative reinforcement occurs whenever a behavior is followed by the termination of an unpleasant situation. In stuttering, a sudden movement may terminate a moment of stuttering, which means that behavior is reinforced and is likely to occur more frequently in the future when the stutterer is jammed up. All of us may develop habits through negative reinforcement in our daily routines. For instance, if you are trapped in a long line at the cash register in the bookstore, you may bail out and discover that the register upstairs in the CD and DVD section has no line at all. If so, your escape behavior is reinforced, making it more likely that you will again go upstairs to the other register the next time you are stuck in the long line.

Operant conditioning is a major tool for all clinicians. It is a component of every stuttering treatment program. It's a very powerful tool that affects the frequency of the behavior you are interested in, especially in the environment in which you use it. For example, when you are working with a preschool-age child who stutters, one effective approach is to help parents arrange a situation in which the child is fluent, then praise her to reinforce her fluency. After that has been done many times, the frequency of the child's fluent utterances will increase. Remember that the environment in which the operant conditioning takes place is important. Therefore, to increase the child's fluency where it counts most, the clinician teaches the parents to elicit fluency and praise it in their home. With a child, very mild punishment might be used occasionally to help her learn to use fluent speech instead of stuttering, but it must be done with great care and careful monitoring of the effect. Whenever punishment is used, reward is also an important part of a treatment plan. Much reward and little punishment is a good motto. Van Riper (1973) pioneered the use of mild self-punishment to be used by adults who stutter, using a procedure he called "cancellation." Van Riper taught clients to stop talking immediately after they had one of their typical tense stutters and then in silence, plan an easier, more relaxed way of stuttering on the word. That silent pause was mildly punishing, and thus, the frequency of tense stutters decreased. Uttering the word easily after the pause was rewarding, and the frequency of relaxed stutters increased.

Van Riper also developed another operant conditioning technique he called a "pullout." He taught clients to stop in the middle of tense stutters and hold onto the sound that they were stuttering on until they could relax the muscles that were so tense they prevented saying the word. The client then finished the word in a relaxed, slow manner. By finishing the word and continuing the conversation, the client rewarded himself for an easier stutter—the behavior the client was doing just before he rewarded himself. This increased the frequency of relaxed stutters. This technique teaches a person who stutters to escape from a tense block, not by pushing or squeezing with excess tension, but by reducing the tension and finishing the word with a relaxed, nearly normal-sounding production. The reason we say that negative reinforcement is used is because a reward is given for removing the negativity of the situation. In this case, the individual himself stays in the negative situation of holding onto a moment of stuttering but then allows himself to escape only when he loosens the stutter and ends the word slowly and loosely. This act rewards the slow, relaxed production of the sound or sounds he's stuttering on, because immediately after the slowing and relaxing, the word is released, and he can continue talking.

A third operant conditioning-based tool that Van Riper developed to modify stuttering is called a "preparatory set." Van Riper had noticed that stutterers tended to begin their stuttered utterances by putting themselves into jammed up postures or other inappropriate speech gestures. Therefore, he taught his clients to pause momentarily before the word on which they expected to stutter and put their speech mechanisms into relaxed normal states. They then would say the word in a slow, relaxed way that would be reinforced by completion of the word and the experience of not getting stuck.

By combining these three operant-based techniques with classical conditioning to reduce clients' negative emotions, Van Riper had a therapeutic package that effectively taught stutterers to stutter in such easy ways that they sounded like normal speakers.

Avoidance Conditioning

My stuttering in high school, described earlier, was peppered with dozens of "ums." I usually said "um" three or four times before I even tried to say a word on which I expected trouble. Sometimes my classmates, in a curious and friendly way, would count the number of "ums" I had in a row and tell me later what my record was. Once they counted 17 "ums" as I was trying to say "Yugoslavia." These "ums" were the result of avoidance conditioning. I first learned to use "um" as an escape behavior. When I was hopelessly stuck on a word, I could sometimes release it by quickly saying "um" and trying the word again. Then I began to say "um" even before starting a word I expected to be difficult. This sometimes prevented a stutter from occurring, and I was on my way to a serious case of avoidance conditioning. Because I rarely tried to say a difficult word without saying "um," I never learned that I might do better without it.

There are many types of avoidance behaviors that people who stutter learn. They include avoiding speaking situations, avoiding certain words and substituting easy words for hard ones, and using extra sounds, words, or phrases, such as "um," "well," and "you know," to get a running start on a difficult word. One politician I worked with cringed every time he'd see himself on television hemming and hawing and dodging difficult words, looking and sounding like a politician. He successfully learned to be open about his difficulty and stutter mildly on words he really wanted to use.

Avoidance conditioning is a big part of everyday life. The example in which you learned to escape from a long line in the bookstore by going to a cash register in the CD section can also be used to describe how avoidance conditioning may be common in your life. Perhaps after escaping from long lines at the front register several times, you might have started to avoid that register altogether and just go straight to the register in the CD section. Although many avoidance behaviors are first learned as escape behaviors, many are not. Think about why you put on your seat belt when you drive or don a helmet when you get on a motorcycle or snowboard. You may never have had an accident, but public safety spots on TV make us imagine what can happen if you don't take these precautions to avoid brain damage or death.

Clinically, you will need to help people who stutter reduce their avoidance behaviors using a number of approaches. It is often difficult to get rid of avoidance behaviors, because the person doesn't dare to find out what would happen if he didn't do them. It's like the man who was referred to a psychiatrist for habitually snapping his fingers. "Why do you do that?" the psychiatrist asked. "Because it keeps the elephants away," the man replied. The psychiatrist then said, "But you don't need to. There are no elephants for miles around." "Well, then," the man replied, "it works, doesn't it?"

This patient might be helped if the psychiatrist could convince him to stop snapping his fingers in the office where the psychiatrist could give him protection and reassurance. This would enable the patient to see that no elephants came even though he didn't snap his fingers for at least an hour. You can use similar techniques to help a high school student learn to tackle difficult words without saying "um." For example, you could highly praise him for starting a feared word without saying "um" but beginning it slowly and deliberately with a "preparatory set" instead and using a "pullout" if stuttering occurs. I have always found it important to teach a client what *to do* when he is afraid he will stutter before teaching her what avoidance behaviors *not to do*.

Fortunately, some individuals who stutter will stop using avoidance behaviors without having to work directly on them. Directly improving fluency, for example, will often decrease avoidances. This is particularly true for children, who may be avoiding a few words or speaking situations, but have not developed a widespread pattern of avoidance. For them, learning how to speak more fluently will reduce their fear of stuttering enough so that they are motivated to approach all the speaking opportunities presented to them.

SUMMARY

- During the preschool years, rapid and differential changes in a child's body—especially in speech structures—may make it difficult for a child to coordinate the rapid movements necessary for fluency.

- A child's cognitive development may not only compete with speech production for resources but may also provide the intellectual ability for a child to compare herself with others, which may lead to embarrassment and shame about stuttering.

- In younger children with immature brains, speech pathways may not be buffered from the effects of emotional arousal, resulting in more disfluency. Some children may be especially vulnerable to the effects of emotion on speech because they can be easily emotionally aroused. Self-conscious emotions develop soon after age 2, and the emotional distress of these children in reaction to stuttering may produce increased physical tension, particularly in the larynx.

- As language develops rapidly, the increasing length and complexity of children's utterances may sometimes exceed their speech production abilities. Selecting words, encoding phonology, planning syntax, and working out the complex prosody for an entire utterance all occur just as the child is starting to speak. It is no wonder, then, that most early stuttering occurs on the first words of sentences.

- There is some evidence that delays in language acquisition, and especially phonological development, may be associated with increased risk of persistent stuttering.

- Parents of children who stutter may, as a group, show slight tendencies to be demanding and perfectionistic. This may be the result of having a child with a speech difficulty or a manifestation of the genetic background that also results in a child having a vulnerable temperament. Research in this area is equivocal, however, with many studies finding no differences between the parents of children who stutter and those of children who don't.

- There is no clear evidence that parents of children who stutter converse using faster rates, more questions, more interruptions, and more long, complex utterances than do the parents of nonstuttering children. Several studies have found differences between these groups of parents, but many have not. Despite the lack of research support, many clinicians believe that it is therapeutically helpful for parents to slow their speech rates and speak in shorter sentences when talking to their children who stutter.

- There is a wealth of clinical anecdotes suggesting that difficult events in a child's life, such as parents' divorce or the arrival of a new baby in the family, may trigger stuttering. However, there is little empirical support for these anecdotes.

- Classical conditioning may cause stuttering to spread to many different contexts and to be consistently present rather than episodic. Operant conditioning can increase the frequency of escape behaviors. Avoidance conditioning can increase the frequency of behaviors that stutterers use to postpone or evade expected stutters. All three types of conditioning are important contributors to the establishment of secondary stuttering behaviors and are also critical to the treatment of stuttering.

STUDY QUESTIONS

1. The effect of a child's development on fluency has been likened to the effect of multiple tasks for a computer. Explain this analogy.
2. It has been said that children usually do not learn to walk and talk at the same time. What does this suggest about how motor development might affect fluency?
3. There is a high incidence of stuttering among individuals with cognitive impairment. What might this suggest about the relationship between cognition and fluency?
4. What aspects of social and emotional development might threaten fluency?
5. What evidence is there that emotional arousal might increase disfluency?
6. What is the possible connection between atypical hemispheric localization and the effects of emotion on fluency?
7. Why would children's speech and language development be likely to put greater pressure on fluency than would their physical or cognitive development?
8. What aspects of parents' behavior might put pressure on a child who is disfluent?
9. Identify several characteristics of parents' speech that may create difficult models for a disfluent child to emulate.
10. Name several life events that have been suggested to increase a child's disfluency.
11. The communicative failure and anticipatory struggle view proposes that experiencing a communication failure may cause a child to anticipate difficulty speaking and begin to stutter as a result. What characteristic of the child may be another important factor?
12. Johnson and associates' (1959) revised view of stuttering suggested that it results from an interaction among the following three factors: (a) the extent of the child's disfluency, (b) the listener's sensitivity to that disfluency, and (c) the child's sensitivity to his own disfluency and to the listener's reaction. Relate these factors to constitutional, developmental, and environmental factors in stuttering.

SUGGESTED PROJECTS

1. Record a natural speech sample from someone who stutters and analyze the relationship between the occurrences of stuttering and the linguistic level of the utterances in which they occur.
2. Develop an experimental protocol to assess the relationship between linguistic variables and stuttering. For example, compare the variables of length of utterance, syntactic level of utterance, and phonological complexity of utterance on the likelihood of the utterance being stuttered.
3. Design a therapy activity for someone who has a classically conditioned fear of dogs. One way to do this would be to develop a hierarchy of situations that progress from easy and nonthreatening to gradually more realistic encounters with dogs. At each level of the hierarchy, have the client engage in some "approach" behavior (like talking to the dog) that will counteract the old tendency to avoid dogs.
4. Study the effect of your speech rate on other people by designing and carrying out an experiment in which you vary the speed at which you talk. Record conversations in which you talk slowly for several minutes and then talk rapidly for several minutes. Measure the effect on your conversational partner's speed of talking. You will need to practice varying your rate beforehand.
5. In the section called Speech and Language Development, research on language abilities of children who stutter is reviewed. Some studies found that children who stutter have poorer language abilities, and other studies did not. Review these studies and suggest what might be causing this disagreement in the literature.

SUGGESTED READINGS

Andrews, G. & Harris, M. (1964). *The syndrome of stuttering.* **London: W. Heinemann Medical Books.**

These authors present data from longitudinal studies of 1,000 families in Newcastle, England. The interpretation of results presents evidence that both genetic and environmental influences are at work to create stuttering. This book gives an early version of the "capacities and demands" view that stuttering is due to a lack of capacity for some aspect of speech and language processing.

Ayres, J. J. B. (1998). Fear conditioning and avoidance. In W. O'Donohue (Ed.), *Learning and Behavior Therapy.* **Boston: Allyn and Bacon.**

This chapter provides a good update of the animal learning literature on fear conditioning. Several findings appear to be relevant to stuttering. First, some responses to fear may be part of an animal's hardwiring (perhaps laryngeal tension is a natural response to fear of speaking in some individuals). Second, some individual animals freeze in response to fear rather than learn an effective coping response (are some children who begin to stutter more predisposed to tense blockages than others?). Third, for a fear-conditioned response, reducing fear without teaching a new response to fear leaves the animal vulnerable to relapse (it may be important to reduce stutterers' fear of stuttering as well as teaching them a coping skill they can use when fear is present).

Bernstein Ratner, N. (1997). Stuttering: A psycholinguistic perspective. In R. Curlee & G. Siegel (Eds.), *Nature and Treatment of Stuttering: New Directions* (2nd ed.). Boston: Allyn & Bacon.

This is an insightful review of the many connections between language and stuttering. The author's background allows her to use linguistic theories and evidence from child language studies to discuss how language influences the loci of stuttering in speech, how parent-child interactions may affect stuttering, how language development may be important in stuttering onset, and the role of feedback on speech, language, and stuttering development.

Bloodstein, O., & Ratner, N. (2008). Inferences and conclusions. In Bloodstein, O., *A Handbook on Stuttering*. Clifton Park, NY: Thompson-Delmar Learning.

This chapter presents the communicative failure and anticipatory struggle view of stuttering onset. Bloodstein musters the evidence he has summarized in earlier chapters of this handbook to argue convincingly that stuttering develops from an interaction between the child and his environment.

Crystal, D. (1987). Towards a "bucket" theory of language disability: Taking account of interaction between linguistic levels. *Clinical Linguistics and Phonetics, 1*, 7–22.

A theoretical discussion of interaction among levels of speech and language, with an illustrative case of a child whose stuttering increases when language demands are greater. The article makes a clear argument for the influence of speech and language development on stuttering.

Johnson, W., et al. (1959). *The onset of stuttering*. Minneapolis, MN: University of Minnesota Press.

This book presents extensive data on parents' perceptions of the onset of their child's stuttering, compared with other parents' perceptions of their child's normal disfluency. Johnson eloquently lays out his view of stuttering as the product of an interaction between the child's disfluency, his sensitivity, and the listener's reactions.

Kagan, J., Reznick, J. S., & Snidman, N. (1987). The physiology and psychology of behavioral inhibition in children. *Child Development, 58*, 1459–1473.

This article discusses the findings that behaviorally inhibited children show high levels of laryngeal tension. Neurophysiological mechanisms are also discussed as well as possible genetic and environmental contributions. Recommended for those interested in the hypothesis that behavioral inhibition may be a component in some stuttering.

Paden, E. P. (2005). Development of phonological ability. In Yairi, E., & Ambrose, N., *Early Childhood Stuttering*. Austin, TX: Pro-Ed.

This chapter focuses on the phonological development of children who stutter with particular emphasis on comparisons between children who recover without intervention and those who persist in stuttering. The author brings to light several aspects of her research that are intriguing puzzles for future researchers to solve.

Watkins, R. V. (2005). Language abilities of young children who Stutter. In Yairi, E. & Ambrose, N. *Early Childhood Stuttering*. Austin, TX: Pro-Ed.

Although current evidence reviewed in this chapter suggests that language abilities of children who stutter and those who don't are similar, language factors appear to play an important role in stuttering. The author discusses several interesting relationships between language and stuttering, including the role of language factors in the occurrence of stuttering in an utterance and the finding that early onset of stuttering is often associated with advanced language skills.

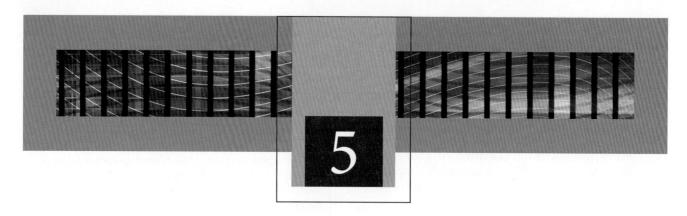

Research Findings on Developmental, Environmental, and Learning Factors in Stuttering

| CHAPTER OBJECTIVES

After studying this chapter, readers should be able to discuss research findings on developmental, environmental, and learning factors in stuttering in greater depth

Like Chapter 3, this chapter describes in detail the research studies that provide evidence about factors important in understanding stuttering that were summarized in the previous chapter—in this case, Chapter 4. Note that not every topic discussed in the previous chapter is covered here, because in some cases, the research is minimal.

PHYSICAL AND MOTOR SKILL DEVELOPMENT

In the main section of this chapter, I suggested that developmental factors may influence stuttering in young children. Here, I will make the case that speech motor skill

development in all children puts great demands on neural resources needed for fluent speech, and it may present a special challenge for children who stutter because of differences in brain structure and function.

One problem posed by physical development in children is rapid change in the vocal tract between ages 2 and 5 years. During this time, structures in a child's head, neck, and torso undergo their most accelerated growth; moreover, different structures grow at different rates (Kent & Vorperian, 1995, 2007). As children's speaking mechanisms change day by day—the shape, size, and biomechanical properties of muscles and bones are different today from the way they were yesterday—children somehow manage to continue to produce intelligible speech. Callan, Kent, Guenther, and Vorperian (2000) propose that children maintain a stable speech output in the face of almost daily changes in their speech structures by using feedback to continuously update the motor commands they send to their muscles to produce specific sounds. What their brains told their muscles to do yesterday must be adapted to the new size, shape, and biomechanical properties of the vocal tract today. Auditory feedback, integrated with proprioceptive and other muscle feedback, helps children discover errors in their motor commands and adjust the commands to the new dimensions.

The theory behind this hypothesis may be important for understanding theories of stuttering discussed in Chapter 6 (e.g., Neilson & Neilson, 1987, 1988), so I will spend a little extra time explaining it. A key assumption about learning to speak is that from the day he is born, a child is learning the relationship between what his brain tells his muscles to do (motor commands) and what sounds come out of his mouth (perceptual target). He begins this learning with his earliest cries and babbles. As he begins to attend to the speech around him, he develops a sensory memory of those sounds and then practices the motor commands needed to produce them. In doing so, he develops "sensory-motor neural maps" that he uses to generate these motor commands in a reliable way (Kent & Vorperian, 1995, 2007). These maps are sometimes called "inverse internal models" of the relationship between the sensory-motor target that the child wants to hit and the motor plan needed to hit it. They are called "inverse" because the child's brain selects the target to hit (the sound he wants to make) and instantly calculates how to hit it with movements of articulators, larynx, and breathing apparatus, given their current positions. As the child's vocal tract changes and matures, he maintains and updates the relationships between motor commands and acoustic output from the information provided by the auditory feedback of his own speech, as well as feedback from the touches and movements of his articulators involved in producing that speech.

Evidence from brain imaging studies presented in Chapter 2 (Cykowski, Fox, Ingham, Ingham, & Robin, 2010; Sommer, Koch, Paulus, Weiller, & Buchel, 2002) suggests that bidirectional pathways connecting sensory integration areas with speech motor planning areas are less dense in individuals who stutter. Thus, the pathways that were designed to build and update the sensory-motor models of the sounds and words they want to say may be inefficient in children who stutter. These pathways not only help the child as he learns to speak accurately during development, but they are used for every utterance. When these children plan to speak and need quick access to the stored inverse internal models, this access may be slow in coming, and stuttering may result.

SPEECH AND LANGUAGE DEVELOPMENT

This section contains research and commentary about the phenomenon that the first appearance of stuttering frequently happens when a child is rapidly developing speech and language.

Many writers have eloquently commented on the connection between the onset of stuttering and language acquisition. Peggy Dalton and W.J. Hardcastle (1977), for example, commented that "it is tempting to see the ever-increasing demands on linguistic competence and articulatory proficiency as major factors in the onset of some disfluency." Joseph Sheehan (1975) said, "The age of onset of stuttering is consistently related to certain stages in the developmental sequence. Most notably, the 'period of resonance,' or high readiness in language learning...is also the period during which stuttering develops and flourishes" (p. 142). Andrews and colleagues (1983) pointed to the demands placed on speech by rapidly developing language, noting

that "stuttering [has] a maximal frequency of onset at a time when an explosive growth in language ability outstrips a still-immature speech-motor apparatus" (p. 239).

Many studies have found that greater length and complexity of language is associated with more stuttering. This is a developmental factor because stuttering may first appear when—in those children predisposed to stutter—their language matures and they use longer and more complex utterances. For example, research on natural conversational speech of children who stutter has shown that more complex utterances contain more stuttering (Brundage & Bernstein Ratner, 1989; Gaines, Runyan, & Meyers, 1991; Logan & Conture, 1995; Yaruss, 1999). Some research suggests that utterance length may have a greater effect on stuttering than does complexity (Logan & Conture, 1995; Wilkenfeld & Curlee, 1997; Yaruss, 1999). Experimental studies, in which children were asked to produce both more and less complex utterances, show that both stutterers (Bernstein Ratner & Sih, 1987; Stocker & Usprich, 1976) and nonstutterers (Gordon, Luper, & Peterson, 1986; Haynes & Hood, 1978; Pearl & Bernthal, 1980; Yaruss, Newman, & Flora, 1999) increase their disfluencies as language complexity is increased. Unfortunately, there is little longitudinal research that directly bears on the question of how and when emerging language is associated with normal disfluency or stuttering.

One of the few descriptive studies of this phenomenon was Norma Colburn's analysis of the disfluencies of four nonstuttering children using data originally gathered by Lois Bloom for her work on normal language development. Published reports of her analysis (Colburn & Mysak, 1982a, 1982b) suggested that these children's normal disfluencies did not emerge when they first learned a new language construction but as they began to master it and started using it regularly. Explanations suggested for this result include the possibility that a child who has not completely automatized the use of a new construction allocates fewer resources than are necessary for its production (Kent & Perkins, 1984) or that when a child masters the new construction he produces it at an increased rate, thereby straining capacity (Starkweather, 1987).

A single-case study by Frank Wijnen (1990) was used to explore the relationship between syntax acquisition and normal disfluencies. Weekly speech samples were obtained from a boy from age 2 years, 4 months to 2 years, 11 months. The number of repetitions, revisions, and incomplete phrases was assessed in relation to the length and complexity of utterances. It was reported that disfluencies were randomly distributed initially, but eventually clustered on function words and sentence-initial words and then declined. Although speech rate was not measured (increased rate might have accounted for some of the increase in the child's disfluencies), the number of disfluencies was not highly correlated with length of utterance. Instead, Wijnen concluded that the eventual decline in the child's disfluencies was associated with his development of a routine type of sentence (pronoun + verb + some other word) and that learning this routine involved so much of his processing capacity that speech production was shortchanged and initially caused the disfluencies. This preliminary study needs to be followed up with many more cases to test the hypothesis that the process of first learning to make sentence productions more automatic through routinization of several sentence types is related to increased normal disfluency. With a larger sample size, multiple regression analyses could be used to determine which of many possible factors best predict instances of or increases in disfluency.

Having looked at the evidence of an association between increasing sentence complexity and/or sentence length and the frequency of stuttering in children, let's consider what may be specifically interfering with fluency as the child acquires language. I'll begin by recounting what the child acquires during this period of time. Between ages 2 and 3, a child's vocabulary jumps from 50 to well over 500 words; in fact, toward the end of this year, five to seven new words may be learned each day (Studdert-Kennedy, 1987). At the same time, the child's single-word utterances develop into successive single-word pairs with sentence-like intonations and durations, then to multi-word sentences (Branigan, 1979). Thus, the child's speech graduates from a simple "syllable-timed" prosody for single words to complex prosodic rhythms that span multiple words (Allen & Hawkins, 1980). As the child expands sentences, he also overhauls his language storage system. At first, his shelves are stocked with whole words in the form of articulatory routines or gestural patterns; then, he must change strategies and begin to stock, not whole words, but segments that can be combined in various ways to form a multitude of words (Kent, 1985; Nittrouer, Studdert-Kennedy, & McGowan, 1989; Sternberger, 1982). During these same early preschool years, the child also progressively learns active, negative, and passive constructions as well as present, future, and past tenses. At the same time, he increases the length and linguistic complexity of his sentences together with the rate of his utterances as he increasingly tries to synchronize the rates and rhythms of his speech with those of his family, with whom he has a growing urge to communicate.

This huge array of language and speech production tasks is a challenge even to the fluency of nonstuttering children. Normal disfluencies of children also increase from ages 2 to 4, peaking when they tackle the task of producing long, complex sentences (Ito, 1986). It is not surprising, then, that children who are predisposed to stutter because of genetic or congenital factors tend to begin stuttering during this same period.

I would like to move from *what* may interfere with a child's fluency to consider *how* it may occur. Imagine that a child's brain has a limited amount of space that is chock full of highly interconnected networks of neurons (Kinsbourne & Hicks, 1978). Because the child's brain is immature but tightly packed, neural networks may not be well insulated from one another. The insulation of axons is provided by myelin sheaths, fatty protective coatings that develop slowly throughout childhood. Thus, in a younger child, myelinization is incomplete, allowing "cross talk" among axons of different neural networks, creating interference in the transmission of information. In Chapter 3, I described early speculations by Karlin (1947) about delayed myelinization as a cause of stuttering and more recent findings of Cykowski and colleagues (2010) that delayed myelinization in key neural pathways may result in disruption of appropriate sensory-motor integration for fluent speech.

Another challenge to the child developing language may be introduced by different neuronal groups maturing at different rates. Neuronal groups working on vocabulary may be more efficient than those working on syntax, or vice versa. In addition, structures—such as the corpus callosum—that link prosodic functions of the right hemisphere with syntactic functions in the left may be slower to develop than other structures involved in speech-language production. All these differences may account for why a young child may have trouble synchronizing the tasks required for speech, some of which are simultaneous while others are sequential. As a child grows, however, his brain gains more functional space with expanded neural networks that can function more independently from one another. As different groups of neurons mature and become more efficient, they can synchronize their actions more easily. Thus, when the child becomes a teenager, he can rub his tummy and pat his head with less disruption of either task.

Returning now to the realm of speech and language production, when a young child is at the one-word stage of language development, the amount of simultaneous activity in different neural networks may be relatively small. As I indicated earlier, the child's task is to select a word from a small shelf of whole words and then produce it with simple prosody. But when the child moves to the two-word stage and beyond, he must select several words to make each sentence, and his chosen words must be assembled from a large storehouse of smaller segments rather than a storehouse of whole words. He must also work out a grammatical plan for the sentence and align it with a complex rhythm that spans the entire sentence. Some of the planning for the later parts of the sentence is going on at the same time he is beginning to produce the first words of the sentence, putting greater stress on developing cognitive factors such as memory. Clearly, these simultaneous but different tasks, involving interconnecting neural networks that are not fully mature, will sometimes interfere with each other. Think of the errors we all make when we try to do too many different things at the same time. The hesitations, pauses, and repetitions in the speech of normal children who are learning to talk in sentences may be the equivalent of the stops and starts and confusion that children show when simultaneously performing tasks that interfere with each other.

Delayed and Deviant Speech and Language Development

When assessed on such measures as the ages when they said their first words or uttered their first sentences, the size of receptive vocabulary, mean length of utterance, and expressive and receptive syntax, children who stutter often score lower than their nonstuttering peers (Andrews & Harris, 1964; Arndt & Healey, 2001; Bernstein Ratner & Silverman, 2000; Berry, 1938; Darley, 1955; Kline & Starkweather, 1979; Murray & Reed, 1977; Ntourou, Conture, & Lipsey, 2010; Okasha, Bishry, Kamel, & Hassan, 1974; Wall, 1980; Westby, 1979; Williams, Melrose, & Woods, 1969). However, other studies have not found language differences (e.g., Johnson, 1955; Miles & Ratner, 2001; Peters, 1968; Seider, Gladstien, & Kidd, 1982; Watkins, Yairi, Ambrose, & Grinager, 1999).

Young children who stutter have also been shown to have difficulty achieving age-appropriate speech. In the clinic, we often observe children in the early stages of stuttering who have multiple articulation or phonological errors and speech that can be difficult to understand. Research has repeatedly confirmed the finding that stutterers have roughly two and a half times the incidence of articulation disorders as that found in same-age nonstutterers (Andrews & Harris, 1964; Berry, 1938; Bloodstein, 1958; Bloodstein & Ratner, 2008; Kent & Williams, 1963; Williams, Silverman, & Kools, 1968). Nevertheless, several studies have found no differences in the articulation abilities of children who do and do not stutter (Ryan, 1992; Seider, Gladstien, & Kidd, 1982).

At least two excellent, critical reviews of the research on language, phonology, and stuttering have been published. Nippold (1990) suggests, for example, that research does not clearly support the hypothesis that children who stutter are also likely to have language or articulation difficulties. Rather, she proposes that there may be subgroups of children who stutter who have language or articulation problems related to their stuttering. Bernstein Ratner (1997) and Bloodstein and Ratner (2008) concurred and noted that the differences found between groups of children who stutter and children who don't stutter have been very subtle. They suggested that future research should use more sophisticated tests of language and phonology and look for subgroupings, not only in children but also in adults who stutter. Although not strictly a review of the literature, Watkins (2005) summarizes this research and gives an excellent overview of the many findings related to language and stuttering in the Illinois Stuttering Research Program. Her chapter suggests that there is no strong evidence that children who stutter have language delays or language difficulty; on the contrary, many children in their studies showed advanced language abilities near the onset of stuttering.

Findings of deficits in articulation and language performance, at least in some children who stutter, can be interpreted in several ways. Some authors have suggested that children who have articulation or language difficulties will start to believe that speaking is difficult. Their anticipation of such difficulty is hypothesized to lead to hesitation and struggle and then to stuttering (Bloodstein, 1995, 1997; Bloodstein & Ratner, 2008). An alternative view is that stuttering, language disorders, and articulation errors all result from a common deficit, which might be passed on genetically. Because specific regions and pathways of the brain are responsible for speech and language-related functions, delayed development of (or damage to) these areas may result in language, articulation, or fluency problems in any combination. Small differences in how the brain processes such functions could tip the balance toward any of these disorders.

The literature on disfluencies of language-impaired children who are not considered stutterers provides support for a slightly different hypothesis about the relationship between language deficits or delays and stuttering. Several studies of language-impaired children have found that they—or a subgroup of them—evidence high frequencies of the types of disfluencies that are seen more often in children who stutter than in normal children, even though they wouldn't be considered stutterers (Boscolo, Ratner, & Rescorla, 2002; Hall, Yamashita, & Aram, 1993; Hodge, Rescorla, & Ratner, 1999). These authors speculate that the excess disfluencies result from difficulties in formulating and executing utterances just beyond the limits of their language abilities. Thus, when language resources are strained, fluency is sacrificed in order to meet the demands of language production. Perhaps these children need extra time to meet these demands, and part- and whole-word repetitions provide the needed time, or this may be what results when a speech production system is spinning its wheels, waiting for elements of the language plan to be ready for execution. These findings suggest that the association between stuttering and language delay or deficit may emerge from the demands of normal development on weak language formulation/production systems and result in high frequencies of stuttering-like disfluencies. Other factors, such as a vulnerable temperament, environmental pressures, or a traumatic life event, may turn these disfluencies into real stuttering.

In addition to the evidence that children who stutter have a higher incidence of language or articulation problems, researchers are finding evidence that articulation or language delays and disorders may be related to whether or not a child recovers from stuttering. This is reflected in the research of Conture, Louko, and Edwards (1993), Paden (2005), St. Louis (1991), and Yairi, Ambrose, Paden, and Throneburg (1996), whose findings suggest that children who stutter and also have phonological or language differences are more likely to persist in stuttering or take longer in treatment. As part of a large ongoing study of children identified and assessed close to the onset of stuttering, Yairi and colleagues (1996) found that children who later recovered from stuttering without treatment had higher scores on the Preschool Language Scale (Zimmerman, Steiner, & Pond, 1979) than the children who did not recover. It is noteworthy, however, that the children who later recovered as well as those whose stuttering persisted scored above the norms on this test. A more recent study of an extended cohort of these same children (Watkins, Yairi, & Ambrose, 1999) did not replicate the study's initial finding. Specifically, lexical, morphological, and syntactic analyses of the cohort's spontaneous language close to the time they began to stutter showed no differences between recovered and persistent groups of children. However, in looking at the phonological development of both groups near onset of their stuttering, Paden, Yairi, Ambrose, and Grinager (1999) found that the children who recovered from stuttering scored significantly higher on the Assessment of Phonological Processes-Revised (Hodson, 1986) than did those who did not recover. Thus, it appears that among factors measured near the onset of stuttering, a child's phonological status, but not expressive language status, may predict recovery. Children with delayed phonology are at risk for stuttering to persist.

COGNITIVE DEVELOPMENT

The studies reviewed here are not directly concerned with cognitive development but do show the link between cognitive abilities and stuttering. First, there is strong evidence that people with cognitive deficits, especially when deficits are relatively severe, have a high incidence of stuttering (Van Riper, 1982). An explanation has been suggested by Starkweather (1987), who noted that developmentally delayed individuals are slower in their overall acquisition of speech and language. Their extended period of acquisition may make them more vulnerable to speech breakdown because competition between language acquisition and motor speech production for limited neurological resources occurs over a relatively long period of time.

Individuals who have had traumatic brain injury, which usually affects cognitive functions such as memory and attention, also have an increased risk for fluency disorders (Jokel, De Nil, & Sharpe, 2007; Theys, van Wieringen, & De Nil, 2008). This may occur for more than one reason. In the first place, typically rapid and complex speech and language production depend on fully functioning perception, attention, working memory, and executive functions. When these processes are compromised, breakdowns in spoken language are likely to result. As an example, consider the effect of a faulty working memory on rapid retrieval of vocabulary or syntax. If some components of language are mistimed in relation to others, repetitions of words or syllables may result, just as an engine with an unsteady fuel supply will stop and start, stutteringly.

Yet another link between cognition and stuttering is found in a study by Yairi and colleagues (1996) indicating

that poorer cognitive skills are associated with lack of ability to recover from stuttering. Of the study's 32 children who began to stutter, 12 continued to stutter for 36 months or more. The two groups of stutterers, those who recovered and those who did not, were compared with a control group of nonstuttering children on an intelligence test—the Arthur Adaptation of the Leiter International Performance Test (Arthur, 1952). The group of children who continued to stutter scored significantly lower than the nonstuttering control group, although their mean score was not below the norm for the test. However, the children in the recovered group were statistically identical to the control group. Thus, some abilities associated with cognition may be related to a neural resilience allowing recovery from stuttering. In other words, children with slightly higher cognitive functioning may have the extra resources needed to reorganize their speech and language processing, allowing them to develop a workaround for the problem causing them to stutter.

ENVIRONMENTAL FACTORS
Parents

In the 1930s and 1940s at the University of Iowa, Wendell Johnson developed the "diagnosogenic" theory of stuttering (1942). This theory, which is described more fully in the next chapter, proposes that a child's parents misdiagnose normal disfluencies as stuttering. Their reaction to the "stuttering" then causes the child to try to avoid these normal interruptions of speech and struggle in a way that becomes real stuttering. Johnson's diagnosogenic theory generated a great deal of research on parents of stutterers. Were they different from the parents of nonstutterers? Were they unusually critical? Did they have unreasonably high standards of speech?

One of the first studies of parents of stuttering children was conducted by John Moncur (1952). He interviewed the mothers of both stuttering and nonstuttering children about their parenting practices and concluded that mothers of stuttering children tended to be more critical, more protective, and more domineering toward their children than the mothers of nonstuttering children. Not long afterward, Frederick Darley, a student of Wendell Johnson, investigated the attitudes of stutterers' parents in more detail. Using interview techniques based on Alfred Kinsey's studies of sexual behavior, Darley (1955) questioned the parents of 50 stutterers and 50 nonstutterers. Although there was a great deal of overlap in the attitudes of both groups, parents of children who stuttered had significantly higher standards and expectations, particularly with regard to speech. They had greater sensitivity to speech deviations and believed in early intervention for disfluencies, and their overall drive and need for domination was greater as well.

Johnson and his research associates (1959) expanded Darley's study to the parents of 150 stuttering and 150 non-stuttering children. Again, there was much overlap between both groups, but parents of children who stutter were reported to be more perfectionistic and to have higher standards of behavior than the parents of children who did not stutter. These studies by Moncur, Darley, Johnson, and others were largely responsible for the widespread belief that parents are a key factor in precipitating the onset of stuttering. Parents could transmit a culture's "competitive pressure for achievement or conformity," which may be the environmental factor most likely to be linked with stuttering (Bloodstein, 1987).

Let us digress for a moment from the Iowa studies that found competitive pressures to be common in the homes of stutterers. Different results were found in England. Gavin Andrews and Mary Ann Harris (1964), whose work was described in Chapter 2, collected and analyzed data from families in Newcastle, England. Andrews and Harris compared the medical and home visit records of parents of stutterers with those of parents of nonstuttering children and concluded that both groups of parents, most of whom were mothers, were generally similar in personality but differed in some key traits. The parents of stutterers were lower in intelligence, had poorer school records when they were younger, had poorer work histories, and provided poorer housing for their children. There was no evidence, however, that they criticized or pressured their children. This finding is a far cry from the reports of excessively high standards in the homes of children who stutter in Iowa.

Why are these results so different from those of the Iowa studies? There may be many reasons, but two come readily to mind. First, stuttering may emerge in children under many types of stress. In industrial England, the greatest stress may have come from social and economic disadvantages, but the greatest stress in Iowa may have been the high standards of upwardly mobile parents. Second, these different results may reflect differences in these researchers' expectations and theoretical biases of several decades ago. Americans tend to believe that everyone is created equal, and American researchers, especially those conducting studies in the heartland of the United States during the 1950s, would be predisposed to look for causes of stuttering in the environment rather than the child's heredity. In contrast, many British people at that time may have believed that inheritance plays a major role in determining one's life outcomes, and researchers in the United Kingdom would have been inclined to consider parents' intelligence and social class as likely causes of stuttering.

The hypothesis that lower class homes provide stress that may precipitate stuttering did not originate in England. John Morgenstern (1956), who investigated stuttering in Scottish children, found that stuttering was more prevalent in the lower class homes of skilled manual, weekly wage earners compared to homes in the Iowa studies. This, however, was a social stratum in Scotland that was upwardly mobile and may have expressed families' ambitions through high speech standards for their children. Here, we have a combination of forces if

Morgenstern's hypothesis was correct. The stress of lower class homes lies not in their deprivation but in the cultural pressure to perform well and rise above humble beginnings.

Studies of parents of children who stutter compared to parents of children who don't present mixed results. Some have reported that parents of children who stutter are more rejecting or anxious than are parents of children who do not stutter (Flugel, 1979; Zenner, Ritterman, Bowen, & Gronhovd, 1978), but others have found either small or no differences between the two groups of parents (Goodstein, 1956; Goodstein & Dahlstrom, 1956). In his thorough review of the home environments of children who stutter, Yairi (1997b) concluded that the mix of diverse findings boils down to the likelihood that children who stutter grow up in unfavorable environments—homes that may stress children. But he also noted that even though many studies suggest that parents of children who stutter may be somewhat anxious, overprotective, socially withdrawn, and prone to negatively evaluate their children, there is no evidence that these parental tendencies cause stuttering. Yairi went on to point out that since a child's risk for stuttering is often inherited, the parents of these children may themselves stutter, have stuttered in the past, or had contact with other family members who stuttered. Thus, their negative traits may be a result of their own experiences with this disability.

Speech and Language Environment

Several clinical researchers have examined parent-child conversational interactions, seeking to determine if parents of children who stutter talk to their children differently than parents of nonstuttering children. A review of many such studies was published by Nippold and Rudzinski (1995). In the following paragraphs, we highlight some of the important studies in this area. Susan Meyers and Frances Freeman (1985a, 1985b) compared the speech of mothers of stuttering children with that of mothers of nonstutterers. They found that mothers of stutterers spoke more rapidly than did the mothers of nonstutterers. This may be critical, since a mother's high speech rate may encourage a child to try to speak faster than his optimal speed (e.g., Jaffe & Anderson, 1979). The possibility that rapid speech rates may lead to stuttering is consistent with Johnson and Rosen's (1937) finding that adult stutterers were more likely to stutter when they spoke more rapidly than their habitual rates. Children who stutter may be even more vulnerable to fluency breakdowns during rapid speech than adults who stutter by virtue of the fact that children's natural rates of speech are slower and their temporal coordination less than those of adults (e.g., Kent, 1981). Also, remember from Chapter 2 that Kloth, Janssen, Kraaimaat, and Brutten (1995), Kloth, Kraaimaat, Janssen, and Brutten (1999) found that children at risk for stuttering who developed stuttering spoke faster than those at risk who didn't develop stuttering.

However, several studies subsequent to those of Meyers and Freeman (1985a, 1985b) failed to find speech rate differences between parents of children who stutter and parents of children who don't stutter. For example, Kelly and Conture (1992) found no differences in the speaking rates of mothers of these two groups of children, Kelly (1994) found no differences in the rates of fathers of the two groups, and Yaruss and Conture (1995) found no differences in the articulatory rates (the rate at which each individual phrase is spoken, in contrast to "speaking rate," which includes pauses between phrases) between mothers of stuttering children and mothers of nonstuttering children. However, the latter researchers did find a significant correlation between children's severity of stuttering and parent-child differences in speaking rate; greater differences in parent-child speech rates were associated with more severe stuttering in the children. These results could have been obtained if more severely stuttering children talk more slowly than other children and their parents have speech rates similar to other parents in the study. It is also possible that greater parent-child differences in rate make a child who already stutters more severe.

In general, earlier studies found differences between parents' speaking rate but later ones didn't. Why might this be so? Zebrowski (1995) discussed this disparity in her review of the conversational patterns of families of children who stutter. She suggested that differences in measurement techniques and the fact that Meyers and Freeman (1985a, 1985b) had a larger number of severe stutterers in their sample might account for the differences in the studies. We think it is possible, also, that parents of children just beginning to stutter have become increasingly aware of the importance of speaking slowly because of publicity aimed at stuttering prevention. Such parents may try to speak more slowly than is typical for them while they are under the scrutiny of clinical researchers, thus adding to the likelihood that more recent studies may not find differences in the speaking rates of parents of stutterers and nonstutterers.

Another suspected parental stress, in addition to rapid speech rates, is the frequency with which parents interrupt their children. One of Meyers and Freeman's reports (1985a) presented some unexpected evidence about interruptions. The mothers of both stuttering and nonstuttering children interrupted most frequently when a child was disfluent. It seems possible that such parental interruptions, some of which may have been elicited by the child's disfluencies, may in turn elicit changes in the child's speech. Some children might increase tension and rate, thereby developing the struggled behaviors of stuttering. Others might suppress disfluencies to avoid interruptions and eventually be "taught" by parents not to be disfluent.

In a later study, Kelly and Conture (1992) found no significant differences in the interruptions of mothers of stuttering children and those of mothers of nonstuttering children. However, a closer inspection of their data revealed a correlation between the duration of "simultalk" (one person talking at the same time another is talking) of the mothers of children who stutter and the severity of their stuttering. Thus, mothers of more severe stutterers did more simultalk when their children were talking than did mothers whose children stuttered less severely. In a later study of fathers, Kelly (1994) found no differences in the interruptions of fathers of children who stutter and those of fathers whose children don't stutter. Moreover, the correlation between these fathers' simultalk and severity of stuttering was not significant.

Another variable of children's speech and language environments that has been studied is the extent to which parents ask questions. Meyers and Freeman (1985a) found no significant difference in the number of questions asked by mothers of children who stutter compared to that of mothers of children who do not. Langlois, Hanrahan, and Inouye (1986), however, did find significant differences when making a similar comparison. Langlois and Long (1988) then conducted an experimental treatment of a 4-year-old who stuttered, in which the mother was taught to reduce the number of questions she asked, among other changes. After 16 treatment sessions in which the mother had markedly reduced her number of questions and given her child more speaking turns, the child no longer stuttered. This finding is especially interesting because it is tempting to assume that asking questions results in more stuttering. However, subsequent studies tested this assumption and failed to support it. In a study of eight stuttering children in conversations with their parents, Weiss and Zebrowski (1992) found that the children stuttered less when they answered questions than when they made assertions. This appeared to be related to the fact that questions were often answered with brief responses, but assertions were often longer responses. A more direct test of the effect of parents asking questions was carried out by Wilkenfeld and Curlee (1997), who used a single-subject ABAB design to vary an adult's verbal behavior (questions versus comments) in conversations with a child who stuttered. Their results with three children who stuttered demonstrated that stuttering did not appear to be related to whether the adult asked questions or commented but was more likely to occur in either condition when the child's utterances were longer.

It is becoming evident that findings about speech rates, interruptions, and questions in the conversations of parents with their children who stutter are equivocal. But what about the linguistic complexity of their speech? Miles and Ratner (2001) conducted a study of the overall complexity of the language of parents of children who stutter, gathering samples of conversations from 12 mother-child pairs involving stuttering children and 12 involving fluent children. All children were between 27 and 48 months of age, and the stuttering children were within three months of the onset of their stuttering. Mothers' utterances were assessed for syntactic complexity, lexical diversity and rarity, and mean number of utterances per turn. No significant differences between the mothers of the stuttering children and the mothers of the fluent children were found.

Two recent studies have taken a different approach to examining the effects of parents' verbal behavior on children's stuttering. The complexity of mothers' language was examined in relationship to whether or not their children recovered from stuttering. Kloth and colleagues (1999) studied 23 children who stuttered, 16 of whom had recovered after four years and seven of whom had not. The complexity of the mothers' language was measured in terms of mean length of utterances in words in conversations with their child, both before and immediately after the onset of stuttering. They found that the language of the mothers of children who persisted in stuttering was significantly more complex than that of the mothers of children who recovered both before their children began to stutter and again after stuttering began. In another study of persistent and recovered stutterers, Rommel, Hage, Kalehne, and Johannsen (2000) assessed the complexity of the language of 71 mothers soon after their children had begun to stutter, rather than before stuttering began. They followed these children for three years and found that one of the more powerful predictors of whether or not a child would recover were "the linguistic demands to which the child is exposed" (p. 181). More specifically, these researchers found that the more complex the mother's syntax (mean length of utterance or MLU) and the greater number of different words she used in talking to her child, the more likely that her child would not recover over the following three years. The language abilities of the children had no predictive value (Rommel et al., 2000). The findings of these two studies support the hypothesis that the language environment of a child who stutters may influence recovery.

Nippold and Rudzinski's (1995) review of research on parents' speech and children's stuttering, covering studies published through the mid-1990s, makes it clear that there was only weak support for the hypothesis that parents of children who stutter have more demanding verbal interaction styles than do other parents. However, the findings by Kloth and colleagues (1999) and Rommel and colleagues (2000) about recovered and persistent stuttering in children suggest that earlier researchers were asking the wrong questions. Asking if the parents of children who stutter talk faster, interrupt more, ask more questions, or use more complex language than do other parents suggests that earlier studies had assumed that such parent behaviors causes stuttering in otherwise normal children. However, given the strong evidence cited in Chapters 2 and 3 that stuttering has a neurophysiological basis, it is unnecessary to look for a cause of stuttering in demanding parental speech patterns. It may be that parents of children who start to stutter have relatively typical speech and language patterns when talking to their children. The problem may be that these typical patterns don't particularly nurture the growth of fluency in children just starting to stutter, and thus, these children persist in stuttering. On the other hand, parents of children starting to stutter who simplify their language and slow their speech rates may facilitate their child's recovery from stuttering.

This ends the summary of the research findings on developmental, environmental, and learning factors associated with stuttering. I would like to remind the reader that the most recent article or book cited in this chapter is 2010. More up-to-date findings will be uncovered by using databases such as PsycINFO, PubMed, and Google Scholar.

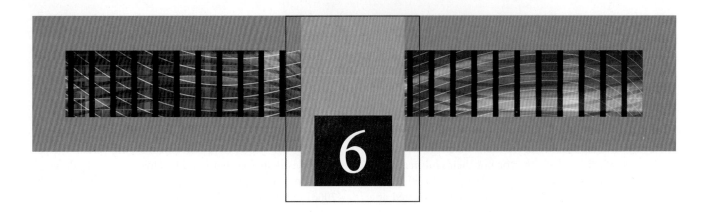

6

Theories about Stuttering

CHAPTER OBJECTIVES

After studying this chapter, readers should be able to:
- Explain what a theory is and what hypotheses are
- Identify five perspectives about constitutional factors in stuttering
- Identify three perspectives about developmental and environmental factors in stuttering
- Describe the author's integrated view of stuttering

KEY TERMS

Theory: An explanation of some phenomenon; regarding stuttering, a theory might explain why some people stutter and others don't
Hypothesis: A specific and testable proposition derived from a theory
Hemispheric dominance: In general, the phenomenon that one hemisphere of the brain (left or right) takes the lead or is stronger for a particular function. In the context of this chapter, hemispheric dominance refers to the fact that the left side of the brain is usually more specialized for speech and language than the right side
Inverse internal models of the speech production system: A concept about how your brain functions when you learn to talk as a child and as you are talking as an adult. The basic idea is that as a child hears speech in his environment, he stores auditory images of the sounds and words. During babbling, he learns how to send motor commands to his muscles to make those sounds and words

These connections create the internal model for speech production. They are called *inverse* because they start out as the auditory images or targets but get "inverted" to become the motor commands needed to hit those auditory targets

Sensory targets: These are essentially the auditory targets mentioned in the last definition, but actually the targets contain not only auditory information but also information about the movements of the articulators (kinesthetic and proprioceptive information)

"Covert repair" hypothesis: An explanation of stuttering as the result of the brain's stopping production of speech when it detects an error in the plan that the brain has made to produce a word

Multifactorial, dynamic disorder: Stuttering may be seen as multifactorial because many factors (e.g., genetic, emotional, cognitive, social, environmental) interact to create it. It is also dynamic because the overt signs of stuttering are seen as surface manifestations of an ever-changing neurophysiological process underlying the disorder

Diagnosogenic theory: A belief that stuttering is caused by the misdiagnosis of typical disfluencies as stuttering

Capacities and demands: A view of stuttering (often called the demands and capacities model) that suggests that stuttering results when the demands (e.g., pressure to talk rapidly) put on a child's speech are greater than the child's capacity for fluency (e.g., capacity to manage the complex components of spoken language production at a high rate)

Communicative failure and anticipatory struggle: A view of stuttering that supposes that stuttering begins when a child experiences problems with communication (e.g., having many repetitions or being told he must try harder to say sounds correctly) and then develops a fear of having difficulty, which then causes tension and fragmentation of speech

Primary stuttering: Early stuttering, near the onset of the disorder, that is characterized by loose, easy repetitions.

For those children who begin stuttering in this fashion, it is assumed that at first they are not aware of their stuttering and do not react to it

Secondary stuttering: Stuttering characterized by tension and struggle and sometimes by avoidances. In some views, this type of stuttering is thought to be a reaction to primary stuttering, as the child becomes self-conscious and frustrated by her difficulty with speaking

Myelination: The development of an insulating sheath around nerve fibers, increasing the speed and integrity of neural transmission. Myelination occurs primarily before age 5 and is achieved in left-hemisphere frontotemporal tracts before the right-hemisphere tracts

Sensory-motor modeling: The process of building "maps" that code the motor commands to hit the auditory (and kinesthetic and proprioceptive) targets that the speaker intends; a bidirectional process

Behavioral inhibition system: A view developed by psychologist Jeffrey Gray (1987) that humans are endowed with a hard-wired protective response to frustration and fear; the body's response in this situation is freezing, flight, or avoidance

Autonomic reactivity: The tendency of the autonomic nervous system to respond quickly and strongly to various stimuli. The sympathetic part of the autonomic nervous system is responsible for the flight-or-fight response and causes the heart, respiratory system, and other organs to be ready for action

Anomalous neural organization: Brain structure and function that differs from the typical. This often (but not always) causes problems because structures not well suited for certain activities (such as speech and language) are used and because subcomponents of speech and language may be located at some distance from each other, and neural transmission of information may not be efficient

What are theories, and what can we learn from them? A **theory** puts together findings in a systematic way so that past phenomena are explained and future ones are predicted. A theory about tsunamis explains how they are caused by earthquakes on the ocean floor and predicts that when a large undersea earthquake occurs again, another tsunami will occur. A theory about stuttering would take the many facts, findings, and observations that you have been reading about in the first five chapters and put them together to explain why one person stutters and another does not. A complete theory would also explain why a person stutters on some words and not others or in some situations and not others and why stutterers do the things they do when they stutter. When a theory can explain these things well, it can lead to effective treatment. When we know what causes stuttering, we will have a better chance of being able to modify it and perhaps even prevent it.

Scientists often use the word "theory" to mean a formal set of **hypotheses** that explain the important causal relationships in a phenomenon. These hypotheses are then tested, and the theory may be thrown out, improved, or partially confirmed as a result. The field of stuttering research and treatment hasn't developed far enough to have a formal theory of stuttering, although there are a number of informal theories that might be called theoretical perspectives or theoretical models.

In this chapter, I present several theories of stuttering as well as my own attempt to integrate research and clinical findings. I have organized the theories by the areas covered in Chapters 2 to 5—constitutional, developmental, and environmental factors. These models change every few years as more data are gathered on stuttering and new information is generated in related areas. Without a doubt, the explanations of stuttering I summarize in this chapter, including my own, will be superseded by others in a few years.

Theoretical Perspectives About Constitutional Factors in Stuttering

Anomalous Brain Organization

Inefficient Sensory-Motor Processing

Theoretical Perspectives on Developmental and Environmental Factors

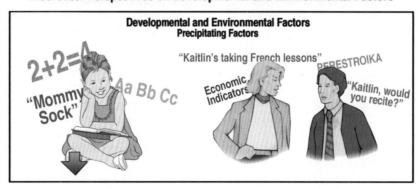

An Integration of Perspectives on Stuttering

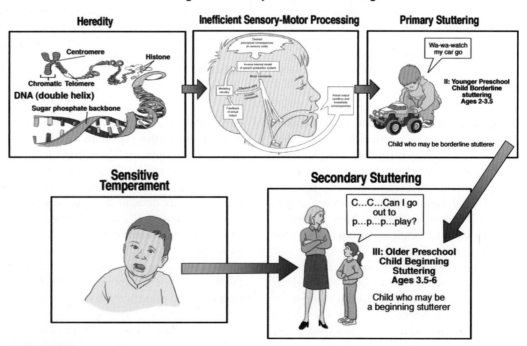

Figure 6.1   An overview of theories about stuttering.

THEORETICAL PERSPECTIVES ABOUT CONSTITUTIONAL FACTORS IN STUTTERING

I have chosen several contemporary views of constitutional factors to discuss in the following sections. Although the views differ, they are not mutually exclusive. If linked together, they provide us with some interesting notions about what factors might be inherited or acquired and how that might result in stuttering.

Stuttering as a Disorder of Brain Organization

Many studies of both normal speakers and brain-damaged patients have demonstrated that the left hemisphere is dominant for language in most people. This means that areas in the left hemisphere are specialized for processing language and that the right hemisphere is subservient to the left, playing a minor role in the production and comprehension of language.

One early theory of stuttering suggested that it is caused by lack of **hemispheric dominance** (the Orton-Travis theory of stuttering referred to in Chapter 2). The theory came about in this way. In an atmosphere of intense scientific curiosity and collaboration among researchers at the University of Iowa in the 1920s, Samuel Orton, a neurologist, and Lee Edward Travis, a psychologist and speech pathologist, observed that many stutterers seemed to have been left-handers whose parents changed them into being right-handed (Travis, 1931). They suspected that this change led to conflicts in the control of speech in which neither hemisphere was fully in charge, creating neuromotor disorganization and mistiming of speech, in turn resulting in stuttering. Travis and Orton's treatment derived from this theory was simply to switch stutterers back to being left-handed. This approach, as you might guess, turned out to be fruitless. Furthermore, there was never convincing evidence that high numbers of stutterers were originally left-handed. Consequently, the original cerebral dominance theory of stuttering languished for many years. But in the 1960s, evidence began to accumulate that stutterers may not, after all, have normal left-hemisphere dominance for language. In the 1970s and early 1980s, more published studies supported this finding.

In 1985, a new version of the cerebral dominance theory of stuttering was proposed. Two neurologists, Norman Geschwind and Albert Galaburda, proposed that many disorders, including stuttering, dyslexia, and autism, resulted from delays in left-hemisphere growth during fetal development that led subsequently to right-hemisphere dominance for speech and language (Geschwind & Galaburda, 1985). The delay in left-hemisphere growth that resulted in these predominantly male disorders was thought to be caused by a male-related factor. Geschwind and Galaburda hypothesized

that these delays might result from fetal exposure to excess testosterone during embryonic development. So far, however, no evidence has been found to support their hypothesis about testosterone. In fact, Neilson, Howie, and Andrews (1987a) provided some evidence against this hypothesis, but the idea of a delay in left-hemisphere development continues to be of great interest.

Geschwind and Galaburda's theory suggests that a delay in left-hemisphere growth and development may affect speech and language for the following reasons. Various left-hemisphere structures that evolve during embryonic development appear to be especially suited for speech and language functions. As these structures develop, specialized nerve cells that are genetically programmed to sprout the neural connections for speech and language processes disperse from their point of origin in the "neural tube," where the central nervous system is formed. These nerve cells normally migrate to previously developed structures in the left hemisphere that are appropriate for their specialized functions. But if development of left-hemisphere structures is delayed, cells migrating from the neural tube may not receive the "homing beacon" they need to reach the left hemisphere. Instead, these specialized cells receive signals from the more developed right hemisphere and migrate there instead. These specialized cells then organize themselves as "networks" of neural activity in the right hemisphere for processing of speech and language. However, because the right hemisphere is not designed by its architecture and interconnections for this function, speech and language operate inefficiently there, like the Internet search engine Google trying to access information through the postal service.

Although speculation about atypical cerebral localization in stutterers has received some support from research, especially from the recent brain imaging studies reviewed in Chapters 2 and 3, details of how stuttering behaviors result from abnormal localization are another issue requiring other theories that will be described in a later section of this chapter.

William Webster has proposed another version of the view that stuttering results from anomalous cerebral organization. As I noted in the discussion of studies of nonspeech motor control in Chapters 2 and 3, Webster (1993a) studied the effect of interference on one task (sequential finger tapping) caused by another task (turning a knob in response to an auditory signal) done simultaneously by the other hand. He concluded that people who stutter have normal localization of speech and language in the left hemisphere but that their left-hemisphere structure for speech planning and sequencing, the supplementary motor area (SMA), is especially vulnerable to disruption by activities in other areas of the brain. Webster suspected the SMA because it is strongly connected to the motor cortex as well as to subcortical motor areas and is known to be involved in the initiation, planning, and sequencing of motor activities. The left SMA, located near the corpus callosum, receives input coming across this bridge from the right hemisphere as well as input from the left hemisphere itself. Because of its location and its multiple inputs from both hemispheres, the left SMA might be highly susceptible to disruption by excess activity from either hemisphere. Webster further suggested that individuals who stutter often may have overactive right hemispheres and speculated that overflow of right-hemisphere activation, especially from right hemisphere–regulated emotions (e.g., fear), would disrupt SMA functions in planning, initiating, and sequencing speech motor output.

Stuttering as a Disorder of Timing

Several authors believe that the known facts about stuttering point toward a disorder of timing. For example, Van Riper (1982, p. 415) stated that "when a person stutters on a word, there is a temporal disruption of the simultaneous and successive programming of muscular movements required to produce one of the word's integrated sounds…." Building on Van Riper's view, Kent (1984) marshaled several lines of evidence to support a hypothesis that stuttering arises from a deficit in temporal programming. He speculated that this deficit reflects the inappropriate localization of speech and language functions to the right hemisphere that results in an inability to create the precise timing patterns needed to perceive and produce speech efficiently. Like a conductor of a symphony orchestra who determines when each section plays, as well as its speed or tempo, mechanisms in the brain control the rate at which we speak and the order of movements for producing sequential sounds. Just as a conductor integrates the timing of an orchestra's several sections, the brain must coordinate complex timing relationships for phonemes, syllables, and phrases of speech.

Kent (1984) suggested that the inability to perform precise timing functions consistently may stem from a stutterer's left hemisphere being less well developed than the right hemisphere (cf., Geschwind & Galaburda, 1985). Because the left hemisphere is specialized for processing brief, rapidly changing events such as those needed for fine motor control of verbal output, a person who stutters may be disadvantaged when trying to process at the speed required for normal speech.[1] This central timing function, Kent points out, must not only regulate left-hemisphere aspects of speech production but must also integrate the production of rapid, left hemisphere–generated speech segments with the slower prosodic elements of speech.

Kent also noted that emotion may play an important role in disrupting the timing of the speech of someone who stutters. As I indicated earlier, the right hemisphere is believed to be heavily involved in the regulation of certain

negative emotions. The stutterer's deficit, then, may be that his timing functions for speech are arranged so that they are (1) less efficient than those of nonstutterers and (2) vulnerable to interference by right-hemisphere activity during increased emotion. How this deficit causes the repetitions, prolongations, and blocks we hear in stutterers' speech is not explained in this theory.

Stuttering as Reduced Capacity for Internal Modeling

Another view of constitutional factors in stuttering was advanced by Megan and Peter Neilson, whose research on stutterers' tracking abilities was reviewed in Chapter 2. The Neilsons proposed that the repetitions of beginning stutterers are the result of a deficit in their ability to create and use **"inverse internal models of the speech production system"** (Neilson & Neilson, 1987). This rather complicated sounding model can be easily understood if we go back to an assumption about how children learn to speak.

During the first year of life, infants store up perceptions of the speech sounds they hear around them and begin to play with speech sounds, trying to imitate what they hear. Gradually, as they grow older, children learn how to make these sounds accurately. Some scientists, like the Neilsons, believe that too much of the brain's neural resources would be required if children had to remember each of the movements needed to produce each sound of their language in every possible phonetic context. Instead, children are thought to develop a mental "model" of the relationship between their speech movements and sounds they hear. Just as someone beginning to play a trombone must learn the relationship between the movements of the trombone "slide" and the sounds that result, experienced trombonists have established mental models of the relationship of their arm movements to the sounds produced and are able to move the slide to produce a desired sound without having to think about it in any deliberate way.

A child, then, develops a mental model of the relationship between speech sounds and motor commands. The mental model in the brain might be called a sensory-motor model for speech, which the Neilsons call an "inverse internal model" of how speech is produced. It is an "inverse" model because it transforms or inverts sensory targets (i.e., heard speech sounds) into the motor commands needed to produce them. As infants learn to produce the sounds they hear, they constantly use and refine their sensory-motor model for speech. They plan a word or sentence in terms of what it should sound like (the target) and then rely on their sensory-motor model to generate the motor movement commands that will produce the speech targets they are trying to hit.

The process of learning to speak is something like learning to drive a car. At first, keeping the car on the road requires constant vigilance. But as we learn the relationships between

---

[1]This notion of the left hemisphere being specialized for more rapidly changing signals has recently been challenged by Boemio, A., Fromm, S., Braun, A. & Poeppel, D. (2005).

turning the wheel, stepping on the accelerator, and going where we want, the linkage becomes automatic, even when driving a stick-shift vehicle in stop-and-go traffic. Moreover, the linkage is refined as we encounter different driving conditions and different cars (e.g., cars with loose steering wheels and sticky accelerators). Just as drivers establish sensory-motor models for driving, children develop sensory-motor models for speaking.

Figure 6.2 is a schematic depiction of how the brain may transform desired sensory (perceptual) targets into motor commands for speech. In the figure, the desired output (the word or phrase, e.g., that a child intends a listener to hear) is fed into the internal inverse model of the speech production system. Here, the desired output is entered as sensory code of its expected auditory and kinesthetic results, which is "inverted" by the model to generate its output as movement codes or motor commands. Experience, practice, and vocal play help the child to acquire these inversions or transformations. Moreover, this internal model is continually updated as a child's speech and language skills mature and the speech production system changes with age. The internal model's motor commands are sent to the muscles of the speech production system, whose coordinated contractions produce the acoustic output that result in a planned utterance. Concurrently, ongoing planning and feedback of this process are fed into the modeling circuitry.

Let us retrace our steps for a moment; when motor commands are sent to muscles, a copy of these commands, which is called the "efference copy" by motor physiologists, is also sent to the modeling circuitry. Here, efference copy is transformed into its hypothetical output, which is a model, or template, of the output that should be produced based on the motor commands. This hypothetical output is continuously compared with feedback on the current positions and movements of the speech mechanism so that the inverse internal model can update its ongoing motor commands, if necessary, to produce the desired output more accurately. These components of the speech production process are assumed to involve the corticocerebellar structures and pathways that are commonly described in neural models of speech output (e.g., Neilson & Neilson, 1987; Neilson, Neilson, & O'Dwyer, 1992; Neilson & Neilson, 2005a, 2005b).

The Neilsons and their coworkers have used the inverse internal model of the speech production system to understand the performance of stutterers in experiments that tested their ability to track an auditory tone that changed unpredictably (Neilson, Quinn, & Neilson, 1976). The subjects heard an unpredictably changing "target" tone in one ear and a "cursor" tone, which they could control with a handheld device, in the other ear. Their task was to track the pitch of the target tone with the cursor tone as accurately as possible. The Neilsons' experiments found that stutterers were poorer than nonstutterers in tracking auditory tones that went up and down in pitch. Stutterers were still poorer than nonstutterers even after practicing the task. These findings suggested to the Neilsons that if stutterers had difficulty

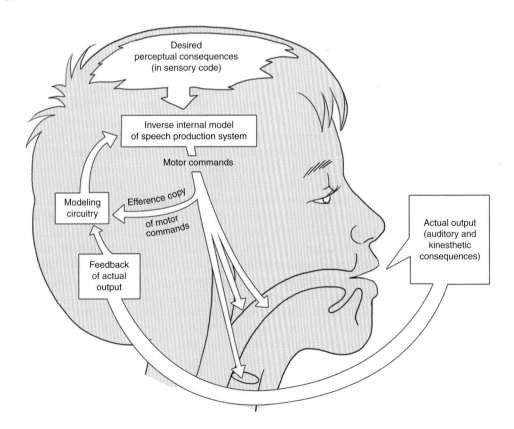

Figure 6.2 Schematic of the inverse internal model theory of speech production.

learning the relationships between the sounds they want to say and the movements required to produce them as young children, they would also, therefore, have difficulty making the sensory-to-motor and motor-to-sensory transformations required by the tracking tasks.

However, this difficulty would not always result in stuttering. When circumstances don't call for much of the brain's functional capacities in speech and language areas, stutterers should be able to compensate for their slight weaknesses. On the other hand, when large portions of the brain's functional capacity are allocated for language tasks, such as choosing new or unfamiliar words or constructing complex sentences, the diminished neural capacity cannot be accommodated, and more repetitions would result. As these researchers put it, "whether one will become a stutterer depends on one's neurological capacity for these sensory-to-motor and motor-to-sensory transformations and the demands posed by the speech act" (Andrews et al., 1983).

How do these intermittent deficits in available functional neural capacity result in the symptoms of stuttering? This theory attempts to account only for the core behaviors of early stuttering, that is, repetitions and prolongations. According to the theory, repetitions and prolongations result from inadequate transformations of **sensory targets**, transformations that should generate the motor commands for speech. A speaker with reduced functional neural capacity may begin to speak but be unable to plan and carry out the rest of his utterance without disruption. Repetitions or prolongations may occur if a speaker is attempting to push ahead with speech while his brain is still planning the syllables that follow and how to link them with the initial sound.

Recently, other researchers have also used the concept of inverse internal models to explain the behaviors of stuttering. The Neilsons' view was echoed in the perspective described in Guenther (1994), which was later adapted by Max, Guenther, Gracco, Ghosh, and Wallace (2004) to propose a theoretical model of stuttering based on unstable or insufficiently activated internal models. One of their hypotheses parallels the Neilsons' proposition that some children are predisposed to stutter because of the difficulty learning the relationships between their motor commands and the desired acoustic output. This difficulty would result in an inaccurate inverse internal model of the speech production system (Fig. 6.2), which would generate output that would not match the desired perceptual consequences. The speech production system would then "reset" itself to try again, producing repetitions (one for each mismatch). This resetting process would continue until the child's error-correction process could update the model sufficiently to make the output match the consequences. If this could be done quickly, only one or two repetitions would occur; if not, many repetitions would occur. The Max team's proposal has other hypotheses and an extensive review of the literature to support them.

Their proposal is particularly effective in relating various stuttering phenomena to aspects of the model. For example, the findings that stutterers' movements are slower during fluent speech (see Chapters 2 and 3) and the evidence that slow speech can induce fluency are both explained by the possibility that a slower rate of speech production would allow the stutterer more time for feedback to update the internal model. With a properly updated internal model, the actual speech acoustic output would match the intended perceptual consequence. Therefore, the system would not produce the repetitions that are thought to be a result of inaccurate speech output that doesn't match the intended perceptual consequences. In other words, slower speech makes corrections possible while a syllable is being produced rather than after it is completed. Note that if this hypothesis is accurate, errors would be found in the stutterer's unsuccessful repetitions.

Recent work by Cykowski, Fox, Ingham, Ingham, & Robin (2010) has updated this perspective on stuttering as a deficit in using inverse internal models for speech. Specific pathways in the brain used for sensory-motor integration—within the superior longitudinal fasciculus (SLF III)—have been found to be less efficient in adults who stutter compared to adults who do not. This new information will be described in detail when we present an integrated model of stuttering in the last section of this chapter.

Stuttering as a Language Production Deficit

Many researchers have been intrigued by the influence of linguistic factors on stuttering. For example, stuttering often begins when a child enters a period of intense language development. Similarly, stuttering is most frequent when the load on language functions is heaviest (e.g., in longer utterances, at the beginnings of sentences, and on longer, less familiar words) (Bloodstein, 2002). These factors have prompted several theorists to propose that stuttering reflects an impairment in some aspect of spoken language. I use the term "spoken language" because these theorists believe the major problem is not in the motor execution of speech, but rather in the planning and assembly of language units, such as phonemes, that occur before speech is produced.

Herman Kolk and Albert Postma (1997) developed the **"covert repair" hypothesis** to explain stuttering from a language production point of view. They believe that both stuttering and normal disfluencies result from an internal monitoring process that we all use to check whether what we are about to articulate is exactly what we mean to say. Perhaps this may be clearer if we imagine for a moment that language production is like a factory making bicycles (Fig. 6.3). The factory must monitor the quality of its bicycles by checking them at different stages. Some quality control checks occur after the bicycles leave the factory, when factory workers

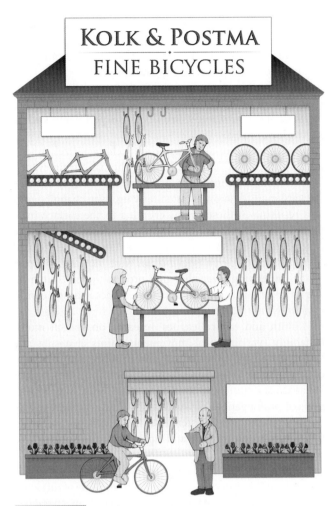

KOLK & POSTMA
FINE BICYCLES

Figure 6.3 Quality control in a bicycle factory as an analogy for part of the language production system in the brain.

themselves ride the bicycles and tell the factory about any defects they find. In speech and language production, this is like a speaker's auditory feedback (the sound of your own words as you are speaking them).

The bicycle factory might also use another quality control process, one that occurs inside the factory before the bicycles are shipped out. This is like our internal monitoring process of speech and language. Without being aware of it, we check the "phonetic plan" for what we are about to say before we articulate it. This allows us to detect potential semantic, syntactic, lexical, and phonological errors before they are produced. Just as the production line in a bicycle factory would have to be halted when a defect is detected, speech production is interrupted when our internal monitor detects an error in our phonetic plans. Repairs need to be made before production can continue. Kolk and Postma (1997) believe that the halting of production and the repair process cause the disfluencies of both normal speakers and individuals who stutter.

To Kolk and Postma (1997), the most common stuttering disfluencies (repetitions, prolongations, and blocks) are the result of correcting or "repairing" the phonological (rather than semantic, syntactic, or lexical) errors detected in the phonetic plan before they are spoken. In the case of part-word repetitions, if a speaker detects an error in the final part of a syllable (e.g., the /p/ in "cup"), he restarts the phonological encoding process ("cu-cu-") and keeps going until the phoneme is encoded correctly and the entire syllable can be produced. In contrast, prolongations are thought to occur when the phoneme of a word or syllable preceding the error is a continuant (e.g., the /l/ in the word "lip" when the error involves the vowel). In this case, the continuant, /l/, is prolonged until the speaker successfully encodes the vowel, /i/, following /l/.

Blocks are thought to result from errors in the initial sounds of words or syllables. When an error is detected, speech production is halted for repairs, but the speaker may try to plunge ahead, building up muscle tension, unaware of the automatic error detection and repair that is in progress. Kolk and Postma (1997) suggest that stutterers are prone to have more phonological encoding errors because they are constitutionally slower in encoding and need more time than a typical conversational rate gives them. In various articles, Kolk and Postma lay out the evidence supporting their views and suggest, among other things, that the benefits of a slower speech rate on stuttering are derived from the greater amount of time that stutterers have for phonological encoding.

Several years before Kolk and Postma (1997) published their covert repair hypothesis, an innovative language production view of stuttering was published by Wingate in *The Structure of Stuttering: A Psycholinguistic Approach* (1988). In this book, he reviewed linguistic and neurological research on stuttering and hypothesized that stuttering results from a dyssynchrony of functions in the left and right hemispheres, as well as subcortical structures. These different areas, Wingate suggested, are responsible for different components of language planning and production, such as consonants, vowels, and prosody. He theorized that when speakers produce the initial portion of a syllable, the consonant, vowel, and prosody must be synchronously blended. If some component lags behind at this critical moment, the result is a disruption in speech production that we observe as stuttering. Returning to our imaginary bicycle factory, it is as if the wheels, gears, and frame all must be assembled at the same time on a high-speed assembly line. If one component is delayed, production is halted. However, Wingate does not explain how this halt appears in speech as a repetition, prolongation, or block.

Perkins, Kent, and Curlee (1991) proposed another theory of stuttering as a deficit in language production. These authors suggested that stuttering results from a dyssynchrony between two components of language production. The "paralinguistic" component is a right hemisphere–controlled social-emotional process that is responsible for vocal tone and prosodic functions. The other component is linguistic and involves a left hemisphere segmental system that is responsible for the content and structure of language (semantics, syntax, and phonology). The two components must be integrated before spoken language is produced. If one lags behind the other for whatever reason, the resulting dyssynchrony produces disfluency.

Perkins, Kent, and Curlee (1991) add two elements to this dyssynchrony that must also be present if the resulting disfluency is stuttering, rather than just a normal disfluency. First, the speaker must experience time pressure either from an outside source or an inner feeling, so that he continues trying to speak even though the dyssynchrony in paralinguistic or linguistic processes has resulted in an incomplete or anomalous speech motor program. Second, the speaker must experience a feeling of "loss of control," which arises from being unaware of why he cannot say the word.

In our imaginary bicycle factory, Perkins, Kent, and Curlee's theory might be characterized as a production line that stops automatically whenever one of the two major subcomponents of a bicycle is not ready for assembly. However, the boss in this factory demands that the production line move rapidly, and the workers panic if the production line grinds to a halt. They frantically keep trying to restart production even though they don't know what the problem is or how to fix it.

Stuttering as a Multifactorial Dynamic Disorder

For almost 25 years, Anne Smith has been carrying out a systematic program of research on stuttering, developing a theory that at the core of stuttering is a motor speech disorder, the appearance and severity of which are influenced by a multitude of cognitive, linguistic, and psychosocial factors (e.g., Smith, 1999; Smith & Goffman, 2004; Smith & Kelly, 1997; Zimmerman, Smith, & Hanley, 1981). In arguing for the multifactorial nature of stuttering, Smith quotes Van Riper (1982) who makes the point that not only are there multiple factors acting in concert that determine if individuals stutter but that different individuals will have unique combinations of factors—different amounts of various factors—that determine their own stuttering fate.

Portraying stuttering as a **multifactorial dynamic disorder,** Smith thinks it is inappropriate to search for a single underlying "cause" of stuttering but instead thinks it's important to look for which factors interact in stuttering and determine *how* they interact. A good example of the way this view is manifest in Smith's research is the finding that when a group of individuals who stutter produce utterances that are longer and more linguistically complex, their speech motor coordination becomes more variable (movements of articulators are less regular when standard deviations are computed for many repetitions of a phrase), compared to a group of nonstutterers (Smith, Sadagopan, Walsh, & Weber-Fox, 2010). Despite the greater variability in their coordination, the individuals in the stuttering group did not overtly stutter as they produced the utterances in this experiment. Exactly how this greater variability does result in stuttering from time to time will probably await further study of other factors that can be manipulated in these experiments, such as psychosocial stress.

The multifactorial, dynamic view characterizes stuttering as a "dynamic" disorder because the "stuttering events" of repetitions, prolongations, and blocks are seen as only the outward manifestation of an underlying, ever-changing process resulting in these events erupting to the surface from time to time.[2] So in the experiment described above, there may be increasing speech motor instability as linguistic load increases, and if psychosocial stress were increased (as part of the underlying, ever-changing process), some stuttering events might surface. Perhaps this would occur in some individuals but not others.

Smith and her colleagues' research on speech motor instability (variability of movements) hints at a substrate that might be related to early or primary stuttering, but what can explain the secondary reactions of tension and struggle? What causes stuttering to change from brief, easy repetitions or prolongations of words and syllables that are hardly noticed by the child or listeners to the long, tense blockages that frustrate, embarrass, and upset both the speaker and often his audience?

Smith and her colleagues have done some important research on this aspect of stuttering as well. Some of this work has indicated that some moments of stuttering are characterized by rapid (5 to 12 Hz), rhythmic, oscillatory neural input to the muscles of speech so that they contract in a rapid, tremor-like way (Smith, 1989). Not every stutterer's muscles show these tremors during stuttering, however, and they may not appear in younger children who stutter but only in older children whose stuttering has persisted for some time. In one study, Kelly, Smith, and Goffman (1995) found that these neural oscillations were present in the stutters of the three older children in their study (ages 10 to 14 years) but were absent in the stutters of the seven younger children (ages 2 to 7 years). The researchers noted that such tremors may appear in the stuttering of only those individuals who have stuttered for some time and have developed maladaptive reactions. As Kelly, Smith, and Goffman (1995) pointed out, it is also possible that these tremors are evoked or magnified by autonomic arousal or the emotion that arises in response to the expectation or occurrence of speech difficulties.

---

[2]See Guitar, Guitar, Neilson, O'Dwyer, and Andrews, 1988 for early evidence in line with Smith and Kelly's view. This study found that electromyographic signals reflecting muscle contractions closely reflected whether moments of stuttering were clearly audible vs. subtly present versus not evident at all.

Several writers have linked stress with stuttering and suggested that the tiny tremors that appear in everyone's muscles may be amplified by emotion to a level that interferes with talking (Fibiger, 1971, 1972; Van Riper, 1982; Weber & Smith, 1990). The effects of emotion on tremor may provide a physiological explanation of how the mild disfluencies of young children become the more severe blockages we see as beginning stuttering evolves into advanced stuttering. Even mild disfluencies may trigger emotional responses in some children that result in increased tremors that block speech. Emotional responses may also explain the unusual cases of severe blocks at the onset of stuttering, especially when stuttering begins during conditions of stress and strong emotion. The interaction of very strong emotion with a child's vulnerable speech motor system may create sudden severe stuttering because it amplifies tremors in the speech musculature. Such tremors may be analogous to the quivering lip of a toddler who is about to burst into tears when frightened by a barking dog or by a screaming parent. Just how magnified tremors block or slow the forward movement of speech is not known, but Van Riper's (1982, p. 126) description of tension and tremor may give us some clues. He suggested:

> What usually seems to happen is that tremors begin when the stutterer creates a fixed closure, invests its antagonistic musculatures with tension, and then suddenly produces an increase of air pressure behind or below the closure. At the moment this increase occurs, the antagonistic musculatures become suffused with a sudden burst of further tension and the stuttering tremor comes into being. Then it persists…

Why stutterers would create fixed closures is a mystery. Perhaps it is one of the body's responses to fear that Gray (1987) described as a behavioral inhibition system, which I will discuss later in the section on secondary stuttering and temperament.

THEORETICAL PERSPECTIVES ON DEVELOPMENTAL AND ENVIRONMENTAL FACTORS

The three views presented in this section represent three different conceptualizations of how developmental or environmental stresses (or both) result in stuttering. One view is called the "**diagnosogenic**" view because it proposes that stuttering begins when parents mistakenly diagnose normal disfluency as stuttering. The other two views look more broadly at circumstances under which stuttering might arise. For example, the communicative failure and anticipatory struggle view assumes that some form of communication difficulty precipitates stuttering, whereas the **capacities and demands** view presumes that almost any developmental or environmental pressure may precipitate it. As you read this section, keep in mind that these three views differ not only in their concept of the roles that development and the environment play but also in their specificity. The first view (i.e., diagnosogenic) proposes that specific factors create stuttering; the last view (i.e., capacities and demands) describes how many different variables may interact to produce stuttering. The specificity of the remaining view (i.e., communicative failure) lies somewhere in between the two others.

Diagnosogenic Theory

In the 1930s, Wendell Johnson and other researchers at the University of Iowa began studying the onset of stuttering in children. As Johnson examined the speech of young stutterers and nonstutterers, he noticed a similarity. The most common disfluencies of both groups were repetitions. As Johnson contemplated this observation, he was struck by the possibility that all of these children may have had the same disfluencies to begin with but that those who became stutterers developed more serious disfluencies by overreacting to their repetitions. But why? Johnson speculated that perhaps their parents or other listeners mislabeled their repetitions as stuttering and in so doing, made the children so self-conscious that they tried to speak without any disfluency. Their efforts to avoid all disfluencies may have become what is generally regarded as stuttering (Johnson et al., 1942).

Johnson's hypothesis came to be called the diagnosogenic theory, meaning that stuttering was caused by its diagnosis or in this case, misdiagnosis. It was the most widely accepted explanation of stuttering throughout the 1940s and 1950s. It pinpointed environmental factors as the sole cause of stuttering by placing the blame on the negative reactions of parents and other listeners.

Johnson and his associates continued gathering data on the disfluencies of stuttering children and their nonstuttering peers to further support the diagnosogenic theory. The results of several studies were summarized in a landmark book, *The Onset of Stuttering* (Johnson & associates, 1959). Table 6.1, taken from Johnson's book, gives an overview of the similarities and differences in the disfluencies reported by stutterers' and nonstutterers' parents. Johnson interpreted these data as showing similarity between the disfluencies of stuttering and nonstuttering children; both groups of children were reported to show at least some of each type of disfluency. He suggested that the same disfluency types that parents of nonstuttering children considered normal were reported by parents of stuttering children as the earliest signs of stuttering. Johnson used this as evidence to support the diagnosogenic hypothesis that the problem was parents' interpretation of their child's disfluencies, or as some often put it, "the problem was not in the child's mouth but in the parent's ear."

It should be noted that later authors interpreted the data in Table 6.1 quite differently than Johnson did. The data were seen as evidence that the two groups of children were different at the onset of stuttering. McDearmon (1968), for

Table 6.1	Percentage of Parents of Stutterers and Nonstutterers Who Reported Child Was Performing Each Speech Behavior When They First Thought Child Was Stuttering						
Group	Repetition			Other Nonfluency			
	Syllable	*Word*	*Phrase*	*Sound Prolongation*	*Silent Intervals*	*Interjections*	*Complete Blocks*
Control (nonstutterers)							
Fathers	4	59	23	3	36	30	0
Mothers	10	41	24	4	41	21	0
Experimental (stutterers)							
Fathers	57	48	8	15	7	8	3
Mothers	59	50	8	12	3	9	3

From Johnson, W., et al. (1959). The onset of stuttering. *Minneapolis: University of Minnesota Press. Copyright © 1959 by the University of Minnesota. © 1987 Edna Johnson. Reprinted with permission of the University of Minnesota Press.*

example, argued that these findings showed that the disfluencies of normal children were notably different from those in the stuttering children. Syllable repetitions, sound prolongations, and complete blocks were reported to have occurred much more frequently in the stuttering children, whereas phrase repetitions, pauses, and interjections were reported more frequently in the nonstuttering control group. This reinterpretation of Johnson's evidence and new findings about genetic and constitutional factors in stuttering have caused the diagnosogenic view of stuttering to be largely abandoned.

To illustrate the diagnosogenic view, I take an example from a master's thesis that Johnson directed (Tudor, 1939). At that time, the diagnosogenic theory had not been formally proposed, but undoubtedly Johnson and others must have entertained the possibility that labeling a child as a stutterer would create more hesitancy in his speech. This thesis was an exploration of that idea. Johnson's student, Mary Tudor, screened all the children at a nearby orphanage for speech and language disorders. Tudor selected six children who were normal speakers, but she told these children that they should speak more carefully because they were making errors when they talked. She warned them that they were showing signs of stuttering. She also cautioned caregivers that these children should be watched closely for speech errors and corrected when they slipped up. After several months, Tudor went back to the orphanage and found that a number of these children showed stuttering-like behaviors. Although

she tried to treat them, at least one child was reported to have continued stuttering for some time thereafter (Silverman, 1988). Tudor was remorseful about these results and regretted conducting this experiment (Zebrowski, personal communication). Nonetheless, it reinforced Johnson's strong conviction, which he held throughout his career, that if a child is made self-conscious about his normal disfluencies, he may begin to stutter.

Communicative Failure and Anticipatory Struggle

The theoretical view of **communicative failure and anticipatory struggle**, developed by Oliver Bloodstein (1987, 1997; Bloodstein & Ratner, 2008), proposes that stuttering emerges from a child's experiences of frustration and failure when trying to talk. The child's original difficulty in talking *may* be the typical disfluencies of childhood, but other frustrations might instead be the provocation for stuttering. Many types of communication failure may lead the child to anticipate future difficulty with speech and thus increase tension. It is common, Bloodstein noted, to find delays in the development of articulation and language, cluttering, and other speech problems in the histories of children who begin to stutter. Table 6.2 lists some of the circumstances that Bloodstein suggested might cause some children to believe that speaking is difficult. If a child cannot make himself understood or is penalized for

Table 6.2	Experiences That May Make Some Children Believe Speaking is Difficult

1. Normal disfluencies criticized by significant listeners
2. Delay in speech or language development
3. Speech or language disorders, including articulation problems, word finding difficulty, cerebral palsy, and voice problems
4. Difficult or traumatic experience reading aloud in school
5. Cluttering, especially if listeners frequently say, "slow down" or "what?"
6. Emotionally traumatic events during which child tries to speak

the way he talks, he may begin to tense his speech muscles and fragment his speech, reactions that become the core behaviors of the child's stuttering. And these behaviors in turn result in more frustration and failure in communication, which the child anticipates with dread.

Other aspects of the child's "internal" and "external" environments and his development also play important parts. The child's personality may be perfectionistic, or he may harbor needs to live up to parental expectations. His family may have high standards for speech, find any speech abnormality unacceptable, or otherwise pressure the child to conform to standards beyond his reach. The presence or absence of these sorts of developmental and environmental pressures may cause some children to interpret an articulation difficulty, language problem, or disfluency as a failure, whereas other children only shrug it off.

This perspective on stuttering accounts for the wide variability of disfluency among children. Most normal children experience temporary frustration when learning to talk as they produce the mild fragmentations of speech we associate with normal disfluency. Children who stutter for just a few weeks may encounter unusual difficulty when first learning to talk but soon master the fundamentals and feel successful. Children who become chronic stutterers may be those who repeatedly experience communication failure and grow up in an environment fraught with communicative pressure.

Here is a case that illustrates some of the environmental pressures that some children who begin to stutter may experience. Susan grew up in the oil fields of Oklahoma, where her parents set themselves apart from the rest of the community by their aloof manner and precision of speech. They raised their children to feel that they were more cultured than their neighbors; in fact, Susan's father would often say, "We speak better than other people." Unfortunately, Susan's speech development was delayed. When she did begin talking in sentences at about age 3, she began to stutter with mild repetitions. When she started school, she worried that her father was embarrassed by her speech. Then she tried to speak better and began to push out the words instead of repeating the first parts of them. She soon developed severe secondary stuttering.

Although we have no way of knowing for sure, Susan's critical father may have been a major factor in the onset of her stuttering. However, many children grow up in families that are critical of speech but don't develop stuttering. Perhaps both a constitutional deficit, which led to her delayed speech development, and family pressure for perfect speech were necessary to produce Susan's stuttering. Neither may have been sufficient by itself to create stuttering, but together they may have been enough to tip the balance.

Capacities and Demands

A third interactional view of stuttering onset is proposed by the capacities and demands theory. Others have called this a "demands and capacities" view, but I prefer to put capacities first, because they exist in children before demands are placed on them. This view suggests that disfluencies as well as real stuttering emerge when a child's capacities for fluency are not equal to speech performance demands. Earlier in this chapter, I briefly discussed a narrow version of this view in describing the reduced capacity for internal modeling theory of stuttering. Andrews and colleagues (1983) stated that "whether one will become a stutterer depends on one's neurological capacity … and the demand posed by the speech act" (p. 239). These authors indicated that some demands come from the rapid development of language between ages 3 and 7 years. Other demands may come from fast-talking parents, whose speech rates may be hard for a child to keep up with. Demands for speech performance sometimes come from within the child, sometimes from outside stimuli, and sometimes from both.

Joseph Sheehan (1970, 1975) expressed an early variation of the capacities and demands view when he wrote that, "a child who has begun to stutter is probably a child who has had too many demands placed on him while receiving too little support" (Sheehan, 1975, p. 175). The demands that Sheehan pinpointed were primarily those of parents who have high standards and high expectations for their child's behavior. The support he refers to appears to be the environment's capacity to provide love, care, and encouragement. In addition, he believed that, "there are persisting reasons for retaining the possibility that some kind of physiological predisposition for stuttering exists" (Sheehan, 1975, p. 144). Thus, Sheehan, who is best known for a theory that stuttering is learned, professed the view that stuttering is precipitated by the demands of the environment interacting with a predisposition to stutter.

Starkweather (1987) added considerable detail to the concept of capacities and demands as an explanation of stuttering onset and development. The normal child's capacities, he points out, include the potential for rapid movement of speech structures in well-planned sequences that are coordinated with the rhythms of his language. Demands on the child include those of her internal environment, such as her increasingly complex thoughts to be expressed, which require more sophisticated phonology, syntax, semantics, and pragmatic skills. The external environment often places demands on the child's fluency through parents' interactions. Parents may ask questions rapidly, interrupt frequently, and use complex sentences choked with big words. They may show impatience about the child's normal disfluencies and may make the child feel that she meets their expectations only when she performs at high levels. These kinds of interactions can stress any child but are likely to push a slowly developing child to try to speak beyond her capacity for fluency.

Because a child's capacities develop in spurts and environmental demands fluctuate, stuttering may wax and wane in rapid cycles. A child may be highly fluent for a day or a week when he has mastered new speech and language skills and when external demands are low. But his stuttering may suddenly flare up if his capacities become strained by his efforts to use more advanced syntax or if the demands of the external environment suddenly increase when his fast-talking, interrupting, big-city cousins arrive for the Fourth of July holiday weekend.

The capacities and demands view provides a way to account not only for the day-to-day variability of stuttering within an individual but also the great differences between one individual who stutters and another. As Adams (1990) pointed out, some children may grow up in an environment with normal levels of demand but have limited speech production capacities. Others may have normal capacities for speech production but grow up with excessive demands for rapid, fluent speech.

Treatment based on this model would begin with a careful evaluation of the child's capacities and the demands in her environment. Therapy would be designed to enhance capacities, decrease demands, and provide support for the child and her family while these changes are taking place. Starkweather and his colleagues have used this approach to formulate a sensible and effective program of stuttering prevention (Gottwald, 2010; Gottwald & Starkweather, 1984, 1985; Starkweather & Gottwald, 1990; Starkweather, Gottwald, & Halfond, 1990). Figure 6.4 depicts the ratios of capacities and demands in a child predisposed to stutter. In one view, the demands are greater than the child's capacities and stuttering occurs. In the second, the demands are lessened, and although capacities stay the same, stuttering is diminished.

To illustrate the capacities and demands view more fully, the following case is from my own experience. Gina was a bright, happy 7-year-old. Her mother had been a severe stutterer as a child, but through treatment and her own perseverance, she had largely recovered. When Gina began the second grade, she had no history of stuttering or any problem with school. Some time before Christmas that year, however, when her class was learning to read, Gina began to dislike school, and her mother soon discovered that she was having problems academically. After some testing, it was discovered that she had a learning disability that had not been apparent before; however, once reading was required, it became obvious. As Gina struggled to cope with her reading problem throughout the rest of the second grade, she began to stutter. Over the course of the next two years, she stuttered noticeably but did not receive therapy. She was, however, given extra help for her reading disability. By the fourth grade, Gina was making headway with reading, and her stuttering had diminished to an inconsequential level without treatment.

Although there are various ways to account for the onset of Gina's stuttering and recovery, a capacities and demands view would see it this way: Gina was predisposed to stutter,

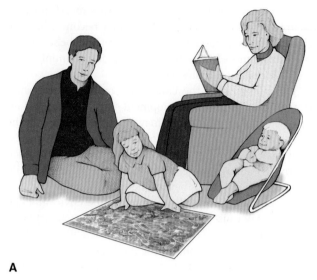

A

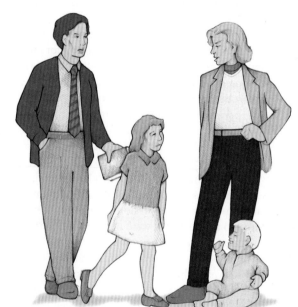

B

Figure 6.4 Two different ratios of capacities and demands and their hypothesized effects on fluency.

but it lay dormant until she was faced with the challenge of reading. Reading, at least when first learned, involves a highly conscious use of linguistic processes, in contrast to the more automatic linguistic processing used in listening and speaking. Consequently, learning to read puts a heavy demand on the pool of available resources that are also used for speech and language processing. Such demands may result in a reduced capacity (i.e., fewer available resources) for speech production, which may result in disfluency for a vulnerable child. In this case, Gina did not seem to develop a persistent fear of speaking as a result of her stuttering. Thus, when she overcame her initial reading difficulty and reading became more automatic (i.e., demanded fewer resources), her available capacity for speech processes increased, and she "outgrew" her stuttering.

Once again, the reader is reminded that the capacities and demands view is a model for describing relationships that appear again and again but are not well understood. As such, its major function is to help students and clinicians organize the complex interrelationships of variables associated with stuttering into a set of principles that may guide its treatment and suggest hypotheses for research.

AN INTEGRATION OF PERSPECTIVES ON STUTTERING

In this section, I will try to draw together some of the theoretical views just described coupled with my own speculations to provide a description of the etiology of stuttering that may guide your assessment and treatment. Figure 6.4 depicts the major components of this perspective.

A Two-Stage Model of Stuttering

Many years ago, a child psychiatrist who stuttered, Charles Bluemel, observed that stuttering begins in most children as repetitions, of which they are hardly aware and to which they don't react. He thought that over time, many of these children become aware of their disfluencies and react to them by increasing the tension and tempo of their repetitions. These repetitions then become fast, irregular, and halting as children are bothered by them and do what they can to stop them. As they tense further, the repetitions become blocks and sometimes prolongations. This can happen overnight in some children and over a period of months for others. Bluemel (1932) called the beginning behaviors **"primary" stuttering** and the later reactions **"secondary" stuttering**. Recently, Bloodstein (2001) concluded that this division of stuttering into primary and secondary phases is an appropriate description of the early development of stuttering. This view of stuttering as having two separate stages or components seems useful to me also and suggests the possibility that each component may have a different etiology. In fact, I think each may have a constitutional basis.

There are reasons to be cautious about embracing this apparently simple view. For example, primary and secondary stages of stuttering may overlap in children because the forces that create these stages wax and wane and make it hard to place them in one phase or another. Moreover, there is evidence that some children begin stuttering in the secondary phase (Yairi & Ambrose, 2005). Despite these exceptions, I will lay out an integrated view of stuttering on the presumption that there are, for most children, two stages of stuttering, and I will describe how the exceptions themselves can be explained in this view.

A Perspective on Primary Stuttering

In Chapters 2 and 3, we reviewed studies of brain structures and functions, sensory-motor coordination, central auditory processing, and hemispheric dominance. These studies support the view that individuals who stutter have differences in the way their brains process sensory information and produce motor output. Many of the brain imaging studies point to structural and functional anomalies in the language- and speech-generating areas of the left hemisphere with possible compensatory activity in homologous areas of the right.

The etiology of these differences in people who stutter appears to be either the result of inheritance or early brain damage. Either of these factors would affect how the brain grows during embryonic development or how the brain responds to injury. Let's look more closely at this process.

The development of speech and language networks in the brain begins soon after conception with the proliferation, migration, and differentiation of neural cells, a process guided by genetic predisposition and affected by external events, such as experience, injury, and disease (Chase, 1996). As neural cells continue to proliferate and differentiate, millions of synapses are formed, and pathways of communication emerge when clusters of cells send information back and forth in response to stimulation. Cells that communicate readily among themselves become self-organizing, functional neural circuits that perform various tasks. For example, after birth as an infant interacts with the outside world, groups of circuits in the infant's brain bind together to form "maps" or representations of the outside world to help them process incoming sensory information and produce appropriate motor responses (Edelman, 1992).

If there are anomalies in speech and language areas of the left hemisphere due to inheritance or injury, the developing brain will deal with them in a number of different ways. The most common is by extensive anatomical reorganization, including growth of new fibers, new synapses, and entire new cortical tracts (Hadders-Algra & Forssberg, 2002). This reorganization would attempt to establish the functional circuits necessary for the development of spoken language in whatever structures are available. If reorganization involves relocation of these circuits to areas that have not naturally evolved to serve these circuits, or if reorganization entails neuronal groups being placed at some distance from each other, these circuits will be both inefficient and vulnerable to disruption by other brain activities occurring in nearby areas. Vulnerability to disruption may occur if new circuits or even the original ones are insufficiently myelinated (insulated by a protective sheath), an outcome that would result in less-efficient transmission of neural signals. In fact, several researchers (Karlin, 1947; Cykowski et al., 2010) have suggested that inadequate **myelination** itself may be the reason why neural circuits for speech in language are

An Integration of Perspectives on Stuttering

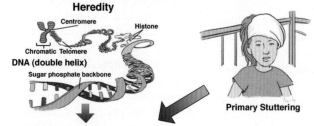

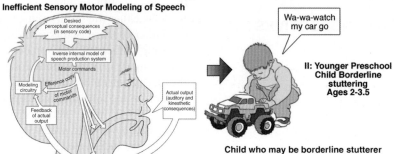

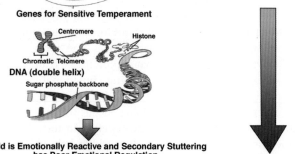

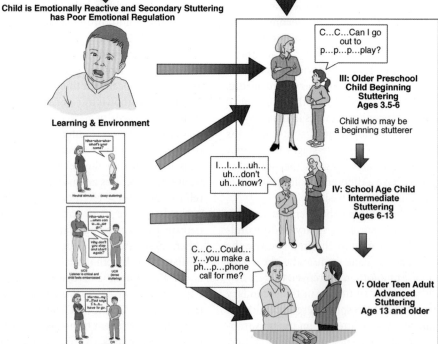

Figure 6.5 Integrated perspective on stuttering.

inefficient or vulnerable to disruption in the brains of those who stutter.

Which neural circuits underlying spoken language may be inefficient or vulnerable to disruption? One of the functions that often seems to be atypical in stuttering is sensorimotor processing, particularly auditory-motor processing. Because auditory processing plays a major role in infants' use of the sounds of adult speech and the sounds of their own babbling, a dysfunction in this area would obviously have an influence on the development of interacting neuronal circuits for speech and language production. The sounds of adult speech give infants auditory targets to aim for when they are learning to speak. The sensorimotor activity in babbling helps a child develop internal models that specify what articulatory gestures are needed to produce desired auditory targets (Guenther, Ghosh, & Tourville, 2006; Hickok & Poeppel, 2007; Neilson & Neilson, 1987, 2005a, 2005b). Moreover, the auditory information from babbling allows the child to adapt his internal auditory-articulatory model to his rapidly growing speech production mechanism (Callan, Kent, Guenther, & Vorperian, 2000). Because these circuits are self-organizing, they may develop a variety of solutions to the auditory processing problem. Some individuals may use homologous right-hemisphere structures for auditory processing, others may continue to use inefficient areas of the left hemisphere, and still others may try to do both.

Four of the brain imaging studies described in Chapters 2 and 3 suggest problems in the very pathways that would be expected to support **sensory-motor modeling** for speech. The findings of Sommer, Koch, Paulus, Weiller, and Buchel (2002), Chang, Erickson, Ambrose, Hasegawa-Johnson, and Ludlow (2008), Watkins, Smith, Davis, and Howell (2008), and Cykowski and colleagues (2010) suggest that individuals who stutter have less dense bidirectional fiber tracts between sensory and motor areas. If these fiber tracts are less dense, they are probably less efficient for rapid transmission of signals. Let's step through the process of speech production to see why this matters. Remember that according to the inverse internal model theory of speech production, when individuals plan to generate a word or phrase, they use the inverse internal model system (see Fig. 6.2) to generate motor commands (including making an efference copy—a copy used to rapidly produce a hypothetical output of the motor commands for error-correction purposes) based on the sensory target they are trying to produce. However, this inverse internal modeling system depends on continuous back-and-forth communication between sensory and motor areas. Sensory areas supply information about the current tension in muscles and positions of speech structures, while motor areas use this information to plan and carry out the motor commands to speech system muscles to produce speech output. Then sensory areas analyze both the efference copy of the motor plans as well as the actual speech output to correct errors and update the internal model.

Rapid information flow between sensory and motor areas is critical for accurate and fluent speech. If there is a delay in the information needed to generate the motor plans and execute them, repetitions may occur. This often happens after the speaker produces the first sound, syllable, or word. This sound or syllable of the utterance is usually fluent because it can be based on already obtained sensory information about the resting state of the speech system structures. But new information is needed to go forward—information required for production of the next sound, syllable, or word. However, that information is often delayed because it depends on rapid updating of information about the new state of the speech system (sensory analysis) and the rapid analysis of the sound just produced (comparison of efference copy of motor commands and feedback of actual output). Again, see Figure 6.2 for a description of the process.

This description of dyssynchrony in the assembly of components of speech and language production is intended only as a possible explanation of primary stuttering, which is a stage of stuttering characterized by relatively relaxed repetitions and occasional prolongations that typically occur, as Bloodstein (2001, 2002) has suggested, at the beginnings of phrases or sentences. As indicated in the paragraph above, the first sound or syllable may be fluent but the second is often a repeat of the first, li-like this. Most children who begin to stutter outgrow their primary disfluencies as their speech and language systems mature or as they develop effective ways to work around the problem. Other children, however, react to their primary stuttering by increasing the speed and tension of their disfluencies. They go on to develop the characteristics of secondary stuttering: blocks, escape behaviors, and avoidance reactions. Why? And why do some children begin to stutter with blocks rather than repetitions? The answer, I think, can be found in the temperament of these children, interacting with the processes of learning.

A Perspective on Secondary Stuttering

In earlier sections I mentioned that several authors have suggested that the speeding up, tension, struggle, escape, and avoidance behaviors of secondary stuttering are a reaction to the simple repetitions of sounds and syllables that often characterize stuttering when it first begins. I now want to make the case that the child's temperament and emotional responses interacting with learning can explain the behaviors of secondary stuttering.

Temperament

This section focuses on the personality or temperament of children and uses both "sensitive" and "reactive" to refer to the same thing: a behavioral and emotional style characterized by being easily aroused by novel stimuli, as well as a tendency to withdraw when confronted by unfamiliar people or situations. Kagan (1994a, 1994b) often uses "inhibited" to describe the same traits. There is evidence, which was discussed in Chapters 2 and 3, that individuals who stutter tend to have more sensitive or reactive temperaments (Anderson, Pellowski, & Conture, 2001; Embrechts & Ebben, 1999; Fowlie & Cooper, 1978; Guitar, 2003; LaSalle, 1999; Oyler & Ramig, 1995; Wakaba, 1998). If so, such reactivity may explain why some children who stutter eventually respond to their disfluencies by tightening their muscles. Research on normal children who have sensitive temperaments indicates that they respond to novel, threatening, or unfamiliar events by increasing their physical tension, particularly in the larynx (Kagan, Reznick, & Snidman, 1987). If children who stutter have more sensitive temperaments than their peers, they may be more likely to increase their laryngeal tension in response to primary stuttering, which they experience as threatening because it seems out of their control. This may be the mechanism that causes many children's disfluencies to change from easy, relaxed repetitions to tense repetitions and progressively more involved secondary behaviors.

The increases in physical tension just mentioned may be part of a larger defensive response that is triggered more easily in individuals with reactive temperaments. In describing his **behavioral inhibition system**, Gray (1987) proposes that when individuals experience frustration or fear, their innate response is freezing (i.e., widespread muscular contractions that produce tense and silent immobility), flight (i.e., speeded up activity to escape), or avoidance. Gray (1987) indicates that these unconditioned responses may occur rapidly without intervening autonomic arousal, arising from the central nervous system substrate underlying the increased muscle tension, increased tempo, and escape behaviors and avoidance behaviors that characterize secondary stuttering. It is notable also that Gray suggests that the way that individuals' behavioral inhibition systems affect behavior is influenced by temperament. The more reactive individuals are, the more they will engage in freezing, flight, or avoidance responses when experiencing fear.

Further evidence of a neurological substrate underlying the characteristics of secondary behavior is provided by the research of Davidson (1984), Kinsbourne (1989), and Kinsbourne and Bemporad (1984), which was described in Chapters 2 and 3. They propose that the right hemisphere is specialized for emotions that accompany avoidance, withdrawal, and arrest of ongoing behavior, whereas the left hemisphere is specialized for emotions that are associated with approach, exploration, and release of ongoing behavior. Thus, it can be argued that individuals who stutter and are more reactive are more prone to behaviors regulated by right-hemisphere emotions. This argument is supported by the findings of Calkins and Fox (1994) and Davidson (1995)

who reported that sensitive children are right hemisphere–dominant for emotion. Their research may also explain why secondary behaviors develop in the forms they do in many stutterers. Those beginning stutterers who develop secondary behaviors may be more sensitive individuals whose innate defensive mechanisms, the behavioral inhibition system of Gray (1987), are triggered more easily because of their right-hemisphere dominance for emotions. It is possible that some of the excess activity seen in the right hemisphere of those who stutter, described in Chapters 2 and 3, may be related to activation of behavioral inhibition. These stutterers, especially those whose behaviors at onset are characterized by tension and struggle, may not be likely to spontaneously outgrow their stuttering.

The notion of greater emotional reactivity in children who stutter is supported by a study of 65 children who stuttered and 56 children who did not by Karrass and colleagues (2006). They found that compared to nonstuttering children, children who stutter have greater emotional reactivity, less emotional regulation, and poorer attention regulation. These authors suggest that this combination of traits contributes to the development of stuttering in a "reverberant" fashion. Reacting to what I would term "primary stuttering," these children have a strong emotional response to their primary stutters and they are unable to regulate this emotion. This in turn makes them stutter more (and more severely), and they have even stronger emotional responses to the more severe stutters and on and on.

The importance of emotion in secondary (persistent) childhood stuttering is also supported by recent genetic evidence. As I indicated in Chapters 2 and 3, mutations in several genes, including GNPTG, have been linked to persistent stuttering, and it is also known that this same gene influences the development of the cerebellum and the hippocampus (Kang et al., 2010). The cerebellum is known for its role in motor control and in emotional regulation (e.g., Schmahmann & Caplan, 2006). The hippocampus is also a structure which influences emotion and is a key component of Gray's behavioral inhibition system, described above. Thus, many lines of evidence converge on the link between secondary stuttering and emotion.

I've described many of the temperamental and emotional factors related to secondary stuttering as though they were completely within the child. But of course the child interacts with a complex environment, and this influences temperament and emotion, which in turn influence stuttering. An example that comes to mind is a girl and her mother in a study of parent-child interaction that we published many years ago (Guitar, Kopff-Schaefer, Donahue-Kilburg, & Bond, 1992). We computed correlations between several variables in the mother's talking and the girl's primary stuttering and secondary stuttering. What we found led us to surmise that different aspects of the mother's conversation affected the two types of stutters differentially. The mother's speech rate was highly correlated with the girl's primary stutters but not with her secondary stutters. On the other hand, the mother's nonaccepting comments were highly correlated with the girl's secondary stuttering but not her primary stuttering. We speculated that when her mother made nonaccepting comments to her, the girl reacted with negative emotion, triggering secondary stuttering. We also speculated that when the mother talked fast, the girl tried to keep up, but because of an inefficient speech processing system, she stuttered with the easy repetitions of primary stuttering.

Learning

It has been evident for some time that learning plays a major role in persistent stuttering—stuttering that continues beyond the primary stage and usually grows more severe. In the last section of Chapter 5, I described the major types of learning involved in stuttering, but I did not deal with the question of why some children seem more vulnerable to this learning than others. One answer to this puzzle was given by Brutten and Shoemaker (1967) in their influential book, *The Modification of Stuttering*. They proposed that individual differences in conditionability and in **autonomic reactivity** are a constitutional predisposition in stuttering. My own understanding of the role of learning, described in the following paragraph, is in agreement with theirs and adds some detail from recent literature about emotional learning.

The perspective given earlier that some children who stutter are more temperamentally reactive and thus are more prone to physical tension, rapid escape behaviors, and avoidance suggests that these children will also be more emotionally conditionable. That is, the physiology that predisposes these children to be temperamentally reactive involves the limbic system, especially the amygdala, which is that part of the limbic system that stores emotional memories. This is what makes learning for them under conditions of strong emotion so indelible.

Emotional events are etched into the brain more strongly than neutral ones. Think about how well you can remember what you were doing when you found out about a very exciting or upsetting event. Many people can remember vividly what they were doing when they heard about the planes crashing into the twin towers of the World Trade Center in New York City on September 11, 2001. The strength of emotional memories is enhanced even further in people with more reactive limbic systems, which may account for why some people suffer posttraumatic stress syndrome and others do not. Children with reactive limbic systems are more likely to react to the multiple repetitions of primary stuttering with tension, escape, and avoidance and are also much more likely to store their memory strongly (e.g., LeDoux, 2002). Such reactions and memories can snowball. The child's natural fear response to a repetition that feels out of control is to tense his muscles. This increased tension soon makes the stutter last longer, which increases his feeling that he is helpless

and triggers a bigger fear response. Stuttering experiences become even more traumatic as the child increases physical tension because of his initial negative emotion, which causes repetitions to become tense prolongations or blocks. These new, tense forms of stuttering can be more unpleasant to the child and can provoke expressions of anxiety and alarm from his parents. The child's stronger feelings of "stuckness" and his concern about his parents' alarm are likely to generate more activity in the limbic system, thereby creating stronger memories that will trigger these more tense forms of stuttering more quickly whenever he experiences primary stuttering. The child's reactive amygdala mediates the storage of unpleasant memories of stuttering, largely on an unconscious level. At the same time, another part of the limbic system, the hippocampus, stores information about the situations in which stuttering occurs (e.g., who the child was talking to, what word was being said, where it happened). These contextual cues cause stuttering to spread rapidly from isolated experiences to more and more repeated experiences in similar contexts and eventually to many other situations.

Children with reactive temperaments are not only more likely to learn to increase tension when they anticipate or experience stuttering but are also more likely to engage in other components of the behavioral inhibition system. These include increases in tempo, other aspects of escape behaviors, and a wide array of avoidances. Thus, these children quickly develop secondary symptoms, such as eye blinks and changing words, to avoid or escape stuttering.

Emotional conditioning occurs rapidly in these children, but unlearning is a much slower and more difficult process. There is evidence that emotional memories are stored permanently, and even when new behaviors replace them, the original emotions and learned behaviors may reappear under stress (Ayres, 1998). When clinicians work with individuals who have secondary stuttering, they need to keep in mind the strength and persistence of behaviors learned through fear conditioning. New behaviors will have to be learned as new responses to the stimuli that elicited the old responses. Because emotional conditioning may produce cortical as well as subcortical changes in the brain, cognitive therapy may be a useful adjunct to behavioral therapy in older children and adults.

Two Predispositions for Stuttering

This view of primary and secondary stuttering proposes that there are two constitutional predispositions: one for primary stuttering and one for secondary stuttering. As may be evident, the most common occurrence is for a child to have a predisposition for primary stuttering that is resolved through neural maturation or reorganization—this accounts for the 70 percent or so of children who spontaneously recover. It is also possible for a child's primary stuttering to continue into adulthood and for secondary behaviors never to emerge;

these adults may simply be considered highly disfluent, rather than stutterers. Some children, of course, do acquire secondary behaviors in response to their primary stuttering, and I would hypothesize that these children have the second predisposition, a reactive temperament, which leaves them prone to the tension, escape, and avoidance behaviors that characterize secondary stuttering. I believe that neither of these predispositions is "all or nothing;" that is, a child may have a little or a lot of either. For instance, an adolescent may have a substantial amount of repetitions in his speech but only occasionally show tension, escape, or avoidance behaviors. Or a child may start stuttering suddenly at age 3, with severe stutters marked by struggle, tension, escape, and avoidance. Perhaps that child has only a little predisposition for primary stuttering but a substantial predisposition for secondary stuttering. This continuum for stuttering agrees with most clinicians' observations that we see a wide range of severity, from mild to very severe, with some stutterers having little avoidance and others having a great deal. I also notice that outside the clinic, there are many individuals whose "stuttering" is so mild that they don't recognize it in themselves and other lay persons don't notice it either.

The possibility of two predispositions for stuttering may also shed light on such phenomena as neurogenic stuttering, which are the disfluencies that sometimes appear in persons with neurological diseases or injuries. The changes in the brain that may occur as part of a neurological problem may give rise to a dyssynchrony in speech and language production processing that is similar to that of primary stuttering. On the other hand, the changes in temperament that sometimes occur with brain injury (e.g., Kinsbourne, 1989) may, in a few cases, give rise to disfluencies that are more characteristic of secondary stuttering.

There is support in genetic research for two (or more) predispositions in individuals who do not naturally recover from stuttering. After an analysis of many children who stutter for some period of time in their lives, Ambrose, Cox, and Yairi (1997) concluded that persistent and recovered stuttering are not two different forms of the disorder. Both persistent and recovered stutterers appear to have genetic factors related to the onset of stuttering. Those children who persisted in stuttering (i.e., continued to stutter for more than three years), however, have additional genetic factors, related to the persistency of the disorder. It may be that the additional genetic factors gives rise to a reactive temperament, making it more likely that these children will become frustrated, have other emotional reactions to their stuttering, and thus develop secondary/persistent stuttering. This connection between a child reacting to his stuttering and the persistence of the stuttering is reflected in Van Riper's beliefs that "...most children who begin to stutter become fluent perhaps because of maturation or because they do not react to their … repetitions, or prolongations by struggle and avoidance … [while] those who struggle or avoid because of

frustration or penalties will probably continue to stutter all the rest of their lives no matter what kind of therapy they receive" (Van Riper, 1990).

Indeed, as Ambrose, Cox, and Yairi (1997) suggest, there may be more than two predispositions in stuttering. The factors that cause a child to react with frustration and fear to primary stuttering may also cause another child to react the same way to lack of intelligibility or difficulties in word finding, for example. Communicative failures may lead to anticipatory struggle (Bloodstein & Ratner, 2008), as described earlier in this chapter. However, no matter how many predispositions a child may have, the chance of his actually developing primary or secondary stuttering is enhanced or diminished by both developmental and environmental factors.

Interactions with Developmental Factors

In this section, I describe three ways in which aspects of children's development may interact with the two predispositions to trigger or exacerbate stuttering. In Chapters 4 and 5, I argued that children's physical, cognitive, emotional, and linguistic development may provide the extra demands on resources that precipitate stuttering or worsen it. Now I want to relate these demands to the two predispositions described earlier. You will see elements of the capacities and demands theory of stuttering in this section.

The first interaction is with the demands of language development and a predisposition for primary stuttering. Consider a child who begins to acquire speech with dysfunctional or inefficient speech and language networks. The functional plasticity of the child's brain may allow these pathways to reorganize or repair themselves so that the child processes spoken language more efficiently as he strives to communicate. However, the exponential growth of the child's speech and language at this very time may compete for cerebral resources, straining or exceeding the child's capacity to handle both the demands of reorganization and advancing language at the same time. To see what this may be like, imagine yourself as a student who has let part of the semester slip by without studying. After bombing the first two exams, you resolve to reorganize your study habits and catch up, but just then, your professors decide to pile on even more work than before. Like the child, you may or may not be able to accommodate the professors' increasing demands at the same time you are spending energy to reorganize.

A second interaction will be the maturation of the brain with a predisposition for primary stuttering. Some individuals will have an earlier maturation of the brain or a natural flexibility to respond to anomalies in the wiring for spoken language. Girls, for example, are more likely to recover from early stuttering, probably because of their inherently greater organizational plasticity and their more widely distributed language centers (Shaywitz, Shaywitz, Pugh, Constable, &

Skudlarski et al., 1995). Some males may also be genetically endowed with more flexibility than average for reorganizing their cerebral circuitry and thus may recover more readily than others.

The third type of interaction will occur when a child has normal neural circuitry for spoken language but has a constitutionally inhibited temperament. Typical developmental challenges for most children include some frustration at not being able to speak as fast or with the same complexity as adults and older children in the family. The child may not only be frustrated but embarrassed at his inability to produce more advanced speech and language. Social-emotional development takes the child through some stressful times. All of these typical experiences may produce increased tension and avoidance behaviors associated with speech. Based on my clinical experience, I suspect that some children fitting this description might be hesitant to speak and may be referred for a stuttering evaluation but would not manifest the typical signs of stuttering. Their hesitancies may consist of long pauses, phrase repetitions, or both when their right-hemisphere proclivity toward avoidance, withdrawal, and arrest of ongoing behavior manifests itself while they are speaking. Such hesitancies may diminish in time as myelinization of connections between and within the hemispheres progresses and the left hemisphere has increasingly modulating effects on right hemisphere–regulated emotions.

Interactions with Environmental Factors

Here, I would like to consider the influence of the environment on anomalous speech and language neural networks (predisposition for primary stuttering) and on constitutional predispositions for inhibited temperaments (predisposition for secondary stuttering).

Interactions of Anomalous Neural Networks with Environmental Factors

As a child's developing central nervous system adapts to the inherited or acquired differences in her neural substrates for speech and language, the environment plays a role through various listeners' responses to the child's emerging speech and language skills. Obviously, a child's family will have the most opportunities to provide acceptance and support. The accommodations they can provide, such as slower speech rates, fewer interruptions, and dedicated one-on-one listening time, may foster adaptations of the child's inefficient, dyssynchronous neural networks. At least this environment will not stress the child's speech and language production system and will probably enable the child to develop her own adapted rate of speech and language output. In contrast, an environment with many interruptions, rapid conversational give and take, demands for recitations, and little time for the child to talk may "overdrive" the child's immature speech and language production system, produce an excess

of disfluencies, and inhibit the successful adaptation of the child's system to its original anomalous wiring.

Interactions of Temperament with Environmental Factors

The work of Calkins (1994), Kagan and Snidman (1991), and others suggests that families can have a strong influence on temperament. As Calkins and Fox (1994) expressed it, "the child's interactions with a parent provide the context for learning skills and strategies for managing emotional reactivity." In addition, the environmental factors that I have called "life events" can also influence the development of temperament. As noted earlier, Kagan (1994b) suggested that certain life events could cause a child who is not particularly reactive to become more reactive and inhibited.

Implications for Treatment

A supportive environment and specific therapy approaches may ameliorate the conditions that I have just been describing. By judicious control of speech and language processing demands, the environment may support a child's adaptive neuroplasticity, enabling him to improve the efficiency of his speech and language neural networks. Equally important is the family's fostering of the child's adaptation of inefficient neural networks. With appropriate models of slower speaking rates and pausing, the child may develop a rate of speech and language processing that allows him to synchronize the various components of spoken language.

Families may also help a child develop a less inhibited temperament by encouraging positive, assertive behaviors. Therapy, too, can help a child respond to disfluencies with fewer inhibitory responses. Active, positive treatment sessions often lead to improvements in a child's confidence. Training in fluency skills can provide a child with many satisfying speaking experiences, thereby reducing fear of talking. Development of a slower speaking style and the use of proprioception (conscious awareness of movement) may help a child make the best of an inefficient speech production system. Confronting feared words and situations, reducing tension in stutters, and improving eye contact during speech may help shift a child's characteristic emotional valence from "avoidance" (right hemisphere) to "approach" (left hemisphere). In the chapters on treating stuttering, I expand on this theme and suggest a variety of other ways to help individuals overcome or compensate for factors that predispose them to stutter.

Some recent research indicates another way in which treatment may affect the two predispositions for persistent stuttering. Brain imaging studies of adults before and after treatment (De Nil, Kroll, Lafaille, & Houle, 2003; Neumann, Euler, Wolff von Gudenberg, Giraud, & Lanfermann et al., 2003; Neumann & Euler, 2010) suggest that successful treatment is associated with activation of left-hemisphere areas that had not been active before treatment and reductions in activations of right-hemisphere areas that were highly active. These findings parallel evidence from treatment of nonfluent aphasic patients whose recovery was associated with the same pattern (M. Naeser, personal communication, January 5, 2005). Because this relocation of circuitry serving spoken language places it in areas very near to those used by nonstutterers in the left hemisphere (Neumann & Euler, 2010), activity may be less vulnerable to disruption by right-hemisphere emotions, thus affecting the mechanisms for both primary and secondary stuttering.

Accounting for the Evidence

Let us now turn to the research findings and clinical observations for which these views of stuttering must account.

Stuttering Occurs in All Cultures

The fact that stuttering is universal should not be unexpected because it depends less on culture than on basic biological variations of the human brain. Many other disorders, such as dyslexia and specific language impairment, as well as such personality differences as sensitive temperament, are associated with atypical activity of the central nervous system and are also universal.

Stuttering is a Low-Incidence Disorder

The fact that the prevalence of stuttering is relatively low may be a consequence of chronic stuttering resulting from a combination of at least two biological predispositions, the co-occurrence of which does not happen frequently.

Stuttering Does Not Begin with the Onset of Speech

Why does stuttering usually begin only after fluency at the one- and two-word stage has been achieved? My view is that stuttering emerges first from disruptions caused by a child's inefficient neural networks for speech and language processing. Perhaps the task of coordinating all the phonetic, phonological, syntactic, and semantic components of longer utterances is too much for inefficient neural circuitry under stress. Just like normal disfluency, the neural processing circuitry of children who stutter may be adequate to handle one-word utterances. But once children begin to reorganize their language functions from a lexical to a grammatical-rules basis and try out more complicated syntax, their inefficient neural organization breaks down. An added demand on their planning system is that the shift from one- to two-word utterances requires the use of a more complex prosody.

Remember that Kent (1984), Perkins, Kent, and Curlee 1991), and Wingate (1988) suggested that a major source of breakdown is in timing linguistic and paralinguistic components. This demand for complex prosody at the multiword stage at the same time that phonological, syntactical, and lexical demands are added is likely to be a time when an inefficient speech and language system cannot keep up with the demands for rapid and complex speech production. It is as if our imaginary bicycle factory described earlier in this chapter had been producing old style bikes with pedal brakes and no gears (the one-word stage) but is now being asked to produce bicycles with hand brakes and two sets of gears (multiword stage), even as customer demand is requiring faster work on the production line (speech rate increases with longer utterances).

Stuttering Sometimes Begins with Tense Blocks, But Often with Repetitions

There are children who begin to stutter with tense blocks that did not follow a period of repetitions and occasional prolongations. I have recently been working with a 2-year-old girl who showed excessive squeezing and tension in her stutters after only a few hours of stuttering in a repetitive pattern. For most children who stutter, however, tension responses, as well as escape and avoidance reactions, are elicited by the frustration and fear provoked by early stuttering. Speech itself is not threatening, but when a long repetition occurs as a result of the dyssynchrony in the speech and language production system, the child feels that her speech mechanism is out of control. This triggers her tension, escape, and avoidance responses, and as this happens more frequently, learning takes place, and her tension, escape, and avoidance responses are soon triggered without "runaway" repetitions.

Not All Stutterers Have Relatives Who Stuttered

How do we account for both the genetic transmission of stuttering and that evidence of genetic transmission is lacking in some cases? Genetic transmission of stuttering in many cases may be through the two factors I just described: **anomalous neural organization** for speech and sensitive temperament. In some cases of childhood stuttering, genetic transmission may seem unlikely because no other family members seem to be affected. However, it may occur because persistent stuttering appears to require both predisposing factors. Some family members may inherit one factor and some the other, but unless both factors are inherited by the same individual, persistent stuttering does not develop. Another reason for the absence of stuttering in other family members may be that the predisposing factors were the result not of genetic inheritance, but of environmental factors affecting fetal development that created the neural substrate for stuttering. Moreover, such anomalous speech and language circuitry may create language, learning, or phonological problems in other family members. Remember that the unfolding of the genetic blueprint is extensively influenced by environmental factors and by chance. Thus, the anomalous circuitry in one child may result in stuttering, but in an uncle or grandmother, it may have resulted in an articulation disorder or learning problem.

Stuttering Appears as Repetitions, Prolongations, and Blocks

The immediate causes of the core behaviors of stuttering are not entirely clear in my view. All of them reflect an inability to move forward in speech, but the effortless sound and syllable repetitions of many stutterers at onset seem somewhat different from later tension-filled repetitions, prolongations, and blocks. The sound and syllable repetitions of early stuttering more closely resemble the disfluencies resulting from nervous system damage or "neurogenic stuttering" (Rosenbek, 1984). Thus, these early signs of childhood stuttering (less tense repetitions and prolongations) may arise from a breakdown in the inefficient function of neural circuits, perhaps from causes similar to those of neurogenic stuttering. Repetitions may occur simply because there is a lag in the readiness of the next part of a word or sentence, although the impulse or pressure to continue speaking is strong. Signs of stuttering with tension that emerge later than effortless repetitions in many stutterers likely stem from the frustration and fear elicited by a child's difficulty in speaking. In those cases in which the earliest signs of stuttering are characterized by tension and blocking (Van Riper, 1982), an emotional response may be primary. As Van Riper (1982) suggested, these may be children whose onset is very sudden, resulting usually after an emotionally difficult period or traumatic emotional stress.

Stuttering is More Common in Boys than in Girls

I suspect that the reason more boys stutter than girls is that their genetic blueprints for neural organization of speech and language differ between boys and girls and may be more flexible in females (Shaywitz et al., 1995). Neuroplasticity of the human brain is greatest in the first few years of life, and this neuroplasticity probably diminishes after puberty. Neuroplasticity permits reorganization of neural pathways and, in many cases, recovery. Karlin (1947) advanced another explanation of why more girls recover early from stuttering. He postulated that delayed myelinization of nerve fibers in speech processing areas was a possible explanation of stuttering and cited research that myelinization of nerve fibers is more advanced in girls than in boys.

In Many Children, Stuttering Starts as Mild and Develops into a More Severe Form

The course of development of stuttering seems to us to be determined in part by the biological responses of the child to fear and frustration and to autonomic conditioning, to which a child prone to chronic stuttering may be particularly sensitive. Details on the development of stuttering are discussed in Chapter 7.

Many Conditions Reduce or Eliminate Stuttering

Conditions that temporarily ameliorate stuttering, such as singing or speaking in a rhythm, probably improve fluency by giving speech and language processes more time or an external organizing stimulus to aid speech production.

They may also involve other parts of the brain and not those anomalous networks used inefficiently for typically spoken language. Other conditions, such as speaking when alone or when relaxed, often reduce stuttering but do not necessarily eliminate it. Such conditions may calm a person, thereby diminishing the reactivity of limbic circuits, whereas some conditions, such as speaking more slowly, both provide more time and diminish reactivity.

Stutterers Often Have Poorer Performance on Sensory and Motor Tasks

How about differences in performance between groups of stutterers and nonstutterers? As intimated earlier in this chapter, it seems to me that the wide range of performance on language tests, school achievement tests, and tests of sensory-motor ability by groups of stutterers may reflect the wide range of delays and deviations in the neural substrates for these abilities that led to their inefficient processing of speech and language. Among groups of individuals who stutter, there are likely to be some whose neural organization for sensory-motor processing is deviant enough to depress the group mean. In highly selected groups of stutterers, however, such as all males with no medical, neurological, or psychiatric diagnoses and who are right-handed (Ingham, Fox, Ingham, Zamarripa, & Martin et al., 1996), the chance of finding significant differences between this group and a group of nonstutterers is decreased.

In this regard, it is interesting that two independent studies have shown that children whose stuttering is their only disorder show no speech reaction time differences from nonstutterers, whereas children who stutter and have other language or articulation disorders show significantly poorer reaction time scores than children who only stutter and children with typical speech (Cullinan & Springer, 1980; Maske-Cash & Curlee, 1995). Perhaps the coexistence of poorer sensory-motor integration performance and speech and language disorders reflects additional anomalies in neural organization and function in this subgroup of stuttering children. In other words, I propose that children who stutter have at least some degree of inefficient organization of their neural circuitry for speech and language production; those children who stutter and have poorer sensory-motor skills or other speech and language disorders may simply have greater anomalies in their neural circuitry functions, which affect fluency, articulation, language, or other sensory-motor tasks.

Other characteristics of stuttering that I have said should be explained by any view of stuttering, such as the influence of developmental and environmental factors, are explicitly addressed in earlier parts of this chapter. Some characteristics, findings, and observations are explained more easily than others. However, those that are not accounted for in detail (such as the strong effect of rhythmic stimuli on stuttering) should not be ignored. They are a reality and are hard facts that should mold and shape any theoretical view until it is more fully explanatory.

SUMMARY

- Several theoretical perspectives have been proposed to account for constitutional factors in stuttering. They include views of stuttering: (1) as an anomaly of how the brain is organized for speech and language; (2) as a disorder of timing of the sequential movements for speech; (3) as a result of deficits in the internal modeling process used to control speech production; (4) as a disorder of spoken language production; and (5) as a result of physiological tremor in speech musculature. The first four of these views focus on dysfunctions of cortical and subcortical mechanisms that control the planning and production of speech and language to produce the initial repetitions and prolongations of early stuttering; the fifth view targets neuromuscular malfunctions that may explain the tension and tremors of secondary stuttering.

- Theories concerning developmental and environmental factors include (1) the diagnosogenic theory, which implicates the listener's response to the disfluencies of the child; (2) the anticipatory struggle theory, which suggests that a child may develop stuttering as a result of negative anticipation of speaking after he has had frustrating or embarrassing experiences in communicating; and (3) the capacities and demands theory, which postulates that stuttering arises when the child's capacities for rapid, fluent utterances are unequal to the demands within the child himself or within the environment.

- In this chapter, I elaborate a two-stage etiological model of stuttering that I first proposed in a chapter on children's stuttering and emotions (Guitar, 1997) and that owes much to Bluemel (1957) and Brutten and Shoemaker (1967). The first stage is primary stuttering, which involves repetitions and prolongations that are frequently the first signs of stuttering. These signs are thought to be the result of a constitutional factor: a dyssynchrony at some level of the speech and language production process. The second stage is secondary stuttering, which involves the tension, struggle, escape, and avoidance behaviors that are often present in persistent stuttering. These behaviors are proposed to be the result of a separate constitutional factor—a reactive temperament that triggers a defense response from the behavioral inhibition system and that makes the individual more emotionally conditionable than the average speaker.

STUDY QUESTIONS

1. What are the differences between the Geschwind and Galaburda (1985) theory of stuttering and the Webster (1993a) view?

2. Compare Kent's (1984) view of stuttering as a disorder of timing with the Geschwind and Galaburda (1985) theory.

3. Both Neilson and Neilson's view of stuttering and one of Max and colleagues' (2004) hypotheses about stuttering suggest that repetitions occur because of a problem with the internal models used for speech production. What is the difference between the cause of repetitions in each view?

4. The study by Kelly, Smith, and Goffman (1995) reviewed in this chapter suggested that tremors don't appear in younger children who stutter but do appear in older children. Why would this be?

5. Table 6.2 lists experiences that may generate stuttering in some children because the experiences have led children to believe speaking is difficult. Add as many other hypothetical experiences as you can to this list.

6. A capacities and demands view of stuttering in children would lead to a therapy strategy of enhancing a child's capacities. What are some examples of what capacities in a child you could strengthen to reduce stuttering? Describe how you would do this.

7. What is the relationship between a sensitive temperament and a high level of conditionability?

8. I have suggested there may be two predispositions for persistent stuttering—one for primary stuttering and one for secondary stuttering. How, according to this view, would primary stuttering lead to secondary stuttering?

9. There is strong evidence that girls are more likely than boys to recover from stuttering and are therefore less likely to become persistent stutterers. Is this because girls are more likely to recover quickly from primary stuttering or because their primary stuttering is less likely to trigger secondary stuttering?

10. In this chapter, I have suggested that there are two stages of stuttering—primary and secondary. What are the signs and symptoms of each, and what is the suggested etiology of each?

SUGGESTED PROJECTS

1. The view of stuttering as a problem of the "internal modeling" process in speech production is a complex idea. Read the article by Max and colleagues (2004) and make a class presentation about their full theoretical model, explaining it in as clear and simple a way as possible.

2. Read the article entitled "Resources—A Theoretical Stone Soup" (Navon, 1984) and use the arguments in it to evaluate the capacities and demands theory in this chapter.

3. Wendell Johnson's "diagnosogenic" view of stuttering led to a master's thesis that tried to create stuttering in orphans in 1939. In 2003, this thesis was the topic of a controversy that centered on the ethics of trying to induce stuttering in children. Using the Internet, research this controversy, using "Monster Study" as a keyword. Make a presentation or write a paper on the ethics of this research, given the fact that it was conducted more than 50 years ago when the ethical climate was markedly different than it is now.

4. Pick a theory of stuttering—either one described in the first two sections of this chapter or one you have found elsewhere—and evaluate how it can account for the basic facts about stuttering enumerated in Chapter 1.

5. Go to Guitar and McCauley (2010) and read two chapters concerning specific interventions related to a specific age group of people who stutter. Identify which theories addressed here are cited and how they appear to impact the developers of each intervention approach.

SUGGESTED READINGS

Brutten, E. J., & Shoemaker, D. J. (1967). *The modification of stuttering*. Englewood Cliffs, NJ: Prentice-Hall, Inc.

This is a classic book in the field of stuttering. It describes a theory of stuttering that ascribes the initial symptoms of childhood stuttering to the effect of anxiety on fluency and ascribes the later symptoms to learning. The authors go on to suggest therapeutic approaches that derive from their model.

Guitar, B., & McCauley, R. (2010). How to use this book. In B. Guitar, & R. McCauley (Eds), *Treatment of Stuttering*. Baltimore: Lippincott Williams & Wilkins.

This chapter describes in user-friendly language what a theory is and how it can help researchers and clinicians.

Gray, J. A. (1987). *The psychology of fear and stress (2nd ed.)*. Cambridge: Cambridge University Press.

Gray's experimental work and his theoretical model of a behavioral inhibition system are clearly described here. Some of the book (those parts dealing with the effects of pharmacological agents on the brain) is for specialized readers. Much of it, however, is a readable exposition on the biological basis of learning, stress, and fear. Because this is the second edition of a popular book, I hope a new edition will be available soon.

Kagan, J., Reznick, J. S., & Snidman, N. (1987). The physiology and psychology of behavioral inhibition in children. *Child Development, 58,* 1459–1473.

This article discusses the findings of Kagan and his colleagues that behaviorally inhibited children show high levels of laryngeal tension. Neurophysiological mechanisms are also discussed, as well as possible genetic and environmental contributions. This book is recommended for those interested in the hypothesis that behavioral inhibition may be a component in some stuttering.

LeDoux, J. (1996). *The emotional brain: The mysterious underpinnings of emotional life*. New York: Simon & Schuster.

LeDoux, a highly respected brain researcher, brings together a great deal of evidence about how the brain processes experiences that we consider emotional. His explanations of emotional learning are very clear and relevant to stuttering.

Packman, A., & Attanasio, J. (2004). *Theoretical issues in stuttering*. New York: Psychology Press.

The authors review current and past theories of stuttering and evaluate them in terms of testability, explanatory power, parsimony, and heuristic power. This book effectively teaches the reader what a theory should be expected to do.

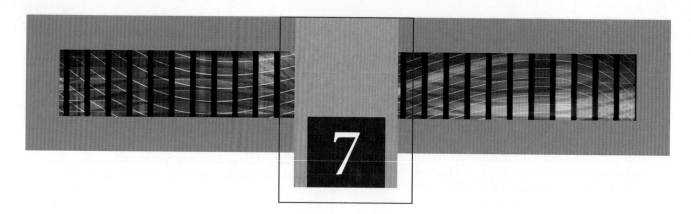

7

Normal Disfluency and the Development of Stuttering

CHAPTER OBJECTIVES

After studying this chapter, readers should be able to:

- Describe and explain the ways in which the age and developmental levels have exceptions and variations
- Describe and explain the (a) core behaviors, (b) secondary behaviors, (c) feelings and attitudes, and (d) underlying processes for the following age and developmental levels:
  - normal disfluency
  - stuttering in younger preschool children: borderline stuttering
  - stuttering in older preschool children: beginning stuttering
  - stuttering in school-age children: intermediate stuttering
  - stuttering in older teens and adults: advanced stuttering

KEY TERMS

Underlying processes: These are speculations about the process that may cause disfluencies or stuttering at each developmental level. For stuttering, these processes help us understand why stuttering often changes from borderline to beginning to intermediate to severe levels

Age/developmental levels: These levels reflect both the age of the individual (e.g., younger preschooler, older preschooler, etc.) and the severity of the stuttering (e.g., borderline, beginning, etc.)

Borderline stuttering: This is the earliest or lowest level of stuttering, usually seen in children ages 2 to 3.5. This type of stuttering is characterized by more frequent part-word and single-syllable whole-word repetitions than typically developing children have, but without awareness or concern on the part of the child

"Within-word" disfluencies: Disfluencies that occur within a word boundary such as repetitions of parts of words, prolongations, or blocks. Stuttered speech is said to contain a higher proportion of within-word disfluencies (as opposed to disfluencies that happen *between words or across words,* such as hesitations, fillers, and repetitions of whole words). Note that disfluencies of typically developing children may also include within-word disfluencies

"Stuttering-like" disfluencies: Short-segment repetitions (i.e., part-word and monosyllabic word repetitions), as well as sound prolongations, and blocks. These are disfluencies that are more typically experienced by listeners as associated with stuttering

Dysrhythmic phonation: A sound prolongation, broken word, or other instance of ongoing phonation being stopped, extended, or distorted

Beginning stuttering: This level of stuttering is usually seen in children between ages 3.5 and 6, although it may occur before and after those ages. It is characterized by more tension and hurry in disfluencies than that seen in borderline stuttering. Stuttering usually consists of repetitions and prolongations, but some children will also exhibit blocks. Escape behaviors appear in this level of stuttering

Intermediate stuttering: Typical of children in their school-age years, this level of stuttering will abound in repetitions and prolongations, but blocks will also be frequent. In addition to escape behaviors, avoidances will appear at this level because there is fear of being "stuck" in a stutter and fear of listener reactions

Starters: Words or sounds used by someone who stutters to get started speaking when blocked or when anticipating a block. For example, a person who stutters might say "My name is, uh, Barry"

Substitutions: The substitution of an "easier" word for a "harder" word on which a stutterer expects to stutter. For example, a stutterer who often stuttered on words beginning with "p" and who had a dog named "Pluto" might always substitute "my dog" for the dog's name when talking about him

Circumlocutions: Rather than stutter on a word, a person who stutters might use a different way of saying something, such as "My father was in the N...n...he served aboard ships in the armed forces"

Postponements: This is like a starter, but usually it just involves waiting a few beats before saying a feared word as in "Back then I voted for Ronald.........Reagan"

Antiexpectancy devices: An unusual way of speaking or acting that seems to reduce stuttering, like laughing and pretending that most things said were a joke. Another example is speaking with an accent that the speaker pretends to have

Avoidance conditioning: A type of learning that occurs when a person avoids something he thinks will be unpleasant. The avoidance is rewarded by the fact that the unpleasantness doesn't happen. Avoidance conditioning is important in thinking about stuttering development and interventions because it can be difficult to combat

Advanced stuttering: This level is characteristic of older teens and adults who have been stuttering since childhood. Their stuttering pattern is quite ingrained, especially behaviors associated with avoidance and ways of coping with blocks

OVERVIEW

This chapter describes the development of stuttering and what it looks like at various ages. It is designed to help you understand why once stuttering has emerged, it often (but not always) progresses from a few relaxed repetitions in preschool children to frequent stuttering accompanied by tension, avoidance, and many negative feelings and beliefs in older children or adults. This chapter will also help you understand how to match treatment procedures to the underlying dynamics of stuttering, as well as to the age of the client. To accomplish these goals, I have organized the content into five levels that reflect not only age groupings but also stages of development of stuttering and important characteristics of each stage of stuttering to guide your selection of a therapy approach (Fig. 7.1)

The five age groupings/developmental levels are given in Table 7.1, along with the four subcategories of stuttering characteristics. The first three subcategories—*core behaviors, secondary behaviors,* and *feelings and attitudes*—were described in a general way in Chapter 1. The fourth, **underlying processes**, is introduced to explain why symptoms may change from level to level. These explanations are hypotheses based on evidence from studies of animal and human behavior about how stuttering behaviors become more severe and complex. This subcategory should help you understand the nature of the symptoms as well as the rationales for the treatments presented in the second section of the book.

Specific age groupings (younger preschool, older preschool, school-age, and teens and adults) are used because age is often critical in selecting the appropriate treatment. Let me give two examples. No matter how severely a preschool child stutters, treatment should always involve his parents, and in my experience, it should focus primarily on increasing fluency rather than modifying stutters. Conversely, a school-age child—whether stuttering is mild or severe—needs an approach that involves teachers and classmates as well as parents. Also, it helps children of this age to discuss their stuttering and their feelings about it. In general, the cognitive-emotional level typically associated with different ages needs to be considered when choosing a therapy strategy.

Age Groupings/Developmental Levels

Normal Disfluency

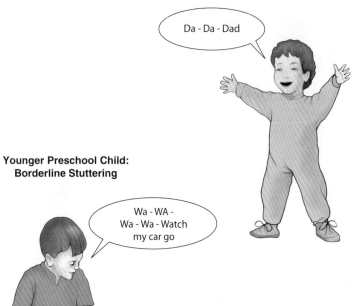

**Younger Preschool Child:
Borderline Stuttering**

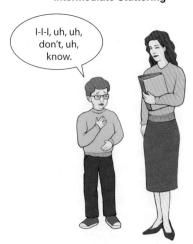

**Older Preschool Child:
Beginning Stuttering**

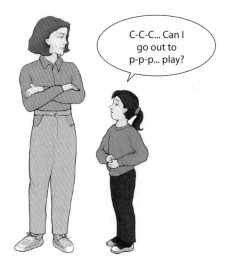

**School-Age Child:
Intermediate Stuttering**

**Adult and Adolescent:
Advanced Stuttering**

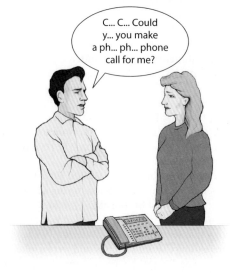

Figure 7.1 Overview of Chapter 7.

Table 7.1	Developmental/Treatment Levels of Stuttering
Developmental/Treatment Level	**Typical Age Range**
Normal disfluency	1.5–6 y, although a small amount of normal disfluency continues in mature speech
Younger preschoolers: borderline stuttering	1.5–3.5 y
Older preschoolers: beginning stuttering	3.5–6 y
School-age: intermediate stuttering	6–13 y
Older teens and adults: advanced stuttering	14 y and above

Exceptions and Variations

The **age/developmental levels** presented in this chapter do not characterize everyone who stutters. For example, some older preschool children may be stuttering so mildly and be so relatively unaware of it that they might best be treated by an approach described for younger preschool children. However, most individuals who stutter will fit reasonably well into their age grouping. Moreover, even though all behaviors of a person may not reflect a single age/developmental level, deciding on a treatment need not be a problem; when some aspects of a person's stuttering seem more advanced than others, strategies can be borrowed from other levels to treat them.

Another qualification of the hierarchy presented here concerns the implication that all individuals who stutter pass through each stage in sequence. This is generally true, but there are exceptions. A child may show only normal disfluencies one day and beginning or intermediate stuttering on another day. She may stop stuttering without apparent reason a week later, or she may continue stuttering unless treated. One 3-year-old boy I knew changed overnight from borderline to severe beginning stuttering after a change in his allergy medication. As soon as he resumed taking the original prescription, he became a borderline stutterer again and then recovered completely without treatment. There are many unsolved mysteries in stuttering.

Two clinical researchers who wrote extensively about the development of stuttering, Van Riper (1982) and Bloodstein (1960a, 1960b, 1961a), agreed that a simple sequence of stages could never capture every stutterer's pattern. Bloodstein (1960b) proposed a series of four stages of stuttering development, which he described as "typical, but not universal" (Bloodstein, 1995, p. 53). He also cautioned that although stuttering near onset is often characterized by

repetitions without awareness or by a lack of concern, some children at this stage show considerable effort and strain in their stuttering as well as crying from frustration at their inability to produce speech easily (Bloodstein, 1960a).

Van Riper (1982) also noted the presence of forcing and struggle in some children at the onset of stuttering, and like Bloodstein, he was struck by the fact that most children, especially in their early years, oscillate between remissions and recurrences of their stuttering, between mild stuttering and normal disfluency, or between more advanced and less advanced stages of development.

In addition to such swings in the progression of stuttering development, there may also be different paths of development, which different stutterers may follow. After searching his clinical files on many individuals whom he had followed for several years, Van Riper (1982) found that his data suggested there are subgroups of stutterers who are characterized by different onsets and different trajectories of development. He proposed that there are four distinctive "tracks" that an individual may follow. The most common consists of children whose stuttering begins as repetitions between 2 and 4 years of age, progresses to include prolongations, then gradually develops into blocks with more and more tension as well as fears and avoidances. The next most common track comprises children whose onset is a little later and is sometimes accompanied by delayed speech development, articulation problems, or very rapid speech. An interesting aspect of this track is that these children seem to have had difficulty hearing their own speech, perhaps as a result of auditory processing problems. This is particularly interesting in light of recent findings from brain imaging studies of adults who stutter (e.g., Foundas et al., 2001), indicating that some have anatomical anomalies that might produce difficulty with higher-level auditory processing. A third less common track includes children who have sudden onsets of stuttering with a great deal of tension that results in tight, laryngeal blocks. Finally, a fourth track consists of individuals whose disfluency appears to have psychogenic components. (An expanded discussion of psychogenic disfluency is presented in Chapter 15.) This track is characterized by late onset, a stereotyped pattern of stuttering that changes very little with age, and few avoidances. Van Riper's four tracks serve as a warning to us that there is much diversity in the evolution of stuttering.

Keeping these variations, exceptions, and limitations in mind, I now begin a detailed description of the levels of stuttering development and treatment, starting with a group of behaviors that is really not stuttering at all, but a part of normal speech.

NORMAL DISFLUENCY

Children vary a great deal in how disfluent they are as they learn to communicate. Some pass their milestones of speech and language development with relatively few disfluencies.

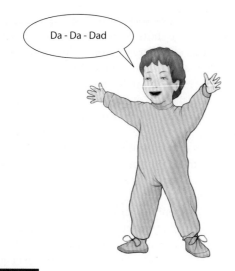

Da - Da - Dad

Figure 7.2   Child who may be normally disfluent.

Table 7.2	Categories of Normal Disfluencies
Type of Normal Disfluency	**Example**
Part-word repetition	"mi-milk"
Single-syllable word repetition	"I...I want that"
Multisyllabic word repetition	"Lassie...Lassie is a good dog"
Phrase repetition	"I want a...I want a ice-ceem comb"
Interjection	"He went to the...uh...circus"
Revision-incomplete phrase	"I lost my...Where's Mommy going?"
Prolongation	"I'm Tiiiiiiiimmy Thompson"
Tense pause	"Can I have some more (lips together, no sound) milk?"

Others stumble along, repeating, interjecting, and revising as they try to master new forms of speech and language on their way to adult competence. Most are somewhere between the extremes of exceptional fluency and excessive disfluency, such as the 2-year-old shown in Figure 7.2.

Children also swing back and forth in the degree of their disfluency. Some days they are more fluent and other days less fluent. Such swings in disfluency may be associated with language development, motor learning, or other developmental or environmental influences mentioned in the preceding chapters. In the following sections, I discuss factors that may influence disfluency, specific behaviors that I categorize as normal disfluency, and the reactions that some children may have to their disfluency. I also highlight aspects of normal disfluency that distinguish it from early stuttering, because one of my aims in this chapter is to prepare you to make this differentiation.

Core Behaviors

Normal disfluencies have been cataloged by several authors, and there is general agreement among them about what constitutes disfluency (Bloodstein, 1987; Colburn & Mysak, 1982a, 1982b; Williams, Silverman, & Kools, 1968; Yairi, 1982, 1983, 1997a; Yairi & Ambrose, 2005). Table 7.2 lists eight commonly used categories of disfluency.

Some of the major distinguishing features of normal disfluency—features that differentiate it from stuttering—are the amount of disfluency, the number of units of repetitions and interjections, and the type of disfluency, especially in relation to the age of the child.

Let's begin with the amount of disfluency. This is often measured as the number of disfluencies per 100 words or syllables, rather than "percent disfluencies." Percent disfluencies implies that the disfluencies are associated with the

production of particular words. For example, if you said that a child had 10 percent disfluent words, it would be assumed that 10 percent of the words spoken were spoken disfluently. However, many disfluencies, such as revisions, interjections, or phrase repetitions, are associated with several words or occur between words. For example, a child may say "Mommy, can you … can you … um … can you buy me that?" It's inaccurate to say that some of these words were spoken disfluently, because the disfluencies were the repetition of the phrase "can you" and the interjection of "um." Were the disfluencies on the words spoken or did they occur because the child was having trouble formulating the remainder of the sentence? In this case, we say that the child spoke six words ("Mommy can you buy me that?") and had two disfluencies (a phrase repetition and an interjection). Hence, we calculate the number of disfluencies that occur when the child speaks 100 words. More details on counting disfluencies are given in Chapter 8.

Although many researchers have measured disfluencies per number of words spoken, a good argument can be made for measuring disfluencies per number of *syllables* spoken. Andrews and Ingham (1971) first recommended the practice of assessing frequency of stuttering in relation to syllables spoken because some multisyllable words may have more than one disfluency, like "S-S-S-Sept-t-t-tember" or "di-dinosa-sa-saur." These examples would be one disfluency each if disfluent *words* were counted, but two if disfluent *syllables* were counted. In line with this, Yairi (1997a) noted that as children get older, they are more likely to use multisyllable words. To keep the count equitable between younger and older children, Yairi has assessed disfluencies in children as the number per 100 syllables attempted (Hubbard & Yairi, 1988; Yairi & Ambrose, 1996; Yairi & Lewis, 1984).

When the frequency of all of a child's disfluencies is measured, we need to know how many of these disfluencies are normal. Some of the earliest research on disfluency was conducted by Wendell Johnson at the University of Iowa. He assembled a team of researchers in the 1950s to examine the evidence for his "diagnosogenic" theory of stuttering. As indicated in Chapter 4, Johnson hypothesized that at the time a child is first "diagnosed" a stutterer by his parents, the child's disfluencies do not differ from those of nonstuttering children. One of the research team's projects was to record children identified by their parents as stutterers and compare the disfluency in their speech with that of nonstuttering children (Johnson & associates, 1959). One part of this study compared 68 male children who stuttered with 68 male children who didn't. The results showed that although there was some overlap, the stuttering children had more than twice the amount of disfluency (on average, 18 disfluencies per 100 words) than did the nonstuttering children (only seven disfluencies per 100 words). Johnson interpreted the findings as showing that the two groups were essentially the same because there was so much overlap in both amount and type of disfluency. Other researchers (e.g., McDearmon, 1968) have reinterpreted these data as indicating there are two different groups, as I discussed in the last chapter.

Other researchers who have examined the disfluencies in nonstuttering children put the amount of their disfluencies at about the same level as Johnson and his colleagues reported (DeJoy & Gregory, 1985; Hubbard & Yairi, 1988; Wexler & Mysak, 1982; Yairi, 1981; Yairi & Ambrose, 1996; Yairi & Lewis, 1984; Zebrowski, 1991). Bringing all these studies together, we can estimate that normally speaking preschool children have on average about seven disfluencies for every 100 words spoken. If measured in terms of syllables, it would be closer to six disfluencies per 100 syllables. This figure may be a little high if children are examined throughout their preschool years (Yairi, 1997a); however, many children at age 2 or 3 go through a period of increased disfluency, which will reach this level.

The range in frequency of normal disfluency is important to note also, especially if the frequency of disfluency is used to make clinical decisions. Johnson and associates (1959) and Yairi (1981) found that, although many nonstuttering children have only one or two disfluencies per 100 words, at least one child in their samples had slightly more than 25 disfluencies per 100 words. Thus, the frequency of disfluencies is not a definitive clinical measure by itself.

Another distinguishing characteristic of normal disfluency is the number of units that occur in each repetition or interjection. Yairi's (1981) data suggest that normal repetitions typically consist of only one extra unit. For example, a child might say "That my-my ball." Interjections are likely to be just a single unit, such as "I want some ... uh ... juice." Instances of multiple repetitions were occasionally observed in these children, but they were the exception. The rule is one and sometimes two units per repetition or interjection, which agrees with the findings of Johnson and associates (1959) that average nonstuttering children have one- or two-unit repetitions.

Another major characteristic of normal disfluency is the type of disfluency that is most common. Johnson and associates (1959) found that interjections, revisions, and whole-word repetitions were the most common disfluency types among the 68 nonstuttering males, who ranged in age from 2.5 to 8 years of age. Yairi's (1981) study of 33 typically developing 2-year-old children found that there were two clusters of common disfluency types. One cluster involved repetitions of speech segments of one syllable or less (one-syllable words or parts of words were repeated). The second cluster consisted of interjections and revisions.

The most common disfluency type seems to change as a child grows older. In a follow-up to his earlier study, Yairi (1982) found that as children matured between 2 and 3.5 years, they gradually increased their frequency of revisions and phrase repetitions but decreased their frequency of part-word repetitions and interjections. He suggested that these data indicate that as nonstuttering children mature, part-word repetitions decline, even if other disfluency types increase. Thus, an increase in part-word repetitions as a child is observed longitudinally may be a sign that warrants concern.

Although the research is far from complete, we can characterize normal disfluency types as follows:

- Revisions are common in normal children and may continue to account for a major portion of their disfluencies as they grow older.
- Interjections are also common, but usually decline after 3 years of age.
- Repetitions may also be a frequent type of disfluency around 2 to 3 years of age, especially single-syllable word repetitions having fewer than two extra units. Repetitions are also more likely to involve longer segments (e.g., phrases) as a child grows older.

Table 7.3 summarizes the major characteristics of normal disfluency.

Secondary Behaviors

A normally disfluent child generally has no secondary behaviors. He has not developed any reactions to his disfluencies, such as escape or avoidance behaviors. Although research

Table 7.3	Characteristics of Normal Disfluency in the Average Nonstuttering Child
1. No more than 10 disfluencies per 100 words 2. Typically one-unit repetitions, occasionally two 3. Most common disfluency types are interjections, revisions, and word repetitions. As children mature past age 3, they will show a decline in part-word repetitions	

suggests that some normal children occasionally display "tense pauses," such tension does not appear to be a reaction to their disfluencies. If a child shows what appears to be normal disfluencies, such as single-word repetitions, but consistently displays pauses or interjections of "uh" immediately before or during disfluencies, he should be carefully evaluated for possible stuttering.

Feelings and Attitudes

A normally disfluent child rarely notices his disfluencies, even though they may be apparent to others. Just as a child may stumble when walking but regains his balance and keeps walking without complaint, a typically developing child who repeats, interjects, or revises usually continues talking after a disfluency without evidence of frustration or embarrassment.

Underlying Processes

First, let's review the behaviors for which we are trying to account. Normal disfluency occurs throughout childhood and adulthood. It may begin earlier than 18 months of age and peak between ages 2 and 3.5 years. It slowly diminishes, thereafter, but also changes in form. Some types of disfluency, such as repetitions, decrease after 3.5 years, but other types, such as revisions, may increase. Episodic increases and decreases in disfluency are also common throughout childhood. What causes these changes? Why are there ups and downs and changes in form? Like most natural phenomena, multiple forces probably have an impact on fluency at any given moment, but some may predominate at certain times. In Chapters 4 and 5, I talked about developmental and environmental influences on stuttering and normal disfluency, and I will review these influences as I discuss studies of normally disfluent children.

Certainly, the development of language is likely to be one major influence on fluency. As my earlier review showed, children tend to be most disfluent at the beginning of syntactic units (Bernstein Ratner, 1981; Bloodstein, 1974, 1995; Silverman, 1974) and when the length or complexity of their utterances increases (DeJoy & Gregory, 1973; Gordon, Luper, & Peterson, 1986; Pearl & Bernthal, 1980). These findings suggest that disfluency is greatest when a child is busy planning long or complex language structures yet must, at the same time as he is planning, begin to produce them, a process that places a heavy load on cerebral resources. It seems likely that producing newly learned language structures would be hardest of all and could result in more frequent disfluencies on a child's most recently acquired forms. However, evidence gathered from four children between 2 and 4 years of age suggests that normal disfluency may be greatest on structures that have been learned but perhaps not fully automatized, thereby requiring more cerebral resources than are allocated to their production (Colburn & Mysak, 1982a, 1982b).

Pragmatics may influence disfluency, too. Studies by Davis (1940) and by Meyers and Freeman (1985a, 1985b) indicate that children's disfluency increases under certain pragmatic conditions, such as when interrupting, when directing another's activity, or when responding to requests/demands to change their own activity. Mastering such pragmatic skills, especially those involving more complex social interactions, creates yet another challenge for a developing child. The pressures of language acquisition, interacting with other factors, can be seen as competing for cerebral resources, which leaves fewer remaining resources available for fluent speech production.

In addition to language acquisition, another likely influence on disfluency is speech motor control. As they mature between 2 and 5 years of age, most children learn to produce almost all the segmental and super-segmental targets of their native language, as well as to increase their speech rates as they produce longer and longer utterances. These maturational changes must keep the average child fairly busy, although the demanding nature of these changes may not be obvious. The child is automatically scanning his parents' and older siblings' speech, acquiring information about talking. He is also continuously modifying his own productions to make them more and more like the speech he hears. This period—from 2 to 5 years—also encompasses an intensive refinement of nonspeech motor skills. It is at this age that children are learning to skip, run, jump, and take part in numerous games requiring skill and speed. Thus, children are mastering a myriad of other motor tasks at the same time they are acquiring the ability to speak in rapid, complex, fluent sequences.

In general, the view of stuttering described in Chapter 6, suggesting that a breakdown in speech fluency may occur when some of the neural pathways critical for sensorimotor control of speech production are immature or inefficient, may fit a nonstuttering child as well. Remember the dyssynchrony hypotheses we discussed in Chapter 6? Even normal disfluencies may be the product of a child learning to integrate all the subcomponents of spoken language at increasingly faster rates with increasingly greater options for vocabulary, syntax, and prosody.

Besides the continuing demands of normal development, there are also episodic stresses in a child's environment that may temporarily increase normal disfluency. An experiment by Hill (1954) demonstrated that conditioned fear could elicit disfluency in normal adults' speech. It is easy to imagine, therefore, that there are many psychological stresses in a child's life that would also increase disfluency. Clinically, I have observed many situations that seem to increase normal disfluency. Among them are the stress of a move from one home to another, parents' separation or divorce, the birth of a sibling, and other events that may decrease a child's sense of security.

We have also seen increases in normal disfluency during periods of excitement, such as holidays, vacations, and visits by relatives. Disfluency increases especially when excitement combines with competition to be heard, such as during dinner table conversations when everyone is talking at once or after school when several children are competing to tell Mom what happened during the day. As we speculated in Chapter 6, emotions may have an especially strong influence on fluency in young children. This happens after interactions between right and left hemispheres develop during the child's first two years (Fox & Davidson, 1984), and overflow activity from emotional arousal in the right hemisphere may disrupt vulnerable, immature language production networks in the left.

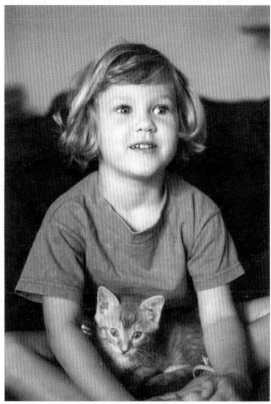

A video clip with an example of a child with normal disfluency is available on *thePoint*.

Summary

1. Between ages 2 and 5, many children pass through periods of increased disfluency. Repetitions, interjections, revisions, prolongations, and pauses are commonly heard during this period.

2. When the average child is between 2 and 3.5, disfluencies reach seven per 100 words spoken and may occur even more frequently in some normally disfluent children.

3. Repetitions are probably the most common type of normal disfluency in younger children, whereas revisions are more common normal disfluencies in older children.

4. Despite the fact that children's disfluencies may occasionally attract some adult attention, normally disfluent children seem generally unaware of the disfluencies in their own speech and don't react to them or engage in secondary behaviors to escape or avoid them as a consequence.

5. Some factors thought to contribute to increases in normal disfluencies include the demands of language acquisition, inefficient speech-motor control skills, interpersonal stress associated with growing up in a typical family, and threats to security from such events as relocation, family breakup, or hospitalization. Disfluencies may also increase under the ordinary daily pressures of competition and excitement while speaking.

YOUNGER PRESCHOOL CHILDREN: BORDERLINE STUTTERING

Stuttering in preschool children between the ages of 2 and 3.5 resembles normal disfluency, but differs in several important ways. The most obvious—the thing that gets parents' attention—is that these children have more disfluencies. We will discuss other key differences in the following sections. Sometimes diagnosis is difficult, because a child may drift back and forth between normal disfluency and **borderline stuttering** over a period of weeks or months. Some children with borderline stuttering gradually lose their stuttering and grow up without a trace of stuttering. Others develop more stuttering symptoms and progress through levels of beginning, intermediate, and advanced stuttering. Still others may continue to show borderline stuttering throughout their lives but may never seek treatment because their disfluency is so mild. A speech sample of a younger preschool child with borderline stuttering is depicted in Figure 7.3.

In describing the behaviors of borderline stuttering, I will begin to define my view of how stuttering differs from normal disfluency. The distinction between stuttering and normal disfluency has been of great interest to theorists for many years. Some theorists (e.g., Johnson, 1955; Johnson et al., 1942) suggested, as was noted previously, that a stuttering child developed symptoms only after his parents

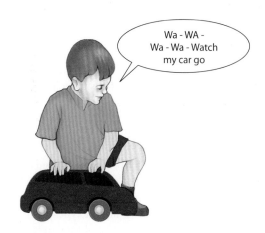

Figure 7.3 Child who may be a borderline stutterer.

mislabeled his normal disfluencies as stuttering. That is, a child's first "stuttering" symptoms were actually just normal speech disfluencies.

An opposing view maintains that there are objective differences between the speech of a normal child and the speech of a child who is stuttering, even before a parent or someone else labels the behaviors as stuttering. Although I hold this latter view, I also agree that there is much overlap between the disfluencies of stuttering children and the disfluencies of normally disfluent children. Moreover, as previously stated, these children often go back and forth between stuttering and normal disfluency over a period of months. For this reason, we use the term "borderline" to indicate that these children are neither entirely normally disfluent nor definitely stuttering.

Core Behaviors

There is no single core behavior that distinguishes borderline stuttering from normal disfluency. However, many researchers and clinicians have suggested three elements that are useful for making this distinction. The *frequency of disfluencies* is one important aspect to consider. As we indicated in our description of normal disfluencies, nonstuttering children between 2 and 5 years may go through periods of increased disfluency. Even so, their level of disfluency averages about seven per 100 words. Typically, if children have many more disfluencies per 100 words (e.g., more than 10), we consider them borderline.

Another feature that can help identify borderline stuttering rather than normal disfluency is *the proportion of certain types of disfluencies*. The study we cited earlier by Johnson and colleagues (1959) suggested that compared to nonstuttering children, those who stutter had significantly more sound and syllable repetitions, word repetitions, phrase repetitions, broken words (i.e., phonation or airflow is abnormally stopped within a word), and prolonged sounds. There were no significant differences between the groups in their number of interjections, revisions, or incomplete phrases.

More information on types of disfluencies was provided by Young (1984), who reviewed a large number of studies that had assessed which types of disfluencies were identified as stuttering and which were not. His summary impression was that repetitions of parts of words, and to a lesser extent prolongations, are the disfluency types that are likely to be classified as stuttering. Bloodstein and Ratner (2008) and Conture (1982, 1990, 2001) generally concurred with other writers, suggesting that **"within-word" disfluencies** (i.e., part-word repetitions and audible as well as inaudible prolongations including blocks) are the types of disfluencies most frequently heard in stuttering children.

Yairi and colleagues (e.g., Yairi, 1997a, 1997b; Yairi & Ambrose, 1996) proposed that children who stutter can be distinguished from normally disfluent children using a grouping of **"stuttering-like" disfluencies**. Included in this grouping were short-segment repetitions (part-word and monosyllabic word repetitions); tense pauses (stoppage of speech with evident muscular tightening both within and between words); and a category introduced by Williams, Silverman, and Kools (1968) called **"dysrhythmic phonation"** (any distortion, prolongation, or break in phonation within a word). Yairi (1997a, 1997b) notes that when many previous studies of stuttering and nonstuttering children are reanalyzed using this grouping, the proportion of stuttering-like disfluencies in nonstuttering children is always less than 50 percent of the total number of disfluencies. Thus, if a child has more than 50 percent stuttering-like disfluencies, he might be considered to be stuttering.

In summary, we can say that one measure that will help us distinguish a child with borderline stuttering from a normally disfluent child is a higher proportion of part-word and monosyllabic whole-word repetitions and prolongations compared with multisyllabic word and phrase repetitions. In the next section, we see that children who show the types of tension in their disfluencies that have been labeled blocks, broken words, and dysrhythmic phonations are beginning rather than borderline stutterers.

The *number of times a word or sound is repeated* in a part-word or monosyllable word repetitive disfluency appears to be another sign that distinguishes children who stutter from their normally disfluent peers. In Yairi's (1981) sample of 33 nonstuttering children, repetitions typically involved only one or two extra units of repetition (e.g., one extra unit would be li-like this). Other studies comparing stuttering and nonstuttering children (Ambrose & Yairi, 1995; Johnson & associates, 1959; Yairi & Lewis, 1984; Zebrowski, 1991) have found that the repetitive disfluencies of nonstuttering children average 1.13 extra units and that of stuttering children, 1.51. Thus, the frequent occurrence of repetitions having more than one extra unit is a warning sign of borderline stuttering.

We have said that borderline stuttering consists primarily of effortless repetitions and occasional prolongations. However, as Van Riper (1971, 1982) and Bloodstein (1995) note, these young children are often highly variable in their stuttering. Although they usually show the core behaviors of borderline stuttering, they may have brief periods of normal fluency as well as days when they show signs of more advanced stuttering.

Secondary Behaviors

A younger preschool child with borderline stuttering has few, if any secondary behaviors. The degree of tension may sometimes seem to be slightly greater than normal, but these children don't seem to increase tension and struggle like older preschool children do. Children with borderline stuttering also do not exhibit accessory movements before, during, or after stutters. In fact, there is often nothing in their behavior to indicate that they are aware of their stutters. Some children with predominantly borderline stuttering may go through periods in which their stuttering suddenly escalates to the level of beginning stuttering, with tension and some other secondary behaviors, but then it falls back again to the borderline level.

Feelings and Attitudes

Because children with borderline stuttering seem to have little awareness of their stutters, they do not show concern or embarrassment. When they repeat a sound or a syllable, even five or six or more times, they usually go on talking as though nothing has happened. One exception, however, is that once in a while children with borderline stuttering might appear surprised or frustrated when they are repeating a syllable several times and are unable to finish a word. Then, they may stop and cry out, "Mommy, I can't say that word," or otherwise demonstrate brief alarm or surprise. But in general, these younger preschool children show little or no evidence of awareness that they have disfluencies that are different from those of their peers, and at this age, peers usually don't react to the stuttering. Table 7.4 summarizes the major characteristics of the younger preschool children's borderline stuttering.

Underlying Processes

I hypothesize that the symptoms of borderline stuttering result from the constitutional, developmental, and environmental factors described in Chapters 2, 3, 4, and 5. The constitutional factors associated with borderline stuttering often first show their effects as an excess of normal disfluencies. As previously stated, environmental and developmental pressures may be great between 2 and 3.5 years, and it is during this period that borderline stuttering typically emerges. The converging demands of expressive language and motor speech development ordinarily peak about this time "when an explosive growth in language ability outstrips a still-immature speech motor apparatus" (Andrews et al., 1983, p. 239). This age is also filled with psychosocial conflicts as

Table 7.4	Characteristics of Borderline Stuttering in a Younger Preschool Child

1. More than 10 disfluencies per 100 words
2. Often more than two units in repetition
3. More repetitions and prolongations than revisions or incomplete phrases
4. Disfluencies loose and relaxed
5. Rare for child to react to his disfluencies

a child copes with security needs as an infant while striving to become more independent as a toddler. The child may be ready to explore but is also fearful. The birth of a new brother or sister may trigger the child's insecurity with the threat of being replaced. An older sibling may turn belligerent toward him because of the older child's own need to express aggression as a prelude to puberty. Just as these stresses wax and wane in strength during preschool years, so does the child's stuttering.

As children mature, certain developmental stresses may taper off. After age 5, children may feel more integrated within themselves and within their families. Articulation and language skills, although still not at adult levels, have been mastered sufficiently for most children to say what's on their minds and to be understood. They have also mastered other motor skills, such as walking and running, as well as riding a tricycle or a bike with training wheels. They may have adjusted to a new, younger sibling as well and made at least temporary peace with an older one.

By now, the capacities of many of the children who had modest predispositions to stutter can easily meet most environmental demands. Therefore, many of those who were borderline stutterers will have acquired normal fluency skills by the time they are 4 or 5 years old. Others may still have many disfluencies at this age, but will eventually outgrow them, perhaps because they are not frustrated by them and do not respond with tension or by rushing. In general, they are functioning well, feel accepted, and can use their resources to compensate for whatever difficulties in speaking remain.

Some children, of course, do not outgrow borderline stuttering. They may continue to stutter, and their symptoms may worsen. They may be children who have substantial predispositions to stutter, which cannot be offset by a "good enough" environment (Winnicott, 1971). Their ability to produce speech and language at the rate and level of complexity used by parents and peers may be insufficient. And their continuing efforts to meet advanced speech and language targets may result in excess disfluency that does not diminish as they pass their third and fourth birthdays. Their frustration tolerance for the repetitions that 2- and 3-year-olds exhibit may be low. Rather than shrugging them off, they may begin struggling to produce flawless speech, thereby placing greater demands on their speech production and emotional resources. Still other children may continue to stutter because environmental and developmental stresses do not diminish. Their insecurity may continue from sibling rivalry, breakup of the family, or a parent's death. They may have language or articulation problems, as well as stuttering, which limit their communication abilities throughout their preschool years.

Deficits in the processes underlying speech and language development, plus the frustration of being unable to communicate easily, may be devastating to fluency. This may result in the increased tension we see in older preschool children with beginning stuttering. A child in this situation is unlikely to outgrow stuttering unless parents and professionals provide extensive support.

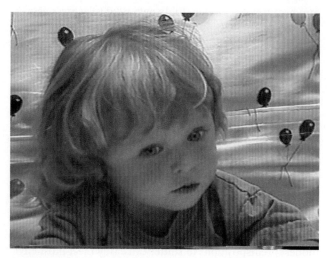

A video clip of a child with borderline stuttering is available on *thePoint*.

Summary

1. Younger preschool children with borderline stuttering usually exhibit a greater amount of disfluency than do normal children—more than seven disfluencies per 100 words.
2. Using another measure of frequency, the proportion of stuttering-like disfluencies may be greater than half of all disfluencies.
3. Children with borderline stuttering are also likely to repeat units more than once in many of their part-word and monosyllabic word repetitions and to have many more part-word and monosyllabic word repetitions and prolongations than multisyllabic word and phrase repetitions, revisions, and interjections.
4. At the same time, their disfluencies, like those of nonstuttering children, are usually loose and relaxed appearing. Also, like nonstuttering children, children with borderline stuttering show little or no awareness of their speaking difficulty. Only rarely do they express frustration about it.
5. Among the underlying processes behind borderline stuttering are probably some of the speech and language-processing anomalies described in the earlier chapter on constitutional origins of stuttering. Such deficits in resources may interact with the demands of speech and language development, the pressure from higher rates of speech, more complex language, competitive speaking situations, and other attributes of a normal home. In addition, some of the psychosocial conflicts described earlier that increase normal disfluency are likely to be active in creating borderline stuttering.

OLDER PRESCHOOL CHILDREN: BEGINNING STUTTERING

In the older preschool child, (Fig. 7.4) stuttering usually has more tension and hurry than stuttering in a younger child. It may have evolved over a period of months or a year or two from borderline stuttering that the child manifested earlier. Or it may appear suddenly in an older preschool child during a time of stress or excitement. The tense and hurried stuttering may alternate with looser, easier disfluencies. Gradually, this more advanced type of stuttering will become commonplace. Soon, the child becomes impatient with his stuttering as it is happening—perhaps even embarrassed—and may begin to use a variety of escape behaviors as a consequence. For example, he may try to end long repetitions by using an eye blink or head nod. Periods of increased stuttering may last for several months, but periods of fluency may last only a few days. As these signs occur more consistently, tension increases and struggle is more evident. Instrumental and classical conditioning processes increase the frequency of struggle behaviors, complicate the child's pattern of stuttering, and spread the symptoms to many more situations.

As mentioned, some children exhibit beginning stuttering at onset, without passing through a stage of borderline stuttering. Van Riper (1971, 1982) described several different profiles of stuttering with tense blockages at onset. Many of the children he depicted as more severe at onset were relatively older (e.g., 4, 5, or 6 years old) when their stuttering first appeared. Onset in these children seemed to be related to one of two factors: delayed language development or emotional events. In a study of the onset of stuttering, Yairi and Ambrose (1992b) described onsets of stuttering that were characterized by the signs I described for

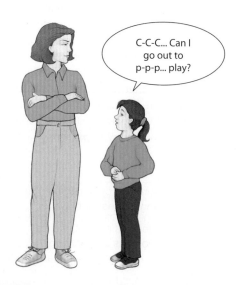

Figure 7.4   Child who may be a beginning stutterer.

beginning stuttering in 28 percent of their sample of 87 children. Many of these children had relatively sudden onsets, with normal fluency changing to beginning stuttering within one day or at most one week.

Core Behaviors

The core behaviors of **beginning stuttering** differ from those of borderline stuttering in several ways. Repetitions begin to sound rapid and irregular. The final segment of a repeated syllable often sounds abrupt; if it is a vowel, it will sound as if it were suddenly cut off or were a neutral or schwa vowel ("uh") that had been substituted for the appropriate one, as in "luh-luh-luh-like" instead of "li-li-li-like." Repetitions are also produced more rapidly, sometimes with an irregular rhythm. Rather than patiently repeating a syllable as a borderline stutterer does, a child with beginning stuttering hurries through repetitive stutters, as though juggling a hot potato.

As symptoms progress, a beginning stutterer increases tension throughout the speech mechanism. Stuttering is sometimes accompanied by a rise in vocal pitch, resulting from increased tension in the vocal folds. Rising pitch may first appear toward the end of a string of repeated syllables, but over time will appear earlier in the repetitions. A child with beginning stuttering sometimes prolongs sounds that he would have previously repeated. Initially, he may prolong the first sounds of syllables, but as stuttering grows more severe, he may also prolong middle sounds, and they too may be accompanied by an increase in pitch.

As beginning stuttering progresses, the first signs of blockages appear. These are significant landmarks, which indicate that a child is stopping the flow of air or voice at one or more places (Van Riper, 1982). He may inappropriately jam his vocal folds closed or wide open, interrupting or possibly delaying the onset of phonation (Conture, 1990). Shutting off the airway is usually heard as a momentary stoppage of sound in a child's speech and is sometimes accompanied by visual cues; the child may seem momentarily unable to move his mouth or may make groping movements with his mouth as he tries to get air or voice going again. When the stoppage of movement, voice, or airflow first begins, it may be so fleeting that we don't notice it unless we are listening and watching carefully. As these blocks worsen, they become so obvious that they may overshadow the repetitions and prolongations that may remain.

Secondary Behaviors

As these older preschool children's symptoms progress, secondary behaviors are added. They are called secondary because they appear to be responses to the runaway repetitions and increased muscle tension that have emerged. In addition, although hard evidence is lacking, the core behaviors of tension and speeding up seem to be "involuntary," to have begun as a reaction that is beyond the stutterer's ability to control. In contrast, the secondary behaviors we are describing seem to have begun "voluntarily." They are—at least initially—deliberate.

Among the earliest of the secondary symptoms are "escape" behaviors, which are maneuvers used to end a stutter and finish a word. Children with beginning stuttering often show escape behaviors after several repetitions of a syllable. They may nod their heads, squint their eyes, or blink just as they try to push a word out. This extra effort often seems to help—in the short run. For the moment, they escape from the punishing repetition, prolongation, or block. Alternatively, they may insert a filler, such as "uh" or "um," after a string of fruitless repetitions. The "um" seems to release the word, perhaps by relaxing the tightly squeezed larynx or by unlocking the lips. The "um" can always be said fluently, and once uttered, phonation and movement for the word often begin. The fillers work like a little push you might give your sled if it were stuck in the snow as you start down a hill; the "um" gets the child going again when he is stuck in a stutter.

A beginning stutterer starts to use escape behaviors earlier and earlier in stutters. The first appearance of these behaviors is usually after a child has repeated a sound quite a few times and is thoroughly frustrated about it. It may sound this way: "Luh-Luh-Luh-Luh-Luh-umLet's go!" Soon, however, the child will not wait until she has tried to say the sound five times. She finds herself about to say a word, feels convinced it won't come out, and then perhaps instinctively uses escape behaviors when she is first starting to stutter: "L-umLet's go!" Such "starters" may even appear before the first sound of the word, in this fashion: "umLet's go!" This is really an avoidance behavior (because it is deployed to avoid a stutter before being stuck in one); they are more common among children with intermediate stuttering, even though it occasionally appears in the speech of a child with beginning stuttering.

Feelings and Attitudes

An older preschool child with beginning stuttering has stuttered many times. He is aware of stuttering when it happens. The feelings a beginning stutterer has just before, during, and after stutters are often strong. Frequently, frustration is a major feeling. The child may stop in the middle of a stutter and say, "Mom, why can't I talk?" However, such momentary frustration grows into momentary fear when a word or sound is stuck for several seconds, and the child feels helpless and out of control.

Although a child with beginning stuttering is conscious that he has some "trouble" when he talks, he has not yet developed a belief that he is a defective speaker. This lack of a negative self-image may be attributed, as Bloodstein (1987) and Van Riper (1982) have suggested, to the "episodic"

Table 7.5	Characteristics of Beginning Stuttering in an Older Preschool Child

1. Signs of muscle tension and hurry appear in stuttering. Repetitions are rapid and irregular with abrupt terminations of each element.
2. Pitch rise may be present toward the end of a repetition or prolongation.
3. Fixed articulatory postures are sometimes evident when the child is momentarily unable to begin a word, apparently as a result of tension in speech musculature.
4. Escape behaviors are sometimes present in stutterers. These include, among other things, eye blinks, head nods, and "ums."
5. Awareness of difficulty and feelings of frustration are present, but there are no strong negative feelings about self as speaker.

nature of stuttering. Sometimes it's there; sometimes it's not. Sometimes a child feels that he has problems when he talks; other times he forgets about it. The essential characteristics of beginning stutterers are presented in Table 7.5.

Underlying Processes

The signs and symptoms of beginning stuttering in the older preschool child can be observed by any experienced clinician. We have seen them in hundreds of children who stutter. But the processes underlying these behaviors are not so easy to see. In Chapters 4 and 5, we suggested that beginning stuttering may result from the interplay between constitutional and environmental factors, especially in a child with a reactive temperament. I will review my hypotheses about the core behaviors of beginning stuttering as well as the learning processes that are likely to perpetuate the core behaviors and a child's secondary reactions.

Increases in Muscle Tension and Tempo

One of the first signs of beginning stuttering in older preschool children is the appearance of extra muscular tension in repetitions and prolongations and increased tempo or rate in repetitive stutters (Van Riper, 1982). Why do these changes occur? Oliver Bloodstein (Bloodstein, 1987; Bloodstein & Ratner, 2008) suggests that facial tension and strained glottal attacks in the speech of young children who stutter may reflect the extra muscular effort that emerges when they anticipate difficulty. Edward Conture (1990) offers a related view. He sees the increased articulatory and laryngeal muscle tension as a child's attempt to control sound-syllable repetitions, which are so distressing to him and his listeners. We have described such tension as a child's effort to control a frustrating and scary behavior of his own body, an attempt to stiffen the speech muscles and brace himself against the perturbations of seemingly involuntary, runaway

repetitions (Guitar, Guitar, Neilson, O'Dwyer, & Andrews, 1988). One can imagine this taking place in the same way that a child who is attempting to ice skate may begin to stiffen in response to rough spots in the ice by stiffening and assuming a less than ideal stance for continued forward movement.

The other early sign of beginning stuttering—increases in the rate of repetitive stutters—is cited by a number of authors as an indication that stuttering is worsening. Van Riper (1982), in describing the developmental course of the majority of children whose stuttering persists, stated that "the tempo changes as the disorder develops. The repetitive syllables become irregular and are often spoken more rapidly than other fluent syllables." Starkweather (1987) explained this increase in the speed of repetitions as a product of the pressure that children feel as they become more aware of the extra time it takes them to produce an utterance.

But why are these increases in tension and tempo so common in the development of stuttering, and why are they so difficult to change in therapy? In Chapter 6, I described my view that children in whom stuttering persists may be especially sensitive to certain kinds of experiences. Faced with frustration or fear, I hypothesized, they would react with elements of their biologically based freezing or flight responses. The signs of beginning stuttering appear to have similarities with such reactions. The excessive muscle tension in stuttering typical of older preschool children can be viewed as a way that the limbic system can cause children to freeze in the face of their frustrating or frightening repetitive disfluencies, transforming them into abrupt, tense repetitions, blocks, or prolongations. As I have mentioned, some children appear to show tense blocks at the onset of their stuttering. These may be children who have high degrees of emotional sensitivity and whose very first manifestation of stuttering may result from fear-based responses to speaking experiences.

Research bears out the speculation that at least some adults who stutter contract their muscles in such a way that movement and phonation are immobilized. Freeman and Ushijima's (1978) and Shapiro and DeCicco's (1982) studies indicate that stuttering is associated with abnormal muscle co-contraction of adductor and abductor muscles in the larynx. Such co-contraction could produce stiffening of the phonatory structures and silencing of vocal output. Other studies of stuttering have demonstrated co-contraction in articulatory structures (Fibiger, 1971; Guitar et al., 1988; Platt & Basili, 1973), which could also produce immobility and silence.

Unfortunately, little research directly supports the notion that the increased rate of repetitions reflects the flight response. We have some preliminary evidence that stutterers have more rapid productions during repetitions than do non-stutterers. An unpublished study (Allen, 1988) carried out in our clinical laboratory indicated that the durations of beginning stutterers' repeated segments and the silences between them were shorter than the durations in similar disfluencies of nonstuttering children matched for age. This finding has been confirmed in the work of Throneburg and Yairi (1994), who also found that the silent intervals and the total durations of repetition disfluencies were significantly shorter in stuttering children compared with those of nonstuttering children controls. Such shortening of segments results in a faster speech rate, at least for the stuttered elements, and may reflect the "great increase in activity" seen in the flight response, although these particular data do not exclude the possibility that stuttering children were more rapid speakers to begin with. It may be relevant at this point to note that Kloth, Janssen, Kraaimaat, and Brutten (1995) found that rapid speaking rate was a predictor of which young children who were fluent at the time of testing but had family histories of stuttering would eventually stutter. The rapid rate in these children might be related to a reactive limbic system, although there is no evidence that speech rate is related to such reactivity.

The possibility that increased muscle tension and rapid repetitions are a result of biologically based freezing or flight responses is highly speculative at this time. If these responses are part of humans' neural wiring designed for survival, this may be a potential explanation of why some children develop stuttering so rapidly and why tension responses are so difficult to change.

Effects of Learning on Stuttering

It is not clear whether the increases in tension and rate are voluntary or involuntary or both, but I have observed repeatedly that these reactions increase with persistent stuttering. This is likely to be the result of classical and instrumental conditioning, which are thought to be the forces at work when stuttering escalates from an occasional tense and hurried repetition to speech that is riddled with tense and hurried repetitions. Learning processes also turn occasional eye blinks or head nods during stutters into stereotyped patterns of blinking and nodding that transform innocuous disfluencies into something so obvious that listeners gape in surprise and parents look away. Let us examine these learning processes more closely so that we can better understand those who come to us for help.

Classical conditioning, I surmise, is responsible for previously "neutral" experiences and situations becoming able to elicit tense and hurried stuttering in a child's speech. This occurs after many experiences in which a child's repetitive stutters have brought on emotions that trigger increases in tension and hurry. Through the repeated pairing of the neutral situations with negative emotions related to stuttering, classical conditioning spreads this change in stuttering behaviors to more and more situations. In few children, tension appears at the onset of the disorder because these children experience a high degree of emotion during a speaking situation. Many children whose stuttering persists may be highly susceptible to classical conditioning because their reactive nervous systems are quick to produce emotions.

If classical conditioning spreads negative emotion to more and more speaking situations, it is *instrumental* conditioning that is responsible for the increase in frequency of escape behaviors in older preschool children's beginning stuttering. This is because the child is rewarded for such things as head nods or eye blinks when they are followed by gratifying releases of the words on which he is stuttering. Instrumental conditioning generalizes escape behaviors to more and more situations and causes escape behaviors to occur earlier and earlier in stutters so that escape behaviors may eventually become "starters."

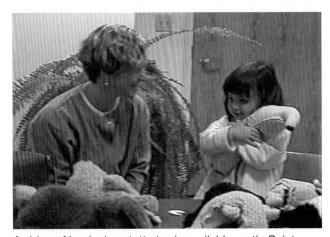

A video of beginning stuttering is available on *thePoint*.

Summary

The principal differences between borderline stuttering seen in younger preschool children and beginning stuttering common in older preschool children are these:

1. The older child with beginning stuttering shows more tension and "hurry" in his stuttering. This is often manifested in abruptly ended syllable repetitions, irregular rhythms of repetitions, evident stoppages of phonation, and momentarily fixated articulatory postures. Older preschool children also evidence such secondary behaviors as escape devices and starters. In addition, these beginning stutterers see themselves as persons who have trouble talking.
2. A major factor underlying beginning stuttering appears to be a child's sensitivity to stress, which may result in frustration, triggering tension responses.
3. Classical conditioning then links such unconditioned response sensitivity to disfluency. When the child is disfluent, he feels threatened, frustrated, or afraid, and this in turn leads to the rapid, tense disfluencies that begin to appear in beginning stutterers. After repeated pairings, disfluency itself, rather than the emotion, elicits increased tension and rate. Classical conditioning also links a child's disfluency to more and more people and places.

4. A third factor in beginning stuttering in older preschool children is instrumental conditioning, which increases and then maintains the use of escape devices. These behaviors are negatively reinforced when a stutterers' frustration is terminated by an escape behavior and are positively reinforced when the stutterer completes his communication.

SCHOOL-AGE CHILDREN: INTERMEDIATE STUTTERING

The school-age child with **intermediate stuttering** (Fig. 7.5), who is typically between ages 6 and 13 years, has two major characteristics that distinguish him from a child with beginning stuttering. First, he is starting to *fear* stuttering, whereas older preschool children with beginning stuttering are usually only frustrated, surprised, or annoyed by it. Second, the school-age child with intermediate stuttering reacts to his fear of stuttering by appearing to *avoid* it, something beginning stutterers don't do with any regularity. These new symptoms emerge gradually as a young stutterer experiences negative emotion more frequently during stuttering. For example, when the school-age child blocks and feels helpless, listeners respond with discomfort, pity, and ridicule. After this has happened frequently, he becomes afraid.

This fear may be attached first to the sounds and words on which he stutters most, and he starts to believe that these sounds are harder for him. Then he begins to scan ahead to see whether he might have to say them. When he anticipates that he will, he tries to avoid them. For example, he may say, "I don't know," to questions or substitute "my sister" for his sister's name when talking about her. Sometimes, he may start a sentence, realize a feared word is coming up, then switch the sentence around to avoid stuttering, and end up producing a maze of half-finished sentences. With tactful questioning, the clinician can verify these avoidances.

A school-age intermediate stutterer's fear of stuttering may be associated with situations as well as words. The youngster may find that he stutters more in some situations than in others. At first, he approaches these situations with dread, but later, he may go to great lengths to avoid them. Van Riper (1982) suggested that the development of such situational fears and avoidances depends on listener reactions. Consequently, counseling or advice for key listeners in a stutterer's environment may help prevent them.

Core Behaviors

What are intermediate stutterers' moments of stuttering like when they don't avoid them? What are the core behaviors? Although they still repeat and prolong, their most notable core behaviors are now blocks. The blocks of children with intermediate stuttering seem to grow out of the increasing tension seen initially in beginning stuttering. A child at the intermediate level usually stutters by stopping airflow, voicing, movement, or all three, then struggling to get his speech going again. His stutters seem to surprise him less than when he was a beginning stutterer. Instead, as evidenced by his voice and manner in certain situations, he anticipates stutters.

I have the impression that the intermediate stutterer's blocks are frequently characterized by excessive laryngeal tension, but he often blocks elsewhere, as well. He may squeeze his lips together, jam his tongue against the roof of his mouth, or hold his breath. Even though he is not highly conscious of just what he's doing during a block, he has a vivid awareness that he is stuck, that he feels helpless, and that the word he wants to say won't seem to come out.

A school-age child described his feeling of being blocked as like "a rock stuck in my throat." When he was lucky, he said, a little army of men would come into his throat and break the rock into little pieces, breaking the block so that sounds would come out. He was describing the experience of first being totally stuck, then rapidly repeating the first segment of the sound as he fought his way out of the block. A common example is the "…uh-uh-uh-I" that you will hear when someone is blocked on "I" and tries to push through it. At first, there is a moment of silence and then the rapid, staccato first segment of the sound as the stutterer gets his larynx vibrating while maintaining a static articulatory posture. The larynx is still very tense; vibration stops and starts again and again. The vowel—either at the beginning or end of the syllable—is often what Van Riper (1982) called the "schwa" or neutral vowel. In fact, it is only the first, brief segment of the intended vowel, which is cut off too abruptly to be perceived as the sound normally used

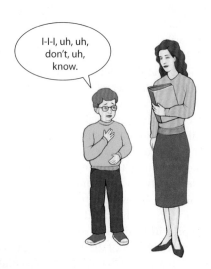

I-I-I, uh, uh, don't, uh, know.

Figure 7.5   Child who may be an intermediate stutterer.

in the word. Inexperienced clinicians sometimes mistakenly categorize these repeated parts of blocks as repetitions, not realizing the stuttering has advanced from repetitions to blocks.

In addition to repetitions of parts of sounds, blocks can have prolongations in them. Sometimes, as he is pushing through a block, a stutterer will momentarily prolong a continuant sound as in "...mmm...mmmm...my." Again, this probably results from the stutterer's larynx vibrating momentarily, then seizing up again, and then vibrating again. I catalog such events as blocks rather than prolongations, because I think the core behavior is a complete stoppage of speech, even though it is mixed with momentary releases of laryngeal vibration. This confusing situation probably results from the fact that the sequence of repetitions, prolongations, and blocks reflects basically similar behaviors along a continuum of increasing tension, particularly in the larynx, as stuttering progresses.

Secondary Behaviors

The blocks just described can be devastating to a child who stutters. He is frustrated not only with his inability to make a sound, but he is often faced with surprised and uncomfortable listeners as well. Even patient listeners may not know what to do. They may interrupt, look away, or fidget, leaving the child or adolescent to conclude that he is doing something wrong and should try to escape or avoid these painful moments.

The escape behaviors that a speaker uses to free himself from stutters are present in preschool children with beginning stuttering, but they occur far more frequently in school-age children with intermediate stuttering. They are often more complex, too. An intermediate stutterer may blink his eyes and nod his head in an effort to escape a block. Sometimes, he may do both, and if he is still unable to say the word, he may resort to yet another device, such as slapping his leg. As these patterns grow more complex, they may also become disguised to look like natural movements and are performed more rapidly.

In addition to escape behaviors, a child at the intermediate level develops both word and situation avoidances, as previously mentioned. Word avoidances appear after he has had repeated difficulty with a particular word or sound and has discovered how to take evasive action before he has to say it. For example, a young stutterer in our clinic had been asked his name by a particularly stern teacher. He blocked severely on it and subsequently became fearful of saying his name, as well as other words starting with the same sound. He could usually think up synonyms for other words but found it awkward to substitute anything different for his name. So he learned to get a running start in saying his name by beginning with "My name is..." whenever he was asked his name. This permitted him to avoid stuttering about half of the time. It is a subtle form of avoidance that many clinicians call "starters." More obvious examples of avoidances are given in the following paragraph.

Van Riper's (1982) catalog of word avoidance techniques included **starters** (beginning a word by saying another word or sound, such as "well" or "uh" just before saying it); **substitutions** (substituting a word or phrase for another when stuttering is expected, as in "he's my unc-unc-unc ... my father's brother"); **circumlocutions** (talking all around a word or phrase when anticipating stuttering, as in "well, I went to ... yes, I really had a good time there, I saw the Empire State Building"); **postponements** (waiting a few beats or putting in filler words before starting a word on which stuttering is expected, as in "My name is.......... Bill"); and **antiexpectancy devices** (using an odd manner or funny voice to avoid stuttering when it's anticipated). I had a client in Australia who could only tell jokes fluently if he put on an accent that sounded like he came from Mississippi or Alabama.

Like escape behaviors, word avoidance techniques often become more rapid and more subtle with time. Indeed, some stutterers can disguise word avoidances to look like normal behavior. For example, they may put on pensive facial expressions and appear to search for a word while postponing their attempt to say a feared sound. Experienced clinicians learn to pick up subtle cues in the rate and manner of speaking that tip them off to the use of such avoidances. Such avoidances can be explored by the clinician and client at the appropriate moment in treatment.

Situational fears and avoidances also begin to appear in the school-age intermediate stutterer. Past stuttering in specific places or with specific people are the seeds from which situational fears grow. In school, stutterers usually have trouble reading aloud or giving oral reports. Most people who stutter, and even many nonstutterers, dread those classes in which teachers call on students by going up and down the rows. As in an earlier example, the students' fears steadily mount as a teacher goes down the row, getting closer and closer to calling on them. Then, if called on, they may take a failing grade rather than give the oral report. In contrast, other school situations, especially casual ones like gym class or lunch period, are likely to hold little fear or expectation of stuttering for them.

Situational fears quickly generate situation avoidances. The student who fears giving answers in class may try to slouch low in his seat in hopes of being overlooked. A stutterer who is afraid of making introductions will contrive ways of having other people make them. In junior high school, I coped with my fear of ordering in restaurants by ducking into the bathroom when the waitress approached our table, leaving my friends to order a cheeseburger for me. Every stutterer has his own pattern of situation avoidances, which may provide an important focus for therapy in many cases.

Feelings and Attitudes

Students with intermediate stuttering have gone well beyond the momentary frustration and mild embarrassment experienced by those with beginning stuttering. They have felt the helplessness of being caught in many blocks and runaway repetitions. The anticipation of stuttering and subsequent listener penalties have been fulfilled many times. These experiences pile up like cars in a demolition derby to create an entanglement of fear, embarrassment, and shame that accompanies stuttering. These feelings may not be pervasive or dog a stutterer all the time. However, stuttering has now changed from an annoyance to a serious problem.

A major influence on such students' feelings is the cognitive development, begun at age 3 or 4, that enables him to compare himself with his peers. Once he begins school, peers have a greater and greater influence on him. He may stutter more as he encounters new people and new situations, and as he does, peers may begin to ask him why he talks the way he does and to make comments about his stuttering or tease him about it. As a result, increasingly negative self-awareness about his speech leads to feelings of embarrassment, shame, and guilt.

A student with intermediate stuttering shows his increasingly negative feelings about stuttering in many ways. He may look away from listeners when he is stuttering and flush with embarrassment immediately afterward. He may become stiff and uneasy at the prospect of speaking. His stuttering pattern includes an increasing number of avoidance devices, and he is beginning to evade situations in which he feels he may stutter. These are all signs that his feelings and attitudes are becoming suffused with fear. Table 7.6 gives the characteristics of intermediate stutterers.

Table 7.6	Characteristics of Intermediate Stuttering in a School-Age Child

1. Most frequent core behaviors are blocks in which the stutterer shuts off sound or voice. He may also have repetitions and prolongations.
2. Stutterer uses escape behaviors to terminate blocks.
3. Stutterer appears to anticipate blocks, often using avoidance behaviors prior to feared words. He also anticipates difficult situations and sometimes avoids them.
4. Fear before stuttering, embarrassment during stuttering, and shame after stuttering characterize this level, especially fear.

The emotions I have described, especially embarrassment and shame, may be mixed with hope as treatment begins. Figure 7.6 was drawn by a young man in his first few weeks of therapy. It reflects his extensive negative feelings on the left side; he has drawn himself in a jail cell with tears/rain falling around him and the key just out of reach. On the right side of the drawing, he shows himself after therapy, escaping from jail, running in the sunshine with grass underfoot and a flower in the background.

Underlying Processes

Many of a school-age, intermediate stutterer's symptoms result from the same processes that underlie those of beginning stutterers. There are major differences, however. In intermediate stuttering, classically conditioned tension responses

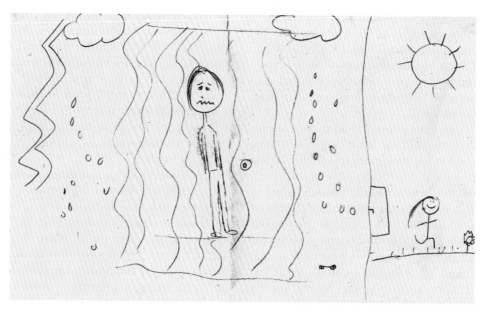

Figure 7.6   A young man's drawing of himself as he begins therapy (*left side*) and his hopes for a happy outcome (*right side*). Drawn by Marcel Etienne.

are more evident, conditioned frustration is now becoming a more intense fear reaction, and avoidance conditioning has become a factor in shaping stuttering behaviors.

Avoidance conditioning transforms *escape* behaviors, such as the use of "um" to escape from a stuttering block, into *avoidances,* such as saying "um" before saying a word on which stuttering is expected. This learning process also leads students with intermediate stuttering to avoid words, to change sentences around, and to avoid speaking situations entirely. Avoidance learning also generalizes from one word to another and from one situation to another.

Avoidance conditioning may proceed very quickly in people with persistent stuttering because they may have a genetic or congenital bias toward right-hemisphere, emotionally based behaviors, as we described in Chapters 2 through 6. The threat of stuttering may elicit "prepared" defensive reactions, such as avoidances of words or situations. Such avoidances are strongly maintained because individuals who have developed them use them when they anticipate stuttering, which decreases or eliminates the fear. Thus, avoidances are maintained by negative reinforcement. By avoiding the stuttering, individuals who stutter never have the opportunity to discover that stuttering is not so painful after all. Therapy must (a) structure situations to help them learn this and (b) give them new behaviors to substitute for the old avoidances.

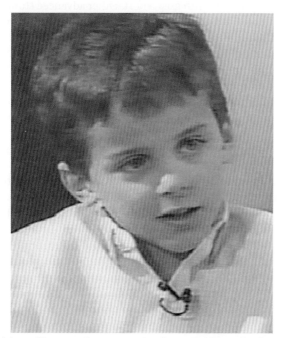

A video of intermediate stuttering is available on *thePoint*.

Summary

Intermediate stuttering in school-age children is differentiated from beginning stuttering in older preschool children by the following:

1. There are increasingly tense blocks, repetitions, and prolongations; the increased tension results from feelings of frustration, fear, and helplessness. These feelings trigger tension responses, which interfere with fluency and in turn produce more frustration, fear, and feelings of helplessness. As tension mounts, this vicious cycle continues; blocks are longer and more noticeable, more listeners react with surprise and impatience, and the student's fear increases in response to these reactions.
2. The increasing presence of fear and anticipation of bad experiences spurs the student to develop avoidance behaviors in addition to the escape behaviors he is already using. Avoidance conditioning is difficult to undo.
3. The child with intermediate stuttering increasingly feels embarrassment, shame, and guilt as he realizes that his speech is markedly different from that of his peers.

OLDER TEENS AND ADULTS: ADVANCED STUTTERING

Individuals whose stuttering has persisted into older adolescence and adulthood (Fig. 7.7) typically have a deeply ingrained pattern of core and secondary behaviors. Often stuttering is a major player in their school, work, and social lives. They may avoid talking in class, decline job opportunities, and limit their social activities from fear of stuttering. This describes me at age 20.

Of course some older teens and adults stutter only mildly or aren't bothered by their stuttering; they carry on their lives seeing it as a minor annoyance. These individuals often don't seek treatment—unless their stuttering suddenly gets in the way of something they want to do. One of my clients who

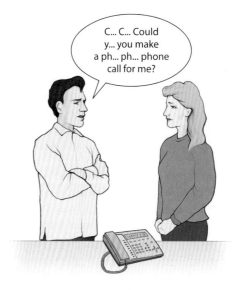

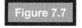 **Figure 7.7** Individual who may be an advanced stutterer.

had relatively mild stuttering was in the U.S. Air Force and wanted to move up from navigator to pilot. This was during the Vietnam War, and I worried that this promotion would put him more at risk. Nevertheless, we worked hard together for six months, and he made the grade.

Treatment of older teens and adults differs from treatment of younger stutterers because the client can take much of the responsibility for therapy including substantial work outside the clinic.

An advanced stutterer's increased capacity for independent work may compensate for another characteristic of this level—a long history of stuttering. Patterns of stuttering with tension, escape, and avoidance behaviors are now firmly established. Emotions such as frustration, fear, guilt, and hostility have built up over many years of being unable to speak like other people and many bad experiences with thoughtless, uninformed, or momentarily startled listeners. Beliefs are usually distorted by the conviction that other people are impatient or disgusted by the speaker's stuttering.

After many years of stuttering, adults and adolescents who stutter increasingly think of themselves as stutterers rather than as people who have occasional difficulty speaking. Except for a few safe situations in which they may be relatively fluent, they have some fear for most speaking situations, and they shape their lives accordingly. They may believe that their stuttering is as noticeable to others as though they had two heads—and nearly as unacceptable.

Core Behaviors

Core behaviors of stuttering in older teens and adults include repetitions and prolongations, but **advanced stuttering** is often distinct in the struggle and tension of blocks—stoppages of sound and movement. Advanced stutterers may block, then release a little sound only to fall back into the block again. It might sound like this: "(silence)…m-m-m… (silence)…m-m-muh…(silence)…my (said with a sudden effort)…name is Barry." Such behaviors may be longer and more struggled in clients with advanced stuttering than in school-age kids who have intermediate stuttering, but they are essentially the same. Blocks may be associated with tremors. During blocks, tremors of the lips, jaw, or tongue may be apparent. As you may remember from the discussion of tremors in Chapters 2, 3, and 6, tremors appear in those who have been stuttering for several years and may occur when stuttering is accompanied by strong emotion.

In a few advanced stutterers, blocks are hardly evident at all. They may have honed their avoidance devices to such a fine edge that core behaviors are scarcely noticeable. If stuttering does become evident, it usually feels devastating. Consequently, much of their energy is spent anticipating blocks that often don't occur and mustering avoidances to keep anxiety at bay. One such individual, a delightful woman I knew and whom I'll call Lenore, said she had stuttered since childhood. Yet,

she almost never had a repetition, prolongation, or block that I could see. She was highly competent at everything she did, but severely limited her life because of her fear that she would stutter. In particular, she often felt she came across as far less articulate than she might have because of the frequency with which she substituted words to avoid stuttering.

Older teens and adults with advanced stuttering, like school-age youngsters at the intermediate level, have repetitions as well as blocks. These are not the easy, regular repetitions of borderline stuttering, but are more like those of beginning stuttering—tense, with a rapid, irregular tempo. They may be repetitions of syllables, luh-luh-luh-like this, or mixed with fixed articulatory postures of tense blocks, l … l … luh-luh-luh … like this. The latter look as if the speaker recoils from a momentary fixation then gets stuck again.

Secondary Behaviors

Advanced stuttering in older teens and adults involves many of the same word and situational avoidances that are seen in intermediate stuttering, but the avoidances are likely to be more extensive. Some behaviors are more obvious than others. When I was in high school, I used several avoidance devices that often didn't work, such as "uh … well … you see" and a gasp of air, followed by a block of long duration filled with unsuccessful escape attempts before I finally released the blocked word with great effort. Other advanced stutterers may approach feared words cautiously and use subtle mannerisms, such as appearing to think just before saying them, so that most listeners don't realize they are stuttering. These stutterers are usually on guard much of the time, scanning ahead with their verbal early-warning systems.

Many advanced stutterers also control their environments carefully so that they can avoid situations in which they are likely to stutter. They may feign sickness when they have to give a speech, use answering machines rather than answering the telephone, or arrange to have their spouses or children deal with store clerks. Often, with careful questioning of advanced stutterers who use avoidances a great deal, you can learn what occurs when avoidances don't work. Even the most skillful avoiders are sometimes caught with their defenses down and become stuck in a block. Core behaviors may also be elicited by asking some stutterers to stutter openly without using secondary behaviors. Stutterers who can do this, especially those who can do it without excessive discomfort, are more amenable to change.

Feelings and Attitudes

The feelings and attitudes of older teens and adults, like their stuttering patterns, have been shaped by years of conditioning. Over and over, they have learned that much of their stuttering is unpredictable. When it is predictable, it comes when they want it least—when they want more than anything to be

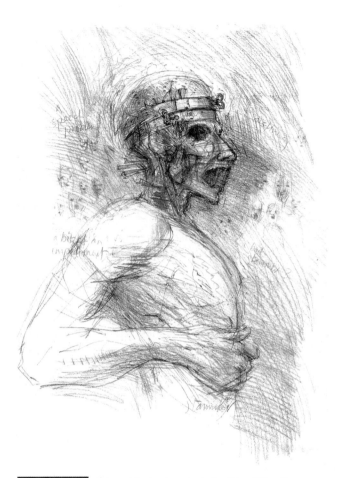

| Table 7.7 | Characteristics of Advanced Stuttering in Older Teens and Adults |

Table 7.7 — Characteristics of Advanced Stuttering in Older Teens and Adults

1. Most frequent core behaviors are longer, tense blocks, often with tremors of the lips, tongue, or jaw. Individual will also probably have repetitions and prolongations.
2. Stuttering may be suppressed in some individuals through extensive avoidance behaviors.
3. Complex patterns of avoidance and escape behaviors characterize the stutterer. These may be very rapid and so well habituated that the stutterer may not be aware of what he does.
4. Emotions of fear, embarrassment, and shame are very strong. Stutterer has negative feelings about himself as a person who is helpless and inept when he stutters. This self-concept may be pervasive.

Figure 7.8 "How I feel when I stutter" by Mike Peace. (Courtesy of Dr. Trudy Stewart.)

fluent. As a result, they often feel out of control. Figure 7.8 reflects one individual's depictions of his own feelings of being out of control when stuttering.

These uncomfortable feelings are often buttressed by a stutterer's perceptions of how others see him. Listeners' reactions look overwhelmingly negative to him. Even when listeners say nothing, their faces appear to say everything. It is as though stuttering is a rattletrap car that always stalls in heavy traffic amid honking drivers. Such experiences gradually shape advanced stutterers' attitudes toward feelings of helplessness, frustration, anger, and hopelessness.

Of course, individuals' responses to stuttering vary greatly. If a person who stutters has many talents and abilities for which he is recognized and if he has an assertive personality, he may be less devastated by stuttering. The former CEO of General Electric company, Jack Welsh, is a good example. But if the individual has a highly sensitive nature, his feelings and attitudes about stuttering may be an important component of his problem. The movie "The King's Speech" suggested that Bertie, who was to become the King of England, George VI, was a sensitive soul who was debilitated by his stuttering until he received some very

confidence-building treatment from Lionel Logue, his unorthodox Australian clinician.

The point is that by the time a stutterer is an adult, he has had years of experiencing stuttering, feeling frustrated and helpless, and has developed techniques to minimize pain. Unless he has strong attributes to compensate, he is likely to feel that stuttering is a big part of who he is to other people. It is a part that he hates, a part on which he blames many other troubles, and a part he wants to eliminate.

Some stutterers, however, who reach the advanced level have become reconciled to their stuttering. If they are in their 20s, 30s, or beyond, there may be some natural resistance to treatment, because stuttering has become part of their identities. After years of doubt and turmoil, they've grown accustomed to themselves as stutterers. To consider treatment is to reject a part of themselves, to open old wounds. Those who risk change, enter treatment, and succeed will find the risk to have been worthwhile. But those who enter treatment and do not succeed may suffer twice from the pain of failure as well as the loss of the denial or reluctant acceptance of stuttering that had been in place before the attempt at treatment but was given up.

Table 7.7 lists the major characteristics of advanced stutterers.

Underlying Processes

Advanced stuttering, unlike lower levels of stuttering, is influenced less by its original constitutional, developmental, and environmental factors than by the older teen or adult's reactions to his stuttering. The effects of home environments, developmental pressures of speech and language, and maybe even some differences in central nervous system function have been diminished by maturation and learning. However, conditioned habits that were learned in response to these early factors are stronger than ever. Their effects have been magnified by years of experience, and the way the brain operates in speech has been modified as a consequence. Moreover, an individual's characteristic patterns of tension, escape behaviors, and word and situation avoidances have become almost automatic through years of practice. For example, he may exhibit a string of avoidance and escape behaviors but only remember that "the word got stuck."

The older teen and adult's stuttering is affected by higher-level explicit learning as well. He has developed a self-concept as an impaired speaker, which carries highly negative connotations for most. Self-concepts begin to be formed during preschool years and are based initially on what one can do, rather than what one is (Clarke-Stewart & Friedman, 1987). More enduring traits are added as a result of social interactions in later childhood, adolescence, and beyond (Roessler & Bolton, 1978). Thus, a stutterer's self-concept at the earliest levels of development is determined, in part, by his perception of how he talks. In a child's early years, his impression of stuttering may be a fleeting awareness that he sometimes has difficulty talking. At later levels of development, the reactions of significant listeners—parents, peer group, other adults—have a major impact. Now his self-concept may become filled with relatively enduring negative perceptions as a result of listeners' impatience and

rejection. A negative self-concept is formed not only by perceptions of listeners' reactions, but it in turn also affects those perceptions.

Researchers studying the psychology of disability suggest that "one's perception of self influences one's perception of others' views of oneself, rendering social interaction more difficult" (Roessler & Bolton, 1978). Applied to clients with advanced stuttering, this suggests that they are likely to project their own rejections of stuttering onto listeners, thereby inhibiting interactions with them. This vicious cycle can only be stopped when an outsider helps a stutterer test the reality of his perceptions.

In addition to working on cognitive aspects of the problem, therapy for advanced stuttering also deals directly with the avoidances such clients have learned so well. As mentioned in the discussion of intermediate stuttering, as avoidance conditioning progresses, individuals fear not only words and situations, but also stuttering itself. By deconditioning this fear and changing such responses, treatment enables stutterers to stutter with less fear by associating the clinician's approval with a calmer, more relaxed way of stuttering. Gradually, tension and hurry fade from disfluencies, they feel more in control, and their fears diminish even further as a result.

Table 7.8	Characteristics of Five Developmental/Treatment Levels			
Developmental/ Treatment Level	Core Behaviors	Secondary Behaviors	Feelings and Attitudes	Underlying Processes
Normal disfluency	10 or fewer disfluencies per 100 words; one-unit repetitions; mostly repetitions, interjections, and revisions	None	Not aware; no concern	Stresses of speech/ language and psychosocial development
Borderline stuttering	11 or more disfluencies per 100 words; more than two units in repetitions; more repetitions and prolongations than revisions or interjections	None	Generally not aware; may occasionally show momentary surprise or mild frustration	Stresses of speech/ language and psychosocial development interacting with constitutional predisposition
Beginning stuttering	Rapid, irregular, and tense repetitions may have fixed articulatory posture in blocks	Escape behaviors such as eye blinks, increases in pitch, or loudness as disfluency progresses	Aware of disfluency, may express frustration	Conditioned emotional reactions causing excess tension; instrumental conditioning resulting in escape behaviors
Intermediate stuttering	Blocks in which sound and airflow are shut off	Escape and avoidance behaviors	Fear, frustration, embarrassment, and shame	Above processes, plus avoidance conditioning
Advanced stuttering	Long, tense blocks; some with tremor	Escape and avoidance behaviors	Fear, frustration, embarrassment, and shame; negative self-concept	Above processes, plus cognitive learning

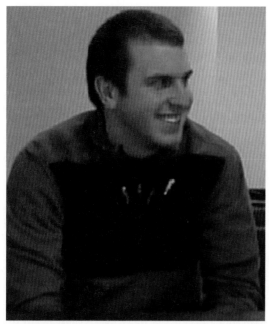

A video of advanced stuttering is available on *thePoint*.

Summary

The diagnosis of advanced stuttering in older teens and adults describes a developmental level and implies a particular treatment orientation as characterized by the following:

1. Treatment may be easier because the client can assume much of the responsibility for generalization beyond the clinic.
2. On the other hand, treatment is more challenging because the client with advanced stuttering has habituated patterns of behavior more deeply than at earlier levels. The advanced stutterer's core behaviors often consist of long blocks with considerable tension and at times visible tremors. Secondary behaviors may consist of long chains of word avoidance and escape behaviors. Situational avoidance is common.
3. Some older teens and adult stutterers may hide and disguise their stuttering well enough to avoid detection by many listeners, but this is at the cost of constant vigilance.
4. Feelings of frustration and helplessness usually accumulate over the years, leading to coping behaviors and a lifestyle that may be highly constraining. Such responses create a self-concept of an inept speaker whose stuttering is unacceptable to listeners. This in turn affects the stutterer's perceptions of the listener's reactions.

SUMMARY

- Table 7.8 summarizes the characteristics of the five developmental/treatment levels described in this chapter.
- Each individual who stutters will have his own course of development, influenced by the interaction of constitutional and environmental factors.
- The clinician needs to use her understanding of the underlying processes to design procedures to treat each individual's core behaviors, secondary behaviors, and feelings and attitudes.

STUDY QUESTIONS

1. In the "exceptions and variations" section of the overview, different types of stuttering onset and development are described. What factors might cause these differences?
2. In discussing normal disfluency, it is suggested that "if a child shows what appears to be normal disfluencies, such as single-word repetitions, but consistently displays pauses or interjections of 'uh' immediately before or during disfluencies, he should be carefully evaluated as possibly stuttering." What might be going on? What might these pauses or interjections signify?
3. The idea of a dyssynchrony in the timing of the elements of spoken language production is suggested as an underlying process of normal disfluency. It is also used to account for primary stuttering. How can both types of disfluency be accounted for by the same process?
4. What is the difference between core behaviors and secondary behaviors?
5. At what ages is normal disfluency likely to be most frequent?
6. Name three influences that may cause normal disfluency to increase.
7. What are three ways in which core behaviors of normal disfluency differ from those of borderline stuttering?
8. Describe the core behaviors of the beginning stutterer.
9. What causes greater muscle tension in beginning stuttering compared to borderline stuttering?
10. Describe why an escape behavior is used by a stutterer. Give examples.
11. What is the major secondary behavior that differentiates the intermediate from the beginning stutterer?
12. Compare the feelings and attitudes of the borderline, beginning, and intermediate stutterers.
13. Describe the role of the listener in the development of the advanced stutterer's self-concept.

SUGGESTED PROJECTS

1. Visit *thePoint* and download the video clips of speakers who are representative of each level of stuttering (normal disfluency, borderline, beginning, intermediate, and advanced), and play them in random order for your class. See how many of your fellow students can correctly identify each level.
2. Make audio or video recordings of a number of nonstuttering students in a class and determine which of them are more disfluent and which are less disfluent. Is there a gradual continuum between more disfluent and less disfluent, or are there two distinct groups? Are any of the more "normally disfluent" students actually borderline stutterers? Should the term "borderline stutterer" be used only for preschoolers?
3. Read Yairi and Ambrose's (2005) chapter on the development of stuttering (see *Suggested Readings*) and compare that perspective with the view presented in this chapter.

SUGGESTED READINGS

Bloodstein, O., & Ratner, N. (2008). Symptomatology. In *A Handbook on Stuttering*. San Diego: Singular Publishing Group, Inc.

The subsection titled, "Developmental Changes in Stuttering" in this chapter describes four stages similar to our levels of stuttering development. Other schemas of developmental changes are also discussed in a clear and logical style.

Gray, J. A. (1987). *The psychology of fear and stress*. Cambridge: Cambridge University Press.

This is a very readable exposition of relatively recent findings about innate fears, conditioning, and brain processes involved with escape and avoidance learning. Gray also describes his concept of the "behavioral inhibition system," a model of the role of conditioning, language, the limbic system, and anxiety on behavior.

Luper, H. L., & Mulder, R. L. (1964). *Stuttering: Therapy for children*. Englewood Cliffs, NJ: Prentice-Hall.

An excellent treatment text that describes four developmental levels of stuttering similar to the levels described here. Although out of print, this book is available for under $10 at http://www.AbeBooks.com.

Starkweather, C. W. (1983). *Speech and language: Principles and processes of behavior change*. Englewood Cliffs, NJ: Prentice-Hall.

This book describes the principles of instrumental, classical, and avoidance conditioning that underlie much of stuttering behavior. It gives a clear account of how these principles create stuttering behavior and how conditioning is used in treatment.

Van Riper, C. (1982). The development of stuttering. In *The Nature of Stuttering*. Englewood Cliffs, NJ: Prentice-Hall.

In this chapter, Van Riper describes four developmental tracks of stuttering, three of which depart substantially from our stages of stuttering development. This chapter gives the reader a good sense of individual variability in stuttering.

Williams, D. F. (2006) *Stuttering recovery: Personal and empirical perspectives*. Mahwah, NJ: Lawrence Erlbaum Associates.

This book is an informal compendium of essays about the experience of stuttering, information about stuttering, and personal anecdotes about the things that happen to you when you stutter.

Yairi, E. & Ambrose, N. G. (2005). The development of stuttering. In *Early Childhood Stuttering* (pp. 141–195). Austin, TX: Pro-Ed.

This chapter reviews other authors' descriptions of the development of stuttering and presents a different perspective on the changes that occur in stuttering from onset to recovery or persistence. The data provided support the view that 75 to 85 percent of children who begin to stutter will recover without treatment and that stuttering typically decreases in severity and frequency after onset.

2

Assessment and Treatment of Stuttering

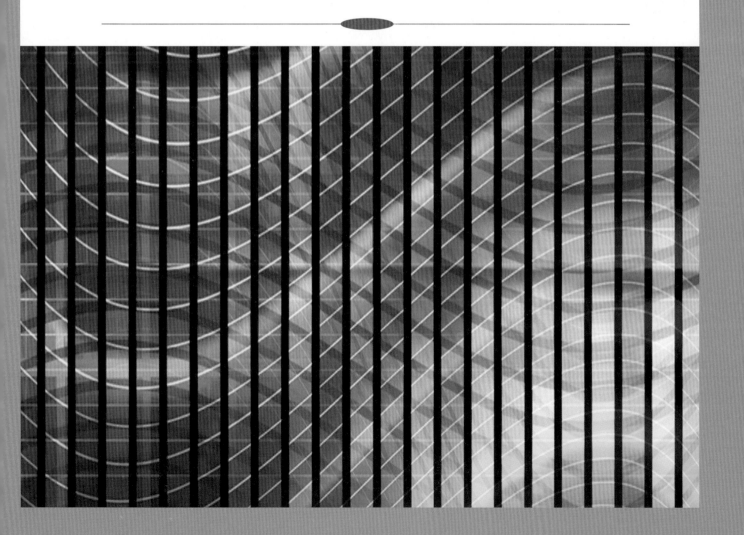

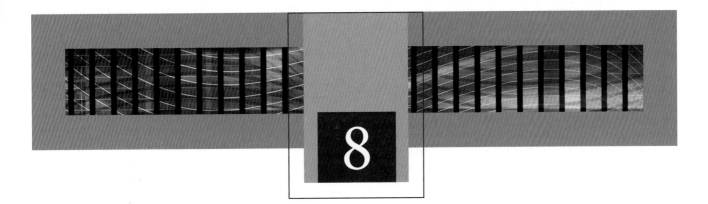

8

Preliminaries to Assessment

CHAPTER OBJECTIVES

After studying this chapter, readers should be able to:
- Understand how to discern the client's needs and plan treatment around them
- Describe how to protect the client's right to privacy and how awareness of the client's right to privacy can facilitate trust
- Explain why multicultural awareness is so important when working with clients from different cultural and linguistic backgrounds
- Describe how a clinician can demonstrate her expertise about stuttering in a way that will engender trust and motivation
- Explain why reliability in a measurement procedure is important and how reliability may be assessed

- Discuss the need for obtaining appropriate speech samples when assessing stuttering
- Explain the advantages and disadvantages of assessing frequency of stuttering and how frequency can be assessed effectively
- Explain why it can be useful to assess different types of stutters that a client may have
- Describe how duration of stutters may be important and how this can be assessed
- Discuss assessment of secondary stuttering behaviors
- Describe four tools to assess stuttering severity and explain when each might be used
- Explain why speech naturalness can be a useful measure
- Explain why assessment of speaking rate may be important
- Discuss at least three ways in which feelings and attitudes can be assessed in each of these age groups: preschool, school-age, and adolescents and adults
- Talk about the need for continuing assessment of clients in treatment

KEY TERMS

HIPAA: Health Insurance Portability and Accountability Act (1996); created national standards to protect the privacy of patient information and still allow access to that information for the safety and proper treatment of patients

Multicultural perspective: An awareness by the clinician of differences in cultures regarding speech, language, and hearing issues as well as differences in styles of interaction between men and women, elders and younger individuals, family and strangers

Bilingual: Having a second language. This applies to individuals who have a single first language that they acquired in infancy and childhood and who then learned a second language or who grew up in a household in which two languages were spoken. Some individuals are multilingual, having learned several languages—either from early childhood or at differing points in time

Empathy: The capacity to understand another's perspectives, beliefs, and emotions. Having this capacity to some degree allows the clinician to undertake appropriate treatment and to develop trust between herself and the patient—a prerequisite for change

Confronting stuttering: Talking about stuttering, emulating it, and being aware of what's happening during the moment of stuttering. These activities can be engaged in by either the clinician or client, when appropriate. These activities and others are thought to reverse the tendency to run away from stuttering that may make stuttering worse

Evidence of reliability: Data that suggest that a procedure or measurement tool produces approximately the same result when used by different individuals or the same individuals at different times

Intrarater reliability: Comparison of results by an individual using a measurement tool at two or more different times

Interrater reliability: Comparison of results by different individuals using a measurement tool

Percentage of syllables stuttered: A common measure of frequency of stuttering obtained by counting the total number of syllables spoken and dividing it into the number of syllables that are stuttered

Types of stutters: The different ways in which an individual may stutter. These include the categories of repetitions, prolongations, and blocks

Duration: The length of time, usually in seconds, that a stutter lasts. From my perspective, this includes the time when forward movement of speech is halted; therefore, the moment of the actual block, prolongation, or repetition is measured as well as the time taken by various starters, postponements, and other secondary behaviors

Severity: Generally a measure of the impediment to communication caused by the stuttering. This may be an overall impression or a compilation of stuttering frequency and duration as well as other behaviors that impede communication

Speech naturalness: The extent to which speech sounds like that of a typical speaker who doesn't stutter. This measure is useful because sometimes treatment leaves the individual technically "fluent" but sounding overly slow or otherwise odd

Speaking rate: How fast a person talks, usually with short pauses included. (Articulation rate is with the pauses removed.) Speaking rate is most often measured in syllables per minute

Feelings and attitudes: Feelings are the emotions experienced by the person who stutters, especially regarding the experience of stuttering and perceived listener responses. They can vary from one time to the next time. Attitudes are more long-lasting; they reflect the stutterer's beliefs about how people perceive him and how he perceives himself in regard to his stuttering

Continuing assessment: Measurement and evaluation of changes the client is making/has made over the short and long term

Assessment operates on many levels, like most human endeavors. On one level, there is information gathering, such as interviewing, measuring speech fluency, and administering tests and questionnaires. This requires careful planning, good observation, and thorough analysis. It begins with clients seeking help and often ends with a plan for treatment. On another level, assessment is a personal encounter. It involves getting to know another person and sometimes his family as well, trying to connect to him, and tuning your antennae to pick up the subtle signals he may be sending out about his needs and how you might help him. On this more subjective level, you are becoming aware of the entire person and family, not just the stuttering. Your clients are also getting to know you and sizing up your ability to help them; thus, this first meeting may be the most critical. Although you will want to show an individual client or family that you know about stuttering and understand its treatment, you will want to spend most of your time listening to their concerns and demonstrating your desire to understand them. The two hats you will wear, that of the humanist and that of the scientist, will become a natural part of your wardrobe as you gain more experience.

THE CLIENT'S NEEDS

It is easy to say we must always consider a client's needs, but it's hard to put this into practice. One reason is that we can develop expectations that function as blinders. Such expectations affect our perceptions of what our clients want, what caused or precipitated their stuttering, what their priorities are, and many other things. Although I know intellectually that every client is different, I have found a tendency in myself, perhaps increasing as I have become more experienced, to jump to conclusions. I sometimes think, "Ah, yes, I understand this kiddo. So much like that child I saw last month." You will find this true for yourself too as you work with more and more clients. We must try to listen carefully to what each client says and see each person with fresh eyes.

We must also be cautious about letting referral information, past experience, and biases cloud our ability to see all aspects of the person clearly. We must be wary of simple explanations and quick judgments about which factors are critical for a client. For instance, if parents tell us that they often ask their child to stop and start again when she stutters, that both parents work long hours outside the home, and that dinner is a noisy and confusing time, we should try not to assume that these pressures at home are a major problem for the child. They may be, but other things may be more critical. We need to ask more questions and explore how the child responds in these and other situations before we decide how to begin helping the child and her family.

Sometimes individuals' or families' requests differ from what we think they need. An adult may say that she wants "completely fluent speech," but we know this is not a likely outcome for a person who has been stuttering for 20 or 30 years. Or a family may want us to treat their 3-year-old child without their having to take part in therapy, although our preferred approach for a child this age involves parent participation. I have found it best not to feel I have to resolve such issues during an assessment session. I make no promises but do make a concerted effort to understand what clients and families want and why. My experience has been that after I work with a family or individual for several sessions, we build up enough trust to work together to make the changes that we mutually decide are appropriate.

I remember seeing a young man who came to our clinic from some distance away for intensive therapy. During the evaluation, he made it quite clear that he didn't want to be treated like a rat in a cage; in other words, he wanted no talk of conditioning, reinforcement, or shaping. In responding to his concerns, I discussed his stuttering with him in terms of what he felt about his stuttering, what he believed his listeners thought, and why he did some of the things he did when he stuttered. Together, we designed an intensive treatment program for him that included plenty of "fluency shaping" and "maintenance" but that made him feel respected as a human and not treated like a laboratory rat. In the process, I also explored with him his concerns about being controlled by others.

In trying to meet a client's needs, I consider the person as well as the problem. The client, no matter what age, will sense quickly whether a clinician is seeing him as an individual or is only seeing his stuttering. An effective clinician is genuinely interested and empathetic; she accepts failures and backsliding as well as victories and progress. The initial evaluation session is a clinician's first opportunity to show the client that she accepts him just as he is, without rejection or fear of his stuttering. This atmosphere helps the client begin accepting himself and his stuttering and take the first critical steps toward more fluent speech and effective communication.

THE CLIENT'S RIGHT TO PRIVACY

All clients should feel they can trust you to protect their privacy and confidentiality. Trust is a vital element of client-clinician relationships. It enables the client to feel that she can safely reveal personal information to you that will help you plan and carry out appropriate treatment. In many cases, the act of expressing feelings in an accepting, secure environment can be therapeutic. For example, a mother whose school-age child was not making progress told her clinician that she was feeling resentment and impatience about her child's stuttering. She talked at some length about this over several sessions, and the clinician listened empathetically. Once she had released these feelings, her child made remarkable progress. Although this example is more about creating an accepting atmosphere for the child, this parent had to trust the clinician to be accepting of her feelings, as

well as not to share this information inappropriately with other family members or the child, or just as inappropriately with fellow student clinicians or others not involved in the child's care.

Federal and state legislation, such as the Health Insurance Portability and Accountability Act of 1996 (**HIPAA**), helps clinicians follow guidelines for protecting clients' privacy. Clinicians should familiarize themselves with these laws and guidelines and ensure that clients give their consent for video recording and observation, and for sharing information about them. You can learn more from the Web site http://www.hhs.gov/ocr/privacy/. When clients perceive that we are scrupulous in guarding their privacy and confidentiality, we gain a level of trust that enhances therapy. This confidentiality extends to children as well. The bond between a child and clinician will be enhanced if the clinician discusses what information the child is willing to have shared with her parent and what not to share. This is especially relevant for school-age children, who should also be consulted about the extent to which they would be comfortable having their parents involved in treatment.

I should mention that there are a few rare circumstances in which confidentiality may be broken. These are the unusual situations when a client discloses plans to hurt himself or others and instances of child abuse disclosed by the child.

CULTURAL CONSIDERATIONS

I have been discussing the need to understand and accept everyone who comes to us for treatment as unique. When people who stutter are from other cultures, our task of really understanding them can be more difficult. The 21st century will be a time of more and more migration among cultures and countries. For example, Vermont has recently become home to immigrants and refugees from 23 different countries. States like California, Florida, and Texas have large refugee populations from all over the world. Many refugees have experienced serious trauma that, in some cases, may have precipitated or worsened stuttering. Thus, it is vital for a clinician working with communication disorders to develop a **multicultural perspective** on assessment and therapy. An underlying principle of this perspective is becoming sensitive to differences in communicative style in other cultures and learning how other cultures view speech and language disorders. You can improve your multicultural sensitivity by reading about cultural issues related to communication disorders in general (Coleman, 2000; Goldstein, 2000; Taylor, 1994) and to stuttering in particular (Conrad, 1996; Cooper & Cooper, 1993; Culatta & Goldberg, 1995; Tellis & Tellis, 2003; Watson & Kayser, 1994). The Stuttering Home Page run by Judy Kuster has a wide variety of interesting papers accessible from a webpage titled "Stuttering in Other Countries/Cultures" (http://www.mnsu.edu/comdis/kuster/nonenglish.html).

Tellis and Tellis (2003) make several important points about the importance of cultural knowledge and sensitivity in assessment and treatment. These authors, as well as Watson and Kayser (1994), suggest that finding out about the client's and/or families' attitudes about stuttering is crucial. Many of the questionnaires to assess attitudes and feelings that will be presented later in this chapter tap into perceptions of the stuttering behaviors and how much stuttering impedes an individual's communication, but don't plumb cultural views of the stigma of stuttering. For example, Tellis and Tellis (2003) report that families from India often feel that stuttering is a reflection on the entire family. This perception may strongly influence family members' responses to the child's stuttering, and it may help to discuss the latest information on the etiology of stuttering and the family's beliefs. The researchers suggest that the clinician ask "open-ended culturally specific questions that address the beliefs, attitudes, and values of the client" (p. 23), in ascertaining how best to work with the client or family.

Some of the multicultural and interpersonal issues relevant to stuttering include:

1. Eye contact. Most treatments for stuttering encourage clients to improve their eye contact when speaking. A major reason for this is that many people who stutter look away from the listener when they stutter, increasing the perceived abnormality of the symptom and further disrupting communication. This is only true in some cultures, however. In contrast, in some cultures, eye contact with a listener may be inappropriate, depending on the status of the listener and the context. Among some Native Americans, for example, not looking at the listener is a sign of respect. Thus, a person who stutters from such a culture may look away from listeners but not necessarily because of shame or embarrassment. The clinician should become aware of situations in which eye contact while speaking is appropriate and when it is not.

2. Physical contact. During an evaluation or in treatment, many clinicians may touch clients to help them identify points of tension or to signal them to make a change in their stuttering as it is happening. However, many individuals may regard being touched during an evaluation as an invasion of their personal space. It is important to ask permission before touching someone. You might say, for example, "I'd like you to try to catch a stutter and keep it going without finishing the word. Is it OK if I touch your arm to signal you to stay in the stutter?"

3. Nature of reinforcers. Some approaches to treatment use praise as a reinforcer that is given immediately after a child has spoken fluently. Cultures differ in the amount and type of praise they give children. A clinician I know working in a suburb of Sydney, Australia, a city rich in new immigrants, adapts her treatment contingencies to fit many different cultures. One family from the Middle East was adamantly against giving verbal praise to their child. Instead, they developed a special signal that the father gave to his son to reinforce fluent speech.

4. Family interactions. Children with borderline stuttering are often helped when families change their interaction patterns. One such change that families can make is to speak more slowly and pause between conversational turns when speaking with the child (e.g., Stephanson-Opsal & Bernstein Ratner, 1988). However, in some cultures, particularly in urban areas of the eastern United States, families speak quickly and often overlap each other while talking. For these families, slowing speaking rate and not interrupting each other may seem so unnatural that they are unable to sustain this new interaction pattern. For their children, an operant conditioning approach in daily one-on-one conversations with a parent may be more appropriate.

5. Intentional stuttering. Sometimes I ask the person I am working with in therapy to stutter on purpose, thereby decreasing her tendency to avoid and be afraid of stuttering. But in some cultures, stuttering is regarded so negatively that stuttering on purpose would be unthinkable, at least in the early stages of treatment. It is important for you to become aware of how stuttering is viewed in different cultures and to understand when and where voluntary stuttering might be helpful and acceptable to your clients. Sometimes, the cultural stigma of stuttering makes it difficult for individuals and families to even discuss it.

Our clinic recently treated a young man from China because he wanted to reduce his accent. Only after months of accent reduction treatment was he willing to talk about his greater problem, stuttering. Until we discussed it, he thought he had been successful in disguising it, even though his stuttering was obvious to most of his listeners.

6. Conversational style. Sensitive evaluations and treatment take into consideration not only the culture's view of stuttering but also the culture's style of verbal and nonverbal interaction. Orlando Taylor (1986) described a number of cultural differences in communication style that are relevant to evaluations of stuttering. For example, interruptions of one speaker by another may be expected among African Americans, so trying to change that style of interaction in a family may meet with resistance. In addition, people from African American and Native American cultures may feel uncomfortable responding to the personal questions often asked in an initial interview, and people from a Hispanic culture may feel it is rude to get down to business before greetings and pleasantries are exchanged.

7. Modes of address. The clinician should find out how to address individuals involved in the assessment and treatment, including proper pronunciation. Also, discuss how they'd like to address you. A family from India that I am working with now prefers to address me as "Dr. Barry."

Table 8.1	Cultural and Interpersonal Considerations in Assessment and Treatment	
Issue	Cultural or Interpersonal Concern	Possible Solution
Eye contact is sometimes a target of treatment.	In some cultures, direct eye contact may be disrespectful.	Discuss with client the appropriateness of eye contact in his culture.
Clinician may touch a client to make a point.	For some individuals, physical contact is unwelcome.	Ask permission before touching a client.
Clinician may use or advocate reinforcers such as candy or praise.	Some families do not choose to use these reinforcers.	Explore with the family what would be acceptable reinforcement for the child.
Clinician may try to change family interaction style.	Family may value their interaction style and not welcome changing it.	Clinician should talk with family about rationale for suggesting change but should accept that family may prefer not to change interaction style.
Clinician may try to teach client to use voluntary stuttering.	Some clients may find stuttering so unacceptable that they will terminate treatment rather than use voluntary stuttering.	Clinician should proceed slowly and tactfully in helping client learn and adapt voluntary stuttering. Some clients will never use it, which is reasonable but may require a work-around.
Clinician may not use appropriate conversational style with client.	Some mode of conversational style (such as asking personal questions) may offend some clients.	Clinician should become aware of conversational style preferences when client is from different culture than her own.
Clinician may not use appropriate mode of address.	Clients may be offended by insensitive mode of address (use of first name) or mispronunciation of name.	Clinician should become sensitive to client's preferred way of being addressed and proper pronunciation of client and family names.

These cultural considerations are summarized in Table 8.1.

It may not be possible for a clinician to know all relevant aspects of each new client's culture. But clinicians can be aware of the importance of culture in a person's response to stuttering, as well as the differences in communication styles between their own cultures and those of their clients. Such awareness can come from reading about a client's culture and discussing it with the client, if appropriate.

Similar sensitivity should be extended to different social classes within the clinician's own culture. Understanding and respecting class differences in such areas as vocabulary and values are crucial. Sometimes working with people from other cultures increases our respect for class differences within our own culture. When I worked in Australia, I often attended grand rounds in a Sydney hospital. One particular case presentation involved a working-class Australian woman who had been mutilating herself with needles. Some of the staff and medical residents were highly unsympathetic to her condition, but a psychiatrist, renowned for his work in other cultures, shifted their attitudes. He spoke passionately about how we fail to understand people when we are blinded by our own values and beliefs and that trying to learn about this woman's circumstances would go a lot further in helping her than our simple condemnations of her self-mutilating behavior.

Some clients will not only be from a different culture or different social class, but they will also speak a different language, one that the clinician may not understand. In this case, an interpreter is necessary. Because interpreters are often from the same culture as that of the client, they may help not only in translating, but also in providing information about important aspects of the culture to aid the clinician's understanding. In the process of translating sensitive or complex messages, interpreters sometimes need to change the clinician's message to the client. When a message is rephrased by an interpreter to a more culturally appropriate style, therapeutic interaction will be facilitated. However, if an interpreter doesn't understand the intent of a question or statement, he may inadvertently convey wrong information. A friend of mine who was working with non-English–speaking Haitian immigrants in Boston understood just enough French to realize that the interpreter was providing wrong information to a client. She rectified the situation by giving the interpreter a brief overview of what she wanted to discuss with the Haitian family and why certain elements were vital, which immediately improved communication.

Special considerations apply when clients are both bicultural and **bilingual**. Bilingual clients, in fact, are not uncommon; there is evidence of an increased risk for stuttering in bilingual individuals (Howell & Van Borsel, 2011;

Karniol, 1992; Mattes & Omark, 1991; Roberts & Shenker, 2007; Van Borsel, Maes, & Foulon, 2001). In these cases, one challenge for clinicians is to determine if the "stuttering" is really stuttering or is simply an increase in disfluency as a result of limited proficiency in a second language. Making this determination may be aided by careful observation of whether there are secondary symptoms (such as eye blinks or signs of increased tension) and cognitive or emotional responses to the suspected stuttering. For example, does the client feel ashamed of her disfluencies? Does she anticipate them? Are they consistently on the same words or same sounds? Another clue is that the disfluencies may be stuttering if there is a history of stuttering in the client's family.

There is some debate in the literature about the extent to which stuttering occurs in one or more languages of a bilingual speaker. The excellent review of stuttering and bilingualism by Van Borsel, Maes, and Foulon (2001) discusses the evidence on this issue, concluding that although stuttering may occur in one or both languages, it is more likely to occur in both. In some speakers, stuttering may be more severe in one language than another, so that careful analysis of stuttering in both languages will enable the clinician to decide whether to apply treatment to both. Analysis of stuttering in a language not spoken by the clinician is likely to be more accurate if a native speaker of that language, such as a family member or friend of the client, can work with the clinician to identify stutters. In adults, the client herself will be able to help identify stuttering in the language unfamiliar to the clinician. This topic is more thoroughly discussed in the many good chapters on multilingual aspects of stuttering in Howell and Van Borsel (2011).

THE CLINICIAN'S EXPERTISE

During an assessment, the clinician has a chance to demonstrate not only her **empathy** with a client's feelings but also her mastery of evaluating and treating stuttering. Adolescents and adults who stutter and their family members often come with feelings of frustration, fear, and helplessness. They are looking for someone they can trust and someone who can successfully guide them through the often difficult process of recovery. One of the first things a clinician can do to establish trust and credibility is to show that she not only knows about stuttering, but is comfortable asking questions about it, duplicating it in her own speech, and exploring it empathetically. This provides both clients and family members with an ally, someone who is unafraid of the problem that is so troubling to them.

This process can begin with the clinician asking an older school-age, adolescent, or adult client to teach her how to stutter the way the client himself stutters. This may take some coaching and cajoling, but it will convey the clinician's willingness to stutter and her interest in the client's pattern of stuttering. This same credibility can be achieved in the evaluation of a preschool child if the clinician asks about the types of stutters that the child has and demonstrates various possible types such as repetitions, prolongations, and blocks. With a younger school-age child, once she has gotten to know the child a little—this may take a few sessions of working together—the clinician can tell the child she has worked with other kids who stutter but needs to learn about his particular way of stuttering. Then she can ask him if it's OK if she interrupts him when he stutters to have him show her how to stutter like him. This requires tact, a sense of timing, and even humor to be sure the child feels comfortable **confronting stuttering**, but it can convey her expertise and thus engender trust.

The clinician's statements and questions also convey her expertise. For example, as she interviews an older child, she can show that she knows about stuttering by making empathetic comments, such as "Giving reports in front of class can sometimes be hard for kids who stutter." This allows the child to respond without the pressure of a direct question but also lets the child appreciate that the clinician is someone who has experience with stuttering. When talking with families, the clinician can intersperse questions with such statements as "When children keep repeating a sound that won't come out, their voices sometimes rise in pitch as the repetition continues." The family can then confirm whether or not they have noticed this in their child's speech and at the same time recognize that the clinician is knowledgeable about children's stuttering. Obviously, these kinds of comments and questions are easier for experienced clinicians, but even beginning clinicians can rely on their reading, their all-too-brief practicum experiences, and their intuition to convey their interest and understanding.

Because it has risks as well as rewards, the approach to interviewing clients and families that was just described should be used carefully. By making comments based on past experience, we may inhibit some individuals and families from telling us about experiences that differ from those offered by the clinician. It is an art to find the balance between showing understanding and leading the witness. As your clinical judgment develops, you will learn which clients will be helped by this approach and when.

I would also caution that demonstrating your expertise should be secondary to acquiring an understanding of clients' needs. A clinician's first task is to discern what an individual or family would like from the clinician. The second task is to understand the stuttering problem. In the normal course of accomplishing these two tasks—with attentive listening, empathetic comments, and perceptive questions—the clinician's expertise will emerge naturally.

ASSESSMENT OF STUTTERING BEHAVIOR

Assessment of stuttering behaviors is a broad area that can be divided into several different targets for evaluation, such as frequency, type, duration, and severity. In some situations, it may also be important to assess speech naturalness, speech rate, and concomitant or associated behaviors. The importance of each of these is slightly different depending on the age of the client and the type of treatment you expect to use. Before describing how to assess stuttering, I will clarify what behaviors are considered stuttering. As I mentioned in Chapter 7, a number of authors (e.g., Conture, 2001; Yairi & Ambrose, 1992a) have discussed which types of disfluencies distinguish stuttering from nonstuttering children. Borrowing from their discussions, I have concluded that the following behaviors should be counted as stutters: part-word repetitions, monosyllabic whole-word repetitions, sound prolongations, and blockages of sound or airflow. The latter category (blockages of sound or airflow) can sometimes be quite subtle, occurring in the middle of a word (as in "co-oookie" in which a glottal stop appears to break the word in half) or before a word. I also count successful avoidance behaviors as stutters if they are unequivocally an avoidance. See the section on assessing frequency for a further description of deciding on unequivocal avoidances.

Reliability

Whenever a procedure is used to assess a behavior or a trait, it is important to know how reliable the procedure is. For example, if a police officer pulls you over for speeding because her radar gun has clocked you going 40 miles per hour in a 25-mph zone, you might want to know how reliable her radar gun was. When this happened to me several years ago, I went to court to contest the ticket. Many factors, I figured, could affect the accuracy of the radar gun's measurement of my speed: the weather, the age of the gun, and whether it was adjusted properly. Fortunately, the judge asked the officer for **evidence of reliability** of the radar gun to prove that it could repeatedly, dependably, and consistently measure the speed of a car. Unfortunately, the officer was able to provide the judge with evidence of her radar gun's recent reliability check, and I shelled out $85 for the fine.

Reliability is obviously an important characteristic of a procedure to measure stuttering. Many factors affect the measurement process, and some of these influences may result in data that are not representative of a client's true performance. In addition, it appears that stuttering is a particularly changeable behavior, making it difficult to measure. This phenomenon and its consequences are described by Cordes (1994) in her seminal article about reliability:

"Perceptions, judgments, and observations are affected by variables attributed to the observers, to the instrumentation or coding procedures, to the situation or conditions of observation, to the subjects being observed, and to interactions among all of these. Consequently, researchers using direct observation methods are currently expected to provide evidence that their findings are not simply the results of situational influences or observer idiosyncrasies. They are expected, in other words, to provide evidence that their data are reliable" (p. 264).

The same caveat is true for clinical work. Despite our good intentions, observations of clients' stuttering before treatment and after may be influenced by our desires to see them improve. Measurements may also be affected by random fluctuations in stuttering apart from treatment effects, by the setting in which the client is assessed, by length and type of sample taken, and by the particular dimension of stuttering, such as frequency, severity, duration, or type that is chosen for assessment. It is important for clinicians to learn to assess stuttering reliably and to provide evidence that they have done so. It is also part of the clinician's responsibilities to know the reliability of the standardized measures he uses to assess stuttering and to choose those measures that are most reliable.

When human judgment is involved, as it always is with measures of stuttering, reliability is checked first by demonstrating that the observer makes the same judgment when observing the same behavior a second time from a video recording, usually several weeks later so that the second observation is fresh and not affected by memories of the earlier judgment. This is called **intrarater reliability**. Reliability is also checked by comparing the original judgment with the judgment of a second observer who rates the sample independently of the first observer. This is called **interrater reliability**.

Remeasurement of the data does not have to include the entire sample that is used, although doing so would certainly be the most rigorous approach (e.g., O'Brian, Packman, & Onslow, 2004). It is common for clinical researchers in stuttering to remeasure a randomly selected portion (10–25 percent) of samples taken (e.g., Hakim & Bernstein Ratner, 2004; O'Brian, Packman, & Onslow, 2004). When reliability of judgments is to be established for measurements made on clients who increase their fluency over the course of a treatment regimen, samples should be randomly selected from various points in therapy to include both less fluent and more fluent samples.

Measures of reliability are usually selected according to what behavior is being measured. In situations where evaluation and treatment depend on accurate identification of stuttering moments (such as whether a word or syllable is stuttered or not), reliability can be measured using what is commonly called "point-by-point agreement." A videotaped sample (e.g., 400 syllables of conversational speech) can be transcribed, and each stutter can be identified and marked on the transcript by an original judge or rater. Sometime later, the rater can return to the sample and again identify stutters by marking a fresh copy of the transcript. The two transcripts are then compared syllable by syllable, and the rater determines how many syllables are agreed upon as stuttered and how many are agreed upon as fluent. This total is termed "number of agreements." The number of disagreements (syllables that were determined to be stuttered in the first rating but not stuttered in the second rating or vice versa) is totaled and termed "number of disagreements." The reliability measure is then the number of agreements divided by the total number of agreements plus disagreements, multiplied by 100. Cordes (1994) notes that 80 percent agreement is commonly thought of as the lower limit for a sample to be considered reliable. Figure 8.1 gives an example of a point-by-point assessment of reliability.

When clinical research is carried out, some authors (e.g., Cordes, 1994) are concerned that point-by-point agreement can be affected by the fact that some agreements might happen by pure chance. To deal with this, it may be useful to report both percentage of agreement for stutters and percentage of agreement for fluent syllables or words. Alternatively, the agreement calculation can be corrected by a procedure that takes into account the effects of chance, such as the kappa statistic (Cohen, 1960; Cordes, 1994).

Point-by-point agreement is appropriate when it is important to judge whether stuttering is present or absent on each syllable. It is also a good tool for new clinicians to use to assess their ability to accurately judge stuttering. However, other procedures are called for when assessment requires quantification rather than presence or absence. An example would be measurement of the duration of stutters. An appropriate measure of reliability would be percent error, obtained by remeasuring at least 10 percent of the data. In this case, it is appropriate to begin by (1) obtaining the absolute differences between each first judgment and each second judgment (change all negative numbers to positive); (2) summing those absolute differences together; (3) dividing by the total number of them to get the average; and finally (4) dividing the average absolute difference by the average of the first judgments. Table 8.2 shows an example.

A third method of assessing reliability can be used when measuring the amount of stuttering in cases when point-by-point agreement is not critical. One example would be when you are assessing frequency of stuttering as a measure of week-by-week progress. This procedure involves calculating both the correlation between the first

---

Observer 1:

You wish to know all about my grandfather. Well, he is nearly ninety-three years old; yet he still thinks as swiftly as ever. He dresses himself in an old black frock coat, usually several buttons missing. A long beard clings to his chin, giving those who observe him a pronounced feeling of the utmost respect. When he speaks his voice is just a bit cracked and quivers a trifle. Twice each day he plays skillfully and with zest upon our small organ. Except in the winter when the snow or ice prevents, he slowly takes a short walk in the open air each day. We have often urged him to walk more and smoke less, but he always answers, "Banana oil!" Grandfather likes to be modern in his language.

Observer 2:

You wish to know all about my grandfather. Well, he is nearly ninety-three years old; yet he still thinks as swiftly as ever. He dresses himself in an old black frock coat, usually several buttons missing. A long beard clings to his chin, giving those who observe him a pronounced feeling of the utmost respect. When he speaks his voice is just a bit cracked and quivers a trifle. Twice each day he plays skillfully and with zest upon our small organ. Except in the winter when the snow or ice prevents, he slowly takes a short walk in the open air each day. We have often urged him to walk more and smoke less, but he always answers, "Banana oil!" Grandfather likes to be modern in his language.

There are approximately 14 syllables upon which the observers did not agree. There are approximately 156 syllables upon which they agreed were either stuttered or were fluent. The simple point-by-point agreement (rather than the kappa statistic) would be calculated as agreements (156) divided by agreements plus disagreements (170), or 92 percent.

Figure 8.1   An example showing how to calculate point-by-point agreement. An initial observer has marked the reading passage by underlining syllables on which stuttering was judged to occur. A second observer has marked the second passage. Point-by-point agreement can be calculated by comparing the total number of agreements with the agreements plus disagreements.

Table 8.2	An Example of Assessment of Reliability by Calculating Percent Error of Duration Measurements		
	Time 1	Time 2	Absolute Difference
	3.5	3.0	0.5
	4.0	4.0	0.0
	0.5	0.7	0.2
	0.4	0.3	0.1
Mean	2.1		0.2

Duration of stuttering (in seconds) measured by an observer at Time 1 and remeasured at Time 2. Percent error = 0.2/2.1 = 9.5 percent.

Table 8.3	Assessing Interrater Reliability by Calculating Correlations and *t* Tests	
Observer 1		Observer 2
12		11
10		9
15		10
4		6
8		5
2		2
14		12
7		9
3		4
6		6
5		3
1		3

Measures are percentage of syllables stuttered measured by Observer 1 and Observer 2.
Pearson $r = 0.90$; paired $t = 0.92$; df = 11; $p = .38$. These calculations suggest that there is substantial interrater reliability because the ratings are highly correlated, and there is no significant difference between the means.

rating and a second rating for multiple samples, as well as test of significant differences between the means of the ratings, such as a paired samples *t* test. Correlations and *t* tests should be done for both intrarater and interrater reliability. Correlations should be above 80 percent, and *t* tests should show no significant difference between the samples. Table 8.3 depicts correlations and *t* tests for a sample of 12 original and re-rated samples.

As a final comment about reliability, I would suggest that although different measures of reliability can be used for different purposes, beginning clinicians should establish their reliability using a point-by-point agreement procedure, both during their initial training and to recheck their reliability periodically as they gain more experience. This may help them develop relatively consistent and agreed-upon definitions of what a stutter is and is not.

A summary of reliability measures is given in Table 8.4.

Table 8.4	Measures of Reliability		
Type of Reliability	Brief Description		When to Use
Point by point	Transcript of speech sample made; original judge and another observer marks whether a syllable is stuttered. Reliability is assessed by counting the number of syllables that were agreed upon by both observers as stuttered and dividing that number by total number of syllables in sample (agreements plus disagreements).		Use when it is important to ascertain whether stuttering has occurred on each individual syllable, as in an experiment that punishes individual stutters. Also useful for new clinicians to assess their accuracy at judging stuttering.
Percent error	Experiment assesses the difference between the first observer's judgment and the second observation on at least 10 percent of sample. Expressed as absolute difference (all numbers made positive). Then these differences are averaged (average absolute difference), and this figure is divided by the average of the first observer's measures.		Use when assessing reliability of a continuous variable like duration of stutters.
Correlation and *t* test	Pearson product-moment correlation employed to see the extent to which initial observations of behavior are related to second observations. In addition, *t* test is used to assess whether the mean of the second observations is not significantly different from the mean of the initial observations.		Use when an overall measure of variable (e.g., percent syllables stuttered) is used and when it is not important to show agreement on individual syllables.

Speech Sample

The size and number of samples depend on the purpose of the assessment. In a first assessment, it would be wise to have at least two samples: one recorded in the clinic and one recorded in the client's typical environment. Before I see a preschool child for an evaluation, I ask parents to send in a video of the child in conversation at home. Video recording is common in some homes so that the presence of a video camera will probably not make most children self-conscious. I sometimes ask parents to leave the camera on a tripod in a familiar place for several days so the child is used to it when the recording is actually done. When video recording is not possible, audiotaping is still useful. With a school-age child, a sample collected in the school would be important; practically speaking, a sample could be most easily recorded in the therapy room. A second sample from home would also be very helpful, but it is not always obtainable. When evaluating an adolescent or adult, I recommend that a sample be taken in the treatment room and a sample be taken from work or home. It is often convenient for adolescents or adults to audiotape telephone conversations. I often urge clients to buy a small digital audio recorder for recording work done outside therapy; Sony has one for $20.

An important consideration in obtaining samples is that stuttering varies. It differs in frequency and severity from month to month, week to week, day to day, and from situation to situation within the same day. Such variability affects both children and adults but is most apparent with younger stutterers. Sometimes a preschool child is stuttering severely, and then three weeks later during the evaluation, the child is entirely fluent. Therefore, it is important to discuss with the client or family whether the sample you have obtained is representative of the stuttering and if not, whether more samples should be taken, maybe in other situations and at other times.

After the initial sample, when further assessment is done to measure progress in therapy, it is crucial to ensure that any reduction in stuttering is not confined to the therapy room. Thus, ongoing assessments should include measures taken in the client's real world, outside the treatment situation.

For any sample in which severity of stuttering is to be rated or any sample for research purposes, videotaping is essential. Many subtleties of stuttering would be missed if only an audiotape were used; thus video recording allows better assessment of observer reliability than audio recording. Sometimes online (while the client is talking) scoring can be done without either video or audio recording. For example, online scoring is appropriate when the clinician samples frequency of stuttering at the beginning of every session for clinical rather than research purposes.

The length of the sample must be long enough for it to be representative of the speaker's typical stuttering. A sample that's too short won't include enough stuttering to see the range of severity and types of stuttering, and a sample that's too long would take time away from other assessment activities and would be tedious to score. For a client who reads, I usually like to take a sample of 300 to 400 syllables of conversational speech (where there is likely to be more variability) and 200 syllables of a reading passage (where there is likely to be less variability). Using a typical figure of 1.5 syllables per word (Williams, Darley, & Spriestersbach, 1978), these samples would be equivalent to approximately 200 to 265 words and 130 words, respectively.

When obtaining a reading sample, it is important to ensure that the reading passage is at or below the client's reading level. A client's stuttering is likely to worsen when reading a passage that is difficult, giving a false impression of typical stuttering during reading. Reading passages in the *Stuttering Severity Instrument-4* (SSI-4) (Riley, 2009) are designed for third, fifth, and seventh grade levels, as well as for an adult reading level. You can also write your own passages and check them for grade level using the Tools option on Microsoft Word, which uses the Klesch-Kincaid Reading Level statistics, or you can use the Fry Readability Graph available at http://school.discovery.com/schrockguide/fry/fry.html.

When obtaining a speaking sample, it would be wise to select topics that are not emotional unless it is desirable to elicit a maximal amount of stuttering, as you might do with a client who says she stutters but is not demonstrating any during the evaluation. I usually ask children and adolescents to talk about their favorite weekend or afterschool activities, sports, hobbies, or pets. With adults, I ask them to talk about their favorite activities, sports, hobbies, work, or school.

When making a formal assessment or when first learning to assess stuttering, it is very useful to make a written transcript of the spoken material, including all words and even those nonmeaningful utterances, such as "uh." However, you should not indicate on the transcript which syllables are stuttered, so that you, at a later date, or another rater, on a separate occasion, can rescore a copy of the transcript to check for reliability without being influenced by the notations indicating which syllables were stuttered. Using your recording of the spoken material and an unmarked transcript, you can note where the stutters are, with details of how the individual stuttered. Write out each element of a repeated sound or syllable, the sounds that were prolonged, and the sounds on which blocks occurred. Describe escape and avoidance behaviors accompanying each moment of stuttering. Mark those moments of stuttering that seem longer than most. For a complete assessment, you will want to return to the longer stutters and time how long each one was to determine the average length of the three longest stutters. You will also want to count the words or syllables spoken, although it is often most accurate to count syllables from recordings because some speakers omit syllables in longer words. This can be done with software, such as the Computerized Scoring of Stuttering Severity (CSSS) software that accompanies the SSI-4.

Assessing Frequency

Frequency of stuttering is a simple, reliable measure (Andrews & Ingham, 1971) that can be used for a variety of purposes. It is important in an initial assessment to help distinguish a normally disfluent child from a child with borderline stuttering. It is a vital part of composite ratings, such as the SSI-4 (Riley, 2009), that provide a multidimensional view of stuttering. Frequency of stuttering is also useful as a "snapshot" measure of progress during treatment. In the first place, it is highly correlated with severity (Young, 1961). If used alone, however, frequency has the limitation that it doesn't reflect the duration of stutters or physical tension associated with stuttering. Decreases in these variables are often signs of improvement.

Frequency of stuttering is most commonly reported as percentage of syllables stuttered, although some use percentage of words stuttered or number of stutters per 100 words. I prefer to use **percentage of syllables stuttered**, following the logic of Minifie and Cooker (1964), because it can capture instances when a speaker stutters on more than one syllable of a multisyllable word. Moreover, when counting syllables and stutters online, syllables can be counted more easily than words by counting the syllable beats as the client talks. When counting stutters, I assume that each syllable can be stuttered only once. Thus, multiple repetitions, like "Where is my ba-ba-ba-basketball?" are counted as only one stutter. "Where is my…my…uh…well ba-ba-ba-ba-basketball?" is also one stutter, because I assume that the repetition of "my" and interjections of "uh" and "well" are postponements associated with the stutter that was anticipated and actually occurred on "basketball." If a speaker appears to have a habit of using a particular word or sound as an avoidance behavior, I will count a word as stuttered even if no overt stuttering occurred. For example, a speaker may say "Where is my… uh…uh…uhbasketball?" In this case, the speaker appears to be using "uh" to postpone starting the word "basketball" on which he anticipates stuttering. And he keeps saying "uh" until he feels he can say "basketball" fluently, then rushes to say "basketball" after saying the last "uh." When I am fairly certain that a speaker has used a sound or word as a (successful) avoidance behavior like this, I count the word as stuttered. Note that I do not count each utterance of the sound or word that is used as an avoidance; instead I count the next word in the utterance as stuttered. When I am in doubt about whether an avoidance has occurred on a word, I count it as fluent.

When assessing the speech of someone who can read, I find it helpful to compare the frequency of stuttering in reading to that in speaking. If stuttering is markedly greater in the reading task, this may be because the speaker is avoiding words he expects to stutter on in the speaking task, but he can't do this when reading. In most cases, I talk about my hypothesis with the client to see if he agrees.

A variety of instruments designed for counting stutters are available. A free online counter that counts stuttered syllables, fluent syllables, and calculates percent syllables stuttered and speech rate is available at http://www.natke-verlag.de/silbenzaehler/index_en.html (recommended by Julie Pera). You could also use two electronic hand-held counters—one in each hand, available at http://tallycounterstore.com/electronic_tally_counter.html for under $15 (recommended by Jennifer Code). Some clinicians using the Lidcombe Program for Early Intervention (Chapter 10) prefer to use a hand-held counter called a TrueTalk (http://www.synelec.com.au/synergy/). My own preference is to use a TrueTalk, which counts syllables and stutters, as well as time during which the counter buttons are pressed. Output includes total syllables spoken, percent syllables stuttered, time elapsed, and stutters per minute. This device can be used with one hand and held discretely at your side when assessing a client's speech while you are standing, sitting, or walking.

Assessing Types of Stutters

When assessing the speech of preschool children, it is often useful to count the total number of disfluencies, both those that are considered **types of stutters** and those considered normal. As you will remember from Chapter 7, disfluencies that are not considered stutter-like include multisyllable word repetitions, phrase repetitions, interjections, and revisions in which a phrase is incomplete. When both types of disfluencies (stutter-like and not) are counted, you can use the proportion of total disfluencies that are stutter-like to help you decide whether a child is stuttering or normally disfluent. As I indicated in Chapter 7, Yairi (1997a, 1997b) surveyed a number of studies and proposed that if less than 50 percent of a child's disfluencies are stutter-like, the child is more likely to be normally disfluent. Caution must be used with any single measure used alone. Conture (2001) noted that a child he had recently evaluated was, in his opinion, stuttering severely even though the child's proportion of stutter-like disfluencies was only 34 percent of the total disfluencies. Clearly, Conture had relied on several other measures of stuttering in concluding that the child was a severe stutterer.

Another measure involving the type of disfluencies that a child produces is the number of stutter-like disfluencies per 100 words. In summarizing his findings on disfluencies in stuttering and nonstuttering children, Yairi (1997b) noted that children who stutter have more than three stutter-like disfluencies per 100 words, whereas normally disfluent children have fewer. In this same chapter, Yairi reviewed research about the gradual decline in some types of disfluencies as children grow older. Perhaps the most important finding is that part-word repetitions show a steady decline in normally disfluent children by age 4 and thereafter. Thus, if a child shows a plateau or increase in part-word repetitions in later preschool years, the child may be showing stuttering rather than normal disfluency.

Assessing Duration

In a thorough assessment, measures of the **duration** of a client's longest blocks can give us important information about how much stuttering may be interfering with communication. Van Riper (1982, p. 208) noted in his inimitable prose that "The duration of the individual moments of stuttering is one of the basic components of any adequate index of severity. Like tapeworms, longer stutterings are worse than shorter ones."

A common practice is to average the duration of the three longest stutters in a speech sample (Myers, 1978; Preus, 1981; Riley, 2009; Van Riper, 1982). One way to do it is use a digital stopwatch while watching a videotape of the client speaking. With a little practice, you can turn the stopwatch on at the moment the stutter begins and turn it off when it ends and measure the moment of stuttering to the nearest half-second. Any delays in starting the stopwatch at the beginning of stutters are compensated for by similar delays when you stop it at the end. I recommend using duration as part of a more complete assessment of severity, such as the SSI-4 (Riley, 2009), when making an initial assessment of a client's progress and when you want to give a detailed description of a client's stuttering in a report. The software accompanying the SSI-4 provides a means to automatically calculate the mean of the three longest stutters by holding down the mouse key for the duration of each stutter as it is being counted.

Assessing Secondary Behaviors

Stuttering feels like being in the grip of an unseen hand damming up the flow of your speech. Or as one of my young clients said, it is like having "a rock jammed in your throat." You struggle to keep going, squeezing your lips, blinking your eyes, or twisting your shoulders in the process. Such behaviors add to the abnormality of stuttering and reflect an important aspect of its development. Reducing or eliminating these behaviors may be a vital goal for therapy.

Secondary behaviors are also referred to as "concomitant," "associated," or "accessory" behaviors. They are most often escape behaviors that are used to break out of a stutter once it has started, but secondary behaviors may also be avoidance behaviors that are used in an attempt to keep from stuttering (see Chapters 1, 4, and 7 for further discussion of these terms). These behaviors may be physical movements (e.g., eye blink), extra sounds (e.g., "uh"), or changes in the way speech is produced (e.g., pitch rise). They are often signs that stuttering has progressed to a more advanced stage (i.e., escape behaviors distinguish beginning from borderline stuttering), but they may in a few cases appear very close to the onset of stuttering.

Conture (2001) briefly reviewed the limited research on secondary behaviors and noted that most are just more frequent and more exaggerated versions of behaviors seen in normal speakers. Zebrowski and Kelly (2002) suggested that the most common behaviors involve the eyes, particularly blinking, squeezing, lateral and vertical eye movements, and loss of eye contact. These authors and Shapiro (1999) also pointed out that the presence of secondary behaviors can be an important diagnostic sign that may distinguish normally disfluent children from those who are beginning to stutter.

Some clinicians enumerate these secondary behaviors as part of their assessment, particularly when they will use a treatment approach that helps the client gradually modify her stuttering behaviors. Standardized measures, such as the SSI-4 (Riley, 2009), include ratings of these behaviors as part of an overall severity assessment. We will consider this assessment next.

Assessing Severity

Measures of **severity** may be the most clinically relevant assessment of overt stuttering behaviors. Severity reflects an overall impression that listeners may have when they listen to an individual who stutters. Thus, it is an important measure for assessing the outcome of treatment. It is also an important yardstick of progress during therapy because many treatments gradually reduce the severity of stuttering rather than eliminate it.

The most commonly used measure of severity is the SSI-4, which was first published in the *Journal of Speech and Hearing Disorders* (Riley, 1972). A recent version, the SSI-3 is illustrated in Figure 8.2, and the most current version is available with forms and a manual from PRO-ED (http://www.proedinc.com). In my mind, it is the best measure of severity available, but like its predecessors, the SSI-4 has some drawbacks. The sample of children and adults on which it was normed is not well described, its reliability is not strong, and its validity has not been convincingly demonstrated (McCauley, 1996). Despite these limitations, the SSI is easy to use and captures the severity of overt stuttering behaviors as a composite of three important dimensions: frequency, duration, and physical concomitants. The SSI-4 is one of the few measures of stuttering that has standardized procedures for gathering and scoring speech samples and is the only measure that includes the three dimensions just cited.

The total overall score for the SSI is the sum of the three subcomponents measured.

1. Frequency is assessed as the percentages of syllables stuttered on a speaking task and a reading task. For nonreaders, the speaking task is given twice the weight in the scoring procedures. Riley originally used percentage of words stuttered but currently uses the percentage of syllables stuttered, which is converted to a "task score" on the form.

SSI-3

Stuttering Severity Instrument–3

TEST RECORD AND FREQUENCY COMPUTATION FORM

Identifying Information

Name _____

Sex M F   Grade _____ Age _____

Date _____ Date of Birth _____

School _____

Examiner _____

Preschool ___ School Age ___ Adult ___ Reader ___ Nonreader ___

FREQUENCY Use Readers Table or Nonreaders Table, not both.

READERS TABLE				NONREADERS TABLE	
1. Speaking Task		**2. Reading Task**		**3. Speaking Task**	
Percentage	Task Score	Percentage	Task Score	Percentage	Task Score
1	2	1	2	1	4
2	3			2	6
3	4	2	4	3	8
4–5	5	3–4	5	4–5	10
6–7	6	5–7	6	6–7	12
8–11	7	8–12	7	8–11	14
12–21	8	13–20	8	12–21	16
22 & up	9	21 & up	9	22 & up	18

Frequency Score (use 1 + 2 or 3) [ ]

DURATION

Average length of three longest stuttering events timed to the nearest 1/10th second		Scale Score
Fleeting	(.5 sec or less)	2
Half-second	(.5– .9 sec)	4
1 full second	(1.0– 1.9 secs)	6
2 seconds	(2.0– 2.9 secs)	8
3 seconds	(3.0– 4.9 secs)	10
5 seconds	(5.0– 9.9 secs)	12
10 seconds	(10.0–29.9 secs)	14
30 seconds	(30.0–59.9 secs)	16
1 minute	(60 secs or more)	18

Duration Score (2 – 18) [ ]

PHYSICAL CONCOMITANTS

Evaluating Scale

0 = none
1 = not noticeable unless looking for it
2 = barely noticeable to casual observer
3 = distracting
4 = very distracting
5 = severe and painful-looking

DISTRACTING SOUNDS	Noisy breathing, whistling, sniffing, blowing, clicking sounds	0 1 2 3 4 5
FACIAL GRIMACES	Jaw jerking, tongue protruding, lip pressing, jaw muscles tense	0 1 2 3 4 5
HEAD MOVEMENTS	Back, forward, turning away, poor eye contact, constant looking around	0 1 2 3 4 5
MOVEMENTS OF THE EXTREMITIES	Arm and hand movement, hands about face, torso movement, leg movements, foot-tapping or swinging	0 1 2 3 4 5

Physical Concomitants Score [ ]

TOTAL OVERALL SCORE

Frequency _____ + Duration _____ + Physical Concomitants _____ = [ ]

Percentile _____

Severity _____

---

10 9 8 7 6 5 4 3 2 1   98 97 96 95 94

For additional copies of this form (#6722), contact PRO-ED, 8700 Shoal Creek Blvd., Austin, TX 78757

Figure 8.2 The Stuttering Severity Instrument-3. *(Continued)*

**Percentile and Severity Equivalents of
SSI-3 Total Overall Scores for Preschool Children (*N* = 72)**

Total Overall Score	Percentile	Severity
0– 8	1– 4	Very Mild
9–10	5–11	
11–12	12–23	Mild
13–16	24–40	
17–23	41–60	Moderate
24–26	61–77	
27–28	78–88	Severe
29–31	89–95	
32 and up	96–99	Very Severe

**Percentile and Severity Equivalents of SSI-3
Total Overall Scores for School-Age Children (*N* = 139)**

Total Overall Score	Percentile	Severity
6– 8	1– 4	Very Mild
9–10	5–11	
11–15	12–23	Mild
16–20	24–40	
21–23	41–60	Moderate
24–27	61–77	
28–31	78–88	Severe
32–35	89–95	
36 and up	96–99	Very Severe

**Percentile and Severity Equivalents of
SSI-3 Total Overall Scores for Adults (*N* = 60)**

Total Overall Score	Percentile	Severity
10–12	1– 4	Very Mild
13–17	5–11	
18–20	12–23	Mild
21-24	24–40	
25–27	41–60	Moderate
28–31	61–77	
32–34	78–88	Severe
35–36	89–95	
37–46	96–99	Very Severe

Figure 8.2 *(Continued)*

2. Duration is assessed by measuring the length of the three longest stutters, calculating their mean duration, and finding the appropriate "scale score" on the form.
3. Physical concomitants are assessed by adding the scale values of each subcomponent (i.e., distracting sounds, facial grimaces, head movements, and movements of the extremities) and deriving a total score.

The values for frequency, duration, and physical concomitants are then added together to provide a total overall score. Percentiles and severity ratings (e.g., mild, moderate, and severe) based on total overall scores are given on the form. Clinicians should carefully read Riley's directions on administering this measure in the manual of the SSI-4 before using it.

Clients should be video recorded, and the SSI should be calculated from the recording because duration measures and assessment of physical concomitants cannot be done easily online, and the frequency count will be more accurate if equivocal stutters are replayed repeatedly until a decision can be reached. The CSSS software accompanying the SSI-4 allows computer-aided calculation of stuttering frequency and duration for the overall severity score.

A relatively new measure of severity, the *Test of Childhood Stuttering* (TOCS) (Gillam, Logan, & Pearson, 2009), can be used with children ages 4 to 12. It can be obtained from PRO-ED (http://www.proedinc.com). The TOCS consists of several subparts:

1. A Speech Fluency Measure which is comprised of (a) rapid picture naming; (b) modeled sentences; (c) structured conversation; and (d) narration.
2. An Observational Rating Scale to be used by the clinician, teacher, or caregiver. This component provides information from the observer about (a) how often the child has various stuttering behaviors, and (b) how often the child has negative responses to his stuttering, such as showing such secondary reactions as concomitant physical behaviors and avoidance of speaking.
3. A Supplemental Clinical Assessment which allows a more detailed analysis of the stuttering frequency, duration, types, and associated behaviors, as well as speech naturalness. This measure can help to decide if the child stutters and how severe the child is. It can also be used for pre- and post-treatment assessment.

In a review of TOCS in Mental Measurements Yearbook, Shapely and Guyette (2010) comment favorably on the instrument's validity and reliability, but suggest caution in interpreting the test's index scores and percentile ranks because of limited sample sizes used in standardization and in validity and reliability assessment.

Another measure of severity, which captures frequency, duration, and perhaps secondary behaviors, is the *Scale for Rating Severity of Stuttering* (Johnson, Darley, & Spriestersbach, 1952, 1963; Williams, 1978). This early scale, shown in Figure 8.3, is more subjective than the SSI, relying

on an overall impression of a speech sample to rate the sample with one of eight values (0–7). Raters are encouraged to treat each of the eight intervals between the scale values as equal, although there is some debate about whether this is truly an equal-interval scale (Berry & Silverman, 1972). Although it has been shown to be reliable when a group of raters is used, the reliability of the Scale for Rating Severity of Stuttering for use with single raters is questionable. Williams (1978) cautions that the scale gives only a rough measure of severity because of its limitations. But he also notes that it has clinical utility because it captures the listener's impression of a client's speech and may therefore convey information about what the client faces every day when he is speaking. Ratings by a number of real listeners in the client's environment, as well as the client herself, would increase the value of this information. Any scale, including this one, has real risks if used as a single measure of therapeutic progress by a clinician. Unconscious bias and familiarity with the client may lead to improved ratings in the absence of change. Progress should be assessed with a variety of tools, including the SSI-4.

A fourth measure of severity is the Lidcombe Program's Severity Rating Scale, which was developed by Onslow, Costa, and Rue (1990) as part of an operant treatment program for preschool children. This is simply a 1-to-10 scale that parents use to make daily ratings of their child's stuttering (1 = no stuttering, 2 = extremely mild stuttering, through 10 = extremely severe stuttering). The scale, in a format that allows for a week's ratings, is shown in Figure 8.4. At the beginning of treatment, parents are trained to accurately rate their child's severity using observations of the child's speech in the clinic. The clinician and parent compare their ratings and discuss any differences between them until the parent's ratings are within one scale value of the clinician's. Throughout treatment, a sample of the child's speech that is long enough to ensure that any stuttering in the child's speech is observed is taken at the beginning of each clinic meeting. Both the clinician and the parent rate this sample, ensuring continued agreement.

This severity rating scale has also been used with school-age children who stutter. These older children often rate themselves in a version of the Lidcombe Program developed for older children. Research on this severity rating scale has shown it to be a valid and reliable tool for conveniently obtaining information on a child's stuttering outside of the treatment environment (Onslow, Andrews, & Costa, 1990; Onslow, Harrison, Jones, & Packman, 2002).

ASSESSING SPEECH NATURALNESS

In recent years, clinical scientists have been concerned that treatments that produce fluency may not always result in natural-sounding speech. As Schiavetti and Metz (1997) warned, "Some stutterers may reduce their number of stutters at the expense of a speech pattern that is stutter-free but not really fluent." Thus, some stuttering treatments may get rid of stuttering but leave an individual with speech that

Scale for Rating Severity of Stuttering

Speaker_____ Age ____ Sex____ Date_____

Rater _____ Identification _____

Instructions:

Indicate your identification by some such term as "speaker's clinician," "clinical observer," "clinical student," or "friend," "mother," "classmate," etc. Rate the severity of the speaker's stuttering on a scale from 0 to 7, as follows:

0   No Stuttering

1   Very mild–stuttering on less than 1 percent of words; very little relevant tension; disfluencies generally less than one second in duration; patterns of disfluency simple; no apparent associated movements of body, arms, legs, or head.

2   Mild–stuttering on 1 to 2 percent of words; tension scarcely perceptible; very few, if any, disfluencies last as long as a full second; patterns of disfluency simple; no conspicuous associated movements of body, arms, legs, or head.

3   Mild to moderate–stuttering on about 2 to 5 percent of words; tension noticeable but not very distracting; most disfluencies do not last longer than a full second; patterns of disfluencies mostly simple; no distracting associated movements.

4   Moderate–stuttering on about 5 to 8 percent of words; tension occasionally distracting; disfluencies average about one second in duration; disfluency patterns characterized by an occasional complicating sound or facial grimace; an occasional distracting associated movement.

5   Moderate to severe–stuttering on about 8 to 12 percent of words; consistently noticeable tension; disfluencies average about two seconds in duration; a few distracting sounds and facial grimaces; a few distracting associated movements.

6   Severe–stuttering on about 12 to 25 percent of words; conspicuous tension; disfluencies average three to four seconds in duration; conspicuous distracting sounds and facial grimaces; conspicuous distracting associated movements.

7   Very severe–stuttering on more than 25 percent of words; very conspicuous tension; disfluencies average more than four seconds in duration; very conspicuous distracting sounds and facial grimaces; very conspicuous distracting associated movements.

Figure 8.3   Scale for rating severity of stuttering.

sounds odd, unusual, or unnatural. Martin, Haroldson, and Triden (1984), one of the first investigative teams to report on this problem, found that unsophisticated listeners rated the stutter-free speech of individuals who stutter speaking under DAF (delayed auditory feedback) as significantly more unnatural than the general speech of nonstutterers. Ingham, Gow, and Costello (1985) used the same rating scale and found that the fluent speech of treated stutterers was judged to be more unnatural than that of nonstutterers. Both investigations used a nine-point, equal-appearing interval scale to rate speakers based on judges' intuitive sense of what sounded "natural," **speech naturalness**. The judges in these

and most subsequent studies exhibited satisfactory levels of interrater reliability and agreement, although individual rater reliability was only marginally satisfactory.

Clinically, we need to be sure that clients sound as natural as possible after treatment. Otherwise, they are likely to abandon their fluency skills in favor of old, familiar stuttering patterns because of their own and listeners' negative reactions to their post-treatment speech. Can we rate our clients' naturalness reliably? Schiavetti and Metz (1997) indicated that clinicians who have learned to be consistent raters of speech naturalness may rely on the relative values of their ratings. Thus, they can judge when a client sounds less natural than other clients they have

Figure 8.4 The Severity Rating Scale. Rate the speaker on a 10-point scale, where 1 = no stuttering and 10 = extremely severe stuttering (the worst stuttering the speaker has produced) for the entire day. Put an X in the appropriate box at the end of each day.

treated and take appropriate steps to improve that client's naturalness before releasing her from treatment. The SSI-4 incorporates a naturalness rating as part of the assessment.

ASSESSING SPEAKING AND READING RATE

Many clinicians believe that **speaking rate** often reflects the severity of stuttering (e.g., Shapiro, 1999; Starkweather, 1985, 1987). Van Riper (1982) described studies that found correlations that ranged from 0.68 to 0.88 between reading rate and severity. If a client's speaking rate is well below average for her age, communication will be affected; listeners may become impatient or lose the thread of what the speaker is saying. Speech rates that are too fast will also affect communication. A subgroup of individuals who stutter also have the disorder of cluttering, which is rapid, often unintelligible speech (see Chapter 15). Thus, it is useful to measure the client's rate in standard speaking and reading tasks. Table 8.5 gives average speaking rates for children and adults.

Rate can be measured as either words or syllables per minute, depending on the clinician's preference. Some clinicians find it easier to calculate rate by using words per minute because words are easily observable units on the page. Others note that syllables per minute can be calculated more rapidly than words because clinicians can use the

"beat" of syllables to count them online (i.e., while a speaker is talking). The syllables-per-minute approach also accounts for the fact that some speakers use more multisyllabic words than others and might be penalized because such words take longer to produce than one-syllable words. I recommend using syllables for these reasons.

No matter which method is used, the following rules can be used for counting words or syllables. Count only those words or syllables that would have been said if the person

Table 8.5	Speaking Rates for Children and Adults	
Age (y)	Range in Syllables per Minute	Reference
3	116–163	Pindzola, Jenkins, and Lokken (1989)
4	117–183	"
5	109–183	"
6	140–175	Davis and Guitar (1976)
8	150–180	"
10	165–215	"
12	165–220	"
Adult	162–230	Andrews and Ingham (1971)

had not stuttered. Thus, if a person says, "My-my-my, uh, well my name is Peter," this should be counted as four words or five syllables because it is apparent that the extra instances of "my," the "uh," and the "well" are part of the stuttering. If a person says, "When I went to Boston, I mean when I went to New York…," and it does not appear that the person was postponing or using a "trick" to avoid stuttering, this would be counted as 13 words or 14 syllables because stuttering did not interfere with the utterance. Only true words (or syllables in true words) are counted; "uh" or "um" are not counted. "Oh" or "well" are counted, unless they are used as a postponement, starter, or other component of stuttering. These distinctions may seem difficult to remember, but the main rule of thumb you should use is that you are counting syllables or words that convey information to the listener.

When syllables per minute are calculated, it is often easiest to use an inexpensive calculator to count syllables cumulatively as they are spoken, although this takes some practice. Before the speaker begins, push the "1" key, then the "+." When the speaker starts speaking, press the "=" key for each syllable spoken or read, and the cumulative total will appear in the readout window. It is easier to count syllables by reading a transcript of the conversational sample aloud slowly and pushing the "=" key for each syllable spoken; inexperienced raters should learn to count syllables first from a transcript. Experienced raters can assess conversational speech rate directly from recordings by pressing the "=" key for each syllable spoken. Some calculators will count cumulatively when the "1" is pressed, followed by repeated presses of the "+" button; I have not found an expensive calculator that will count cumulatively (a cheap one will), but the calculator that came with my PC software will count cumulatively with the 1, +, = maneuver.

Some clinicians have found that they are able, with practice, to count syllables per minute as the client is speaking by using graph paper with small boxes. As the client is talking, they put a dot in each box for each syllable spoken. They also use this method to assess frequency of stuttering, by putting a check instead of a dot for each syllable stuttered.

When words per minute are calculated, a transcript is made of a client's five-minute sample of conversational speech, and her five-minute reading sample is marked to indicate where she finished. The total number of words is counted, and this figure is divided by five to give a per-minute conversation or reading rate.

It is important to measure these samples accurately with a stopwatch or another timing device. In measuring the amount of speaking time in a conversational sample, I stop the stopwatch whenever the client is not talking but allow it to run during moments of stuttering. Short pauses of less than two seconds are incorporated into the five minutes, but formulation pauses longer than two seconds are excluded. With a little practice, starting and stopping a stopwatch during pauses and turn-switching becomes easy and natural.

The CSSS software that comes with the SSI-4 allows the clinician to count number of stutters and number of fluent syllables and assess total sample duration in seconds. By totaling the stuttered and fluent syllables and dividing that by the sample duration in minutes (minutes + number of seconds divided by 60) you can get overall speech rate in syllables per minute.

ASSESSING FEELINGS AND ATTITUDES

The feelings or emotions of individuals who stutter, as well as their beliefs and attitudes about themselves, about communication, and about stuttering, are all components of stuttering. For most people who stutter, the experience of stuttering and the reactions of others to their stuttering have a notable effect on their behavior and on their response to therapy. Therefore, assessment of these aspects of stuttering is important. In this section, I focus on formal measures of **feelings and attitudes** that can be administered throughout therapy to assess progress. As clinicians gain more experience, they will develop informal procedures to supplement formal measures. I will describe these in the next chapter, as well as in appropriate treatment chapters.

Assessment of Preschool Children

There are not many instruments to assess feelings and attitudes of preschool children who stutter, but two are worth noting. The first is the KiddyCAT (Hernandez, 2001; Vanryckeghem, Brutten, & Hernandez, 2005; Vanryckeghem, Hernandez, & Brutten, 2001), which was designed to assess communication attitudes of preschool children who stutter. It consists of 12 yes/no questions asked by the clinician after some practice items. An example is "Do you think that Mom and Dad like the way you talk?" The questions are asked in a play environment, such as putting a marble in an egg carton after each response. Higher scores indicate more negative attitudes about speech. In a sample of 45 children who stutter (ages 0–3 to 5–6) and 63 children who don't (ages 2–3 to 3–6), the mean scores were 4.35 (SD = 2.78) for children who stutter and 1.79 (SD = 1.78) for children who don't. This difference is statistically significant ($p < .001$).

Another assessment tool for attitudes and feelings of preschool children who stutter takes an indirect approach by surveying parents about the impact of stuttering on the child and themselves (Langevin, Packman, & Onslow, 2010). The survey—The Impact of Stuttering on Preschoolers and Parents (ISPP)—consists of 20 questions covering (a) child-related questions (e.g., "Has your child ever been frustrated when stuttering?"); (b) questions about playmates (e.g., "Has your child ever been teased by other children about his stuttering?"); and (c) parent-related questions (e.g., "Has your child's stuttering ever affected you emotionally?"). One of the purposes of this tool, according to the authors, is to help decide whether to enroll the child in treatment or to delay treatment to see if stuttering resolves. This survey awaits further testing to assess validity and reliability. The ISPP is shown in Figure 8.5.

THE IMPACT OF STUTTERING ON PRESCHOOLERS AND PARENTS (ISPP) QUESTIONS

Response options were (a) "Yes," "No," and "Don't Know" for questions 1–10 and 11–14, and (b) "Yes" or "No" for questions 16–19. For "Yes" responses, more information was most often solicited.

Part I. Child-related questions:

1.   Has stuttering ever caused any changes in how easy it is for your child to talk with other children? If you answered YES, was it easier or more difficult?

2.   Has stuttering ever caused any changes in your child's self-confidence? If you answered YES, did your child gain or lose self-confidence?

3.   Has stuttering ever caused any changes in your child's general talkativeness? If you answered YES, did your child become more or less talkative?

4.   Has stuttering ever caused any changes in how much your child plays with other children? If you answered YES, did your child play with other children more or less?

5.   Has stuttering ever caused any changes in the way your child plays with other children? This question refers to a broad range of possible changes in the way children play. For example, a child may change from being more or less assertive, may use gestures to communicate in play, or may give up when he/she can't get or keep a playmate's attention. If you answered YES, please comment on the way your child's play changed.

6.   Has stuttering ever caused any changes in your child's general mood? If you answered YES, please comment on how your child's general mood changed.

7.   Has stuttering ever caused any changes in your child's quality of life? If you answered YES, please comment on the changes.

8.   Has your child ever been frustrated when stuttering?

9.   Has stuttering ever caused your child to become withdrawn?

10. If you think stuttering has affected your child in any way other than in the ways referred to above, please summarize.

Part II. About playmates:

11. Has your child ever been teased by other children because of his/her stuttering? If you answered YES, can you please describe what children do or did when they tease(d)?

12. Has stuttering ever caused a change in how much children play with your child? If you answered YES, did children play more or less with your child?

13. Has stuttering ever caused a change in the way children play with your child? Again, this question refers to a broad range of possible changes in the way children play with your child. For example, playmates may become more empathetic and watch out for your child, they may not wait for your child to say what he/she wants to say, or they may become more bossy or directive. If you answered YES, please describe the change.

14. Have other children ever reacted in any other way to your child's stuttering? If you answered YES, please describe how the children react(ed).

15. Is there anything else about how children react to your child or your child's stuttering that you wish to share?

Part III. Parent-related questions:

16. Has your child's stuttering ever affected you emotionally?

17. Has your child's stuttering ever affected how you communicate with your child?

18. Have you ever not known what to do or say when your child was stuttering?

19. Has your child's stuttering ever affected the relationship between you and your child insofar as it would be affected by a breakdown in communication?

Figure 8.5   The impact of stuttering on preschoolers and parents.

A number of clinicians have suggested that a preschool child's sensitivity or reactivity to new situations may be an important consideration in therapy and possibly predictive of chronicity (Conture, 2001; Guitar, 1998). I have found that the *Behavioral Style Questionnaire* (BSQ) (McDevitt & Carey, 1978, 1995), which is administered to parents, provides some information on this dimension. Some research indicates that the BSQ may be able to identify those children who have a more inhibited, sensitive temperament (Anderson,

Pellowski, Conture, & Kelly, 2003; Conture, 2001). The BSQ has relatively high mean test-retest reliability for the 3 to 7 years scales (0.81) and a moderate internal consistency for this age range (0.70) (McDevitt & Carey, 1995).

Assessment of School-Age Children

There are several tools available for assessing attitudes about speaking or about stuttering in children. Figure 8.6 depicts

Establish rapport with the child, and make sure that he or she is physically comfortable before beginning administration. Explain the task to the child, and make sure he or she understands what is required. Some simple directions might be used:

"I am going to ask you some questions. Listen carefully, and then tell me what you think: true or false. There is no right or wrong answer. I just want to know what you think." To begin the scale, ask the questions in a natural manner. Do not urge the child to respond before he or she is ready, and repeat the question if the child did not hear it or you feel that he or she did not understand it. Do not reword the question unless you feel it is absolutely necessary, and then write the question you asked under that item.

Circle the answer that corresponds to the child's response. Be accepting of the child's response because there is no right or wrong answer. If all the child will say is "I don't know," even after prompting, record that response next to the question. For the younger children (kindergarten and first grade), it might be necessary to give a few simple examples to ensure comprehension of the requited task:

a. Are you a boy?   Yes   No

b. Do you have black hair?   Yes   No

Similar, obvious questions may be inserted, if necessary, to reassure the examiner that the child is actively cooperating at all times. Adequately praise the child for listening, and assure him or her that a good job is being done.

It is important to be familiar with the questions so that they can be read in a natural manner.

The child is given 1 point for each answer that matches those given below. The higher a child's score, the more probable it is that he or she has developed negative attitudes toward communication. In our study, the mean score of the K through fourth grade stutterers (N = 28) was 9.07 (S.D. = 2.44), and for the 28 matched controls, it was 8.17 (S.D. = 1.80).

Score 1 point for each answer that matches these:

1. Yes	11. No
2. Yes	12. No
3. No	13. Yes
4. No	14. Yes
5. No	15. Yes
6. Yes	16. No
7. No	17. No
8. Yes	18. Yes
9. Yes	19. Yes
10. No	

Figure 8.6 A-19 Scale of Children's Attitudes by Susan Andre and Barry Guitar (University of Vermont; reprinted from Susan Andre, with permission). *(Continued)*

A-19 SCALE

Name_____   Date _____

1. Is it best to keep your mouth shut when you are in trouble?	Yes	No
2. When the teacher calls on you, do you get nervous?	Yes	No
3. Do you ask a lot of questions in class?	Yes	No
4. Do you like to talk on the phone?	Yes	No
5. If you did not know a person, would you tell your name?	Yes	No
6. Is it hard to talk to your teacher?	Yes	No
7. Would you go up to a new boy or girl in your class?	Yes	No
8. Is it hard to keep control of your voice when talking?	Yes	No
9. Even when you know the right answer, are you afraid to say it?	Yes	No
10. Do you like to tell other children what to do?	Yes	No
11. Is it fun to talk to your dad?	Yes	No
12. Do you like to tell stories to your classmates?	Yes	No
13. Do you wish you could say things as clearly as the other kids do?	Yes	No
14. Would you rather look at a comic book than talk to a friend?	Yes	No
15. Are you upset when someone interrupts you?	Yes	No
16. When you want to say something, do you just say it?	Yes	No
17. Is talking to your friends more fun than playing by yourself?	Yes	No
18. Are you sometimes unhappy?	Yes	No
19. Are you a little afraid to talk on the phone?	Yes	No

Figure 8.6   (Continued)

a scale that a graduate student and I developed many years ago, called the A-19 Scale (Guitar & Grims, 1977). It consists of questions that we have found will distinguish between children who stutter and children who do not. Thus, if treatment is effective, a child's attitude about communication may change, although this has not been established by research.

In addition to the A-19, the Communication Attitude Test (CAT), which was developed by Brutten and his colleagues, has been shown to be a reliable and appropriate tool to measure the attitudes of children and adults who stutter. In a study by De Nil and Brutten (1991) 70 children who stuttered and 271 children who didn't (ages 7–14) were administered the CAT. The children who stuttered had significantly more negative communication attitudes ($p <.01$), and this difference increased with age. Vanryckeghem and Brutten (1997) replicated this finding with children (ages 6–13). In 1992, Vanryckeghem and Brutten affirmed the CAT's test-retest

reliability using 44 school-age children; results indicated correlations of 0.86, 0.81, and 0.76 for retesting after 1, 11, and 12 weeks, respectively, indicating that it is appropriate to administer it to a child several times. In a study of 143 children who stuttered (ages 7–13), Vanryckeghem, Hylebos, Brutten, and Peleman (2001) examined the relationship between negative attitudes as measured by the CAT and negative emotions elicited by the questions on the CAT, as measured by a 1-to-5 scale filled out by the children. The authors found a high positive correlation ($r = 0.89$) between negative attitudes and negative emotions. Both negative attitudes and negative emotions increased with age. In summary, the CAT is a well-researched tool that can be used to determine the presence of negative attitudes in individuals ages 6 and older. It is now part of a larger assessment battery (Behavior Assessment Battery for School-Age Children Who Stutter, Brutten & Vanryckeghem, 2007), which also contains the Speech Situation Checklist that evaluates a child's reactions to a range of situations, as well as the Behavioral Checklist which assesses a child's coping responses to his disfluency.

It is important that a trusting relationship with the child has been developed before administering either the A-19 or the CAT to a school-age child.

The *Overall Assessment of the Speaker's Experience of Stuttering* (OASES) is a questionnaire designed to assess the impact of stuttering on a person's life. It is based on the World Health Organization's *International Classification of Functioning, Disability, and Health* (World Health Organization, 2001) and focuses on feelings about stuttering, reactions to stuttering, communication in daily situations, and the extent to which stuttering interferes with daily living. A new version is adapted for use with children ages 7 to 12. A more detailed description is given in the next section on adolescents and adults, and a sample for adults is shown in Figure 8.7.

Although not strictly a measure of attitude, the Teachers Assessment of Student Communicative Competence (TASCC) (Smith, McCauley, & Guitar, 2000), which is depicted in Figure 8.8, is useful in assessing a child's communicative functioning in the classroom. I have listed it here because one of the subscales purports to measure approach/avoidance in the classroom based on questions about the child's class participation and volunteering to talk. Other areas that the teacher rates the child on include intelligibility, comprehension, appropriateness of communication, and pragmatic/nonverbal communication skills. I have found the TASCC to be helpful in getting information about how a child's communication is changing over the course of treatment. The measure was tested on 69 students in grades 1 through 5 in Maine, Vermont, Texas, Virginia, and Idaho and showed high internal consistency. Cronbach's coefficient alphas (a measure of a test's reliability) for the five subscales ranged from 0.77 to 0.95, respectively, suggesting that the TASCC items were related measuring a similar construct (Smith, McCauley, & Guitar, 2000). Redundancy analysis was used to remove redundant items and combine some that were similar, leaving a 50-item scale.

Further pilot work (Sequin, 1999) on the TASCC was conducted with 14 children who stuttered, paired by gender and ethnic background with 14 who did not stutter. Scoring of each pair of participants was obtained from teachers of children in grades 1 to 5; the participants included eight Caucasian pairs, two Hispanic pairs, and four African American pairs. Three of the pairs were females and 11 were males. The children who stuttered had significantly lower communicative competence scores ($p = .0001$) than the control children; the "approach/avoidance attitude" subscale showed the greatest difference between the groups. A second pilot study (Pierson, 2004) compared TASCC ratings of eight children who stuttered and eight children who did not (grades 1–5) matched for age, gender, grade, cultural background, and academic performance. Again, the children who stuttered had significantly lower communicative competence scores ($p = .002$).

The approach/avoidance attitude subscale was not found to be significantly different between the groups, but these three scales were, with the differences between the groups in this rank order: intelligibility > appropriateness of communication > clarification/repair (of output)/comprehension (of input) > pragmatic/nonverbal communication. Clinically, I have found it useful to know what subscales are most deviant for a child. In one instance, a child who was rated deviant on the intelligibility subscale benefited from learning to speak more slowly and loudly, even when he stuttered.

Assessment of Adolescents and Adults

A variety of questionnaires can be used to assess various aspects of a stutterer's feelings and attitudes about communication and stuttering. I typically use the Modified Erickson Scale of Communication Attitudes (S-24) (Andrews & Cutler, 1974) to obtain information about a client's communication attitudes (Fig. 8.9). This questionnaire has been normed on both stutterers and nonstutterers. A colleague and I (Guitar & Bass, 1978) studied a sample of 20 individuals treated by a fluency-shaping program and found that if communication attitude as measured by the S-24 does not change during treatment, the likelihood of relapse within 12 to 18 months increases. Ingham (1979) disputed this finding, but Young (1981) confirmed it using a reanalysis of the original data. Later data by Andrews and Craig (1988) also supported the relationship between normalizing attitudes on the S-24 and long-term treatment outcome.

I also use a questionnaire to assess a client's tendency to avoid stuttering, which is the avoidance scale of the Stutterer's Self-Rating of Reactions to Speech Situations (SSRSS) (Johnson et al., 1952); this questionnaire assesses a client's tendency to avoid specific speaking situations (Fig. 8.10). Research suggests that clients with avoidance scale scores higher than 2.56 before treatment may be more likely to have appreciable levels of stuttering one year after treatment with fluency-shaping therapy than clients with lower scores (Guitar, 1976). Thus, I suggest that clinicians use a client's avoidance scale score to guide them in choosing whether to focus more on ways of enhancing fluent speech or to combine shaping fluency with an approach that modifies stuttering as well as the fears and avoidances associated with stuttering.

Sometimes I also use the Perceptions of Stuttering Inventory (PSI) (Woolf, 1967) to examine a stutterer's perception of the presence of struggle, avoidance, and expectancy of stuttering (Fig. 8.11). Woolf suggests that the PSI can be used to help a stutterer view her problem more objectively, to develop treatment goals, and to assess progress. I find that the avoidance section of the PSI complements the avoidance scale of the SRSS because the SRSS focuses more on situations, whereas the PSI deals more with stuttering behaviors.

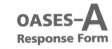

OASES™

OASES–A
Response Form

Ages 18 and above

Overall Assessment of the
Speaker's Experience of Stuttering

J. Scott Yaruss, PhD, CCC-SLP, BRS-FD
Robert W. Quesal, PhD, CCC-SLP, BRS-FD

Name: _____

Birth Date: _____/_____/_____ Test Date: _____/_____/_____

ID Number: _____ Age: _____ Sex: ☐M ☐F

General Instructions:

This form includes four sections of questions that examine different aspects of your experiences with stuttering. Please complete each question in each section by circling the appropriate number. Please think about how you are *currently* feeling or speaking when answering each question. Some of the questions do not apply to everyone. If one of the questions does not apply to you, please check the "Not Applicable" box and go to the next question.

For Office Use Only

Instructions for Clinicians: Calculate Impact Scores for each of the four sections on the OASES–A by first summing the number of points in each section (A) and then counting the number of items completed in each section (B). Divide the total number of points (A) by the number of items completed (B) to obtain the Impact Score. Impact Scores range between 1.0 and 5.0. Using the Impact Scores on the left-hand side of the table, determine the Impact Rating for each section.

				Impact Rating				
Section	**A** **Points**	**B** **Items Completed**	**A ÷ B =** **Impact Score**	**Mild** **1.00–1.49**	**Mild/Moderate** **1.50–2.24**	**Moderate** **2.25–2.99**	**Moderate/Severe** **3.00–3.74**	**Severe** **3.75–5.00**
I	_____	_____ (min = 18)*	_____	☐	☐	☐	☐	☐
II	_____	_____ (min = 28)	_____	☐	☐	☐	☐	☐
III	_____	_____ (min = 23)*	_____	☐	☐	☐	☐	☐
IV	_____	_____ (min = 23)*	_____	☐	☐	☐	☐	☐
Overall (Total)	_____	_____ (min =92)*	_____	☐	☐	☐	☐	☐

*Note: Reduce this number by the number of items marked "Not Applicable," if any.

PEARSON

Copyright © 2010 NCS Pearson, Inc. All rights reserved.

ⓦ PsychCorp

Product Number 30403

Figure 8.7 Overall assessment of the speaker's experience of stuttering. (Reprinted with permission from NCS Pearson, Inc. © 2010.)

Another measure of attitude that has been shown to predict long-term outcome is the Locus of Control of Behavior Scale (Craig, Franklin, & Andrews, 1984), which assesses the extent to which a client believes he controls his own behavior (i.e., whether the control is "internal" or "external")

(Fig. 8.12). Scoring adds the points for each item, and higher scores reflect greater perceived "externality" of control. Because the values of items 1, 5, 7, 8, 13, 15, and 16 are reversed to minimize the effect of social desirability in responding, the scores on these items are transposed (e.g., you change a

TEACHER ASSESSMENT OF STUDENT COMMUNICATIVE COMPETENCE (TASCC)

Student's Name _____ Age _____ Gender _____ Ethnicity _____

Below are a series of items that describe a student's communicative competency. Use the following scale to rate a student in your grade whom you consider to have communication competency issues. For each item, circle the number that best describes the student's communication. Please answer each item as well as you can, even if the item does not seem to apply to the student.

1 = Never   2 = Seldom   3 = Sometimes   4 = Often   5 = Always

Item	1	2	3	4	5
1) Student remains attentive when others communicate with him/her	1	2	3	4	5
2) Student verbally relates thoughts in an age-appropriate meaningful manner to adults	1	2	3	4	5
3) Student adjusts style and content of speech according to communication partner and situation	1	2	3	4	5
4) Student appears to nonverbally relate feelings in an age-appropriate meaningful manner (e.g., facial glare, smile)	1	2	3	4	5
5) Student demonstrates age-appropriate nonverbal requests for message repetition (e.g., makes a "puzzled" face)	1	2	3	4	5
6) Student participates in age-appropriate turn-taking in conversations and class discussions	1	2	3	4	5
7) Student demonstrates age-appropriate verbal requests for message repetition (e.g., "Could you say that again?" or "What?")	1	2	3	4	5
8) Student uses appropriate voice inflection when speaking (e.g., intonation with questions)	1	2	3	4	5
9) Student uses appropriate eye contact when speaking to adults	1	2	3	4	5
10) Student gets the listener's attention before the student introduces a topic	1	2	3	4	5
11) Student uses age-appropriate opening and closing communication comments in conversations with peers (e.g., "Hello, see you later.")	1	2	3	4	5
12) Student's speech is understandable even when the topic is unknown	1	2	3	4	5
13) Student participates in story-description/retell interactions	1	2	3	4	5
14) Student verbally relates thoughts in an age-appropriate meaningful manner to peers	1	2	3	4	5
15) Student sticks up for his/her own views when confronted by group pressure	1	2	3	4	5
16) Student's overall speech is understandable (e.g., clear voice, clear articulation)	1	2	3	4	5

Figure 8.8   Teacher assessment of student communicative competence. *(Continued)*

17) Student nonverbally expresses frustration toward peers when appropriate	1	2	3	4	5
18) Student responds within an appropriate time frame to remarks, questions, requests	1	2	3	4	5
19) Student joins into conversations with peers easily	1	2	3	4	5
20) Student uses vocabulary that is relevant to the conversation	1	2	3	4	5
21) Student appropriately engages in group discussions	1	2	3	4	5
22) Student uses appropriate rate of speech for situation	1	2	3	4	5
23) Student initiates topics of conversation in one-to-one situations with adults	1	2	3	4	5
24) Student initiates topics of conversation in one-to-one situations with peers	1	2	3	4	5
25) Student adjusts vocal intensity to account for distance and noise variables	1	2	3	4	5
26) Student freely volunteers answers to questions in class	1	2	3	4	5
27) Student uses speech effectively in directing peer's actions when intended	1	2	3	4	5
28) Student's speech is understood by unfamiliar listeners	1	2	3	4	5
29) Student uses appropriate eye contact when speaking to peers	1	2	3	4	5
30) Student uses age-appropriate humor within peer conversations	1	2	3	4	5
31) Student uses age-appropriate verbal communication to gain attention	1	2	3	4	5
32) Student nonverbally expresses frustration toward adults when appropriate	1	2	3	4	5
33) Student uses a variety of age-appropriate (or better) vocabulary	1	2	3	4	5
34) Student seems to understand age-appropriate humor within peer conversations	1	2	3	4	5
35) Student clarifies and/or rephrases when verbal communication is not understood by the listener	1	2	3	4	5
36) Student uses age-appropriate (or better) sentence length when answering questions in class	1	2	3	4	5
37) Student is able to shift to different topics within conversations	1	2	3	4	5
38) Student links his/her words together with age-appropriate (or better) grammatical structures	1	2	3	4	5
39) Student follows three-step instructions with minimal need for repetitions or visual cues	1	2	3	4	5
40) Student's speech is understood even when the speech becomes more complex (e.g., longer sentences, change in topic)	1	2	3	4	5

Figure 8.8 *(Continued)*

41) Student verbally or nonverbally indicates that he/she understands the speaker's message	1	2	3	4	5
42) Student is able to integrate information presented auditorily (e.g., lessons, stories, a sequence of directions) and comprehend the meaning	1	2	3	4	5
43) Student identifies characters/people in conversations	1	2	3	4	5
44) Student uses age-appropriate (or better) sentence length when having a conversation	1	2	3	4	5
45) Student uses the environment to get a message across when the student's verbal communication is not understood (e.g., points to relevant objects or people)	1	2	3	4	5
46) Student seems to understand nonverbal communication (e.g., gestures)	1	2	3	4	5
47) Student uses age-appropriate nonverbal communication to gain the attention of adults	1	2	3	4	5
48) Peers and adults seem to understand what the student says to them	1	2	3	4	5
49) Student interacts with a variety of peers and adults	1	2	3	4	5
50) Student uses age-appropriate nonverbal communication to gain the attention of peers (e.g., wave, gentle tap)	1	2	3	4	5

TASCC SUBSCALES

The TASCC is divided into five subscales. The following information indicates which items, distributed randomly, belong to which subscales.

Subscale	Item #s
I. Intelligibility	8, 12, 16, 22, 25, 40, 48
II. Appropriateness of Communication	2, 3, 6, 10, 11, 13, 14, 18, 20, 27, 30, 31, 33, 36, 37, 38, 44
III. Comprehension (of input) and Clarification or Repair (of output)	7, 34, 35, 39, 41, 42, 43, 46
IV. Pragmatic/Nonverbal	1, 4, 5, 9, 17, 29, 32, 45, 47, 50
V. Approach/Avoidance Attitude	15, 19, 21, 23, 24, 26, 49

Figure 8.8 *(Continued)*

MODIFIED ERICKSON SCALE OF COMMUNICATION ATTITUDES (S-24)

Name: _____   Date: _____   Score: _____

Directions: Mark the "true column with a check (✓) for each statement that is true or mostly true for you and mark the "false" column with a check (✓) for each statement which is false or not usually true for you.

	TRUE	FALSE
1. I usually feel that I am making a favorable impression when I talk.		
2. I find it easy to talk with almost anyone.		
3. I find it very easy to look at my audience while speaking to a group.		
4. A person who is my teacher or my boss is hard to talk to.		
5. Even the idea of giving a talk in public makes me afraid.		
6. Some words are harder than others for me to say.		
7. I forget all about myself shortly after I begin a speech.		
8. I am a good mixer.		
9. People sometimes seem uncomfortable when I am talking to them.		
10. I dislike introducing one person to another.		
11. I often ask questions in group discussions.		
12. I find it easy to keep control of my voice when speaking.		
13. I do not mind speaking in front of a group.		
14. I do not talk well enough to do the kind of work I'd really like to do.		
15. My speaking voice is rather pleasant and easy to listen to.		
16. I am sometimes embarrassed by the way I talk.		
17. I face most speaking situations with complete confidence.		
18. There are few people I can talk with easily.		

Figure 8.9   Erickson S-24 Scale of Communication Attitudes. (Reprinted from Andrews, G. & Cutler, J. (1974). Stuttering therapy: The relation between changes in symptom level and attitudes. *Journal of Speech and Hearing Disorders, 39*, 312–319, with permission. Copyright 1974, American Speech-Language-Hearing Association.)

| 19. I talk better than I write. |
| 20. I often feel nervous while talking. |
| 21. I find it hard to talk when I meet new people. |
| 22. I feel pretty confident about my speaking ability. |
| 23. I wish that I could say things as clearly as others do. |
| 24. Even though I knew the right answer, I have often failed to give it because I was afraid to speak out. |

Data on the "Modified Erickson Scale of Communication Attitudes"
I. Answers (Andrews & Cutler, 1974)
Score 1 point for each answer that matches this:

1. False	13. False
2. False	14. True
3. False	15. False
4. True	16. True
5. True	17. False
6. True	18. True
7. False	19. False
8. False	20. True
9. True	21. True
10. True	22. False
11. False	23. True
12. False	24. True

II. Adult Norms (Andrews & Cutler, 1974)

	Mean	Range
Stutterers	19.22	9–24
Nonstutterers	9.14	1–21

Figure 8.9   (Continued)

5 to a 0, a 4 to a 1, and so on) before totaling the score. This scale is given just before treatment and again immediately after treatment. Studies have shown that clients who did not decrease their locus of control scores more than 5 percent from pretreatment to post-treatment are in danger of relapse (Craig & Andrews, 1985; Craig et al., 1984).

Andrews and Craig (1988) reported that two measures of attitude, combined with a measure of stuttering behavior, are useful in predicting relapse after fluency-shaping treatment. They found little relapse among those stutterers who met the following three goals by the end of treatment: (1) no stuttering on telephone calls to strangers; (2) a score of 9 or below on the Modified Erickson Scale of Communication Attitudes; and (3) locus of control score reductions greater than 5 percent. Their assessment of relapse was based on a single telephone call with a stranger 10 to 18 months after treatment, and relapse was considered to be more than 2 percent of syllables stuttered during the call.

STUTTERER'S SELF-RATING OF REACTIONS TO SPEECH SITUATIONS

Name_____ Age_____ Sex _____
Examiner _____ Date _____

After each item put a number from 1 to 5 in each of the four columns.

Start with the right-hand column headed "Frequency." Study the five possible answers to be made in responding to each item, and write the number of the answer that best fits the situation for you in each case. Thus, if you habitually take your meals at home and seldom eat in a restaurant, certainly not as often as once a week, write the number 5 in the Frequency column opposite item No. 1 "Ordering in a restaurant." In like manner respond to each of the other 39 items by writing the most appropriate number in the Frequency column.

Now, write the number of the response that best indicates how much you stutter in each situation. For example, if in ordering meals in a restaurant you stutter mildly (for you), write number 2 in the Stuttering column.

Following the same procedure, write your responses in the Reaction column and, finally, write your responses in the Avoidance column.

Numbers for each of the columns are to be interpreted as follows:

A. Avoidance

1. I never try to avoid this situation and have no desire to avoid it.
2. I don't try to avoid this situation, but sometimes I would like to.
3. More often than not I <u>do not</u> try to avoid this situation, but sometimes I do try to avoid it.
4. More often than not I <u>do</u> try to avoid this situation.
5. I avoid this situation every time I possibly can.

B. Reaction

1. I definitely enjoy speaking in this situation.
2. I would rather speak in this situation than not speak.
3. It's hard to say whether I'd rather speak in this situation or not.
4. I would rather not speak in this situation.
5. I very much dislike speaking in this situation.

C. Stuttering

1. I don't stutter at all (or only very rarely) in this situation.
2. I stutter mildly (for me) in this situation.
3. I stutter with average severity (for me) in this situation.
4. I stutter more than average (for me) in this situation.
5. I stutter severely (for me) in this situation.

Figure 8.10 Stutterer's Self-Rating of Reactions to Speech Situations. (Reprinted from Johnson, W., Darley, F., & Spriestersbach, D.C. (1952). Diagnostic manual in speech correction. New York: Harper & Row, with permission. Copyright 1952 by Harper & Row. Copyright renewed 1980 by Edna B. Johnson, Frederick L. Darley, and Duane C. Spriestersbach.)

D. Frequency

1. This is a situation I meet very often, two or three times a day or even more, on the average.
2. I meet this situation at least once a day with rare exceptions (except Sunday perhaps).
3. I meet this situation from three to five times a week on the average.
4. I meet this situation once a week, with few exceptions, and occasionally I meet it twice a week.
5. I rarely meet this situation—certainly not as often as once a week.

	Avoidance	Reaction	Stuttering	Frequency
1. Ordering in a restaurant.				
2. Introducing myself (face to face).				
3. Telephoning to ask price, train fare, etc.				
4. Buying plane, train, or bus ticket.				
5. Short class recitation (10 words or less).				
6. Telephoning for taxi.				
7. Introducing one person to another.				
8. Buying something from a store clerk.				
9. Conversation with a good friend.				
10. Talking with an instructor after class or in his or her office.				
11. Long-distance phone call to someone I know.				
12. Conversation with my father.				
13. Asking someone for date (or talking to someone who asks me for date).				
14. Making short speech (1–2 minutes).				
15. Giving my name over telephone.				
16. Conversation with my mother.				
17. Asking a secretary if I can see the employer.				
18. Going to house and asking for someone.				
19. Making a speech to unfamiliar audience.				
20. Participating in committee meeting.				
21. Asking the instructor a question in class.				
22. Saying hello to friend passing by.				
23. Asking for a job.				
24. Telling a person a message from someone else.				
25. Telling a funny story with one stranger in a crowd.				
26. Parlor game requiring speech.				

Figure 8.10   (Continued)

27. Reading aloud to friends.

28. Participating in a bull session.

29. Dinner conversation with strangers.

30. Talking with my barber/hairdresser.

31. Telephoning to make appointment
    or to arrange to meet someone.

32. Answering roll call in class.

33. Asking at a desk for book or card
    to be filled out, etc.

34. Talking with someone I don't know well
    while waiting for bus, class, etc.

35. Talking with other players during game.

36. Taking leave of a host or hostess.

37. Conversation with friend while walking.

38. Buying stamps at post office.

39. Giving directions to a stranger.

40. Taking leave of a girl/boy after date.

Totals

Averages (divide total by # of answers)

Figure 8.10 *(Continued)*

As mentioned in the preceding section, the OASES (Fig. 8.7) is an assessment tool based on the WHO's 2001 International Classification of Functioning, Disability, and Health. It is a 20-minute paper-and-pencil questionnaire designed to obtain information about the impact of stuttering on a client's life that is not usually gained by other measures. It is divided into four sections: I. General Information, II. Reactions to Stuttering, III. Communication in Daily Situations, and IV. Quality of Life. An "impact score" for each section as well as a "total impact score" can be calculated and then related to normative data so that a clinician can find out how severely stuttering is impacting a client's life.

The developers of the OASES published data on validity and reliability (Yaruss & Quesal, 2006) on the adult version, indicating that internal reliability within each of the four sections was high (Cronbach's alpha coefficient ranged from 0.92 to 0.97), suggesting that questions within a section were tapping into a homogenous area. In addition, Pearson product-moment correlations between total scores for these four sections were low enough (0.66 to 0.85) to indicate that the different sections were measuring different domains. Criterion-related validity was assessed by comparing an earlier version of the OASES to the Erickson S-24 Scale of Communication Attitudes (Andrews & Cutler, 1974; Erickson, 1969). Correlations suggested one

section (Reactions to Stuttering) was positively and highly correlated with the S-24, whereas the other two sections (Communication in Daily Situations and Quality of Life) were moderately correlated. Test-retest reliability was assessed by giving the OASES to 14 individuals two different times, separated by 10 to 14 days without intervening treatment. Responses were identical for 77 percent of responses and within ± 1 for 98 percent of responses, suggesting that it is appropriate to administer the instrument repeatedly to an individual (e.g., before, during, and after treatment).

A summary of instruments to assess feelings and attitudes is given in Table 8.6.

CONTINUING ASSESSMENT

Assessment is an ongoing process. As treatment progresses, the clinician should continue to ask herself, "Am I using the best approach with this person? Is there something else or something different I should be doing?" She should also decide what measures of progress are important for a client and apply these measures at regular intervals. My own approach is to assess stuttering behavior at the beginning and the end of each semester. In other settings, I often assess a client after every 10 hours of treatment. Although

PERCEPTIONS OF STUTTERING INVENTORY (PSI)

The symbols S, A, and E after each item denote struggle (S), avoidance (A), and expectancy (E). In practice, these symbols are not included in the Inventory, but are listed on a separate scoring key.

<u>S</u> <u>A</u> <u>E</u>

Name _____ Age _____ # _____

Examiner _____ Date _____ % _____

Directions

Here are 60 statements about stuttering. Some of these may be characteristic of <u>your</u> stuttering. Read each item carefully and respond as in the examples below.

Put a check mark (✓) under "characteristic of me" if <u>repeating</u> sounds is part of your stuttering; if it is not characteristic, leave the space blank.

"Characteristic of me" refers only to what you do <u>now</u>, not to what was true of <u>your</u> stuttering in the past and which you no longer do, and not to what you think you should or should not be doing. Even if the behavior described occurs only occasionally or only in some speaking situations, if you regard it as characteristic of your stuttering, check the space under "characteristic of me."

Characteristic
of me

_____ I. Avoiding talking to people in authority (e.g., a teacher, employer, or clergyman). (A).

_____ 2. Feeling that interruptions in your speech (e.g., pauses, hesitations, or repetitions) will lead to stuttering. (E).

_____ 3. Making the pitch of your voice higher or lower when you expect to get "stuck" on words. (E).

_____ 4. Having extra and unnecessary facial movement (e.g., flaring your nostrils during speech attempts). (S).

_____ 5. Using gestures as a substitute for speaking (e.g., nodding your head instead of saying "yes" or smiling to acknowledge a greeting). (A).

_____ 6. Avoiding asking for information (e.g., asking for directions or inquiring about a train schedule). (A).

Figure 8.11 Perceptions of Stuttering Inventory. (Reprinted from Woolf, G. (1967). The assessment of stuttering as struggle, avoidance, and expectancy, *British Journal of Disorders of Communication, 2*, 158–171, with permission.) *(Continued)*

_____	7. Whispering words to yourself before saying them or practicing what you are planning to say long before you speak. (E).
_____	8. Choosing a job or hobby because little speaking would be required. (A).
_____	9. Adding an extra or unnecessary sound, word, or phrase to your speech (e.g., "uh," "well," or "let me see") to help yourself get started. (E).
_____	10. Replying briefly using the fewest words possible. (A).
_____	11. Making sudden, jerky, or forceful movements with your head, arms or body during speech attempts (e.g., clenching your fist, jerking your head to one side). (S).
_____	12. Repeating a sound or word with effort. (S).
_____	13. Acting in a manner intended to keep you out of a conversation or discussion (e.g., being a good listener, pretending not to hear what was said, acting bored, or pretending to be in deep thought). (A).
_____	14. Avoiding making a purchase (e.g., avoiding going into a store or buying stamps in the post office). (A).
_____	15. Breathing noisily or with great effort while trying to speak. (S).
_____	16. Making your voice louder or softer when stuttering is expected. (E).
_____	17. Prolonging a sound or word (e.g., m-m-m-m-my) while trying to push it out. (S).
_____	18. Helping yourself to get started talking by laughing, coughing, clearing your throat, gesturing, or some other body activity movement. (E).
_____	19. Having general body tension during speech attempts (e.g., shaking, trembling, or feeling "knotted up" inside). (S).
_____	20. Paying particular attention to what you are going to say (e.g., the length of a word, or the position of a word in a sentence). (E).
_____	21. Feeling your face getting warm and red (as if you are blushing) as you are struggling to speak. (S).
_____	22. Saying words or phrases with force or effort. (S).
_____	23. Repeating a word or phrase preceding the word on which stuttering is expected. (E).
_____	24. Speaking so that no word or sound stands out (e.g., speaking in a sing-song voice or in a monotone). (E).
_____	25. Avoiding making new acquaintances (e.g., not visiting with friends, not dating, or not joining social, civic, or church groups). (A).

Figure 8.11 _(Continued)_

_____ 26. Making unusual noises with your teeth during speech attempts (e.g., grinding or clicking your teeth). (S).

_____ 27. Avoiding introducing yourself, giving your name, or making introductions. (A).

_____ 28. Expecting that certain sounds, letters, or words are going to be particularly "hard" to say (e.g., words beginning with the letter "s"). (E).

_____ 29. Giving excuses to avoid talking (e.g., pretending to be tired or pretending lack of interest in a topic). (A).

_____ 30. "Running out of breath" while speaking. (S).

_____ 31. Forcing out sounds. (S).

_____ 32. Feeling that your fluent periods are unusual, that they cannot last, and that sooner or later you will stutter. (E).

_____ 33. Concentrating on relaxing or not being tense before speaking. (E).

_____ 34. Substituting a different word or phrase for the one you had intended to say. (A).

_____ 35. Prolonging or emphasizing the sound preceding the one on which stuttering is expected. (E).

_____ 36. Avoiding speaking before an audience. (A).

_____ 37. Straining to talk without being able to make a sound. (S).

_____ 38. Coordinating or timing your speech with a rhythmic movement (e.g., tapping your foot or swinging your arm). (E).

_____ 39. Rearranging what you had planned to say to avoid a "hard" sound or word. (A).

_____ 40. "Putting on an act" when speaking (e.g., adopting an attitude of confidence or pretending to be angry). (E).

_____ 41. Avoiding the use of the telephone. (A).

_____ 42. Making forceful and strained movements with your lips, tongue, jaw, or throat (e.g., moving your jaw in an uncoordinated manner). (S).

_____ 43. Omitting a word, part of a word, or a phrase that you had planned to say (e.g., words with certain sounds or letters). (A).

_____ 44. Making "uncontrollable" sounds while struggling to say a word. (S).

_____ 45. Adopting a foreign accent, assuming a regional dialect, or imitating another person's speech. (E).

_____ 46. Perspiring much more than usual while speaking (e.g., feeling the palms of your hands getting clammy). (S).

_____ 47. Postponing speaking for a short time until certain you can be fluent (e.g., pausing before "hard" words). (E).

_____ 48. Having extra and unnecessary eye movements while speaking (e.g., blinking your eyes or shutting your eyes tightly). (S).

_____ 49. Breathing forcefully while struggling to speak. (S).

_____ 50. Avoiding talking to others of your own age group (your own or opposite sex). (A).

_____ 51. Giving up the speech attempt completely after getting "stuck" or if stuttering is anticipated. (A).

_____ 52. Straining the muscles of your chest or abdomen during speech attempts. (S).

Figure 8.11 _(Continued)_

_____ 53. Wondering whether you will stutter or how you will speak if you do stutter. (E).

_____ 54. Holding your lips, tongue, or jaw in a rigid position before speaking or when getting "stuck" on a word. (S).

_____ 55. Avoiding talking to one or both of your parents. (A).

_____ 56. Having another person speak for you in a difficult situation (e.g., having someone make a telephone call for you or order for you in a restaurant). (A).

_____ 57. Holding your breath before speaking. (S).

_____ 58. Saying words slowly or rapidly preceding the word on which stuttering is expected. (E).

_____ 59. Concentrating on <u>how</u> you are going to speak (e.g., thinking about where to put your tongue or how to breath). (E).

_____ 60. Using your stuttering as the reason to avoid a speaking activity. (A).

Figure 8.11 (Continued)

LOCUS OF CONTROL OF BEHAVIOR SCALE

Directions: Below are a number of statements about how various topics affect your personal beliefs. There are no right or wrong answers. For every item there are a large number of people who agree and disagree. Could you please put in the appropriate bracket the choice you believe to be true? Answer all the questions.

0	1	2	3	4	5
Strongly disagree	Generally disagree	Somewhat disagree	Somewhat agree	Generally agree	Strongly agree

1. I can anticipate difficulties and take action to avoid them..............................( )
2. A great deal of what happens to me is probably just a matter of chance.........( )
3. Everyone knows that luck or chance determines one's future..........................( )
4. I can control my problem(s) only if I have outside support.............................( )
5. When I make plans, I am almost certain that I can make them work..............( )
6. My problem(s) will dominate me all my life...( )
7. My mistakes and problems are my responsibility to deal with.......................... ( )
8. Becoming a success is a matter of hard work; luck has little or nothing to do with it..( )
9. My life is controlled by outside actions and events..( )
10. People are victims of circumstance beyond their control..................................( )
11. To continually manage my problems I need professional help ....( )
12. When I am under stress, the tightness in my muscles is due to things outside my control..( )
13. I believe a person can really be the master of his fate......................................( )
14. It is impossible to control my irregular and fast breathing when I am having difficulties..( )
15. I understand why my problem(s) varies so much from one occasion to the next...( )
16. I am confident of being able to deal successfully with future problems.........( )
17. In my case, maintaining control over my problem(s) is due mostly to luck....( )

Figure 8.12 Locus of Control of Behavior Scale.

Table 8.6	Methods of Assessing Attitudes and Feelings	
Age Group	Measure	Comment
Preschool	KiddyCAT	A 12-item set of questions that are asked of preschool children about their speech. Vanryckeghem and her colleagues have gathered considerable data comparing children who stutter and children who don't. Our own experience suggests caution lest children give answers they think the examiner wants to hear.
	ISPP	A 20-item questionnaire for parents about their child's response to his stuttering and about parents' own feelings about their child's stuttering.
	BSQ	A broad scale completed by parents which may reveal children's sensitivity. Children ages 3–7 who stutter have been shown to be more sensitive than typical children, using this scale.
School age	A-19	This is an informal 19-item questionnaire given to children. Although it has been shown to distinguish between children who stutter and those who don't (kindergarten through fourth grade), it has not been extensively tested. Useful for generating discussion about how the student feels about his stuttering.
	CAT	This questionnaire, assessing communication attitudes, has been shown to be reliable with individuals who stutter, from school-age to adult. It has generated a great deal of research by Brutten and his colleagues.
	OASES	Developed as a measure of the overall impact that stuttering has on a person's life, this instrument is very helpful for planning treatment and assessing the effect of treatment on day-to-day functioning.
	TASCC	This is a 50-item questionnaire filled out by the teacher(s) to give information about how well the child communicates in his classroom(s). Normed on children in first through fifth grades, it can be helpful in assessing ways in which a student's communication is affected by his stuttering.
Adolescents and adults	S-24	A 24-item questionnaire, shown to be reliable for initial testing and retesting attitudes about communication. Several studies have shown that it can be predictive of outcomes for certain treatments.
	SSRSS	This questionnaire assesses the frequency with which an individual encounters speaking situations, his reactions to them, and tendency to avoid them. Also shown to be predictive of outcomes for certain treatments.
	PSI	This questionnaire assesses the individual's own perceptions of his own struggle, avoidance, and expectancy related to his stuttering. May be helpful to understand how much the individual is aware of his stuttering.
	Locus of Control	This scale enables the clinician to estimate how much the client believes that he controls his own destiny. May be predictive of treatment outcome.
	OASES	Assesses the overall impact of stuttering on the individual's life. There are published data on reliability and validity of this (adult) version. Can be used to evaluate whether treatment is having a broad effect on daily functioning versus only providing more fluent speech.

I don't always succeed in these periodic assessments, I try to obtain samples of my clients' speech in nonclinical situations, such as in the classroom or at work. I also do **continuing assessment** when I bring them in for maintenance checkups at increasingly longer intervals after formal treatment is over.

In addition, I assess clients' feelings and attitudes at the beginning and end of treatment and may assess them at other times if I am concerned about progress. If I am working on changing attitudes and feelings, change should be reflected in my measures, or I should try a different approach. Decreases in negative attitudes and feelings should be accompanied by decreases in stuttering severity, and my measures should show this.

SUMMARY

- In an assessment, the clinician has a variety of tasks. These include
1. Gathering data from the client
2. Getting to know the client as an individual

3. Showing an understanding of the client's point of view
4. Demonstrating an understanding of stuttering

- Clinicians must develop skills and sensitivities in working with clients from cultures other than their own.

- Building a relationship with a client begins in the first meeting, which is usually the assessment. A clinician must take this opportunity to demonstrate that she knows about the disorder of stuttering, is unafraid of it, and is accepting of it. At the same time, she must show that she expects change.

- Behaviors counted as stutters include part-word repetitions, single-syllable whole-word repetitions, prolongations, blocks, and unequivocal avoidance behaviors.

- Samples for assessing stuttering should include a variety of situations. The initial sample and samples assessing outcome should be videotaped for more accurate scoring and measurement of reliability. These samples should include speaking and when appropriate, reading.

- Frequency of stuttering is commonly assessed as the percentage of syllables or words stuttered.

- Different types of disfluencies can be assessed to reveal the percentage of stutter-like disfluencies or number of these disfluencies per 100 words. This information may be particularly useful in helping to decide if a preschool child needs treatment.

- Durations of moments of stuttering are useful in quantifying an aspect of the abnormality of a client's stuttering and the extent to which it may interfere with communication. Speaking and reading rates will also help to quantify this aspect of the impact of stuttering.

- Frequency and severity of secondary or concomitant behaviors associated with stuttering can be important measures of how much these behaviors call attention to themselves and distract listeners.

- Three severity scales are the Stuttering Severity Instrument (SSI-4), the Scale for Rating Severity, and the Lidcombe Program's Severity Rating Scale. The commonly used SSI-4 combines an assessment of frequency of stuttering, mean duration of the three longest stutters, and physical concomitants accompanying stuttering.

- Speech naturalness can be reliably and easily assessed. It is thought to be an especially important measure when evaluating treatment outcomes.

- Various instruments have been created to assess emotions and attitudes associated with stuttering. When combined with measures of stuttering behaviors, these measures provide a multidimensional view of the disorder. In some cases, they can aid the clinician in selecting appropriate treatment and in assessing whether a client is ready for dismissal.

- Assessment is an ongoing activity. Measures of progress are important indicators of whether ongoing treatment is effective and should be continued. Measures of outcome are critical for our knowledge of how effective a treatment has been in the long term with each client.

STUDY QUESTIONS

1. What does it mean to suggest that a clinician must play two different roles during an evaluation?
2. Which types of disfluencies are counted as stutters, and which are considered normal?
3. What factors can affect the process of measuring stuttering?
4. Describe the procedures for the two measures of reliability called "point-by-point agreement" and "percent error."
5. Why is it important to obtain several samples of speech from a client when assessing stuttering, whereas a single sample might be adequate for assessing a phonological disorder?
6. Give two reasons why assessment of reliability of measurements of stuttering is important.
7. Describe five dimensions or aspects of stuttering that may be assessed in an evaluation of a client who stutters.
8. To you, what is the most important aspect of stuttering? Defend your choice. How do you measure it?
9. Why is it relevant to assess speech rate for a person who stutters?
10. Discuss the pros and cons of protecting the privacy of conversations between yourself and a teenage client by not sharing their content with parents.

SUGGESTED PROJECTS

1. Research how different cultures react to stuttering and suggest how evaluation procedures in this chapter need to be changed for individuals from a culture that has very different beliefs about stuttering than those suggested in this text.
2. Make or obtain a video of a conversational and a reading sample of a person who stutters. Use two different methods of measuring the stuttering and obtain intraobserver and interobserver reliability assessments for each method. Discuss why one measurement procedure is more reliable than the other.
3. Obtain a videotaped conversational sample of one or more individuals who stutter and identify moments when you think the client has used an avoidance behavior to prevent stuttering. Discuss whether these avoidances should be counted as stutters.
4. Obtain samples of repetitive stutters from normally fluent children and from children who stutter. Compare the repetitions from both groups in terms of length of silent periods between iterations, pitch, and other acoustic variables.
5. Search the literature on assessment of stuttering to determine whether reliable methods have been developed for clients to assess their own stuttering during the progress of treatment.

SUGGESTED READINGS

Brutten, G., & Vanryckeghem, M. (2007). *Behavior Assessment Battery for school-age children who stutter.* San Diego, CA: Plural Publishing.

Conture, E. (2001). Assessment and evaluation. In *Stuttering: Its Nature, Diagnosis, and Treatment.* Boston, MA: Allyn & Bacon.

This chapter is rich with ideas for assessment of children, adolescents, and adults who stutter. It is particularly good in the breadth of coverage of evaluation of children who stutter, reflecting the years of experience the author has had in working with this age group.

Cordes, A. K. (1994). The reliability of observational data: I. Theories and methods for speech-language pathology. *Journal of Speech and Hearing Research, 37,* 264–278.

This article provides an excellent tutorial on the problems associated with establishing reliability of observational data in stuttering.

Howell, P., & Van Borsel, J. (2011). *Multilingual aspects of fluency disorders.* Tonawanda, NY: Multilingual Matters.

An edited book that discusses stuttering in many languages and cultures as well as stuttering and bilingualism.

Rosenberry-McKibbin, C. (2002). *Multicultural students with special language needs: Practical strategies for assessment and intervention* (2nd ed.). Oceanside, CA: Academic Communication Associates, Inc.

This book provides many insights into evaluation of multicultural students.

Wright, L., & Ayre, A. (2000). *The Wright Ayre stuttering self-rating profile.* United Kingdom: Winslow Press Ltd. (www.winslow-press.co.uk)

This assessment tool was designed to be used by clinicians working with adolescent and adult clients who can participate in assessing their own behaviors and feelings. It is intended to go beyond traditional clinician-based assessments to obtain indications of how clients observe themselves.

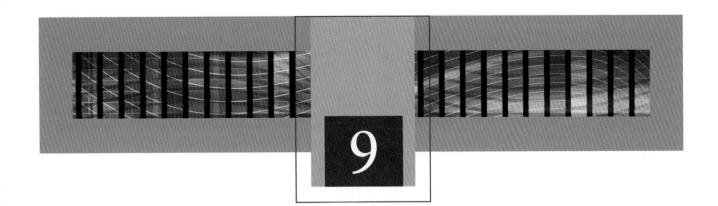

9

Assessment and Diagnosis

CHAPTER OBJECTIVES

After studying this chapter, readers should be able to:

- Plan and carry out an evaluation of a preschool child, school-age child, adolescent, and adult
- Understand how to evaluate the stuttering behaviors of a client
- Understand how to evaluate attitudes and feelings of a client (and when appropriate, the client's family)
- Understand how to determine appropriate follow-up to evaluation of each age level

KEY TERMS

Preassessment: The time before the formal assessment, in which the clinician gathers key information needed for the assessment

Parent-child interaction: Play-based conversation between parent(s) and child that is often used to assess and treat environmental influences on a child's stuttering

Parent interview: A conversation with parent(s) in which parents are encouraged to describe their child's stuttering and their concerns about it. In this interaction, the clinician elicits and gives information relevant to the child's stuttering

Clinician-child interaction: Play-based conversation between clinician and child in which clinician observes child's speech and may seek information about child's feelings about his stuttering, as well as information about child's articulation and language skills

Speech sample: A segment of speech used to assess a client's stuttering. A sample may be limited to 300 syllables. It may be spontaneous conversation or written work that is read aloud. It is meant to be representative of a client's speech in general

Pattern of disfluencies: The types of stuttering and/or typical disfluencies shown by someone who stutters. Examples are whole-word repetitions, part-word repetitions, and prolongations

Risk factors for persistent stuttering: Characteristics within the child or within the environment that are hypothesized to increase probability that child will not overcome his stuttering naturally, that is, without intervention

Closing interview: A conversation at the end of an evaluation session in which the clinician informs the client or family of her findings, makes recommendations for the future, and elicits questions

Individuals with Disabilities Education Act (IDEA '97): A federal law that mandates the procedures for gathering information and deciding on treatment of children in public schools

Teacher interview: A conversation with a child's classroom teacher(s) for the purpose of getting information about the child's speech and performance in the classroom. Such a conversation may also be used to enlist the teacher's help with the child's treatment

Classroom observation: Time spent in the classroom by the clinician to assess how a child's stuttering may be affecting him in his classes

Accepting environment: Behavior by parents and other family members (and teachers and classmates where appropriate) that convey to the child that they accept his speech

Trial therapy: A brief administration of one or more therapy strategies, used for the purpose of determining the effect on the client's speech in an evaluation

Fluency skills: Ways of speaking designed to induce fluency. Examples are slow rate, easy onset of voicing, and light contact of articulators

Individualized Education Program (IEP): A plan, mandated by the Individuals with Disabilities Education Act, that describes how a person with a disability will be educated to meet his individual needs

Stuttering modification: Ways of managing stuttering that are designed to reduce struggle and tension. Examples are cancellations, pull-outs, and preparatory sets

This chapter and the preceding one are bridges between chapters on the nature of stuttering and chapters on treatment. My aim is to show you how to understand a client and his stuttering problem and then use the information you have gathered to determine a treatment approach. Figure 9.1 has a chapter overview, and Figure 9.2 illustrates the components of assessment and diagnosis.

I've organized the assessment procedures in this chapter by age levels: preschool, school-age, and adolescent/adult. I've done this in part because in preparing to evaluate a client, you often know little about him except his age, so you will at least know what section of this chapter to turn to as you plan an evaluation. Another reason for this organization is because each age level requires a different approach and somewhat different procedures. When evaluating preschool children, for example, the clinician must determine

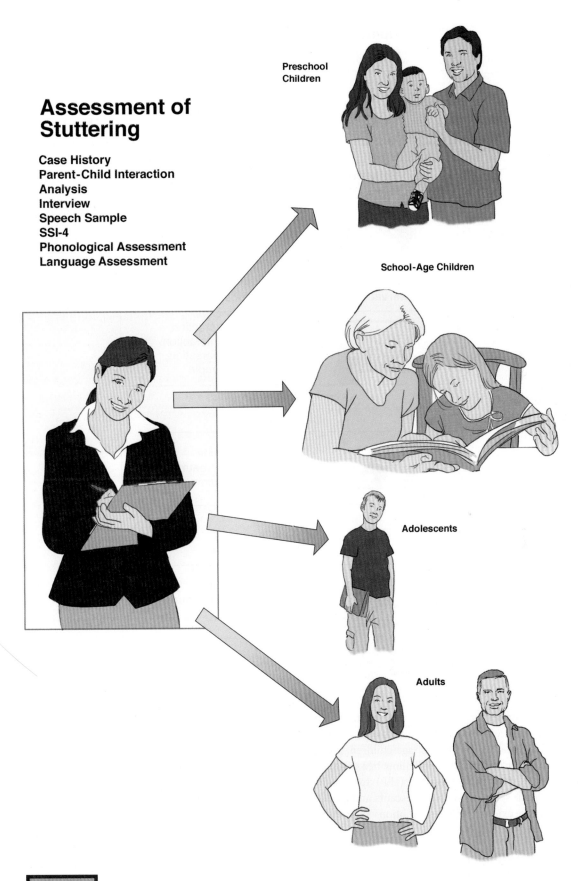

Assessment of Stuttering

Case History
Parent-Child Interaction
Analysis
Interview
Speech Sample
SSI-4
Phonological Assessment
Language Assessment

Preschool Children

School-Age Children

Adolescents

Adults

Figure 9.1 Chapter overview.

Components of Assessment and Diagnosis

Background information

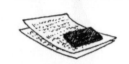 case history, questionnaires,
tapes, review the questions
to be answered

↓

Gather more background information

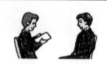 parent interviews,
teacher interviews,
student/adolescent/adult
interviews

↓

Observation of present behavior and feelings

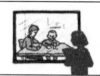 parent-child interaction,
clinician-child interaction,
structured conversation,
and reading sample

↓

Diagnosis

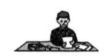 data interpretation,
developmental/treatment
level determination

↓

Meet with client or family to review options for treatment

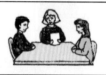 parent counseling,
explanation of treatment
plan

Figure 9.2   Sequence of assessment and diagnosis.

whether they are stuttering or normally disfluent and then whether treatment, if warranted, should focus on the family or on the child's speech. With school-age children, a clinician often follows procedures that will allow her to develop an Individualized Education Program (IEP) for children who are eligible for services. With adolescents and adults, a clinician may more extensively assess emotions and attitudes as well as core and secondary behaviors to determine appropriate treatment.

Within each age level, I have subdivided the sequence of activities you will typically engage in when you evaluate

a client. First, under the **preassessment** sections, I describe the clinical questions guiding the evaluation, as well as preliminary information-gathering activities. Under the assessment sections, I have described the observations, interviews, and measurements at the heart of the evaluation. Under the diagnosis sections, I discuss how to integrate the information you have gathered to decide on a course of action (whether to recommend treatment and if so, the type of treatment). Last, under the Summary and Recommendations sections, I describe the closing interviews, assignments, and the means to assess progress and outcome.

PRESCHOOL CHILD

Preassessment

Clinical Questions

When you assess a preschool child, you first want to answer the question, "Is this child stuttering, or is he normally disfluent?" In the process of trying to answer this, I have found that certain other information is critical: What are the amounts and types of disfluency this child shows in various situations? What kinds of risk factors for stuttering does the child have? Is the child reacting to his speech with frustration, fear, or other emotions? This information will also help you determine the developmental/treatment level of the child's disfluency. To respond to the family's needs and to involve them fully in planning treatment, you need to know the answers to questions like: What are the family's concerns about the child and his stuttering, as well as their preferences, expectations, and availability for treatment? Once you have gathered this information, you will need to decide among options for the child and family—no treatment, watchful waiting, parent-delivered treatment, or clinic-based treatment. You will also want to decide if the child is within the normal range for language, articulation, and voice. Finally, you should determine if a referral to another professional (e.g., a family counselor or a learning specialist) is warranted.

Initial Contact

In your initial contact, the family member who has approached you is forming his or her first impression of you. In many cases, this is the beginning of a helping relationship. You should focus on understanding the other person's point of view, concerns, and hopes. When you can, give realistic reassurance about the prospect of recovery, but in all cases, convey that you are ready to work with the family member as part of a team who will, together, help the child.

Your initial contact is likely to be on the telephone. If it is, listen to the parent's voice and pay attention to the parent's level of concern. Often, the most helpful thing you can do in this conversation is to listen. As you listen carefully, you may need to ask an occasional question to get clarification. When you think you have an initial understanding of the problem, set up an appointment, if appropriate. If you cannot meet with the family for several days or longer, it is important to give them some suggestions to get started. For example, you may want a parent to rate the child's stuttering using the Severity Rating Scale described in Chapter 8. It also may be helpful to have the family set aside a few minutes every day, in which one parent can play alone with the child and give him special attention. Also, consider letting the family know that they can contact you before the first formal meeting if they have new concerns. Prior to an evaluation, I let the family know what will take place in the evaluation and approximately how long it will take. A discussion of fees and payment may also be appropriate.

Case History Form

The case history form, shown in Figure 9.3, is sent to parents several weeks before their child's assessment. It informs the clinician about the parents' current perception of the problem, as well as its onset and development, and the child's medical, family, and school history. This information is used as a starting place for further questions during the parent interview. More about this will be discussed when the actual evaluation is described.

Audio/Video Recording

Along with the case history form, I ask the parents of a preschool child to send me an audio recording or preferably a video recording of their child speaking in a typical home situation. I encourage parents to video five or 10 minutes of themselves playing with their child so I can preview the child's speech soon after the parents have contacted me. In cases in which several weeks go by between the parents' contact and the evaluation, the child's stuttering may have diminished substantially, and I may observe only a fluent cycle of the child's speech. In addition, I can learn from the recording a little about this family's parent-child interactions.

Assessment

Parent-Child Interaction

When possible, I observe one or both parents interacting with the child, preferably at the beginning of the evaluation for several reasons. First, parents may be less affected by my orientation toward stuttering, which they would learn during the parent interview. So observing the **parent-child interaction** first gives me a more natural sample. Second, this interaction gives me an opportunity to see the child's stuttering firsthand. I can note, for example, how much the child seems aware of his stuttering, whether or not there are escape and avoidance reactions, and to what extent the child is reacting emotionally to his stuttering. Third, I can observe how the parents interact with their child. Do they interrupt? Do they correct? Do they talk at a fast rate or use complex vocabulary or advanced syntax? Fourth, if I began the evaluation by talking with the child, he might not talk much, since he doesn't know me. Thus the parent-child interaction will give me at least a larger sample of his speech. Then when I interact with him, I can get a sample of how his speech is with new people. Such observations of the parent-child interaction add to what I have learned from the audio-video sample that the parents have sent before the assessment. Together, the observation of home and live samples provide a basis for planning the parent interview and developing recommendations for treatment.

STUTTERING CASE HISTORY FORM – PRESCHOOL AND SCHOOL-AGE CHILD

Instructions: Please fill out this form in as much detail as possible. You can be assured that this information will be treated as confidential. If information is not available, please specify the reason so that we will know that the question has been considered. **Please return this form prior to your appointment.** Thank you.

Date: _____

Child's Name: _____   Gender: M   F   Age: _____
Address: _____   (years: months)

_____   Telephone: _____
E-Mail Address: _____   Cell Phone: _____
Date of Birth: _____   Place of Birth: _____
Medicaid#: _____   Referring Physician: _____
Child lives with: Own Parents: _____   Other Relative: _____

Foster Parents: _____

If other than own parents, give name/s: _____

_____

Teacher's Name (if applicable): _____

School (if applicable): _____

School Placement or Grade Level (if applicable): _____

Name of person completing this form: _____

Relationship to child: _____

FAMILY

<u>Father:</u>

Name: _____   Age:_____

Is he living with the family? _____   Occupation: _____

Employed by: _____

Education level: _____

Telephone (Home): _____   (Work): _____

Social Security#: _____

<u>Mother:</u>

Name: _____   Age:_____

Is she living with the family? _____   Occupation: _____

Employed by: _____

Education level: _____

Telephone (Home): _____   (Work): _____

Social Security#: _____

Figure 9.3   Case history form for preschool and school-age children. *(Continued)*

Brothers and Sisters:

	(Name)	(Age)		(Name)	(Age)
1.	_____	_____	4.	_____	_____
2.	_____	_____	5.	_____	_____
3.	_____	_____	6.	_____	_____

HISTORY OF STUTTERING

Give approximate age at which stuttering was first noticed: _____

Who first noticed or mentioned the stuttering? _____

In what situation was the stuttering first noticed? _____

Describe any situations or conditions that might have been associated with the onset of stuttering:

_____

_____

Under what circumstances did the stuttering occur after initial onset? _____

_____

What were the first signs of stuttering (check all that apply):

    A. Repetitions of the whole word?   (boy-boy-boy) _____

    B. Repetitions of the first letter?   (b-b-b-boy) _____

    C. Repetitions of the first syllable?   (ca-ca-cat) _____

    D. Complete blocks on the first letter?   (b....oy) _____

    E. Prolongations of the vowel?   (caaaaaaat) _____

    F. Visible attempt to speak (i.e., mouth movement) but no sound forthcoming? _____

    G. Other _____

Was the stuttering always the same or did it occur in several different ways? _____

If it occurred in different ways, how were they different from one another? Describe.

_____

_____

Approximately how long did each block (one word) seem to last? _____

Was the stuttering easy or was there force at the time when the stuttering was first noticed?

_____

Were stuttered words primarily at the beginning of sentences or were they scattered throughout

the sentence? _____

When stuttering first began, was there any avoidance of speaking (i.e., changing word or stopping

mid-stutter, using gestures instead of speech) because of it? Give examples, if any. _____

_____

_____

Figure 9.3   (Continued)

Does or did the child add extra words or sounds to "get started" (i.e., hey mom, hey mom...)?

_____

Does or did the child use a lot of "fillers" when they speak (i.e., uh, um)? _____

At the time when stuttering was first noticed, what was your child's reaction?

      Awareness that speech was different? _____   Surprise? _____

      Indifference to it? _____   Anger or frustration? _____

      Fear of stuttering again? _____   Shame? _____

      Other? _____

What attempts have been made to treat the stuttering problem (either at home or with a professional)? _____

_____

Does the child have articulation or pronunciation problems in addition to stuttering? If so, please describe. _____

Does child have hand preference? Right- or left-handed or use both equally well? _____

Does child have a foot preference for kicking a ball? _____

Does the child seem to be sensitive or have difficulty adapting to new situations? _____

_____

Has the child been diagnosed with ADHD or ADD? _____

DEVELOPMENT OF STUTTERING

Since onset, has there been any change in stuttering symptoms? Check those that are appropriate.

      Increase in number of repetitions per word   _____

      Change in amount of force used—Increased?   _____

                             Decreased?   _____

      Increase in amount of stuttering   _____

      Increase in length of block   _____

      Periods of no stuttering   _____

      Longer periods of stuttering   _____

      More precise in speech attempts   _____

      Lowered voice   _____

      Slower speech rate   _____

      Physical struggle (i.e., facial tension, eye blinks)   _____

      Looking away from the listener   _____

      Increase in pitch during stutters   _____

Describe any of the above things the child does when he stutters (i.e., eye blinks). _____

_____

_____

Figure 9.3 *(Continued)*

Were there any periods (weeks/months) when the stuttering disappeared? _____

Were there any periods (weeks/months) when stuttering increased? _____

Can you give any explanations for these "worse" periods? _____

Are there any situations that are particularly difficult? If so, describe: _____

_____

List any situations that never cause difficulty: _____

_____

Does the child stutter when he or she (check those that apply):

Asks questions?	_____	Uses new words that are unfamiliar	_____
Talks to young children?	_____	Uses the telephone?	_____
Says his or her name?	_____	Reads out loud?	_____
Answers direct questions?	_____	Recites memorized material?	_____
Talks to adults, teachers?	_____	Talks to strangers?	_____
Speaks when tired?	_____	Speaks when excited?	_____
Talks to family members	_____	Talks to friends?	_____

Do you know anyone who stutters? _____ Are they relatives? Friends?

Acquaintances? _____

Do you feel that stuttering interferes with your child's daily life? _____

Social relationships? _____

Success in school? _____

MEDICAL, DEVELOPMENTAL, AND FAMILY HISTORY

Describe mother's health during pregnancy and birth history (i.e., complications): _____

_____

_____

Describe any development problems during infancy or early childhood (i.e., late to walk or talk, feeding problems, food allergies): _____

_____

Do you think the child's speech and language development was unusually rapid or delayed? If so, please describe: _____

_____

List all significant illnesses, injuries, severe fevers, and operations:

Date	Illness	Complications	Treatment	Physician
1.				
2.				
3				

Figure 9.3 *(Continued)*

List any medications your child is on: _____

List all present disabilities: _____

Any chronic illnesses, allergies or physical conditions? _____

_____

Vision normal? _____   Hearing normal? _____

Child's eye color? _____   Hair color? _____

Do other members of the family have speech, language, reading problems, or learning disabilities?

If so, please describe: _____

_____

_____

_____

Are any family members left-handed or use both right and left hands equally well? _____

_____

Does the child or other family members show artistic talent or interest? _____

_____

Do any family members talk very rapidly? If so, who? _____

_____

SCHOOL AND SOCIAL HISTORY

Favorite subjects or activities in school: _____

Difficult subjects: _____

Hobbies: _____   Sports: _____

Leisure time activities: _____

Favorite toys: _____

What specific questions do you have about your child that you would like us to try to answer?

(Use back of sheet if necessary) _____

_____

_____

In addition, what goals would you like to see accomplished as a result of this evaluation?

_____

_____

_____

Signature: _____ Date: _____

Please return these completed forms to us in the envelope provided. Thank you.

Figure 9.3   *(Continued)*

The parent-child interaction can be done formally or informally. Some clinicians observe these interactions in the waiting room. Others who work in preschool or early intervention programs may visit a child's home and arrange to observe parent-child interactions while they sit quietly in the same room. Still others, myself included, videotape the parents and child in a play-style interaction in a treatment room supplied with toys and games. When recording these interactions is possible, this sample of a child's speech can be assessed for severity and types of stuttering behavior, as described in Chapter 8.

Parent Interview

In the last few years, I have talked more freely about stuttering directly with preschoolers, as well as with their parents when their child is within earshot. I think this directness may reduce parents' distress about their child's stuttering, perhaps by reducing everyone's fear of it. When I first meet a child and his parents, however, I hold back a little until I have had a chance to discuss this openness with the parents. The child may be only normally disfluent, or the parents may be reluctant to talk about stuttering in front of the child. The **parent interview** gives me a chance to suggest how, in my experience, openness about stuttering decreases some of the shame a child (and parents) may feel about stuttering. First, I talk to parents without the child present, giving them an opportunity to talk about matters that they feel they would like to share in confidence. If I'm working with another clinician or a student, she plays with and observes the child while I talk to the parents. If I'm working alone and both parents have come to the evaluation, I talk to each parent separately, while the other is with the child. If only one parent is present, I often arrange to have the child playing by himself in a nearby room with the door open.

I begin the interview by letting parents know what I will be doing with them and their child during the remainder of the evaluation, even though I may have touched on this in the first contact. I assure them there will be a time for me to share my assessment and recommendations with them at the end. Sometimes during an initial interview, parents ask direct questions about things they think they may be doing wrong. I let them know that, in my view, stuttering is often the result of many factors acting together and that parents do not cause it (see Chapters 2 to 5 for evidence). I rarely give advice about what they should change or what they should do until after I have finished interviewing the parents and assessed the child directly. I believe that I am more accurate, and parents are more receptive to my recommendations if I delay a discussion of what to do until the closing interview when I have the most information possible. On the other hand, there may be "clinical moments" during an initial interview when parents might be most receptive to suggestions. Many times, for example, parents have asked me whether it's a good idea for them to tell their child to slow down whenever the child stutters when excited. My response is usually to ask them how the child responds to this and to build upon their answer so that we can brainstorm the best way to help the child together.

I begin initial interviews by asking parents to describe the problem their child is having. I ask open-ended questions, such as "Tell me about Justin's speech," or "Please describe Justin's speech and tell me what concerns you." Open-ended questions allow parents to describe their concerns in their own words. This is then an opportunity for me to listen carefully, to be nonjudgmental, and to be comfortable with silence so that parents can express themselves fully. Listening attentively and being comfortable with silence require concentration on the clinician's part, so it is worthwhile to remind yourself of this when you are preparing for an evaluation. When parents have had a chance to describe the problem and appear to have no more to say at that moment, I ask about the first stages of the child's life (the child's birth and development) and then work up toward the present time. In the ensuing conversation, I try to be sure I get information indicated by the questions in the following paragraphs. This interview is not a strict question-and-answer format, but rather a discussion punctuated by both their questions and mine.

1. **Were there any problems with your pregnancy or the birth of this child?**
   Although there is little evidence that stutterers as a group have difficult birth histories, there is an increased incidence of stuttering among individuals who have a known history of brain injury (Boehme, 1968; Poulos & Webster, 1991). Thus, I am seeking to determine whether there is the possibility of congenital brain injury. If a difficult pregnancy or birth is reported, I might examine the child's motor and cognitive development more closely. Because it is completed before the evaluation, the case history form provides preliminary information for potential follow-up.

2. **What was the child's speech and language development like? How did it compare with siblings' development and with your expectations?**
   The first appearance of stuttering may be influenced by the "processing load" that language acquisition has on a child's speech production, as described in the sections on speech and language development in Chapters 4 and 5. Thus, it is important to understand the course of a child's overall speech and language development. I explore the possibility that a child's language acquisition is proceeding so rapidly that his developing motor system cannot keep up. I also examine the possibility that a child's speech and language development are delayed, and he is frustrated and finding it hard to talk. As mentioned in Chapters 2 and 3, there is some evidence that poorer speech and language skills may predict persistent stuttering (Yairi et al., 1996).

3. **Describe the child's motor development compared with that of his brothers, sisters, or with other children.**

I am interested in parents' general impressions. Does their child seem to be developing motor skills like other children his age, or do they think he may be delayed? Some indicators of the normal range of children's gross and fine motor development, as well as their personal-social and speech-language development, can be found in the Denver Developmental Screening Test (Frankenburg & Dodds, 1967) and is shown in Figure 3.2 (child development in the first five years).

In my experience, many children who stutter appear to be slightly advanced in their language and to a lesser extent, slightly delayed in their motor skills. Or, they may be well advanced in language but with completely normal motor skills. In either case, these children seem to benefit from models of speech produced at a slow rate (Guitar, Kopff-Schaefer, Donahue-Kilburg, & Bond, 1992; also see the section in Chapter 11 on indirect treatment). Other children who stutter may be delayed in several areas and may need treatment for language and articulation that is integrated with therapy for stuttering (see the section of Chapter 12 on Treatment of Concomitant Speech and Language Problems).

4. **Have any members of your family had speech or language disorders?**

I ask this general question and then ask more specifically whether family members or other relatives have ever had problems related to stuttering, cluttering, articulation, or language disorders (see Chapter 15 for a description of cluttering). To confirm that a problem was considered significant (and was perhaps diagnosed), I ask if the person ever received treatment. I use this information when we discuss stuttering as a disorder that may have predisposing factors. Handled tactfully, a discussion of predisposing factors may help parents realize that their child's stuttering was not something they caused, which in turn may reduce their anxiety or guilt, making them more effective in facilitating the child's fluency.

If a parent stutters or formerly stuttered the parent may have strong negative feelings about the disorder, including guilt that the parent has passed it on to the child. Such feelings should be discussed in the initial interview and throughout any treatment the child receives. The way in which a parent who stutters handles his or her stuttering is also important, because these behaviors serve as a model for the child. It is my observation that a parent who avoids words or otherwise tries to hide stuttering is communicating an attitude that may move the child to the intermediate level faster than if the parent accepts the stuttering, comments neutrally about it in front of the child, and uses facilitating techniques to handle it.

If any of the child's relatives stutter, it is important to find out whether they recovered. Research cited earlier found that among children who were identified within six months of the onset of stuttering, those with relatives who did not recover from stuttering were more likely to have persistent stuttering than those with relatives who did recover (Yairi et al., 1996). After obtaining this background information, I turn to the onset and development of the child's stuttering.

5. **When did you first notice the child's disfluency?**

I have found that if treatment is begun relatively soon after a child starts to stutter (within 18 months, rather than after several years) we have a better chance of preventing negative feelings from building up for both the parents and the child. Therefore, I praise parents for bringing a child in promptly for an evaluation, if they did so relatively soon after they first realized there may be a problem. Another reason I want to know how much time has passed since onset is that most of the predictive information on chronicity of stuttering is based on children identified within six months of onset. For example, Yairi and colleagues (1996) found that children who naturally recovered began to show a steady decline in their stuttering during the first 12 months after stuttering onset, whereas children whose stuttering persisted for at least three years did not show such a decline. Therefore, knowing how long a child has been stuttering helps me make treatment decisions based on findings that some children are likely to recover without therapy.

6. **Was anything special going on in the child's life when the stuttering started?**

This may provide some leads about the kinds of pressures to which a child may be vulnerable, which can help clinicians determine what changes parents can make to reduce stuttering. Events that may precipitate the onset of stuttering include the birth of a sibling, moving to a new home, family travel, prolonged periods of anxiety or excitement, and growth spurts in a child's language or cognition (see Chapters 4 and 5). Many times, no special circumstances have occurred at the onset of stuttering. Events surrounding the onset of stuttering should be discussed in a way that helps parents feel they are not to blame for the stuttering.

7. **What was the disfluency like when it was first noticed?**

Most stuttering begins with easy repetitions, although some children exhibit prolongations and blocks, as well. Some preliminary information suggests that when repetitions sound quite rapid (i.e., when the pause between repetition units is brief), a child is more likely to be stuttering rather than normally disfluent (Allen, 1988; Throneburg & Yairi, 1994). Rapid-sounding repetitions may be predictive of persistent stuttering (Yairi et al., 1996). However, the length of pauses between repetition units cannot be determined accurately without instrumentation, even though a practiced ear can help clinicians perceive the brevity of pauses between repetition units. This information should be used only to support an overall pattern of findings that will help the clinician decide whether or not to recommend treatment.

8. **What changes, if any, have been observed in the child's speech since stuttering was first noticed?**

   The most interesting changes include the frequency and types of disfluencies and whether and for how long the stuttering diminished greatly or disappeared altogether. As indicated in the discussion of Question 5, children whose frequency of core stuttering behaviors (i.e., part-word and single-syllable whole-word repetitions, prolongations, and blocks) does not decrease during the 12 months after onset are at risk for becoming persistent stutterers. In my clinical experience, if a child's physical tension and struggle during stuttering are increasing, or if stuttering is becoming more consistent and less intermittent, the child is not exhibiting a borderline level of stuttering, and direct treatment should be considered.

9. **Does the child appear to be aware of his disfluency?**

   If a child appears to have no awareness of his disfluencies, I am more likely to categorize him as normally disfluent or as a borderline stutterer than if he notices or seems concerned about his disfluencies. If he shows negative awareness, such as expressing frustration, he may be a beginning stutterer. Note that a child may be aware of his stuttering but not particularly bothered by it; some children are even amused by it when it first occurs, though this quickly changes to frustration. Indicators of a child's awareness include such things as his commenting about his stuttering, either when it occurs or at some other time, and responses to the fact that people have brought it to his attention. Awareness is also indicated if a child stops when he is disfluent and starts again or laughs, cries, or hits himself when he stutters. Even without any of these signs, a child may still be quite aware of his stuttering.

   In some cases, preschool children may show more than just signs of frustration. They may show negative feelings about talking and may fear using certain words. They may even comment that they wish they could speak like someone else. These signs of awareness are indications that treatment is warranted.

10. **Does the child sometimes appear to change a word because he expects to be disfluent on it?**

    Parents are usually able to guess this is happening because they can sense the child's apprehension about saying a word. I also may ask them if the child changes words in midstream; that is, does he start a word, get stuck on it, and then change it or stop talking? Such behaviors are warning signs; they may indicate that the child is moving toward a more serious problem.

11. **Does the child seem to avoid talking in some situations when he expects to be disfluent?**

    Again, this is something that most parents know because they sense the child's fear of talking, and like the word avoidances discussed in Question 10, this behavior may indicate a need for direct treatment.

12. **What do the parents believe caused the problem?**

    In some cases, parents may express ideas about the possible causes of their child's stuttering that I believe are appropriate and accurate. In other cases, parents' beliefs about causal factors appear to be incorrect, and I respond by providing more accurate information. I am particularly sensitive to whether or not parents blame themselves or each other for their child's stuttering. This is usually a good time to let parents know that they are not to blame. I tell them that some children may have slight differences in their neurological organization for speech, which may emerge as stuttering during the normal stresses and strains of growing up and learning to talk (see Chapters 2 to 5). Parents should know that they didn't cause their child's stuttering, but they should also know that they can play a key role in their child's learning to deal with it appropriately.

13. **How do the parents feel about the child's disfluency problem?**

    The kinds of feelings and attitudes we are looking for are: Do they feel concern? Guilt? Do they assume the child will outgrow it? Parental emotions and attitudes are contagious and may influence the child, particularly a sensitive child. If parents feel guilty or highly anxious, it is important to engage them in positive treatment activities as soon as possible. I suggest some beginning activities they can use in the Summary and Recommendations sections.

14. **What, if anything, have the parents done about the child's disfluency problem?**

    This question is aimed at finding out how the parents have responded to the child's disfluencies. For example, have they asked the child to slow down or stop and say the word again? Knowing this will help me to decide what to do in counseling them. If parents are correcting the child, I may get them involved in therapeutic activities immediately so that they can develop appropriate ways of responding.

15. **Has the child been seen elsewhere for the problem? If so, what were the outcomes?**

    This information can be important in planning therapy and counseling parents. For example, if their family doctor told them several years ago that the child will outgrow stuttering, this needs to be addressed because they may now be convinced he will not outgrow it. It is wise to comment positively or neutrally on what other professionals may have said or done. So many children appear to overcome stuttering without treatment that most doctors and nurses believe that their advice to parents to ignore the stuttering will have a good outcome. Some doctors and nurses, however, are learning to distinguish between children who are likely to recover without treatment and those who are not.

If the child has been in other treatment previously, knowing what advice the parents were given can be important. Sometimes, parents have been given excellent advice but were not able to follow it. If so, we need to find out why and help them overcome obstacles to helping their child. Sometimes parents have had their child in successful therapy but have moved away and sought me out to continue the same kind of treatment. In these cases, I try to contact the previous therapist as well as explore with the parents what was done so that we can continue to work in the same direction as before. In some cases, parents come to me seeking a second opinion, and I am able to reinforce what others have said if I agree. In other cases, they may have been advised to ignore the child's stuttering, which may lead me to tactfully discuss the possibility of taking an entirely different direction.

16. **When and in which situations does the child exhibit the most disfluency? The least disfluency?**
This information helps to identify fluency disrupters and fluency facilitators that I will use to help parents facilitate their child's fluency. I have also found it effective to point out whenever possible all of the helpful things the parents are already doing. Just the awareness that their child's stuttering responds to environmental cues and thereby has some logic to it helps most parents feel more competent to manage it.

17. **How does the child get along with his brothers and sisters and other children?**
I usually find that children who stutter relate fairly well to others, but I want to find out if a child's stuttering may be interfering with his relationships. Sometimes, when asking this question, I learn about pressure and competition from siblings or teasing by a neighborhood bully.

18. **What is the child's temperament like?**
Some children who stutter may be more emotionally reactive than most other children, and they may have less capacity for self-regulation (i.e., dealing with that reactivity). More emotionally reactive children with less ability to self-regulate would be more likely to respond negatively to parents' anxieties about their speech. A child with this temperament may benefit from extra help in learning to cope with arousing stimuli. There is good evidence that families can help a child develop a more resilient temperament (Calkins & Fox, 1994).

19. **What is a typical day like for your child?**
It can be helpful to get an idea of how busy and rushed a family is. For one thing, it has been my experience that many children who stutter and their families benefit from having less hectic schedules, particularly if the child thrives in more regular, less intense situations. You can add this information to what the parents told you about when their child stutters most to develop a hypothesis about how much the family's schedule may be affecting the child's fluency. If the child stutters more when things are busy, hectic, and stressed, it may be appropriate to brainstorm with the parents about how everyone can have a little more "down time." Knowledge of the family's schedule will also help you begin to consider treatment recommendations. Some treatments are demanding of parents' time and attention, and their schedule must be considered in working with them to determine the most appropriate treatment approach for their child.

20. **Is there anything else you can think of to tell me that will help me better understand your child's stuttering?**
Sometimes, it is not possible to direct questions to all areas of concern, and this question provides parents an opportunity to provide information that I have not thought of asking about.

Clinician-Child Interaction

One of the most important parts of a preschool child's evaluation is the **clinician-child interaction**. Here, the clinician can see firsthand what the child's speech is like, how he responds to various cues, and how well he can modify his disfluency. I always record this interaction for later analysis because it is difficult to make notes as we interact. Video recording is preferable because visual cues are often critical in determining a child's developmental and treatment level. If audio recording must be used, the clinician should make notes on visual aspects of the child's disfluencies.

I focus my interactions on toys or games that are suitable to the child's age. The Playskool® farm or airport is a good example. I play alongside the child, letting him direct the action, commenting on what he's doing or playing with. I refrain from questions as we begin and talk in an easy, relaxed manner, much as I advise parents to do.

If a child's stuttering is like that described by the parent, I maintain the same speech style throughout the interaction. However, if a child is entirely fluent or normally disfluent and the parents have described behaviors typical of stuttering, I speak more rapidly and ask many questions. Occasionally, I interrupt the child to elicit disfluent speech, which may be more characteristic. I do this to avoid misdiagnosing a child who is stuttering as a normally fluent speaker.

An adult client of mine described an experience that illustrates my concern. When she was 5 years old, she stuttered quite severely, and her parents were understandably concerned. Seeking the best help, her mother took her to a famous Midwestern university speech clinic for an evaluation. For reasons she never understood, she was relatively fluent throughout the entire evaluation. The clinicians observed her temporary fluency and despite her mother's protestations that her daughter stuttered at home, did not diagnose her stuttering and advised her mother to ignore any disfluency. Her disfluency gradually worsened, and she became a severe, chronic stutterer.

I realize that, even by putting pressure on the child, I may not elicit stuttering that the child displays in other settings. Thus, the parents' report and the recording they made before the evaluation are of vital importance for a full understanding of a child's speech.

Talking about Stuttering

Before interacting with a child, I try to determine from talking with a child's parents whether the child is aware of his stuttering. If I think he isn't, I simply observe the child's speech while he and I play. If it seems clear that he is aware of his stuttering, I then try to determine how comfortable the child is in talking about his stuttering. Sometimes, I ask if he knows why he has come to see me. Most children answer noncommittally, but some say something like, "Because I don't talk right." This gives me an opening to discuss the stuttering. It is also an important opportunity to let the child know that he isn't alone and that I know other children who get stuck on words and am usually able to help them.

Some clinicians help a child talk about his stuttering by first talking about another child who stutters (Bloodstein, personal communication, 1990). In discussing stuttering with a child, I usually try to use their vocabulary, such as "getting stuck" or "having trouble on words." If a child seems reluctant to talk about stuttering, I drop the issue for the moment and return to playing. Then, later, I will insert a few natural-sounding disfluencies in my speech and comment that I sometimes have trouble getting words out. I might play some more and then insert a few more disfluencies and ask the child if he ever has trouble like this. As before, the child's response will indicate that either he remains unwilling to discuss stuttering or he will give the clinician an opening to discuss, little by little, his disfluency problem. In summary, the goals of these attempts to discuss a child's disfluency are (1) to see if he accepts himself and his disfluencies enough to discuss them, and (2) to assure him that he is not alone with the problem and that his parents and I may be able to help him.

A Child Who Won't Talk

At times, I encounter a preschooler who is reluctant to separate from his parents. A shy child may start to cry and cling to his parents. I don't force the child to separate, of course. It is more important to have him positively inclined toward therapy than to try to elicit a few stutters. In this situation, I sit quietly while the parent and child play together. After a few minutes, I join in the play, without focusing on the child, and after a few more minutes, I'll comment on what the parent and child are doing or what I'm doing with a tractor or a farm animal or whatever I'm playing with. In most cases, the child will soon say something to me or include me in the play. This interaction, leading to at least a little speech from the child, gives me an opportunity to observe, at close range, any stuttering the child may have. Only after a child gets comfortable with me do I attempt to discuss his trouble talking, and only if I'm sure he is aware of his stuttering.

With some children, I do not attempt to discuss stuttering, and I always take my cue from the child and go slowly in this area. A very shy child, who becomes even shyer if I produce a few easy disfluencies, may be quite turned off to therapy if I invade his space by asking about his stuttering at this point. You can infer many things about a child's feelings from observations rather than direct questions.

A Child Who Is Entirely Fluent

Some preschool children who stutter may be entirely fluent during an evaluation. In such cases, there are several options. First, the recording I asked the parent to send me may include enough stuttering to provide a good sample for analysis. Second, if a child is in a particularly fluent period, I may reschedule his evaluation for a later time. If my recommendations to the parents enable them to change the home environment enough in the meantime so that the child remains fluent, the parents may wish to postpone the evaluation until and if the child's stuttering returns.

Speech Sample

The following sections describe how to analyze samples of a preschool child's speech. You should have more than one **speech sample** to analyze from the recordings that the parents sent in, the parent-child interaction, and the clinician-child interaction. Because you may want to use the SSI-4 (Riley, 1994) as part of your assessment, you need to follow the procedures it recommends for this analysis. Thus, the sample obtained from the clinician-child interaction should include conversation using the pictures in the SSI-4. Riley recommends that as the child talks, the clinician should "interject questions, interruptions, and mild disagreements to simulate the pressures of normal conversation at home and elsewhere" (Riley, 1994, p. 7). The samples should include at least 200 syllables; samples this long or longer make it more likely that you will have an accurate picture of the child's speech. By making transcripts of the samples, you can more easily quantify the variables described in the following section on **pattern of disfluencies**.

Pattern of Disfluencies

By analyzing the child's speech sample, I can try to determine whether or not the child truly stutters and if so, his developmental/treatment level. I analyze the following six variables to begin this determination. The choice of variables owes much to four individuals who have written about the differential diagnosis of preschool stuttering (Adams, 1977; Curlee, 1984; Riley & Riley, 1979).

1. Frequency of disfluencies. This is calculated from the entire sample and is expressed as the number of disfluencies per 100 words (see Chapters 7 and 8 for details). Both normal disfluencies and those associated with stuttering are included in this count. Normally disfluent children usually have fewer than 10 disfluencies per 100 words.

2. Types of disfluencies. I described the following eight types of disfluencies in Chapter 7: part-word repetitions, single-syllable word repetitions, multisyllable word repetitions, phrase repetitions, interjections, revisions-incomplete phrases, prolongations, and tense pauses. Children who are normally disfluent are likely to have more revisions and multisyllable whole-word repetitions, as well as many interjections when they are younger than 3.5 years old. Part-word repetitions, single-syllable word repetitions, prolongations, and tense pauses occur more frequently in stuttering children. Another distinguishing measure is the proportion of total disfluencies that are stutter-like disfluencies (SLDs) (i.e., part-word repetitions and single-syllable repetitions, prolongations, and blocks). Less than half of the disfluencies of normally disfluent children are SLDs, but about two-thirds of the disfluencies of children who stutter will be SLDs (Yairi, 1997a).

3. Nature of repetitions and prolongations. This variable has several dimensions. First, normally disfluent children usually have only one extra unit in their repetitions, li-like this, but sometimes they may have two. As the number of repetition units increase, however, so does the likelihood that the child is stuttering. Second, I listen to the tempo of repetitions. If they are slow and regular, a child is more likely to be categorized appropriately as a normally disfluent speaker. If they are rapid or irregular, it is more likely that the child is stuttering. Third, I look for signs of tension in both repetitions and prolongations. Both visual and auditory cues can help here; tension can be seen in the child's facial expression and heard in his increased pitch or loudness and more staccato voice quality. Children who I would label as normally disfluent seldom exhibit tension in their disfluencies.

4. Starting and sustaining airflow and phonation. The child who we usually categorize as stuttering often has difficulty here. You may observe abrupt onsets and offsets of words, especially repeated words, or momentary pauses with fixed articulator positions at the onset of words. Moreover, transitions between words may seem abrupt, jerky, or broken much of the time.

5. Physical concomitants. I look for physical gestures that accompany a child's disfluencies, such as head nods, eye blinks, and hand or finger movements, especially gestures that coincide with the release of a disfluent sound. I also include such extra noises as a child gritting the teeth or clicking the tongue during disfluencies.

6. Word avoidances. Another sign I sometimes see in a disfluent preschool child, which suggests that he stutters, is word avoidance. This can be blatant, as when a child starts a word and then changes it, as in "pu-pu-pu … dog," or it may be more subtle, as when he says, "I don't know," when it's clear that he does know. I also ask about word avoidances when I interview a child's parents. When a clinician interacts with a child, she may sometimes miss avoidances in a live interaction, and it may take a viewing of the videotape to pick them up. For example, a few years ago I noted on the videotape I watched after an evaluation a very subtle avoidance that I had completely missed during the face-to-face interaction. I had asked the child what he was going to dress as for Halloween. He pursed his lips for a "B," but when he couldn't say the word, he used an avoidance by singing the Batman theme, "Na-na-na-na-na-na-na-nah! Batman!"

In my experience, if a child shows any of the characteristics of stuttering just described, he should be considered at least a borderline stutterer. The presence of tension, stoppage of airflow or phonation, physical concomitants, or word avoidances would place him on a level above borderline. Further details on this placement are given in the sections on diagnosis that follow.

Stuttering Severity Instrument (SSI-4)

Using the 200-syllable or longer samples gathered earlier, you should carefully follow the guidelines in the examiner's manual of the SSI-4 to determine a child's stuttering frequency, duration, and physical concomitants scores. Use of the SSI-4 is described more fully in Chapter 8. Using the definitions of stuttering given by Riley (1994) in the manual, which essentially are what I referred to earlier as "stuttering-like disfluencies," you can use the total overall score to derive a percentile ranking for the child, which compares him to the norms for children who stutter. In addition, rankings that range from very mild to very severe can also be derived from the total overall score. Sometimes, normally disfluent children may be rated as stuttering at the very mild level on the SSI-4. Thus, clinical judgment, informed by your analyses of the types and frequencies of disfluencies, must be used to sort out which children are actually stuttering and which are not. The SSI-4 is not a tool for differentiating stuttering from normal disfluency but for assessing a child's severity.

Test of Childhood Stuttering

As described in Chapter 8, the Test of Childhood Stuttering (TOCS) can be used for children ages 4 to 12 and is thus appropriate for older preschool children. This instrument evaluates the child's stuttering in a variety of speaking situations and provides a more in-depth analysis of the child's stuttering, but takes more time to administer than the SSI-4. I have not used it enough to give an informed opinion about the comparative usefulness of the TOCS and the SSI-4.

Speech Rate

I assess preschool children's speech rate using the speech sample obtained for the SSI-4. Counting and timing procedures were described in the section on assessment of speech rate in Chapter 8. One sample of speech rates for preschool children is given in Table 8.5. If a child is stuttering and his speech rate is substantially below the range for his age, the extent to which stuttering slows his rate of speech may be a problem for both listeners and the child. Children whose rates are substantially above the norms—or who sound like they are talking too fast—may have the disorder of cluttering, which is described in more detail in Chapter 15.

Feelings and Attitudes

If I am evaluating a preschooler, I begin by asking the parents if they think the child is aware of his stuttering, and I explore observations they have made of his reactions to his disfluencies. If they are convinced that the child is oblivious to his disfluencies and I observe those disfluencies to be without much tension and struggle, I don't talk directly to the child about his stuttering. Instead, I rely on what the parents can tell me during the parent interview about their child's feelings. I am also beginning to use the Impact of Stuttering on Preschoolers and Parents questionnaire (see Chapter 8) to gather initial information about the child's (and parents') feelings and attitudes about stuttering. However, if the child shows signs of struggle and tension when he stutters, or if the parents indicate that the child is aware through various examples of his frustration with his stuttering, I explore with the child his feelings about getting stuck on words.

Before bringing up the topic of stuttering, I get to know the child by talking with him during various play activities. Then, as we play, I insert a question about his speech, such as "Do you sometimes get stuck on words?" Both the child's verbal and nonverbal responses to a gently asked question about stuttering tell me a lot. Even beyond what I notice when we are talking, I am often able to learn a great deal by watching the video of my interaction with a child. I find that by playing a video recording of my interaction, I am able to devote my undivided attention to observing key segments of the interaction. The recording often provides a rich payload of information about a child's feelings that may not have been apparent to me in the face-to-face meeting. Some children may be quite comfortable answering my question about getting stuck on words, while others are embarrassed, look away, and don't make clear responses. Still others emphatically deny they have any problem talking. If the stuttering is very mild and the child matter-of-factly says he doesn't get stuck, I may tentatively conclude that he really isn't aware.

Assessment of the feelings and attitudes of a preschooler leads me to conclude tentatively whether a child (1) is unaware of his disfluencies, (2) is occasionally aware of them and even then, is seldom and only transiently bothered by them, (3) is aware and frustrated by them, or (4) is highly aware, frustrated, and afraid of them. The levels of awareness and emotion that a child has about his stuttering are an important consideration in planning treatment, as we shall see.

Other Speech and Language Behaviors

When I evaluate a preschool child's speech for stuttering, I also screen for possible articulation, language, and voice problems. In addition, I make sure that his hearing has been checked recently and if not, arrange to have a hearing screening.

A child's language and articulation problems can usually be detected in the recorded parent-child or clinician-child interactions. When I suspect problems in these areas, I administer formal tests. You may wish to consult Bernthal, Bankson, and Flipsen (2009) for testing articulatory and phonological disorders, and Paul and Norbury (2011) or McCauley and Fey (2006) for assessing language problems. I will discuss the management of concomitant articulation and language disorders in Chapter 12, which deals with treatment of beginning stuttering.

My view of the relationship between language and stuttering, which I described in Chapters 4 and 5, is that one of the pressures on a child who stutters may result from language development that is much more advanced than motor development. Thus, in evaluating a child's language and articulation, I explore the possibility that his language exceeds age expectations. In addition, I observe his language usage and motor abilities and question parents about his general motor development and the intelligibility of his speech.

When language development outstrips motor development, there may be a risk that a child will try to produce long sentences at an adult pace with a speech system that at this age, is better suited to a slower rate. A child's motivation to speak quickly may come from his own eagerness to express complex thoughts, from his parents' pleasure at his adult-like speech, or just from the fact that adult speech rate models affect the child. We have demonstrated this with typically developing children—typical in both language and fluency (Guitar & Marchinkowski, 2001). For a child who stutters and who also has advanced expressive language abilities for his age, rate of speech production may be an important factor to target in treatment. How rate is targeted in intervention depends on the child's level of stuttering. If the child is relatively unaware of his stuttering and does not seem to be reacting to it with escape or avoidance behaviors, and his frequency of stuttering is relatively low, I am likely to use an indirect treatment approach. I would train parents to use a slower speech rate when speaking to the child as part of the treatment, with the expectation that their model of a slower speaking rate will influence the child to speak more slowly, thereby putting fluency within his reach. In such cases, I also explore ways in which the family may be putting pressure inadvertently on the child's language skills by expecting a higher level of language development than the child can achieve.

Verbal activities that some parents enjoy most with their children, such as puns, word play, and teaching the child multisyllable words, may convey to a child that the parents place high value on verbal ability. For most children, this would be an incentive to develop their verbal skills. But for children vulnerable to fluency breakdowns, their parents' pride in their verbal proficiency may stress their ability to perform, resulting in increased disfluency. For those children who are really struggling with stuttering, parents' focus on verbal performance may create in the children feelings of shame at their verbal ineptitude.

It is useful to compare a child's language (syntax) scores with his vocabulary scores. Researchers (e.g., Anderson & Conture, 2000; Conture, 2001) have shown that many children who stutter have a disparity between syntax and vocabulary scores that is greater than that for matched typically developing children. Interestingly, it has also been shown that children who have lower language abilities at the beginning of treatment show greater long-term decrease in stuttering as a result of treatment (Richels & Conture, 2010).

As I review my observations of a child's speech and language, I consider not only the possibility that a child's language is advanced relative to his speech motor abilities, but also the possibility that his motor abilities are markedly delayed. A few children have motor problems that impair their coordination of respiration, phonation, and articulation with language production. Many are aware that speech is difficult for them and have already felt frustration and shame, not just about stuttering, but about the way they speak and how they perform other fine motor tasks. Therefore, to help these children improve their feelings about themselves as talkers, the parents and I work on their speech motor skills. These children seem to benefit especially from models of slow speech as well as activities that teach them to speak more slowly.

In addition to exploring the possibility of language and articulation difficulties, I also assess a child's voice. A hoarse voice may be especially significant in a preschool child who stutters because it may be a sign that the child has increased tension in his laryngeal muscles, perhaps in an effort to cope with stuttering. I look closely at how the child is handling his blocks and listen for signs of excess laryngeal tension, such as pitch rises, increases in loudness, and hard glottal attacks. Because many of the techniques I use in treatment of stuttering result in a more relaxed style of speaking, I usually don't treat voice separately from stuttering. However, if a child has voice problems other than hoarseness, or if hoarseness does not diminish with stuttering therapy, I refer the child to an otolaryngologist and follow treatment approaches such as those suggested by Boone, McFarlane, Von Berg, and Zraick (2009).

Other Factors

In Chapters 4 and 5, I described a number of possible developmental influences on stuttering. In this section, I review them briefly so that they may be recognized if they are important in a particular preschool child's stuttering. Because much of this information can be obtained from a parent interview, you may wish to consult Chapters 4 and 5 for further details on developmental influences before conducting a parent interview.

Physical Development

I like to ascertain whether a child has age-appropriate gross motor skills and whether his oral motor development is typical. Figure 4.2 in Chapter 4 presents information about motor development. Most children learn to walk at about age 1 but usually do not learn to walk and talk at the same time. If a child I am evaluating was delayed in walking but average or advanced in talking, I may explore the possibility that the onset and evolution of his stuttering was associated with his delayed motor development.

Cognitive Development

When I consider a child's cognitive development, I want to learn whether there is cognitive delay, which can be associated with increased disfluency. I also want to know if a child may be going through a period of rapid cognitive growth that might, hypothetically, take a temporary toll on fluency.

Social-Emotional Development

As a child grows, various tensions develop between him, his parents, and his siblings. Between ages 2 and 5, many children may display negativity in ways that are felt throughout the family. When I ask a child's parents about conditions surrounding the onset or worsening of a child's stuttering, I explore social-emotional factors as well as environmental and developmental factors.

In Chapter 4, I described various life events that may affect a child's stuttering. In the parent interview, I examine life events surrounding the onset of stuttering to see if upsetting events or ongoing situations may be linked to the child's stuttering. Some events, like the birth of a sibling, may be happy ones, but they can create disturbances in the psychological balance of a family.

Speech and Language Environment

I have referred to the child's communication environment before, but here I am more explicit. Many children have their hands full trying to compete verbally with fast-talking, articulate adults. Children who stutter may find this particularly hard. If the family has sent, as requested, a video or even audio recording of the parents and child talking, I observe the parent-child interactions carefully for indications of a complicated verbal environment, such as rapid speech models without pauses that may be like rough water to a new swimmer.

Diagnosis

Now let us turn to the task of pulling together the information gathered in an assessment and making a diagnosis of a young client's problems. One of the clinical questions that must be answered is whether the child is truly stuttering. Once you have (tentatively) answered that, you can answer the other clinical questions and describe the child's stuttering, his reactions to it, and an appropriate treatment choice.

Determining Developmental and Treatment Level

In determining an appropriate treatment for the child, I begin by trying to figure out if a preschool child is normally disfluent and if not, his level of stuttering: borderline or beginning stuttering. In the following paragraphs, I briefly review these levels, which were described in detail in Chapter 7.

Typical Disfluency

All of the following characteristics must be met for a child to be considered normally or typically disfluent. The child has fewer than 10 disfluencies per 100 words; these disfluencies consist mostly of multisyllable word and phrase repetitions, revisions, and interjections. When disfluencies are repetitions, they will have two or fewer repeated units per repetition that are slow and regular in tempo. The ratio of stuttering-like disfluencies to total disfluencies will be less than 50 percent. All disfluencies will be relatively relaxed, and the child will seem to be hardly aware of them and certainly will not be upset when he is aware.

A child may be considered to have borderline or beginning stuttering if he has any of the characteristics described in the following paragraphs. Place him at the level—borderline or beginning—that includes the child's most salient characteristics.

Borderline Stuttering

The child I place in this category has more than 10 disfluencies per 100 words, but they are loose and relaxed. They may be part-word repetitions and single-syllable word repetitions, as well as prolongations, and the repetitions may have more than two repeated units per instance. Stuttering-like disfluencies will be above 50 percent (Yairi, 1997a), and the disfluencies may cluster on adjacent sounds (LaSalle & Conture, 1995).

Beginning Stuttering

Beginning stuttering usually occurs in children between 3.5 years old and 6. The key features at this level are the presence of tension and hurry in the child's stuttering. Disfluencies may have some of these characteristics: rapid, abrupt repetitions; pitch rises during repetitions and prolongations; difficulty starting airflow or phonation; and signs of facial tension. Just the occasional appearance of these signs would make me believe the child is a beginning stutterer. A beginning stutterer also shows that he is aware of his stuttering (in some, this may be subtle) and may be frustrated by it. He

may use a variety of escape behaviors, such as head nods or eye blinks in terminating blocks. Occasional avoidance may occur. For example, a child who has developed language to the point of using "I" instead of "me" but begins to stutter on "I" at the beginnings of sentences may begin substituting "Me" for "I" to avoid the frustration of stuttering on "I."

Some children are relatively advanced for beginning stutterers. These are children who avoid words and situations, and their behavior and demeanor clearly suggest some fear and shame about stuttering. For example, they may use a variety of starters to begin sentences and look away or appear embarrassed when they stutter.

Although I use information from all sources to determine a child's developmental and treatment level, I have found that my own observations of parent-child and clinician-child interactions are most useful in making this (tentative) decision. Parents are helpful in describing long-term changes in their child's stuttering, but they frequently miss avoidance behaviors, such as starters, circumlocutions, and postponements, which are critical indicators of this more advanced level of stuttering. Parents' reports do provide, however, as much information about a child's feelings and attitudes as I usually gather in observing interactions in the clinic. Thus, parent reports plus my own observations provide valuable, complementary data. A vital adjunct to direct observations are video recordings of parent-child and clinician-child interactions. I sometimes revise my initial placement of a child in a developmental/treatment level after viewing video of the interactions I have already directly observed.

Risk Factors for Persistent Stuttering

Risk factors are those elements within a child or in his environment that make it more or less likely that he will persist in his stuttering (Guitar & Guitar, 2003) or take longer in treatment. Table 9.1 describes several of these factors. For some **risk factors for persistent stuttering**, there are data which support this connection; for others, only clinician observations provide support. I described much of the evidence for these factors in the chapters on Constitutional Factors in Stuttering (Chapters 2 and 3) and on Developmental, Environmental, and Learning Factors (Chapters 4 and 5). You'll be able to get the information you need to determine a child's risk of persistent stuttering from the case history form, questionnaires, parent interviews, and observations of the child.

Drawing the Information Together

After I have completed the assessment tasks, I consolidate the information I have gathered, develop a tentative diagnosis, and meet with the family in a **closing interview** to discuss my findings and their desires and expectations. If I had been able to get a recording from the parents beforehand, I would have carefully analyzed it before the assessment and would present the results of my analysis in the closing interview.

Table 9.1	Risk Factors for Persistent Stuttering or Extended Treatment	
Factors within Child	**Factors within Environment**	
Family history. If child's family history indicates that one or more relatives had persistent stuttering and did not recover without treatment, the child is more likely to have persistent stuttering (Ambrose, Cox, & Yairi, 1997).	**Others' reactions to stuttering.** Clinical observations suggest that if family is critical or impatient with child's stuttering, persistence is likely. More sensitive children are probably more affected by family's reactions to their stuttering.	
Gender. If child is a boy, persistent stuttering is more likely (Ambrose, Cox, & Yairi, 1997).	**Family communication style.** Studies suggest that when parents' language is more complex, stuttering is more likely to be persistent (Kloth, Janssen, Kraaimaat, & Brutten, 1998; Rommel, Hage, Kalehne, & Johannsen, 2000).	
Speech and language skills. If child's language, phonological skills, or nonverbal intelligence are below normal, he is likely to persist in stuttering (Yairi et al., 1996). However, some studies question whether language skills are predictive of persistence (Watkins, Yairi, & Ambrose, 1999). Also, if there is a disparity between child's vocabulary and syntax, child may be at risk for continued stuttering or extended treatment (Conture, 2001).	**Family expectations.** Clinical observations suggest that high expectations for academic, athletic, and social or verbal performance can stress children who stutter, making the stuttering more likely to be persistent.	
Sensitivity/temperament. Some evidence show that children with inhibited or sensitive temperament may take longer in treatment or not reduce stuttering as much in treatment (Richels & Conture, 2010).	**Life events.** Many writers (e.g., Van Riper) have suggested that stressful events may precipitate or perpetuate stuttering. These may include birth of a sibling, death of a relative, or emotional or physical conflicts in the home or in the environment.	
Reactions to stuttering. If child reacts to stuttering with emotion and secondary behaviors, treatment may take longer. It may be related to temperament because emotional reactivity may cause more learned reactions. (see Chapter 6).	**Family's schedule.** Clinical observations suggest that very busy homes in which children are overscheduled can put stress on a child who stutters. However, if child is successful in hobbies, sports, and other activities this can bolster self-confidence.	

The same is obviously true for the other information I obtained before the assessment, such as the Behavioral Style Questionnaire (McDevitt & Carey, 1995) that was described in Chapter 8. Some data, like my analysis of the recordings of parent-child and clinician-child interactions, may not be completed by the time of the evaluation, but results will be included in my assessment report. Thus, for the closing interview, I rely on a combination of previously acquired quantitative data, some of the quantitative data I acquired as I talked with the child, such as frequency of stuttering, and the qualitative data gleaned from my observations and interview questions.

Prior to the closing interview, I spend a few minutes studying my findings or discussing them with students or colleagues if I have been working with a team. I try to make sure that I have obtained enough information to answer two key questions: What is this child's developmental/treatment level of stuttering, and what is the appropriate treatment? Working with the family, we can decide where to go from here. Last year, I began a practice of writing up a brief, one-page summary of our findings and recommendations prior

to the closing interview. I share a copy of this recommendation sheet with the family so that we will have a common reference as we discuss the evaluation and where to go from here. They can share this with other family members and if appropriate, the family can begin to make some changes immediately, without having to wait for the formal written report, which may take several days to prepare.

Closing Interview: Recommendations and Follow-Up

Before I begin, I remind myself to take the necessary time to listen to the family's questions that may arise at any time during the closing interview. When I begin, I always make some positive comments about the child and the family, then describe to the family characteristics of the child's stuttering that I observed in parent-child and clinician-child interactions and the preassessment recording, if I obtained one. I stay away from jargon and strive to be as clear and straightforward as possible as I briefly describe the child's behaviors, review the more important information that the parents provided in the case history and our interview, and estimate the seriousness of the child's problem. If stuttering is a serious concern, I say so, and if the parents have expressed feelings of guilt about their child's stuttering, I again reassure them that they are not to blame but that they will be crucial in helping to resolve it. Next, after answering questions, I describe appropriate treatment approaches, such as environmental changes, indirect treatment, and direct treatment, which will differ depending on the developmental/treatment level of the child's problem.

Recommendations for Children with Typical Disfluency

If I believe that a child's speech is typically disfluent, I deal with the family's concerns rather than the child's disfluencies. Most families benefit from knowing how I reached my tentative conclusion, so I provide them with information about normal disfluency, such as the following: "During their preschool years, many normal children pass through periods of disfluency. Interjections, revisions, pauses, repetitions, and prolongations are common during these periods, but they usually occur in fewer than 10 of every 100 words. Interjections and revisions are more common than part-word repetitions, and part-word repetitions usually have only one or two repeated units per disfluency. Children who are normally disfluent are largely unaware of their disfluencies, do not react negatively to them, and gradually 'outgrow' them."

In most cases, I use analogies to help the family understand their child's disfluent speech. For example, I may point out that learning to speak is like learning many other skills, such as riding a bike or learning to skate, and that a learner falls down a lot in the early stages. I look for analogies that will

fit the family's experiences to help them understand why their child is disfluent and how valuable an accepting environment can be for a child's self-esteem. Parents who are concerned about their child's typical disfluencies usually feel reassured when they find out that this is not uncommon. In those rare cases when parents are still not convinced that their child's speech disfluencies are not stuttering, I teach them how to slow their speaking rates, pause frequently, simplify their language, and relieve other pressures that we mutually agree to change. Then, I set up another appointment to discuss their progress and the child's speech. If parents really are concerned and seem likely to continue worrying and perhaps correcting their child's speech, a few sessions focused on the normalcy of their child's speech and the changes they have made in the family's environment may be an ounce of prevention.

I keep the door wide open for all parents of normally disfluent children. I reassure them that I am available to talk with them if they become concerned again and will be ready to work with them if their child does begin to stutter.

Recommendations for Children with Borderline or Beginning Stuttering

For those preschool children evaluated less than 12 months after the onset of stuttering, there are guidelines to help decide which children should begin treatment and which can be followed for a period of time without treatment. First, children whose stuttering-like disfluencies (part-word and single-syllable word repetitions, prolongations, or blocks) steadily decrease during the first 12 months after onset are more likely to recover without formal treatment. There are more indicators of the likelihood of recovery without treatment, listed in Table 9.2.

Table 9.2	Factors that May Be Associated with Increased Likelihood of Recovery from Stuttering without Treatment*
Factor	**Comment**
1. Decrease in stuttering-like disfluencies during the 12 months after onset	This is an important predictor of recovery. It applies to children with borderline, beginning, and intermediate-level stuttering.
2. Female	Evidence suggests females are more likely to recover.
3. No relatives who stutter, or relatives have recovered from stuttering	Preliminary evidence suggests that persistent stuttering may run in families.
4. Good language and articulation skills	Both receptive and expressive language skills should be considered. Evidence of early phonological problems may predict persistent stuttering.
5. Good nonverbal intelligence scores	Children with persistent stuttering had normal, but slightly lower nonverbal skills.
6. Outgoing, carefree temperament	Our clinical experience suggests these children who begin to stutter often outgrow it.

*When a young preschool child is assessed within one year of stuttering onset.
Factors 1–5 are based on evidence cited in Andrews et al. (1983), Yairi & Ambrose (1992a, 1992b), and Yairi et al. (1996).

I believe that any preschool child who has borderline or beginning stuttering should be treated or followed carefully for several months. I stay in telephone or e-mail contact with families of children who are close to onset whose stuttering is diminishing, who have other indicators suggesting recovery without treatment is likely, and whose families are not overly concerned. However, if families are highly concerned or the child's stuttering is not decreasing and there are few indicators of recovery, I begin treatment as soon as possible.

My closing interview with these parents is usually the first of many sessions we will spend together. Consequently, I don't need to accomplish everything in this meeting. Because treatment of any preschool child who stutters is often focused on the home environment, we frequently begin our discussion with things the parents can do at home. The chapters on treating preschool children (Chapters 11 and 12) contain more extensive discussions and guidelines for involving the family in treatment, but I will make some initial suggestions here.

In my experience, parents who are active in the ongoing assessment process from the beginning feel more hopeful, less guilty, and more motivated to be involved in treatment (see also Zebrowski & Kelly, 2002). Therefore, in the closing interview, I ask parents of preschool children who will soon start treatment to begin observing and recording the day-to-day variations in their child's fluency. Having them assess fluency in the home environment also gives me a more valid indication of changes in stuttering than if assessments are done only in the clinic. I teach parents to use the Severity Rating Scale (Fig. 8.4; Onslow, Andrews, & Costa, 1990; Onslow, Packman, & Harrison, 2003), which is a form on which they record, at the end of each day, a number from 1 (no stuttering) to 10 (extremely severe stuttering), which is their estimate of the severity of their child's stuttering. Parents begin by rating the severity of the child's stuttering during the parent-child interaction sample just recorded. The clinician also rates the severity of this sample. If the parents' and clinician's ratings differ by more than one point, the parents and clinician discuss the ratings and watch the recording of the interaction to help them come to a consensus. If more than one parent or another family member will be using the Severity Rating Scale, each person should be trained until his or her ratings are within one point of the clinician's rating of each sample. More discussion of using this rating scale is provided in the chapters on borderline and beginning stuttering. In addition to rating the child's severity every day, parents can record comments and questions they would like to discuss when we meet at the next session.

If a child with borderline stuttering is being followed but not formally treated, severity ratings are an important part of the monitoring process. Clinicians can obtain information about the child's stuttering via phone calls or e-mail on a regular basis, and parents can report their severity ratings for each day as well as discuss issues of concern and ask questions. In addition to monitoring the severity of a child's stuttering, it is often helpful to brainstorm with the parents about ways in which the environment might be made as facilitating as possible for their child's speech. I shall discuss this in more detail in the following paragraphs.

For the younger preschool child with borderline stuttering who is being treated (i.e., a child whose parents are very concerned or who has multiple risk factors for persistent stuttering), the closing interview is a time when further appointments may be set up and changes in the family environment can be initiated. Such changes will be determined by the clinician's observations of parent-child interactions, the parent interview, and ideas that parents may have about what they would like to change. In my experience, one of the most powerful ways that parents can facilitate fluency is to set aside 10 to 15 minutes each day, preferably in the morning, for child-directed interactions. This is a one-on-one interaction without other children interrupting. In two-parent homes, parents may need to alternate which one does the one-on-one activity so that the other parent can watch the other children. Or a parent may conduct the session when the siblings are at school or napping. During these interactions, the parent primarily listens to the child and plays whatever games the child chooses. When the parent speaks, he or she should use a slow rate with frequent pauses, somewhat like television's Mr. Rogers. I have found this works best if the clinician models this interaction style and then watches the parent carry it out. More information about changing the family environment is given in the chapter on treatment of the young preschool child with borderline stuttering (Chapter 11).

I also give parents of these children reading material or a video recording to help them better understand stuttering and what they can do to help their child. The book, *Stuttering and Your Child—Questions and Answers* (Conture, 2002), gives many good suggestions and is available from the Stuttering Foundation of America (www.stutteringhelp.org) for very little money. The video, *Stuttering and the Preschool Child-Help for Families* (Guitar & Guitar, 2003, SFA publication no. 70), is also available from the foundation, both through the online store and as a streaming video on www.stutteringhelp.org. Another video, *Preventing Stuttering in the Preschool Child: A Video Program for Parents* (Skinner & McKeehan, 1996; Communication Skill Builders) is highly instructive.

For older preschool children with beginning-level stuttering, I begin treatment as soon as possible. For stuttering at this level, I use a direct approach. Options for therapy should be described to the parents, and with the clinician's guidance, they should make an informed choice. In some cases, the family will be able to make their decision immediately. In other cases, they may need time to consider the possibilities.

If they choose to begin treatment soon, one or more family members should be trained immediately in recording daily severity ratings, and the next session should be scheduled. They should be asked to bring in their severity ratings if the session could be scheduled within a week or two. If it has to be delayed, the clinician should be in contact with the family through e-mail or telephone each week to discuss their severity ratings until formal treatment can begin. Once that begins, parents can bring in their severity ratings each week to discuss them with the clinician.

If treatment cannot begin for several weeks, I ask a parent or another family member to conduct one-on-one interactions with the child as was just described for a child with borderline stuttering. If the family is able to begin treatment immediately, the clinician should start the parents on appropriate activities. Clinicians who carry out therapy themselves with the child will probably have a parent watch the first few sessions before beginning direct activities at home. My own preference is to use the Lidcombe Program (Harrison & Onslow, 2010), which is a parent-delivered treatment. Consequently, if therapy can begin immediately, I describe the first phase of this treatment program to the parents, which is a daily parent-child session conducted at home. Parents engage the child in an activity at an appropriate linguistic level to elicit fluent speech and reinforce fluent utterances. After explaining this to the parent, I model this type of interaction and then observe the parent as he or she tries it. The Lidcombe Program and other direct and indirect approaches are described in Chapter 12.

The closing interview should end when the family seems to have a good understanding of the clinician's findings, and they and the clinician agree what the next steps should be. Because a family may come up with new questions and concerns in the days following the evaluation, it is important to conclude the interview with information about how they can contact the clinician.

SCHOOL-AGE CHILD

Preassessment

Clinical Questions

As with preschool-age children, it is important to begin an evaluation with certain questions in mind. What is this child's frequency of stuttering? What types of disfluencies does he display, and what is the percentage of SLDs? What is the child's severity? What is his speech rate? With rare exceptions, the question of whether the youngster is normally disfluent or stuttering is not an issue. By age 6, most children who stutter do so in ways that are quite different from the normal disfluencies typical for their age. Another question is what emotions and attitudes does the child have about stuttering and about speaking? School children with notable fear and avoidance may need special attention to these feelings

and behaviors. Information about risk factors (e.g., gender, family history) are important but not as critical as they are for a preschool child. By the time a child is in school, natural recovery is less likely than in the preschool years; thus, an absence of risk factors doesn't warrant withholding or delaying treatment.

Information from the child's teachers, the clinician's observations of his speech in class and in the treatment room, and information from his family are all required to assign the child a developmental/treatment level. Questions about treatment of children in the public schools can be answered only in the context of federal and state laws, which are considered in the next section. With any school-age child, it is vital to determine the child's school performance and how stuttering interferes with it.

Public School Considerations

The **Individuals with Disabilities Education Act** (IDEA '97 and changes made in 2004) and individual state laws mandate the procedures that public school clinicians must use for gathering information about a child's disability and deciding on treatment. In most states, a "prereferral prevention/intervention" process is used when a teacher encounters a child who stutters in the classroom (Moore & Montgomery, 2007). Speech-language pathologists are usually members of a team that consults with the teacher and parents to determine if a child's difficulty can be resolved by making changes in the educational setting. An example of such modifications might be discussions between the child and teacher about how the teacher can facilitate the child's class participation. If stuttering continues to be a problem in the classroom after the modifications have been in place for a designated time period, the teacher or parent can refer the child for further evaluation. The next step, evaluation by a multidisciplinary team, is usually taken in response to a referral or as the result of a clinician's identification of a child through screening. As part of this evaluation, the clinician discreetly observes the child in the classroom and confirms (or disconfirms) that the child is stuttering. The clinician then discusses the child's problem with the teacher and the school's special education administrator. Next, the clinician, teacher, or administrator contacts the child's parents to ask permission to do a formal evaluation of the child. If permission is given, the clinician gathers information on as many dimensions of the child's stuttering as possible. Typically, this will include the frequency, severity, and types of stuttering observed in two or more situations, the child's feelings and attitudes about stuttering and speaking, concomitant speech or language problems, and overall communicative performance. The clinician uses standardized tests such as the SSI-4, observations, and interviews with the child and his family as well as with his teachers and others at school who know him. After this information is gathered, a team composed of the clinician, teacher, special education administrator, and the parents meet to decide two issues. The first is whether the child's stuttering problems meet the state's criteria for eligibility, and the second is whether the child's stuttering adversely affects his educational performance. These two issues are discussed in detail later in this chapter, after the sections on the parent, teacher, and child interview.

Initial Contact with Parents

Whether contact is made because the child has been referred to the school clinician or because the parents have made an appointment at a private clinic, the clinician's most important task is to listen and try to understand the parents' point of view. If the school clinician is telephoning the parents for permission to evaluate their child, she should describe the process by which the child was identified and convey her and the school's desire to help the child achieve his potential as an effective communicator. It will be helpful to briefly describe the disfluencies that identified the child as stuttering and to find out if the parents have also noticed them. The clinician should calmly convey her interest in the child and his stuttering in an accepting tone of voice, particularly because parents may fear that they are being blamed for the child's stuttering. It may help also to comment that current views suggest that stuttering may be the result of how the child's brain is organized, although its exact cause is unknown. The evaluation process should be described and permission sought. If the parents agree to an evaluation, this is a good time to ask them to fill out a case history form and if possible, send a video recording of the child's speech. It may be beneficial for the clinician to talk to the child as well and ask his permission to have his parents video record his speech at home. In some cases, the home video is easier to obtain once the clinician has gotten to know the child and has conveyed her acceptance and interest in the child's stuttering.

In cases in which parents have made an appointment for an evaluation at a clinic, the clinician should call the parents and let them know what will take place in the evaluation, get some preliminary information about the child and his stuttering, let them know they will receive a case history to complete and return, and request a video from home prior to the evaluation. As with the school clinician's telephone call, the parents' point of view about stuttering must be understood. Even though they will have a chance to talk over their concerns in person, they may also want to talk and ask questions in this preliminary telephone call.

Case History Form

The form used for this age group is the same one used for preschool children (Fig. 9.3). Some of the questions about speech and language development may be difficult for parents to recall. This is not critical for evaluating a school-age child, but it is important to probe for other speech and language problems that may be contributing factors in the school-age child's stuttering. An important section on this

form deals with how the problem has changed since it was first noticed, what has been done about it, and how others have reacted to it. In addition, the section on educational history lets us know if the child is having problems in school.

Audio/Video Recording

Obtaining a recording (preferably a video recording) of the child speaking at home or elsewhere will help clinicians prepare for the evaluation because they can get a preview of the child's pattern of stuttering, analyze the sample ahead of time, and plan the assessment more carefully. For example, if a sample from home has little or no stuttering, the clinician may want to obtain another sample in a more difficult speaking situation. Up to a point, more varied samples of a child's speech lead to a more valid assessment. If a pre-evaluation sample has lots of avoidance behaviors on it, clinicians can prepare questions to ask the child about what he does when he expects to stutter.

Assessment

Parent Interview

This description of the parent interview assumes that the parents have brought their child to a clinic for the evaluation. When the evaluation is school-based, the clinician can get much of this information by telephone and follow-up with a face-to-face meeting at school.

Begin a clinic-based interview by sharing some positive observations about the child and his family and then describe the course of the evaluation. Before obtaining more background information to fill in gaps left by the case history, ask parents an open-ended question, such as requesting them to describe their concerns about their child's speech. Only after the parents or caregivers have had a chance to express their worries and observations, do I ask follow-up questions. As I do with parents of preschool children, I explore the onset and development of the child's stuttering, his reactions to it, family members' reactions, and any gaps in the case history. I also ask parents of a school-age child about his school experiences. Does he like school? Does his speech seem to bother him there? Do you think he participates less in school because of his stuttering? Is he teased or bullied about his stuttering? Do you think he stutters more at school than at home? Has he gotten therapy at school? Has that helped? Has he liked it?

As I ask parents questions about the child's stuttering at home and school, I listen for responses that may help me understand why the child's stuttering has persisted into elementary school. Here are some of the questions I think about as I try to assimilate the information I am getting from the parent: Is the child sensitive about his stuttering? Are the family and child comfortable talking about stuttering? Is the family supportive of the child and his ways of coping with his stuttering? Is the family motivated to participate in therapy?

I also keep in mind that the parents are probably doing their best, given the expectations with which *they* grew up. One of the most important things clinicians can do in parent interviews is to convey an acceptance of the parents as they are and to point out the helpful things they have done for their child.

Teacher Interview

The more assistance we can get from a child's teachers, the more we can help the child. We need to approach teachers respecting their heavy responsibilities and their concern for their students, including the one with whom we are working. But we also should anticipate that they may neither understand nor know what we do to help a child who stutters. As I conduct a **teacher interview**, for example, I try to sense what they would like to know about stuttering and my treatment approach. The following questions serve as guidelines for the types of things I want to find out.

1. **Does the child talk in class? Does he stutter? What is his stuttering like? How does he seem to feel about his stuttering and about himself as a communicator?**

   Here, I am trying to determine how much the child stutters in class and whether his stuttering keeps him from talking as much as he might otherwise if he did not stutter. I may also get a flavor of how the teacher feels about the child, his communication abilities, and his stuttering.

2. **Does stuttering interfere with the child's performance in school?**

   This question is obviously related to the previous one about the child's stuttering in class. But it also may give us some information about how much the child may avoid speaking, especially volunteering in class. I ask about disparities between his oral and written performance; a large disparity may indicate that he declines to talk or says "I don't know" even when he knows the answers.

3. **Do other children tease him about stuttering?**

   Most school-age children who stutter are teased, and I want to get more information about how much he is teased and how it affects him. I also want to find out about any school policies that relate to bullying since teasing may be just the tip of the iceberg, and many schools are developing strategies for addressing both problems.

4. **How does the teacher feel about stuttering, and how does he or she react to it?**

   I am often able to get this information indirectly, from what he or she said before, but if not, I ask directly. Teachers are also likely to ask how they *should* respond to a child's stuttering, which is an important issue because a teacher's response often influences how the class responds. This and other issues related to the child's speech in the classroom are discussed in the chapter on intermediate stuttering (Chapter 13).

Classroom Observation

In addition to the information obtained from teacher and parent interviews, direct **classroom observation** can help clinicians understand the severity of a child's stuttering and the degree to which it interferes with his academic adjustment. If a child is to receive services in the school, the clinician must establish that the child's stuttering is interfering with his education. One way to verify this is by firsthand observation of a child in the classroom.

You should arrange with the teacher to come to the classroom at a time when the child will have opportunities to participate in class and observe the class as unobtrusively as you can. By observing the class when many students are participating, not just when the child you are evaluating is talking, you will not call as much attention to him. Most school-age children want to be like their peers and dread being singled out. Notice whether the child participates in class discussion. If called on, does he speak in a straightforward manner or does he hesitate or deploy any postponement devices, such as repeating "uh" several times? Does he answer "I don't know?" This is a reply many children who stutter (including me) use to avoid speaking and thus risk stuttering—even when they know the answer. If the child does talk in class and happens to stutter, notice how other children react to his stuttering. Do they giggle and look at each other and make comments under their breaths, or do they seem normally attentive? Because the classroom is the arena where children learn, socialize, and develop communication skills, it should be a target of assessment and treatment.

Child/Student Interview

After I obtain parents' consent to evaluate a child, I arrange for the child to come to the treatment room. Here, I set about to make him feel that my room is an **accepting environment** where he can have fun and also discover how he can make his speech much easier. School-age clients sometimes tell me that it helps just to have someone to talk to about stuttering and other things that are bothering them. This can occur only after a trusting relationship is established, and the initial interview is the beginning of building that relationship.

In our first encounter, it is important for a child to feel that I am genuinely interested in him as well as his stuttering. I usually begin by asking what he likes to do, who his friends are, and who is in his family. Then I tell him a little about myself and how I work with other kids who sometimes get stuck on words. As the child talks, I note whether he stutters or not and how he stutters. When a child's body language and behavior tell me he's comfortable in the session, I talk to him about his speech. The following questions are not asked one right after another but over a session or two. Often, it is more effective to make the question a comment, such as phrasing the first question below as: "Sometimes kids have trouble getting words out. Their words just seem to stick a little bit." Then, leave some silence to see if the youngster will talk about his own speech.

1. **Do you ever think that you have any trouble talking?**
   I rarely see school-age stutterers who are unaware of their difficulty. However, if a child regards his problem as minor or seems genuinely unaware of the problem, I avoid giving it undue emphasis or creating an unfavorable attitude about it. Thus, my first talk with a child is usually low-key, and if he truly doesn't seem to be bothered by his stuttering, although his parents and teachers are, I respect his perception and try to treat it as a relatively minor problem, but I remain aware that the child may be bothered by his stuttering much more than he wishes to let on at first.

2. **What happens when you get stuck on a word? When does it happen? Is it different at different times?**
   I am looking for several things here. One is to learn the words the child uses to describe his stuttering so that I can use them when talking with him about it. I also want to find out if the child is unaware of some of his stuttering behaviors, if they seem to be too painful for him to face, or if he just doesn't like talking about them. Even more important, these questions let a child know that the clinician really wants to understand his problem.

3. **Have you learned to use any helpers or "tricks" to get words out? Do you sometimes avoid certain words?**
   With this question, I can convey that I understand what some people do when they stutter. I can also let a child know that I am nonjudgmental about the "tricks" he uses by conveying my acceptance and interest in his descriptions. In addition, I am also exploring which level the child's stuttering has reached by determining if he is using escape and avoidance behaviors.

4. **Are certain speaking situations more difficult?**
   This is another question that helps me understand what a child is experiencing, while conveying my understanding.

5. **Most kids who stutter get teased or picked on about their speech. Do you ever get teased about your stuttering? What do you do when that happens? How does it affect you?**
   Many children who stutter are teased about their speech but are not willing to talk about it straightaway with someone they don't know well. So this question is a "feeler," and if the child denies being teased, the clinician should not dwell on it now.

6. **How do you feel about your speech?**
   To help a child express feelings about stuttering, I can suggest some possibilities by asking, "Does it make you mad sometimes?" or "Do you wish you didn't get stuck?" Don't be surprised, however, if a child says it doesn't bother him because his feelings may have been rejected, perhaps unintentionally, by adults. Adults may say, for instance, "You shouldn't feel that way," or "Why do you let it bother you?" An effective clinician will show the child that whatever feelings he has are OK and that the clinician is really trying to understand. Real discussions of feelings probably won't begin until a child has learned to trust the clinician deeply. However, in this first interview, I may be able to infer what some of the child's feelings are and from that, understand how far his stuttering has advanced.

   Another avenue to elicit feelings is through drawing pictures. For some children, drawing makes it easier to talk about feelings. The child doesn't have to look directly at the clinician, and his self-consciousness may be decreased by his focus on drawing. I usually suggest to a child that both of us draw whatever we would like, and as we are drawing, I talk about feelings. If this goes well, I bridge the gap between the drawing and talking by suggesting that the child might want to draw a picture of what stuttering is like or what he feels like when he stutters. I have found that this technique can make extensive discussion of feelings much easier for some children. In some cases, children have used their drawings when they talked about stuttering with their class once therapy has helped them feel more comfortable with themselves and their speech.

   Some of the activities in the workbook, *The School-Age Child Who Stutters: Working Effectively with Attitudes and Emotions* (Chmela & Reardon, 2001), are helpful in exploring a child's emotions in both the evaluation and treatment. I shall discuss some of these a little later.

7. **How do your parents feel about your speech? Do they ever say anything or give you advice?**
   This helps me determine what sorts of experiences the child may have been going through at home. One parent may be much less accepting of a child's stuttering than the other. Whatever I find out may help me enlist the parents' participation in treatment.

8. **Can you think of anything else important for me to know about you or about the trouble you sometimes have when you talk?**
   This lets the child know that I am interested in him and that his ideas are important to me.

Speech Samples

Preliminaries

With a school-age child, I video record him talking for 10 minutes about school and other activities in the therapy room. I prefer not to turn on the recorder the moment the child walks into the room. Instead, after talking for a few minutes, I ask the child if he would mind my recording our conversation as we talk. If it's OK with the child, I record a sample that optimally includes 300 to 400 syllables of his speech. For those few children who are reluctant at first, I explain that I need a recording of their speech to understand their stuttering better. In rare cases, I might need to postpone recording until the child is more comfortable with me. After recording the speech sample, I ask the child to read approximately 200 syllables of age-appropriate material. I often use the SSI-4 examiner's manual, which has 200-syllable reading passages at the third, fifth, and seventh grade levels.

If possible, I also obtain a video recording from home for a second sample. In some instances, you may not be able to get a second recorded sample from home or elsewhere. Even if you are not able to record a second sample, write down your impressions of the child's stuttering, including the amount of stuttering and the core and secondary behaviors you observed.

Pattern of Disfluencies

A school-age child is likely to show beginning or intermediate stuttering, so you want to know as much as possible about the amount of tension in the child's stuttering, the escape behaviors he uses, and the extent to which he avoids words and situations. You can obtain this information directly by observation or indirectly through parent and teacher interviews. As with adults or adolescents who stutter, I use this information not only to decide at which developmental/treatment level to place the child but also, when appropriate, to plan the process of unlearning conditioned responses, which, once created, now maintain the child's pattern of stuttering.

Stuttering Severity Instrument (SSI-4)

Samples of conversational speech and reading are needed to calculate scores on the SSI-4. Administration and scoring of the SSI-4 were described in Chapter 8.

Speech Rate

The samples you collect for rating severity with the SSI-4 can also be used to assess the child's speaking rate. The purpose of assessing speech rate is to get some idea of how much the child's stuttering interferes with the rate of speech he normally uses. As I help the child manage his stuttering, I expect a steady increase in his speech rate toward normal levels.

Normal speech rates for school children in Vermont between the ages of 6 and 12 years measured in syllables per minute are given in Table 8.5. These rates were obtained from children's conversations with a clinician about Christmas, hobbies, school, and home activities. They were calculated by including normal pauses in their conversation but excluding pauses longer than two seconds for thought. It is reasonable to expect that children's speech rates in other states will be similar.

Trial Therapy

Trial therapy with a school-age child will help me understand what approach might work with this particular child as well as what may be difficult for him. If the child is able to make significant, though temporary changes in his stuttering in this brief treatment, he will gain hope and motivation for our work together.

I usually begin by asking the child to identify moments of voluntary stuttering in my own speech. I explain that I will be putting stutters in my speech and want to see if he can catch me. It's more fun if I can use a small reward for his successes. I then tell him about my favorite recent movie or television show (something he can later talk about himself) and put in a variety of stutters in my speech. As I talk and encourage him to catch my stutters, I let him know how good he is when he catches one of my stutters without my help and hand him a piece of candy or another reward. After a few successful catches, we switch roles and have him put in some stutters—pretend or real—as he talks about a movie, TV show, or any other handy topic, and I try to "catch him." Each time, I make a positive comment about his stutter and give him a reward. Rewarding stutters of school-age children causes no harm; in fact, it reduces negative emotion, which is a very positive step in treatment.

A next step is to see if he can hold on to a stutter. As always, I first demonstrate what I'm asking the child to do. I have the child signal me by pointing to me when he wants me to stutter and make me hold on to the stutter for several seconds by continuing to keep his finger pointing at me. Then, we reverse roles and I coach him to hold on to either voluntary or real stutters. In so doing, I also coach him, while he's holding on to the stutter, to let it go slowly and loosely when he's ready to move on. Typically, my models, my enthusiasm, and the reinforcements I use enable most children to be able to carry out these activities. Note that if the child cannot do these activities, it suggests a higher level of fear or an inability to focus on the task. These possibilities usually mean that a child needs a slower approach, and I will consider teaching him fluency skills before attempting stuttering modification.

Trial therapy using **fluency skills** simply involves teaching the child one or two of the fluency skills described in Chapter 13 on treatment of stuttering in school-age children. I use a word list and give the child an example by producing each word myself before he tries it, using a slow rate and gentle onset of voicing. The severity of the child's stuttering will determine how slowly I begin the word; my aim is to use modeling of slow rate and easy onset to produce fluency in the child. Once he can say words after me in that slow fashion, I then ask him to say each of several words again, but without my model. If he can do this, I create sentences beginning with those words said slowly and with an easy onset (but with the remainder of the sentence produced at a near-normal rate) and again assess whether he can repeat them fluently with my model and then without.

These exercises help me determine how well the child can make changes in his speech and his stutters. By using a large amount of modeling and appropriate reinforcement, I can often take the child quite far along in the time I have.

Feelings and Attitudes

A fair assessor of a child's feelings and attitudes is the clinician's judgment, which usually improves as she gets to know the child better. Nevertheless, the clinician should be able to get a pretty good indication of a child's feelings and attitudes from the first interview. Some indications will emerge from your discussion with the child about his feelings, and some will emerge from observations of his behavior. Watch how the child responds when asked about his stuttering, and note how much he avoids stuttering. When the child does stutter, observe how calm he is and how consistent his eye contact is.

After the clinician has gotten to know the child a bit, she may want to administer a paper and pencil assessment of attitude. Figure 8.6 in the previous chapter depicts the A-19 scale (Guitar & Grims, 1977), a measure developed to assess children's communication attitudes. This scale consists of questions that were found to distinguish children who stutter from those who do not. Hence, if treatment is effective, a child's attitude about communication may change, although this has not been established by research.

In addition to the A-19, the Communication Attitude Test (Fig. 8.7), which was developed by Brutten, has been tested on nonstuttering children (Brutten & Dunham, 1989) and shown to differentiate them from stuttering children (De Nil & Brutten, 1991). It has also been found to have good test-retest reliability for this purpose (Vanryckeghem & Brutten, 1993).

Many informal methods of assessing feelings and attitudes are given in the workbook, *The School-Age Child Who Stutters: Working Effectively with Attitudes and Emotions* (Chmela & Reardon, 2001). These include such activities as a "Worry Ladder," in which a child lists his worries in a hierarchy, and "Hands Down," which elicits things the child likes and does not like about himself. Although the reliability and validity of these tools have not been determined, they provide useful starting points for communication about feelings and attitudes.

With some children, both formal and informal methods of assessing feelings will be productive during the evaluation. But others will hold back until they have developed a trusting relationship with the clinician. Thus, clinicians should be mindful that information about a child's feelings and attitudes obtained in a first meeting may not be complete or accurate.

Other Speech and Language Disorders

In my discussion of the preschool child, I described the importance of screening language, articulation, and voice. The same abilities should be screened in the school-age child. Conture (2001) suggests using the "Sounds in Words" subtest of the Goldman-Fristoe Test of Articulation 2 (Goldman & Fristoe, 2000) for articulation, the Clinical Evaluation of Language Fundamentals-4 Screening Test (Semel, Wiig, & Secord, 2004) for language, and the Peabody Picture Vocabulary Test 4 (Dunn & Dunn, 2007) and Expressive Vocabulary Test 2 (Williams, 2007) for vocabulary. The child may have a previously diagnosed language or articulation (or to a lesser extent, voice) problem and may be in therapy. If so, the clinician should seek out details of any current or previous therapy. If a child is receiving or has received articulation or language therapy in

the past, the clinician should find out details about the type of treatment the child received and how the child responded. Did his articulation or language difficulties improve? Did his stuttering first appear or worsen during treatment? If so, the clinician should pay particular attention to indications that the child may think of himself as a poor speaker and may believe that speaking is difficult. The interviews and questionnaires I suggested in the previous section on feelings and attitudes will help you explore this possibility, and the therapy approaches described in the chapters on beginning- and intermediate-level stuttering are designed to help a child regain confidence in his ability to speak easily and well.

Other Factors

Other factors can influence the outcome of treatment. We recommend evaluating all factors that may have precipitated or are maintaining a child's stuttering so that they may be included in the child's overall treatment plan.

Physical Development

My main concern in this area is that motor development may be lagging behind language development. A child with speech-motor delays may benefit from therapy that helps him coordinate respiration, phonation, and articulation, thereby reducing stuttering. He may also benefit from procedures that help him learn to stutter easily and openly, rather than becoming tense and frustrated if his fluency breaks down under stress. Such children's treatment should also focus on building self-esteem, which may be low in children who are not well coordinated. One way to help build a child's confidence is to figure out what he is good at or what he would like to improve his mastery of and encourage that. I sometimes make up games, like tossing a ball into a waste basket at greater and greater distances and have the child practice this during breaks from working on speech. Most children will delight in improving their skill at tasks at which they have some success, especially when they can do better than the clinician.

Cognitive Development

I try to find out whether or not cognitive stresses of school may be increasing the general demands experienced by the child, which I'll discuss further in a following section on academic adjustment. If a child has academic difficulty or a learning disability, we may need to adjust our approach to treatment to make sure that he understands our explanations and examples.

Social-Emotional Development

I am interested in how well a child fits in with his classmates, how comfortable he feels about talking and relating to others, and how often he feels a need to hide his stuttering. Some children are friendly and outgoing even though they stutter and are supported by their classmates. These social skills are a positive factor in their prognoses for recovery from stuttering. Other children may be sensitive or self-conscious, and stuttering compounds their self-concern and keeps them from relating easily to others. Such children need help in relating more easily to their classmates. Evaluation of this component can be accomplished through teacher, parent, and child interviews; classroom observation may be helpful, too.

I am also concerned with the extent to which a child's home environment provides support and security. This information comes primarily from parent and child interviews. Parents often provide insight into conditions surrounding the onset of stuttering and conditions under which it gets better or worse. I sift through this information, and with the parents' help, determine whether something can be done to improve the child's self-esteem. For some children, school psychologists have been helpful in building self-esteem and helping them improve their social adjustment.

Academic Adjustment

Parent, child, and teacher interviews allow me to find out how well the child is doing in school and how much he likes it. Stuttering may appear for the first time or worsen when a child is under the stress of learning many new things. For example, reading aloud in class when just learning to read is likely to put substantial demands on a child's resources for language formulation and speech production. The child must make "second-order mappings of meanings and lexical units from speech" (Gibson, 1972) while simultaneously translating the written representation into units appropriate for speech production. Thus, some academic challenges may be more demanding for a child who stutters, and his stuttering in school should be understood in relation to this. In practical terms, clinicians can determine if a child needs extra help in certain academic areas through discussions with his teachers about which speaking situations in school are most difficult for him. If the child has more difficulty in certain academic situations, these should be given extra attention in treatment when planning generalization of more fluent speech.

Diagnosis

At this point in a clinic-based evaluation, the clinician pulls together the information collected from the case history; parent, teacher, and child interviews; speech samples; and classroom observations. This information helps the clinician determine the developmental/treatment level of the child's stuttering, which will give direction for treatment.

Most school children are at beginning or intermediate levels of stuttering. Beginning-level stuttering is characterized by physical tension, hurry, escape behaviors, awareness of difficulty, and feelings of frustration. The intermediate level also involves tension, hurry, escape behaviors, and frustration, as well as avoidance behaviors as a result of fear and anticipation of stuttering. In addition to a child's stuttering behaviors and feelings, current developmental and environmental pressures must be considered in planning treatment. Such pressures can be uncovered from parent, teacher, and child interviews and the speech sample. Some pressures may result from other speech and language disorders, motor problems, or pressures in the child's home. Goals can be formulated with the parents' input for alleviating those pressures that can be changed and helping the child cope with those that can't be changed. Some pressures can be dealt with in treatment, but others may require parent counseling or referral to other professionals.

Closing Interview

The closing interview provides an opportunity to summarize my immediate impressions for the parents and make recommendations about treatment. It also provides an opportunity to discuss the crucial role parents can play in reducing environmental pressures. I point out the many beneficial things they have done about their child's speech and assure them that stuttering was not caused by anything they have done. Although some parents may have created conditions in which a child's predisposition to stutter has been transformed into a serious problem, it does not help to make an issue of this. Rather, we want to convince them that they are in a key position to help.

After describing clearly and simply what I observed about the child's stuttering, I summarize my thinking about appropriate treatment. I do this in only general terms because parents' main concerns at this time are not the details of treatment but the prospects for their child's future. Therefore, I rely on my experience to describe likely outcomes. For example, I might say that a combination of many factors will determine the child's outcome. These include the natural increases in fluency that occur as a child matures, feelings of self-acceptance that a child develops when he finds that people accept him whether or not he has trouble with his speech, and his learning ways to speak more fluently. When I talk about the child's prognosis, I always include some aspect of the parents' role, such as their acceptance of the child's speech or their participation in treatment, as part of the formula for recovery. Sometimes, a key aspect of the parents' acceptance of stuttering is realizing they are not responsible for curing it. If I feel that there is a good chance the child will have some stuttering remaining after therapy, I talk with the parents about this possibility, indicating that many people who have some stuttering remaining lead highly successful lives. A few who come to mind are Malcolm Fraser, a highly successful businessman who founded the Stuttering Foundation; Carly Simon, the singer; and Vice President Joe Biden.

After summarizing my impressions and describing some of the ingredients for recovery, I discuss some of the things the parents can do to promote recovery. Specific suggestions depend on findings from our interviews, but the sections on parent counseling in the chapter on treatment of stuttering in school-age children present general ideas for parents' involvement. Discussion of the family's involvement in therapy is the most important part of the closing interview and in fact may continue for several more meetings. If I treat the child directly and in a clinic rather than in a school setting, I meet with parents weekly as part of treatment. In these meetings, I continue to help them explore how various changes in the home environment can facilitate their child's fluency.

Public School Setting

The sequence dictated by IDEA after a referral for stuttering is made is for the multidisciplinary team to develop an assessment plan and carry it out. After the clinician gathers information using tests, observations, and interviews, she writes a report describing the affective, behavioral, and cognitive aspects of the child's stuttering and his current performance in academic, nonacademic, and extracurricular activities. The assessment report should be brief (e.g., two pages) and understandable by lay readers, such as the child's parents.

Then, an **Individualized Education Program (IEP)** team is appointed to consider the report and other information. The IEP team must decide the two issues mentioned earlier—does the child meet the state's eligibility standards, and does the child's stuttering have an adverse effect on his education? The first of these issues is resolved by the data the clinician gathered, particularly the information about the frequency and severity of the child's stuttering and his feelings and attitudes. The second issue is usually more complex because it is necessary to show that the child does not perform as well as he might in school because of his stuttering. For example, the team can conclude that his stuttering prevents him from participating as much as he might in class or in extracurricular activities with his peers. Evidence of this can be obtained from measures of communicative functioning in school, such as the *Teacher's Assessment of Student Communication Competency* (Fig. 8.9) (Smith, McCauley, & Guitar, 2000), observations of the child in the school, and interviews with teachers and parents. Lisa Scott Trautman (personal communication, July 30, 2003) noted that adverse effects can be shown by demonstrating that the child cannot meet the school district's curriculum objectives because of his stuttering. Examples of such objectives might be that students will be active in class discussions or that students must be able to speak effectively in front of a group.

If the evaluation determines that the student is eligible for services, an IEP team, often headed by the SLP, develops measurable goals and short-term objectives (also called "benchmarks") as well as services to be provided that will help the student improve his performance in all aspects of the educational setting. These goals and objectives are considered in detail in the chapters on treatment of beginning and intermediate stuttering.

ADOLESCENTS AND ADULTS

The assessment of an adolescent or adult can be very rewarding for a stuttering clinician. Although some clients may be discouraged because they have been stuttering for years and skeptical that you can really help them, many are highly motivated to work on their speech and ready to begin this work during the evaluation. Your challenge is to take advantage of this motivation, get them working immediately, and to give them realistic hope that hard work and resolve can change their speech and maybe their lives.

Preassessment

Clinic Versus School Assessment

This section is written as though the evaluation is being carried out in a clinic rather than a school. When the setting is a public school, the evaluation process is determined by the Individuals with Disabilities Education Act (IDEA '97) and the laws of each state. The guidelines for this process were described in the previous section on evaluating a school-age child. For the adolescent, an additional consideration is his participation in the IEP process and his transition beyond high school. When a student reaches age 14, his input is sought by the IEP team, and he gradually becomes an active member of the team, not only with regard to his present situation, but also in terms of his aspirations beyond secondary school. When a student reaches age 16, transition plans are a mandated part of the IEP. At age 18, students take over responsibility from their parents for signing off on documentation.

Case History Form

A case history form is sent to adult clients (those over age 18 years and beyond high school) several weeks before their appointment. A copy of this form is shown in Figure 9.4. Because adolescents are often seen in schools, the clinician encourages them to fill out the form with help from their parents for parts of it.

This form requests information that would be appropriate for most speech-language disorders and can be used with all adult clients referred for speech or language problems. It also allows the clinician to learn ahead of time whether the client referred for stuttering may have a different or

STUTTERING CASE HISTORY FORM – ADULT

Instructions: Please fill out this form in as much detail as possible. You can be assured that this information will be treated as confidential. If information is not available, please specify the reason so that we will know that the question has been considered. **Please return this form prior to your appointment.** Thank you.

Date: _____

Name: _____   Gender: M   F

Address: _____   Telephone: (home) _____

_____   (work) _____

E-Mail Address: _____   Cell Phone: _____

Date of Birth: _____   Place of Birth: _____

Referring Physician: _____

Marital Status: _____

Education Level: _____   Occupation: _____

Employed by: _____

Referred to this Center by: _____

Name of spouse/nearest relative: _____

Address: _____   Telephone: _____

HISTORY OF STUTTERING

Are there other individuals in your family background or immediate family who stutter?

_____

Give approximate age at which your stuttering was first noticed: _____

Who first noticed or mentioned the stuttering? _____

In what situation did this occur? _____

Describe any situations or conditions that you associate with the onset of stuttering:

_____

_____

What were the first signs of your stuttering? (If you don't remember, you might ask your parents or siblings.) _____

_____

Was the stuttering always the same or did it occur in several different ways? _____

_____

If they occured in different ways, how were they different from one another? _____

_____

Figure 9.4   Case history form for adults and adolescents.

Did the first blocks seem to be located in the tongue? lips? chest? diaphragm? or throat?

_____

Approximately how long did each block (on one word) seem to last? _____

_____

Was the stuttering easy or was there force at the time when the stuttering was first noticed?

_____

Were the words that were stuttered at the beginning of sentences, or were they scattered through-out the sentence being said? _____

_____

When stuttering first began, was there any avoidance of speaking because of it? Give examples, if any. _____

_____

At the time when stuttering was first noticed, what was your reaction?

      Awareness that speech was different? _____ Indifference to it? _____

      Surprise? _____ Anger or frustration? _____ Shame? _____

      Fear of stuttering again? _____ Other? _____

What attempts have been made to treat the stuttering problem? _____

_____

DEVELOPMENT OF STUTTERING

Since the onset, have there been any changes in stuttering symptoms? Check those that are appropriate.

      Increase in number of repetitions per word _____

      Change in amount of force used (increased? decreased?) _____

      Increase in amount of stuttering _____

      Increase in length of block _____

      Periods of no stuttering _____

      More precise in speech attempts _____

      Lowered voice loudness _____

      Slower rate of speech _____

      Change in location of force when stuttering, if force is present _____

      Looking away from listener _____

Describe any of the above that apply _____

_____

_____

Figure 9.4 *(Continued)*

Were there any periods (weeks/months) when the stuttering disappeared? _____
_____

Were there any periods (weeks/months) when the stuttering increased? _____
_____

Can you give an explanation for these "worse" periods? _____
_____

CURRENT STUTTERING

Are there any situations that are particularly difficult? If so, please describe. _____
_____

List any situations that never cause difficulty. _____
_____

Answer the following "yes" or "no" as they apply to your stuttering. Do you stutter when you

    Talk to young children? _____ Say your name? _____

    Answer direct questions? _____ Talk to adults, superiors at work, teachers? _____

    Use new words that are unfamiliar? _____ Use the telephone? _____

    Read aloud? _____ Recite memorized material? _____

    Ask questions? _____ Talk to strangers? _____ Speak when tired? _____

    Speak when excited? _____ Talk to family members? _____

    Talk to friends? _____

Do you know any stutterers? _____ Describe your relationship with them. _____
_____

Do you feel that stuttering interferes with your career? _____ Social relationships? _____

Success in school? _____ Success on the job? _____ Daily life? _____

Describe what your stuttering currently looks and sounds like. _____
_____
_____

MEDICAL, DEVELPMENTAL AND FAMILY HISTORY

If possible, describe mother's health during pregnancy and/or your birth history (i.e.,
complications). _____
_____
_____

Describe any development problems during infancy or early childhood (i.e., late to walk, feeding
problems, food allergies, late to talk). _____
_____

Figure 9.4   *(Continued)*

Are you: Right-handed? _____ Left-handed? _____ Both? _____ Is there any evidence of visual, artistic abilities in your family? _____

Were you sensitive as a child? _____

Would you describe yourself as sensitive now? _____

List your history of any significant illnesses, injuries, and/or operations:

Date	Fever	Complications	Treatment	Physician

List all present physical disabilities. _____

Any chronic illnesses, allergies, or physical conditions? _____

Vision normal? _____ Hearing normal? _____ List any medication you take regularly or are taking currently. _____

Describe any learning or reading problems you experienced as a child or are currently experiencing. _____

Do any members of your family have speech or language problems or learning disabilities? If so, describe. _____

SOCIAL HISTORY

Hobbies _____

Leisure time activities _____

Describe any previous theraphy you have participated in to aid your fluency. When? Where? With whom? Length of time? The outcome? _____

Add anything else you would like to include and think might be important: _____

In addition, what goals would you like to see accomplished as a result of this evaluation? _____

Signature: _____ Date: _____

Figure 9.4 (Continued)

additional disorder. The form also gives the clinician information about the extent to which stuttering, if that is the problem, affects a client's life.

Attitude Questionnaires

I assess clients' communication attitudes through observations, interview questions, and questionnaires. Because I want to be able to analyze completed questionnaires before the diagnostic interview, I prefer to send them to clients and ask them to complete and return the questionnaires before the interview. If this is not possible, clients can complete them when they arrive for an evaluation before the initial interview or as a less desirable alternative, after the initial interview. Prior to the interview, follow-up questions based on information from the case history and questionnaires, which are described in the section on feelings and attitudes, can be prepared to further explore a client's attitudes.

Audio/Video Recording

It is important to sample a client's speech in several situations to get an adequate picture of his stuttering. I ask clients to video or audio record themselves talking in one or two different situations outside the clinic and get the recording to me prior to the evaluation. It is usually easy for clients to record themselves talking to someone on the phone, recording only their own voices and not the person on the other end of the line. Some clients can also record themselves talking face-to-face with a friend or family member. If I listen to the recording(s) before an evaluation, I am better prepared to understand the client's stuttering and to plan various trial-therapy strategies.

Assessment

Interview

I begin by welcoming the client and reviewing the procedures I will use to evaluate his problem, such as interviewing him about his stuttering and his feelings and attitudes, video recording his speaking and reading, examining what he does when he stutters, and trying to determine if he can change it. I let him know that after the initial part of his evaluation, I will ask him to wait while I analyze the information I've obtained before meeting with him to share my findings and recommendations. If there are any forms or questionnaires I haven't already obtained from him, I'll have him complete those while I analyze the other data.

I begin our interview with an open-ended question such as, "Tell me the problem that brings you here today," or "Why don't you tell me about your stuttering?" The first question might be used if I don't know what is motivating the client to come for an evaluation at this time; the second question I use when I already know from prior information why the client has come right now.

Once a client has had a chance to describe his speech problem, I ask further questions to try to get a deeper understanding. The following are typical questions that I ask with a brief commentary about why I'm asking them. Sometimes, I group several questions together (e.g., a question to start the client talking about a particular topic and follow-up questions that I ask if the first question doesn't elicit all of the desired information). I ask only one question at a time, listen carefully to the client's response and try to understand the client's underlying feelings.

1. **When did you begin to stutter? How has the way you stutter changed over the years?**
   I realize that in answering the first part of this question, a client may just be reporting what parents told him about his stuttering. The accuracy of his response may be questionable, but at least I'll learn his perception of the onset. The second part of the question—about changes over the years—may reveal what kinds of things affect the way a client stutters. Does he stutter more severely because of a recent job change or a threat to his self-esteem, such as a divorce or loss of employment? Less frequently, I may find out that a client began to stutter in late adolescence or as an adult. If so, I would want to consider the possibility of neurogenic or psychogenic stuttering, which is discussed briefly in the upcoming section on diagnosis and more fully in Chapter 15, on other fluency disorders.

2. **What do you believe caused you to stutter?**
   This may give some insights about a client's motivation. For example, a woman whose speech I once evaluated reported that her mother and several brothers stuttered and that her stuttering was therefore a genetic problem that could not be helped. This led us to confront the issue of whether or not she was likely to change.

   In addition, I sometimes find that clients have misinformation about possible causes of their stuttering. If I can give them more appropriate information, their attitudes about the problem may change, and their motivation may increase. I have met individuals who come to the evaluation believing that their problem is entirely psychological. After I discuss current views of stuttering, they are relieved to know that they are likely able to modify their speech without long-term psychotherapy.

3. **Does anyone else in your family stutter?**
   I might find that a parent stutters, which can be significant because a parent's attitudes about his or her own stuttering may have had a profound effect on the client. Moreover, knowing about other family members who stutter and how they have responded to it may provide a better understanding of the factors related to this client's stuttering, which may be useful in treatment. For example, someone I am interviewing may have had a parent who stuttered but who never talked about it. I might then want to explore whether the individual I am working with feels especially ashamed of his stuttering, feels it gives him an important bond with the parent, or both.

4. **Have you ever had therapy for your stuttering? What did the therapy consist of? How effective do you think it was?**
This information is important in planning therapy. For example, if a client had received a type of therapy that he felt did not help, it would be unwise to use that type of therapy with this client. But if a client has had success with therapy but has regressed slightly or moved away before treatment was finished, using this type of therapy again may be most appropriate. It is important that clinicians be familiar with various types of therapy that clients may have undergone. Most current therapies emphasize either modifying stuttering behaviors (**stuttering modification**) or learning to talk in ways that eliminate stuttering (teaching fluency skills).

5. **Has your stuttering changed or caused you more problems recently? Why did you come in for help at the present time?**
Responses to these questions allow clinicians to see the current problems faced by the client and also obtain some inkling of the client's motivation. For example, a client may have been offered a promotion if he can improve his speech or may have recently learned of the clinic's treatment program and is hoping for some relief from a long-standing problem. The following four questions about the client's pattern of stuttering are closely related to one another.

6. **Are there times or situations when you stutter more? Less? What are they?**

7. **Do you avoid certain speaking situations in which you expect to stutter? If so, which ones?**

8. **Do you avoid certain words on which you expect to stutter? Do you substitute one word for another if you expect to stutter? Do you talk around words or topics so you won't stutter?**

9. **Do you use any "tricks" to get words out? Escape behaviors?**
These four questions will provide information that is useful in planning therapy because they tell us something about the client's most difficult situations, how he feels about them, and how he deals with them. This information may also corroborate what has been learned from the questionnaires that the client completed and will also reveal how aware he is of his stuttering behaviors.

10. **Have your academic or vocational choices or performance been affected because you stutter? How?**
The client's answers can be used to help plan later stages of treatment in which new behaviors and new challenges are attempted. They may also prompt the clinician to refer clients in later stages of treatment to an academic or vocational counselor to help them make more appropriate choices for themselves.

11. **Have your relationships with people been affected because you stutter? How?**
As with question 10, I can use this information to plan a client's hierarchy of generalization, moving from easy to difficult social situations gradually if the client finds social interactions difficult. I also need to know how much a client blames his stuttering for any of the difficulties he has in social interactions. A client may be socially inhibited because he is sensitive and vulnerable to expected listener reactions. Such sensitivity can be assessed by observing his facial expressions and body movements while stuttering as indicators of affect. If he appears to be relatively unaffected emotionally by his stuttering but professes to have difficulty relating to people, he may benefit from counseling or psychotherapy that focuses on resolving this interpersonal difficulty.

The decision to refer an individual for psychotherapy as an adjunct to stuttering therapy can seldom be made in the evaluation session. It may be that a few therapy sessions are needed to learn more about a person and to develop the client's trust before a successful referral can be made. If psychotherapy is recommended too hastily, a client may believe that I think his stuttering is too great a problem for me to handle, perhaps an insurmountable problem or one that I secretly believe is due to a psychological disorder. However, if I work with him and he starts making some progress before I refer, he will likely feel supported and may be more likely to benefit from psychotherapy.

12. **What are your feelings or attitudes toward your stuttering? What do you think other people think about your stuttering?**
A client's responses will be used to help determine some of the foci of treatment, such as desensitization procedures to decrease fear as well as shame or guilt about stuttering. Perceptions about others' views of his stuttering may need to be confronted with various "reality-testing" tasks to find out what people really think.

13. **What are your family's (parents', spouse's, children's) feelings, attitudes, and reactions toward your stuttering and toward the prospect of your being in therapy?**
This information can identify sources that may positively or negatively affect a client's motivation and may be an important consideration in planning therapy.

14. **Is there anything else that you think we ought to know about your stuttering?**
This gives the client a chance to get anything off his chest that he may be holding back or an opportunity to discuss issues that occurred to him only after other questions were asked.

15. **Do you have any questions you'd like to ask me?**
Sometimes an adolescent or adult has questions about stuttering that he has been reluctant to ask, and this may give the clinician an opportunity to answer them. On the other hand, a client may want to ask about the length and type of treatment or other issues that are best dealt with after his assessment is completed. In this case, the clinician explains why she needs to delay responding but will keep the questions in mind to answer during the closing interview.

Speech Sample

In this part of the evaluation, the client's overt stuttering behaviors are assessed. Although I always video record the entire evaluation, if the client has given permission, I pay particular attention to the recording of this section because I will need to analyze it carefully afterward. Clinicians use a variety of procedures for assessing overt stuttering. Next, I shall describe in detail the tool I currently use and then note other available options.

Stuttering Severity

As indicated in the previous chapter, stuttering severity is usually measured using the Stuttering Severity Instrument (SSI-4), a moderately reliable tool that is commonly used to assess the severity of stuttering. To obtain appropriate samples, I have the client talk about a familiar topic, such as his work, school, hobbies, vacations, sports, or entertainment. It is important to get about at least 300 syllables of the client's talking, so five or 10 minutes are usually enough, depending on the client's fluency. Then, I provide the client material at an appropriate reading level, such as the passages in the SSI-4 examiner's manual, and ask him to read aloud for about three minutes to get 200 or more syllables of reading.

As I noted earlier, we often gather more than one sample of spontaneous speech from adults and adolescents. A sample of speech during a telephone conversation in the clinic can be video recorded and scored using the SSI-4. In addition, I use samples the client has brought or sent in. If the sample from another environment is audio recorded rather than video recorded, I score it for both frequency of stuttering and speech rate, as described below.

Other Measures of Stuttering

If I am assessing stuttering many times throughout the course of treatment or assessing samples that I cannot visually analyze, such as those audio recorded by a client in his natural environment, I use a combination of frequency of stuttering (percentage of syllables stuttered) and speech rate (syllables spoken per minute). These measures, which were first described in Andrews and Ingham (1971), together require much less time than the SSI.

Starkweather (1991) has presented a case for capturing the amount of time that stuttering takes. This is done by totaling the duration of all disfluencies and pauses in a sample and dividing this total by the overall time spent in speaking, thereby giving the clinician a measure of how much an individual's stuttering interferes with the rate with which he can communicate information.

As part of a determined effort to improve the reliability of stuttering measures, Ingham and his colleagues (Ingham, Cordes, & Gow, 1993; Ingham, Cordes, & Finn, 1993) developed a time interval system of assessment. They have shown that when judges determine whether or not four-second intervals of continuous speech contain one or more stutters, interjudge reliability is higher than when moments of stuttering are counted; however, the clinical usefulness of this procedure has not been determined.

Speech Rate

In addition to measuring stuttering severity using the SSI, I also assess a client's speech rate. I believe, as many other clinicians do, that speaking rate often reflects the severity of stuttering, as well as its effect on communication. If a client's speech rate is markedly slower than normal, communication may be difficult for him. A description of the procedure for measuring speech rate was given in Chapter 8, "Preliminaries to Assessment."

Normal speaking rates of adults range from around 115 to 165 words per minute, or about 162 to 230 syllables per minute, with a mean of 196 syllables per minute (Andrews & Ingham, 1971). Adults' normal rates for reading aloud are faster, ranging from about 150 to 190 words per minute (Darley & Spriestersbach, 1978), or about 210 to 265 syllables per minute (Andrews & Ingham, 1971).

Pattern of Disfluencies

Throughout my evaluation of adult or adolescent stutterers, I observe the client's patterns of stuttering. For example, I try to roughly determine the proportions of core behaviors that are repetitions, prolongations, or blocks and ask myself a number of questions about the client's stuttering. During blocks, where and how does he shut off airflow or voicing? What are his escape and avoidance behaviors? Does he end the stutters quickly with pushing and tension? Is he able to tolerate being in blocks, or does he speak in unusual or vague ways to avoid stuttering? More details on various escape and avoidance patterns can be found in Chapter 7 on the Development of Stuttering.

As I explore the behaviors that constitute a client's stuttering, I comment on them, question him about how typical this sample of his stuttering is, and ask about the escape and avoidance behaviors we've observed. If a client doesn't seem too uncomfortable confronting his stuttering, I ask him to teach me how to stutter like he does, and we work together, with both the client and myself emulating his various types of stuttering. This does not need to be an exhaustive exploration, because I will do much more in treatment. Here, I am trying to accomplish three tasks: (1) model an "approach" rather than "avoidance" attitude toward stuttering, showing calmness and objectivity about behaviors that the client may feel are shameful and perhaps even terrifying; (2) study the client's emotional reaction when he comes face-to-face with his stuttering and perhaps reduce some of his fear; and (3) teach both of us about what the client does when he stutters so that he can begin to learn how to change it.

Trial Therapy

I try therapy techniques with clients during their assessment sessions for several reasons. First, I try to get an idea of how a client responds to different therapy approaches, which provides me with information I may use in talking with him about possible treatments. Second, trial therapy can help me to make a differential diagnosis between developmental stuttering and stuttering with a neurological or psychological etiology. Third, it gives clients a preview of things to come and provides them with hope and motivation to follow through on treatment.

I begin by asking a client to modify his stuttering, which can be done easily in the context of studying his patterns of disfluency, as described in the preceding section. In fact, this exploration of stuttering with a client is a condensed version of the first stage of treatment that aims to change stuttering to an easier pattern. Once a client is able to emulate his stuttering to a small degree, I carry out trial therapy by coaching him through the following sequence:

1. First I encourage him to stutter, telling him we must have a sample of the behavior we are trying to change. Then I ask him to "freeze" during a moment of stuttering but maintain the level of physical tension and posture of his stuttering as I encourage him to stay in the moment of stuttering. In other words, I ask him to catch a stutter and prolong it. This may require modeling of how to hold a moment of stuttering right on the sound that's being stuttered. This is easier with a continuant sound, like /m/, but will be harder and need more coaching for plosives, such as /b/. You will probably have to model for the client how to prolong the posture required for holding a stutter on a plosive. It is key that you and he identify the exact posture that is associated with the moment of stuttering and hold onto it. It is important that during this activity the clinician praises the client enthusiastically for catching and holding onto a moment of stuttering. This helps the counterconditioning process—pairing a positive stimulus with a behavior about which the client feels negative.

2. Have him become aware of what he is doing that creates the stutter. For example, where is he holding back sound or airflow? Lips? Tongue? Larynx? All three? As you are helping him explore what he's doing when he stutters, use plenty of praise for being able to stay in the stutter. This is an experience charged with fear and frustration for most adolescent and adult stutterers. They need the counterconditioning that you provide by rewarding their maintaining of this stuttering moment. It's similar to treatment for a phobia: staying in contact with a feared object (a spider or even, in some cases, a rabbit) reduces fear if there is reward provided by another person. It has been said that the physical awareness of what the client is doing with his body as he stutters can be an antidote to the fear he might otherwise be feeling (Zebrowski, personal communication, October 18, 2011).

3. Have the client change his behaviors that are maintaining stutters by (a) releasing excess physical tension wherever he can feel it, (b) starting to move rigidly held structures,

(c) getting voicing or airflow going, and/or (d) allowing himself to breathe. I may stop a client's trial therapy here if he is unable to release physical tension or does it only with obvious difficulty.

If a client seems able to make these changes easily, I go one step further. I ask him to hold on to the stutter, which has become voluntary by now, and to prolong the airflow or voicing for several seconds (while I tell him how great it is that he can do this!), and then produce the remainder of the word slowly. (Some of my clients call this "catch and release.") If a client is able to do this with coaching, I ask him to do it while reading without my coaching. This is enough. No matter how much or how little our client is able to do, I want to stop when he is feeling successful.

Another approach to trial therapy is to change the client's habitual way of talking so that stuttering is decreased substantially or prevented. I begin by reducing my own speech rate as I describe the aim of this exercise to the client, which is to produce words very, very slowly. I use a written sentence that begins with a vowel or a glide, going over it word by word, teaching the client to use gradual and gentle onsets of voicing and to stretch each sound, whether vowel or consonant. This is essentially the "prolonged speech" or "fluency-facilitating targets" used by some fluency-shaping approaches, such as the Camperdown Program (O'Brian, Packman, & Onslow, 2010) and the Fluency Plus Program (Kroll & Scott-Sulsky, 2010). The clinician needs to provide a good model for each word and to give feedback frequently. When words are produced slowly enough with each part of the speech production system (respiration, phonation, and articulation) moving in slow motion and without excess tension, then fluency results. After a client is able to produce each word of the sentence in this way, he is then coached to produce the entire sentence, linking each word to the next. Breath supply should be monitored closely, so that pauses for breath are taken whenever the client would take a breath naturally. Again, accurate modeling and frequent feedback are crucial at earlier stages of treatment.

As an example, the sentence, "Apples are a red fruit," should take from 15 to 20 seconds to produce, with a pause for a new breath after the word "a." The /p/ in "Apples," the /d/ in "red," and the /t/ in "fruit," each should be produced without stopping airflow, making these plosives sound like fricatives. If clients are particularly adept at this, they can be taken all the way to saying short sentences in conversational speech that are produced in this slow, fluent manner. However, clients who have difficulty should be coached only through the production of the short, written sentence, and care should be taken to stop this activity before they experience failure.

Feelings and Attitudes

A variety of questionnaires can be used to assess various aspects of a stutterer's feelings and attitudes about communication and stuttering. In Chapter 8, I described those questionnaires that I use regularly. These include the Modified Erickson Scale of Communication Attitudes (S-24) (Andrews & Cutler, 1974), the Stutterer's Self-Rating of Reactions to Speech Situations (Johnson, Darley, & Spriestersbach, 1952), the Perceptions of Stuttering Inventory (Woolf, 1967), and the Locus of Control of Behavior Scale (Craig, Franklin, & Andrews, 1984).

Other Speech and Language Behaviors

As I interact with a client during the interview, I informally assess his comprehension and production of language, his articulation, and his voice. I also screen his hearing. If I suspect that there may be an articulation, language, voice, or hearing problem, I follow up with further evaluations. Adolescent language assessment procedures can be found in Nippold (2007) and Nelson (1998), and procedures for assessment of articulation can be found in Bernthal, Bankson, & Flipsen (2009). I let a client's concern about other disorders guide us in treatment. If, as I have found occasionally, a stuttering client also produces distorted /s/ or /r/ sounds, I discuss it with him. If he is not concerned, I don't believe it is necessary to treat that problem. However, if I believe that an articulation, language, or other problem handicaps a client communicatively, I advise treatment for that problem also. Sometimes I deal with voice problems differently. I have found that some stutterers may be hoarse, but I suspect this may be the result of laryngeal tension related to stuttering. If stuttering treatment is successful, hoarseness may disappear. Again, I take my cue from the client. If the problem bothers him and isn't remediated by treatment, I address it. If hoarseness is of recent origin and not associated with a cold, I may refer him for an otolaryngological examination to rule out serious laryngeal pathology.

Other Factors

In this section, I discuss the evaluation of the following factors: intelligence, academic adjustment, psychological adjustment, and vocational adjustment. Each of these factors can affect the treatment of an adult or adolescent stutterer and therefore must be considered in planning therapy. The factors are considered briefly here, but some are covered in depth in the chapter on other fluency disorders (Chapter 15).

If a client has below-normal intelligence, he may have difficulty following the regimen of a typical therapy program. Usually, clinicians know beforehand if a client scheduled for an evaluation has Down Syndrome or some other condition characterized by below-normal intelligence. An adolescent stutterer who has been identified as developmentally delayed will likely already be receiving special education. Adults, too, are usually identified as mentally handicapped if this is the case, and either the referral source will report this, or a guardian will have filled out the case history form.

Problems of academic adjustment in an adolescent who stutters usually become apparent from either the original referral or interviews with the child's teachers as part of the evaluation process. These interviews are described in more detail in the section on the school-age child. An example of poor academic adjustment relevant to stuttering could be a student's conflict with a teacher who insists on oral presentations that the student is unwilling to do. The IDEA 1997 process mandates a team approach to solving such problems. This process will be described in the chapters on treatment.

The research reviewed in Chapters 2 and 3 suggests that there are no group differences in the psychological health of stutterers and nonstutterers. However, we sometimes see individuals who stutter who do not function well in their environment. They may be unable to achieve a satisfying marriage, unable to hold a job, or are socially withdrawn. Clinicians need to be alert to the effects that adjustment problems may have on treatment. If psychological problems are suspected of interfering with treatment progress, the clinician may wish to refer the client for a psychological evaluation. In such cases, the clinician should take care to ask professional colleagues for recommendations of the most effective psychotherapists in the area.

Psychological problems that are relevant to stuttering also may become apparent during the interview when the onset of stuttering is explored. Sudden onset after a psychological trauma, particularly if onset is in late adolescence or adulthood, may indicate psychogenic stuttering. I have found that if the psychological effects of the trauma have subsided, an adolescent or adult client may respond well to the integrated approach to treatment described in Chapter 14. If it is clear that psychological factors are still affecting the client's speech and behavior or if there is doubt, I refer the client for a psychological evaluation. Unless the disorder is a psychosis, in which case stuttering therapy may not be recommended, clients with psychological problems may respond well to a combination of psychotherapy and stuttering therapy.

Interview with Parents of Adolescent

When I evaluate an adolescent who stutters, I also talk with his parents, sometimes separately from the adolescent, to obtain more background information about the student, to give them an opportunity to express their concerns and feelings privately, and to tell them about the evaluation process and the options for treatment.

I begin the interview by asking the parents to describe the problem as they see it and encourage them to express their fears, concerns, and frustrations, as I listen carefully. I try to get an understanding of how their child functions within the family and usually ask such questions as: "What is his stuttering like at home?" "How does he seem to feel about it—is he embarrassed or does he show fear of talking or anger about his speech?" "How do you feel about it?" "What are your and other family members' reactions to it?" "What do you do when he stutters?" "Has he been seen anywhere else for therapy?" "If so, what were the results?" Even though I am putting some of these questions in groups, I am careful to ask one question at a time and listen carefully to the answer before I ask another question. Although parents may ask what can be done to help their child and what they should do, I prefer to wait until after I have seen the youngster before answering these questions.

Adolescents strive to become more and more independent of their parents, and I have found that therapy works best if an adolescent is treated as an adult. I begin fostering independence by talking first to teenage clients separately from their parents so that they can give me their own views of the situation and how they view the prospect of treatment. After this and after my meeting with the parents, I meet with the parents and teenage clients together to seek mutual agreement about their respective roles in treatment. This is often an important time. It serves to let teens know that I respect their ability to work independently from the parents, and it serves to let the parents know that they can be most helpful by being supportive but not directive.

Diagnosis

After I gather the information just described, I need to determine whether the client stutters and if so, what treatment level is appropriate. Typically, teenage clients are advanced stutterers; however, some are still in the intermediate stage. But first, let us consider the possibility that a teenager turns out *not* to be a stutterer.

In rare cases, teens who are normally but highly disfluent may be referred by teachers, employers, or friends. Most have phrase repetitions, circumlocutions, revisions, and hesitations, which are the types of disfluencies described in Chapter 7 as normal. Such disfluencies are observed relatively infrequently after children's elementary school years; however, some adolescents and adults may simply be at the disfluent end of the continuum of normal fluency. In addition to the differences in type and number of disfluencies, secondary behaviors and negative feelings and attitudes will be absent. Our role in such cases is to explain to the individual and to the referring person (if this is a referral) that this kind of speech is not abnormal and need not be of concern. It may also be emphasized to the referring source that excessive attention to these disfluencies may be more harmful than helpful. If the client or referring person feels strongly that the disfluent speech interferes with communication, a fluency-oriented treatment described in the chapters on treating intermediate and advanced stuttering may be offered to the client.

Another need for differential diagnosis, in addition to identifying cases of normal disfluency, is ensuring that cluttering, neurogenic disfluency, and psychogenic disfluency be identified and distinguished from "typical" or "developmental" stuttering. Moreover, it is also necessary to rule out disfluencies caused by word-finding difficulties that we might find in a person with a learning disability.

Some of the salient features of cluttering in adults and adolescents are rapid, sometimes unintelligible speech, frequent repetitions of syllables, words, or phrases, lack of awareness or concern about their speech, disorganized thought processes, and language problems. Cluttering often coexists with stuttering, and both disorders may respond to a highly structured, fluency-shaping approach for treatment. Evaluation and treatment procedures for cluttering are described in Chapter 15.

Neurogenic disfluency in adolescents or adults is usually the result of stroke, head trauma, or neurological disease. Symptoms are likely to be repetitive disfluencies but may include blockages as well. Because stuttering commonly begins in childhood, if a client reports onset of stuttering after age 12, a neurogenic-based disorder is a possibility. In almost all such cases, onsets of neurogenic-based fluency problems are clearly linked to a well-defined episode of neurological damage. A section of Chapter 15 is devoted to evaluation and treatment of neurogenic stuttering.

Disfluency that begins in adolescence or adulthood can also result from psychological trauma. When late-onset disfluencies are seen that are associated with psychological stress and conflict or the onset of a psychiatric condition, psychogenic disfluency should be suspected. Traditional treatments, such as those described in the chapters on treatment of intermediate and advanced stuttering, may or may not be helpful. The patient should be referred for both psychological and neurological assessments, so that treatment needed in these areas will be identified and provided. See Chapter 15 for more information.

When a clinician determines that stuttering treatment would be appropriate for a client, whether the stuttering had a typical onset during early childhood or has another etiology, the focus turns to a consideration of what level of treatment to select for the client. As I indicated earlier, adult and adolescent stutterers are most likely to be at advanced developmental and treatment levels. Signs of this level include the core behaviors of repetitions, prolongations, and blocks, all with tension; the secondary behaviors of escape and avoidance; and negative feelings and attitudes about communication in general and stuttering in particular.

Determining Developmental and Treatment Level

The determination of a developmental/treatment level for an adolescent or adult stutterer is based largely on the client's age. Intermediate and advanced treatment approaches are well suited for clients whose core behaviors are blocks, who have escape and avoidance behaviors as secondary symptoms, and whose attitudes about speech are relatively negative. A client suited to the advanced-level treatment will usually have more entrenched negative attitudes about speech and himself as a speaker simply because he has been stuttering longer. It's possible that someone who is at the advanced level will have developed an extensive repertoire of avoidance behaviors so that actual stuttering behaviors are rare, but the individual's life is highly constrained by his efforts to avoid and hide his stuttering. The major difference between intermediate and advanced treatment levels is that more independence and responsibility are required of clients at the advanced level. Consequently, clinicians ordinarily place adult clients at the advanced level but determine an adolescent's placement based on how much responsibility he can take for self-therapy.

Intermediate Stuttering

A client whose stuttering is at the intermediate level will probably be younger than mid-teens. His stuttering pattern will be characterized by escape and avoidance behaviors and considerable tension on blocks, prolongations, and repetitions. He will also be avoiding some speaking situations. Moreover, his feelings and attitudes, as revealed in questionnaires and interviews with him and with his parents and teachers, will suggest many negative speech attitudes.

Advanced Stuttering

Individuals who fit into the advanced developmental/treatment level are well into their teens and sufficiently mature to handle the assignments used in advanced treatment. Their stuttering pattern is similar to the intermediate stutterer's, but their patterns of avoidance and escape may be more habituated (i.e., patterns appear to be highly automatized and rapidly performed). They will probably avoid difficult speaking situations whenever possible, and I often find strong negative self-concepts and negative anticipations of listener reactions as well. An advanced stutterer may feel, for example, "I must be awfully incompetent to talk like this," or "People think I'm dumb because I stutter."

Closing Interview

I will assume here that the client is a person with developmental stuttering rather than another type of fluency disorder. By this point in the evaluation, I have a pretty good picture of his stuttering and how I will start therapy. I begin by summarizing my impression of his stuttering pattern (i.e., core and secondary behaviors) and his attitudes and feelings. One of my aims is to let him know I have some understanding of his stuttering and why he does what he does when he stutters. I feel it is important to let him know that, given his level of stuttering, it is no surprise that he would use the various secondary behaviors and avoidance tactics that he does. I accept these behaviors rather than criticize them and let him know that I feel I can work with him and help him discover other ways to respond. I try to ensure that he feels he will not be alone, that I will be working alongside him, and that I will gradually give him more and more responsibility to work on his own.

Then, I briefly describe some therapy options and discuss the possibilities with him. With my guidance, the client and I decide on a treatment approach. Afterward, I give him some written suggestions to begin the process of his taking responsibility for part of his treatment. This will also take advantage of the fact that, as indicated earlier, many clients are highly motivated to change at the time they come for an evaluation. I may not do this with adolescents, but there are exceptions. Some adolescent clients are reluctant to participate in therapy rather than being highly motivated because of their desire to close ranks with their peers and distance themselves from adults. With adolescents, I often end our evaluation session by striking a bargain to try at least four sessions of therapy before they make a decision about treatment. I may also give them the booklet, *Do You Stutter: A Guide for Teens* (Fraser & Perkins, 1987), and the video, *Do You Stutter: Straight Talk for Teens* (Guitar & Guitar, 2003), both available from the Stuttering Foundation. These items will help them learn about therapy and develop realistic and motivating expectations about its potential outcome.

If the client has few avoidances and relatively mild stuttering, I am likely to start treatment with fluency shaping. If the client's stuttering is moderate to severe and/or he has relatively many avoidances and fears, I am likely to start with stuttering modification treatment. See the next chapter for an overview of both approaches. An exception that I may make is when a client has many fears and avoidances, but seems unwilling to confront them. I may begin working with this client using fluency shaping. Some clients who are at first unwilling to "touch the hot stove" of stuttering, will be able to confront and change their stuttering if they first get some fluency through fluency shaping.

At the end of the closing interview, I ask a client if he has any questions about the evaluation. I also try to answer the questions asked in the initial interview that I postponed for response until after the evaluation. Adults and adolescents sometimes ask how long treatment will take. This is a reasonable question, given that they need to budget time and money to undertake treatment, but I have no easy answer for this difficult question. With appropriate cautions about individual differences and unexpected issues, I reply that with hard work and a willingness to tackle difficult situations and to confront fears with my help, I believe that considerable progress can be made within a year of the onset of treatment.

SUMMARY

- In evaluating a client who may stutter, your task is to decide
    (1) if his disfluencies warrant treatment,
    (2) if they do, you should also find out more about his history, current environment, speech behaviors, and reactions, as well as
    (3) what treatment seems reasonable given these findings?
- In assessing a preschool child, the important questions to answer are
    (1) whether the child is stuttering or is normally disfluent,
    (2) what the probabilities are that he will recover without treatment, and

(3) if treatment is warranted, you need to determine if indirect (for borderline stuttering) or direct (for beginning stuttering) is best.

- It is important to obtain some information prior to the formal assessment. This includes a recording of the child's speech at home and a completed case history.
- Key elements of the assessment for a preschool child are
  (1) observation of parent-child interaction
  (2) parent interview
  (3) clinician-child interaction
  (4) analysis of child's speech
  (5) screening of language, articulation, and voice
  (6) determining risk factors
  (7) deciding on the child's need for treatment
  (8) making follow-up recommendations to family
- In assessing a school-age child, the important questions are
  (1) how supportive the parents are of the child's problem
  (2) how the stuttering is affecting the child's performance in school
  (3) how the child feels about his stuttering
  (4) how motivated he is to work on it
  (5) how supportive the child's teachers are
- The assessment of the school-age child may proceed differently if he is being seen in a clinic or at school. If seen at school, the IDEA affects the process and mandates how assessment is carried out. If seen in a clinic, the clinician will have more contact with the family but needs to reach out to the school setting.
- Key elements of the assessment for a school-age child are
  (1) initial contact and formal interview with the child's parents
  (2) interview with the child's teachers
  (3) interview with the child
  (4) analysis of speech
  (5) trial therapy
  (6) assessment of other factors, including academic adjustment
  (7) determination of appropriate treatment
- In assessing an adolescent or adult, the important questions are the client's level of motivation and ability to carry out assignments independently, the severity of stuttering and degree of avoidance, the client's feelings and attitudes about his stuttering, whether the problem is typical "developmental" stuttering or is cluttering, psychogenic, or neurogenic stuttering, and the appropriate type of treatment.
- Key elements of the assessment of an adolescent or adult are
  (1) obtaining preliminary case history, attitude questionnaires, and recordings made outside of the clinic
  (2) interviewing the client
  (3) analyzing the client's speech
  (4) conducting trial therapy
  (5) interviewing parents if client is an adolescent

(6) determining appropriate treatment
(7) summarizing findings and making recommendations in closing interview with client.

- Whether the person is to be treated as a normally disfluent speaker or as someone who stutters depends on your interpretation rather than a score. You must weigh what you see and hear to determine whether they indicate stuttering, normal disfluency, or even another disorder. From the flood of information you have gathered, you must extract the essential characteristics that support your choice of treatment.
- To hone your judgment, make evaluations a continuing process. The procedures I have suggested for assessment and diagnosis in this chapter will give you a good start, but stuttering is highly variable, and no individual can be completely evaluated in just an hour or two. Consequently, you will overlook an important element at times, and sometimes a vital clue will not be present in the samples of behavior you see during an initial evaluation. With good ongoing evaluation of a client, you will be able to change decisions and redirect therapy as additional information and understanding become available. You will also be able to evaluate the effectiveness of your treatment and improve it when needed.

STUDY QUESTIONS

1. How do you determine whether a preschool child is stuttering or is normally disfluent?
2. Why is it useful to obtain audio/video recordings of a preschool child's stuttering before the evaluation?
3. What are some indications that a parent of a preschool child who stutters feels she or he is to blame? How can you help the parent deal with those feelings?
4. What do you tell the parent of a preschool or school-age child who asks you what causes stuttering?
5. What are the variables assessed in the speech of a preschooler to determine his developmental/treatment level?
6. What are the advantages and disadvantages of talking to a child about his stuttering?
7. Compare the involvement of the parent and the teacher in the evaluation of a school-age child.
8. In what various ways do we assess the impact of the school environment on the school-age child who stutters?
9. What are the benefits of obtaining both a reading and a conversation sample with school children and adults?
10. In the section on evaluation of the adult and adolescent, what different pieces of information that you may gather from the interview questions help you to assess the client's motivation?
11. What are two reasons we suggest continuing evaluation after the initial assessment of clients who stutter?

12. Compare the assessment of the feelings and attitudes of a school-age child with the assessment in an adult.
13. What is the role of the Individualized Education Program team in the management of a school-age child who stutters?
14. What are the goals of trial therapy?
15. What are the major questions to be answered in the evaluation of an adult?

SUGGESTED PROJECTS

1. Role-play the part of a clinician in a parent interview, having a friend or classmate play the part of a parent. Practice your listening skills by only listening and asking no questions as the "parent" describes in detail his or her child's stuttering problem. Switch roles, then compare your impressions of the experience both as the parent and as the clinician.
2. Pair up with a friend or classmate who could pretend to stutter or with a person who stutters and practice trial therapy that is appropriate for a school-age child and then appropriate for an adult. Try both approaches, modifying stutters to make them less severe and modifying speech to produce fluency.
3. Pair up with a friend or classmate who doesn't stutter, and have them talk rapidly about a complex topic so he or she produces normal disfluencies. See if they are able to "catch" their normal disfluencies and hold onto them (e.g., turn single repetitions into multiple repetitions or make prolongations longer). Can this be done with normal disfluencies? With only certain types of normal disfluencies?
4. Find Web sites on the Internet that contain helpful information for (1) parents of children who stutter, (2) school-age children who stutter, and (3) adults who stutter.
5. One of the challenges for clinicians is to get a good speech sample from a child who may be somewhat shy or reluctant to talk to someone she doesn't know well. Experiment with different ways of interacting with a child until you find a "best" method. For example, try asking lots of questions, try just playing quietly alongside a child, and try playing with a child and making comments about things you are playing with together.

SUGGESTED READINGS

Conture, E. (2001). Assessment and evaluation. In *Stuttering: Its Nature, Diagnosis, and Treatment*. Boston: Allyn & Bacon.

In this chapter, Conture covers many details of the assessment not dealt with in the chapter that you have just read. Among these are finer points of audio and video recording, general interview procedures, and analysis of the speech sample. Conture also discusses concomitant problems like attention deficit hyperactivity disorder, Tourette's syndrome, neuromotor problems, and word finding problems.

Guitar, B. (2010). Stuttering. In M. Augustyn, B. Zuckerman, & E. Coronna (Eds.), *The Zuckerman Parker Handbook of Developmental and Behavioral Pediatrics for Primary Care*. Baltimore: Lippincott Williams & Wilkins.

This brief chapter for pediatricians summarizes key questions and important information for parents, criteria for referral, and initial treatment strategies.

Richels, C., & Conture, E. (2010). Indirect treatment of childhood stuttering: Diagnostic predictors of treatment outcome. In B. Guitar & R. McCauley (Eds.), *Treatment of Stuttering: Established and Emerging Interventions*. Baltimore: Lippincott Williams & Wilkins.

This unique chapter uses the authors' Communication-Emotion Model of Childhood Stuttering as a rationale for their thorough evaluation of a child's speech and language, as well as emotional factors in the child's life. Variables measured before treatment predict short- and long-term outcomes.

Shafir, R. Z. (2000). *The zen of listening: Mindful communication in the age of distraction*. Wheaton, IL: The Theosophical Publishing House.

This is an excellent introduction to the practice of careful listening. Shafir is a speech-language pathologist who has developed her ability to listen to clients and writes eloquently about the healing powers of mindful listening.

Yairi, E., & Ambrose, N. (2005). Assessment of early stuttering. In E. Yairi & N. Ambrose (Eds.), *Early Childhood Stuttering*. Austin, TX: Pro-Ed.

This chapter gives a thorough description, based on assessment experience with hundreds of children, of how to obtain samples and analyze speech of preschool children who stutter. Information regarding prognosis is given by the experts.

Yairi, E., & Ambrose, N. (2005). Parent involvement and counseling. In E. Yairi & N. Ambrose (Eds.), *Early Childhood Stuttering*. Austin, TX: Pro-Ed.

The authors critically review the literature on ways in which parents can be involved in treatment of early childhood stuttering and conclude that there is little evidence to support any of the approaches.

Yaruss, S. (2002). Facing the challenge of treating stuttering in the schools: Part 1. Selecting goals and strategies for success. *Seminars in Speech and Language, 23*, 153–159.

This volume of "Seminars" is a rich source of information for school clinicians. Experienced clinicians, many of whom work in the schools, have written chapters on a wide variety of topics, including interpreting IDEA '97, doing an evaluation in a school setting, and planning therapy for school-age children.

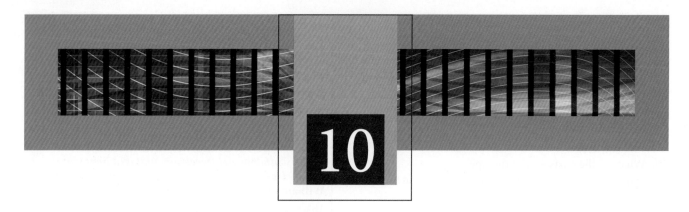

10

Preliminaries to Treatment

Clinician's Attributes
Empathy
Warmth
Genuineness
A Preference for Evidence-Based Practice
A Commitment to Continuing Education
Critical Thinking and Creativity

Clinician's Beliefs

Treatment Goals
Reduce the Frequency of Stuttering
Reduce the Abnormality of Stuttering
Reduce Negative Feelings about Stuttering and about
    Speaking
Reduce Negative Thoughts and Attitudes about
    Stuttering and about Speaking
Reduce Avoidance
Increase Overall Communication Abilities
Create an Environment that Facilitates Fluency

Therapy Procedures
Procedures to Help Clients and Families Deal with Their
    Emotions Associated with Stuttering
Procedures to Reduce the Frequency of Stuttering
Procedures to Reduce the Abnormality of Stuttering
Procedures to Reduce Negative Thoughts and Attitudes
    about Stuttering and Speaking
Procedures to Reduce Avoidance
Procedures to Increase Overall Communication
    Abilities
Procedures to Create an Environment that Facilitates
    Fluency
Motor Learning Principles for Treatment

CHAPTER OBJECTIVES

After studying this chapter, readers should be able to:
- Understand the most important attributes of an effective
  stuttering clinician
- Understand how the clinician's beliefs about the nature and
  development of stuttering affect her choices about treatment
  procedures at different ages
- Understand what important goals are for stuttering therapy
  and how they may vary depending on the client's age
- Understand the therapy procedures used to meet the goals
  selected for a client's treatment

KEY TERMS

Therapy protocol: A detailed plan for carrying out
treatment
Empathy: Ability to put oneself in another's place and to
identify with the feelings that the other person has
Warmth: A feeling of positive regard for another person,
often conveyed by tone of voice or body language
Genuineness: Honesty about life, oneself, and other people;
a sense that the individual is comfortable with herself and
speaks in a straightforward manner in which actions are
congruent with thoughts, beliefs, and attitudes
Evidence-based practice: A commitment to use research
evidence, client goals, and clinician expertise when choosing assessment and treatment tools
Critical thinking: An attitude of mind that encourages
questioning; in the current context, the questioning is about
whether a treatment will be effective for a particular client
Clinician's beliefs: The perspective a clinician takes on
the nature and development of stuttering that leads to her
choices of assessment and treatment strategies

Abnormality of stuttering: Characteristics of an individual's stuttering that make it stand out or be distracting to the listener. Examples are facial tension and facial grimacing, body movements used to release the stutter, and avoidances that make it difficult for the listener to follow what the individual is saying such as "well, um, you see, that is…"

Fluency-facilitating environment: A climate in one or more situations that makes it easier for an individual who stutters to speak more fluently

Emotions related to stuttering: Physiological responses and conscious feelings that arise in a person who stutters, in regard to the act of stuttering or the fact of being someone who stutters

Cognitive behavior therapy (CBT): Treatment based on the notion that persons' perceptions of and thoughts about situations and themselves determine their feelings and behavior. CBT aims to help the persons see situations and themselves more realistically and more compassionately

Before presenting the details of treatment in the next four chapters, I want to provide some background for the **therapy protocols** you can use, as well as how and why you use them. First, I'll describe important attributes of the clinician who works with people who stutter and how his beliefs about the nature of stuttering influence treatment decisions. Then I'll discuss commonly held goals for stuttering therapy and finally the procedures to meet them.

CLINICIAN'S ATTRIBUTES

The clinician is probably the most important ingredient in stuttering therapy other than the client. A clinician's knowledge, skills, and personality have a major influence on outcome. This is true whether therapy's major focus is to change behaviors, thoughts, or feelings—or some combination of these. In this section, I discuss some of the attributes that I think make a clinician effective, and I suggest how these can be developed. Unfortunately, there are no data that I'm aware of to support the importance of these attributes for stuttering therapy. In the field of psychotherapy, Carl Rogers (1961) and others have spent a considerable amount of time and effort measuring the effects of some of these clinician attributes on treatment success. In the field of stuttering treatment, Manning (2010) and Zebrowski (2007) have excellent chapters on the role of the clinician and the importance of the clinical relationship.

Much of my thinking about the treatment process has been influenced by my experiences as a client and later as a student of Charles Van Riper. He was a master clinician of stuttering therapy. Let us begin then with Van Riper's (1975a) description of three important clinician characteristics: empathy, warmth, and genuineness.

Empathy

Empathy, in this context, is the ability to understand the feelings, thoughts, and behaviors of someone who stutters. You might think that this is a little easier for clinicians who stutter. However, Van Riper's own clinician, Bryng Bryngleson, was a fluent speaker who showed an impressive understanding of individuals who stutter. Once, Bryngleson assigned Van Riper the task of voluntarily stuttering to 10 strangers, but he was unable to carry it out. Exhausted from trying again and again and failing over and over, he sought out Bryngleson in his office. Bryng, as he was called, jumped up from his chair and headed for the door, saying, "It's OK, Van, just follow me and watch." Bryng then went into a nearby tobacco store, walked up to the clerk, and pretended to stutter—with the longest, loudest stutter that Van Riper had ever heard, causing the clerk to cower behind the counter. Van Riper was astounded. That single demonstration by his clinician had a huge impact on Van Riper. He felt deeply supported by Bryngleson's acceptance of his failure and Bryngleson's willingness to risk ridicule to help him. Remember this when you wonder how to show your empathy.

You can also develop empathy with all your clients by working on your ability to listen deeply and acceptingly. It will help to observe body language, posture, and the words they use. Van Riper said that he could improve his understanding of a client's feelings if he assumed the same body posture that the client had. You can also get some idea of what clients experience by going out in public like Bryngleson did and stuttering voluntarily, though you don't have to stutter as long or as loud as Bryng did. Reading stories written by people who stutter and parents of children who stutter will also help you better understand the experiences that have shaped their feelings. Good examples of such writings are *Living With Stuttering* (St. Louis, 2001) and *Forty Years after Therapy: One Man's Story* (Helliesen, 2002). I describe these books and others in the suggested readings at the end of this chapter.

Warmth

This attribute has also been referred to as "unconditional positive regard" (Rogers, 1957). Much of it is conveyed in the tone of voice, facial expression, and body language of the clinician. Clients whose clinicians demonstrate **warmth** feel accepted, liked, and nurtured. Warmth creates an environment that supports learning and helps clients make difficult changes. Warmth is also expressed in the comments the clinician makes when a client has done something well. This is sometimes harder than you think. It surprises me when I watch a videotape of one of my therapy sessions, how many opportunities I miss reinforcing the client with a "Good!" or "Well done!" Therefore, I try to watch videos of myself working with a client to discover things that I need to work on. Although it is initially painful for all of us to watch video recordings of ourselves, this is one of the best ways we can improve. Clinicians should become aware of how much or how little enthusiasm they show and warm encouragement they give to their clients. These are important tools of therapy.

Genuineness

A third characteristic of good clinicians that Van Riper (1975a) described is "**genuineness**," which he equated with Rogers's (1961) "congruence." Both terms refer to a clinician's honesty and self-acceptance. She just tries to be who she is, "roughness, pimples, warts, and everything" as Oliver Cromwell said on having his portrait painted. Genuineness allows clinicians to be honest with their clients, not sugarcoating the hard lumps of reality that must be swallowed if real progress is to be made.

For example, Van Riper said to one of his clients with his characteristic bluntness, "Why do you have to have all that junk in your speech? Can't you just go ahead and say the word, starting with the first sound and working your way through it slowly, syllable by syllable?" (Van Riper, 1975b). When a client senses the clinician's genuineness, he gains trust and begins to believe that his clinician means it when she asks about his thoughts and feelings that he can let go and honestly express his frustration, fear, hate, and anger, convinced that the clinician will understand and accept him and his feelings, and be strong enough to be unhurt by them. Clinicians can cultivate their genuineness and strength by being open about their limitations and learning self-acceptance through psychotherapy, spiritual practice, or other experiences that help them accept both their weaknesses and their strengths.

A Preference for Evidence-Based Practice

There are more traits than those three listed above that characterize good clinicians. One is a clinician's desire and ability to base her clinical practice on evidence of its effectiveness, called **evidence-based practice**. In choosing tools and approaches for evaluating and treating someone who stutters, a clinician who wishes to grow looks for evidence of the effectiveness and appropriateness of treatment approaches she is using or considering. She works together with the client or family in the diagnostic evaluation to determine which treatment approach is likely to meet the client's or family's goals most effectively. She measures the client's progress during treatment to assess whether this approach is working with this person. She is flexible, creative, and insightful enough to find ways of altering treatment if it is not working. Many treatments, including some described in this text, have relatively little published data that support their

effectiveness. For example, my approaches to school-age children and adolescents/adults have been derived from years of experimenting, and only now have I developed enough consistency to start collecting data to be disseminated. This does not preclude their being used, but a clinician should be careful to assess how well they work for *her* clients with measures made before, during, and after treatment. In addition, for those clinicians who find them very effective, obtaining research evidence on them to share with others would represent a valuable contribution to the field. Ideas and information on evidence-based practice can be found in Bothe (2004), Frattali (1998), Guitar (2004), Guitar and McCauley (2010), Piertranton (2003), and Sackett, Straus, Richardson, Rosenberg, and Haynes (2000). The American Speech-Language-Hearing Association (ASHA) has provided member access to useful tutorials on evidence-based practice at http://www.asha.org/Members/ebp/web-tutorial/.

An interesting example of an early attempt at evidence-based practice is the data that Van Riper (1958) kept as he experimented with different forms of treatment for stuttering. He attempted to write down in detail what variations he made with his treatment protocols each year and reassessed his clients five years after they had finished therapy. Although he admits his methods are not perfect, the chapter in which he presents 20 years of experiments in stuttering treatment is a fine example of evidence-based clinical practice for its time, some 55 years ago. In this spirit, in the treatment chapters that follow, I suggest ways in which clinicians today can measure client progress.

A Commitment to Continuing Education

Another important attribute for clinicians is the habit of continually updating knowledge gained in graduate school. New methods of evaluation and treatment are developed every year, and new data on treatment effectiveness become available. It is vital for the clinician to keep up to date with the latest and best practices. Journals are the best source of this information, but recent editions of books that review diagnostic and treatment methods for stuttering can also be helpful. New approaches to treatment often require training. Short courses at the annual ASHA convention and workshops offered through schools, hospitals, state associations, and other institutions are excellent sources of such training. However, before adopting a new approach, a clinician should critically analyze the quality of evidence that supports its claim to effectiveness.

Critical Thinking and Creativity

Clinicians should become discriminating consumers and ask, "Which new diagnostic tools and treatment approaches are effective, and which clients are they appropriate for?" This demonstrates **critical thinking**. Some new approaches are not all they are cracked up to be. For example, many years ago, a well-known psychologist and his colleagues (Azrin & Nunn, 1974) suggested that teaching clients simply to take a breath and relax before speaking was an effective treatment for stuttering. Researchers at another clinic tested the approach and found it to be far less effective in their clinic than its developers had suggested (Andrews & Tanner, 1982). Nevertheless, there may be some aspects of relaxation and breathing that are useful for some clients in the hands of a clinician who becomes skilled at integrating these tools into a broader approach.

Another critical question is "Will this approach work for my clients in my environment?" Often a treatment that works under laboratory conditions with carefully selected subjects does not work as well in the real world of a public school, for example. But a clinician may be able to adapt an approach to suit her situation. For instance, an approach developed for very young children in tightly controlled clinical studies with total fluency as its goal may need to be altered so that some degree of easy and open stuttering is an acceptable outcome when used with older children.

CLINICIAN'S BELIEFS

It is important for clinicians to weigh their beliefs about the nature of stuttering against the available data, then develop clinical procedures compatible with the **clinician's beliefs**—procedures supported by data, ideally data collected by the clinician as well as others. My own beliefs about the etiology and development of stuttering that were presented in the first few chapters are reviewed here only in enough detail to illustrate the relationship between beliefs and treatment procedures. I believe that predisposing physiological factors interact with developmental and environmental influences to produce or exacerbate core behaviors that often (but not always) begin as repetitions. When some children experience these early disfluencies as frustrating and/or embarrassing, they increase the amount of physical tension and speed they use when experiencing disfluency. This then creates for these children secondary or coping behaviors as well as negative feelings and attitudes. They learn escape behaviors through instrumental conditioning, speech fears through classical conditioning, and word and situation avoidances through avoidance conditioning. All of these factors and how they contribute to stuttering are reflected in the stages of development I described in Chapter 7.

How does this point of view about the etiology and development of stuttering affect treatment? Let's use the management of school-age children who stutter to illustrate this point. In my view, a child's treatment plan is determined by his developmental level of stuttering, and each advance in level requires new components in treatment. A first grader with beginning stuttering who is not embarrassed or afraid to talk and who doesn't avoid talking requires a different treatment than a fifth grader with intermediate-level stuttering who has developed fears and avoidances in response to his stuttering. In my view, the first grader may be treated with an approach that focuses on increasing fluency and deals only minimally with negative feelings and avoidance behaviors. On the other hand, the fifth grader needs help to reduce the tension and struggle *and* the fears and avoidances. In contrast to these ideas about treatment, a clinician who doesn't believe that fears and avoidances are crucial in understanding and treatment of stuttering might treat both children with the same approach.

Another way in which a clinician's beliefs can affect management is in the assessment procedures she uses. Assessment tools should provide clinicians with information that is essential for planning treatment and measuring progress. In evaluating the children described above, I would evaluate each child's feelings and attitudes about his speech, as well as his use of word and situation avoidances, to accurately determine each child's developmental/treatment level and decide which aspects of the problem to focus on first. Another clinician—for example one who is atheoretical or unconcerned about the etiology and development of stuttering—might simply want to measure each child's frequency and severity of stuttering.

A third way in which a clinician's beliefs about the nature, development, and treatment of stuttering can affect clinical behavior relates to how she counsels the parents of her clients. In counseling the parents of these two school-age children, my beliefs would guide me to describe the etiology of stuttering as being unknown at present, but probably related to the way a child's brain processes speech and language. Using terminology appropriate to the parents, I would talk about brain processing that may predispose a child to stutter, and I would emphasize that this suggests that parents don't cause stuttering. I would also explain that the child's way of processing speech and language can be changed, which means that parents can be vital in helping a child overcome or manage his stuttering. I would also discuss with parents the importance of factors in the environment that might be contributing to the child's stuttering problem and discuss ways of modifying these factors. Lastly, I would use my understanding of the development and nature of stuttering to give parents a general idea of the course of therapy and possible outcome. Clinicians with other beliefs might not go into the nature of stuttering because they feel it is not well-understood and would instead just counsel the parents about their role in the child's treatment.

TREATMENT GOALS

Treatment goals will vary with a clinician's beliefs, the client's age, and the developmental/treatment level of his stuttering. Nonetheless, it is still possible to describe most of the goals that clinicians have for clients who stutter and to suggest which goals are likely to be paramount for which level. Individuals differ in their strengths and weaknesses at the outset of treatment, and these change as treatment proceeds. Thus, a clinician needs to ask herself: "What does this client need? What does he need from me? What does he need from me right now? And why?" (Van Riper, 1975a, p. 477).

As I have said earlier, the clinician is not the only one who determines the goals of treatment. Clients and their families have an important role to play in choosing goals that are paramount for them. Ongoing discussions between clinicians and clients about treatment goals strengthen clients' motivation to achieve them and enhance the relationship between clients and clinicians. The following statement by Donald Baer (1990), an eminent behavioral psychologist, expresses this philosophy.

> "It seems only reasonable to learn that when stutterers are given control of the therapeutic consequences that presumably can change their output, some of them choose different targets than would their therapists or, probably, other stutterers, and some of them target not so much their speech output as they do a private response that they describe as sense of 'imminent loss of control.'" (p. 35)

The selection of goals presented in this section owes much to the *Guidelines for Practice in Stuttering Treatment* (American Speech-Language-Hearing Association, 1995)

Reduce the Frequency of Stuttering

This can be achieved in a variety of ways, but it is important to reduce the frequency of stuttering without creating other behaviors, such as taking deep breaths before speaking that may be distracting to the listener (and speaker) and may therefore hamper communication. This goal is appropriate for all ages and levels of stuttering; note that for preschool children, the goal should be to reduce frequency of stuttering to essentially zero.

Reduce the Abnormality of Stuttering

I think much of the **abnormality of stuttering** comes from the conditioned tension and struggle behaviors that occur during moments of stuttering. It shows up as squeezing of facial muscles as the person is trying to say a word that is blocked. Reducing this tension and struggle is an important goal for school-age, adolescent, and adult clients. In addition, behaviors that occur before the stutter (avoidance) and behaviors that are deployed to terminate the stutter (escape) should be eliminated or at least greatly diminished. These include (1) avoidance behaviors such as the repetition of the sound "uh" before saying a word, and (2) escape behaviors such as eye blinks and head nods used to terminate a block. For some school-age children and older clients, it may not be possible to eliminate their stuttering.

Instead, the stuttering can be changed so that it is easy and comfortable both for the speaker and the listener and doesn't interfere with communication. Van Riper and other experienced stuttering clinicians have suggested that a stutterer may not always have a choice *whether* he stutters but he does have a choice about *how* he stutters. This choice includes stuttering in a way that is easier and briefer than his old habitual pattern. This new way of stuttering reduces fear because it feels and sounds more like normal speech and is often unnoticed by the listener. Once the person has confidence in his ability to stutter this easily, he is less likely to increase muscle tension in response to an actual or anticipated stutter.

Reduce Negative Feelings about Stuttering and about Speaking

Many individuals who stutter appear to have a temperament that is sensitive and somewhat perfectionistic. They are thus vulnerable to feelings of embarrassment, fear, shame, and other negative feelings associated with their stuttering. A cycle can develop in which stuttering gives rise to negative feelings, which in turn increase tension and other struggle behaviors, which then generate more negative feelings. Classical conditioning plays a major role in this cycle. Therefore treatment strategies to deal with classically conditioned behaviors, such as deconditioning and counterconditioning, are crucial in treatment. These and related strategies are discussed in the chapters that describe treatment of school-age children, adolescents, and adults. Reducing negative feelings is an important goal for many clients beyond age 6 or 7, although a few school-age children and even older clients may not have strong negative feelings about being someone who stutters. They may, however, have feelings of frustration about their impediment to speaking easily. Most of these feelings can be changed significantly—either directly or indirectly—through treatments that give the client repeated experiences with effective communication and ease of speaking. One major difference among treatment approaches is whether they deal with clients' negative feelings and emotions directly or indirectly.

Reduce Negative Thoughts and Attitudes about Stuttering and about Speaking

In the chapter on the development of stuttering, I described how people who stutter may acquire negative self-concepts through repeated experiences of stuttering and perceiving—sometimes correctly and sometimes incorrectly—that listeners are impatient or disapproving. As these perceptions become more and more deeply ingrained, they begin to affect a stutterer's expectations in speaking situations. This can lead to more stuttering. If a stutterer expects rejection or disapproval, he may try very hard not to let the stuttering out by adopting fixed, tense articulatory postures that trigger blockages. These are often devastating to the individual who stutters and make him feel helpless and out of control. This then "snowballs" downhill, gathering speed, from negative thoughts to more stuttering to more negative thoughts, on and on. This avalanche of events is at the heart of much chronic stuttering.

Good treatment can roll the snowball back uphill. Clients can be toughened up (desensitized) to the experience of stuttering, decreasing their fears and negative expectations. They can also be shown how to say their feared words without as much struggle. As a result, they will approach speaking opportunities with more relaxed speech muscles and find themselves stuttering more easily or not stuttering at all. This in turn will lead to more positive expectations, which can lead to easier or less stuttering; thus a positive cycle begins to replace the negative one that preceded it.

A different approach is to give the client repeated experiences of being fluent—in many situations, with increasing linguistic and social demands over a relatively long period of time and with much success and little failure. The aim is to replace expectations of stuttering with expectations of fluency. Somehow, through habit change accompanying changes in how the brain produces speech, good quality normal fluency can be established and maintained. This seems to work best, in my experience, with younger clients and when used with adults, with those individuals who have few avoidance behaviors. For those with much avoidance, the strategies described below can help.

Reduce Avoidance

Avoidance behaviors, as you will remember, are evasive maneuvers taken by individuals to keep from stuttering. Sometimes they may occur very close in time to the expected stutter, such as saying "um" or "well" just before attempting to say a feared word. Other times they may be quite separated in time from the expected stuttering, such as *not* volunteering to be in a school play or by driving 20 miles to talk to someone rather than telephoning her. Some stutterers may have an innate predisposition to avoid because of their temperaments, as described in Chapters 2 to 6. Avoidances keep stuttering "hot," because they prevent an individual from learning that it is possible to stutter in an easy fashion and communicate well. Reducing avoidance is usually not the first treatment goal on the list, although it may be one of the most important goals for more advanced levels of stuttering. Usually, before helping clients reduce avoidances, clinicians need to help them reduce negative emotions about stuttering and teach them to stutter more easily. Reducing avoidances is a major goal for older children and adults, but again, some approaches work indirectly by giving them tools to increase fluency, which then, one hopes, reduces fear and thus decreases avoidances.

Increase Overall Communication Abilities

The ability to communicate easily and well varies a great deal from client to client. It may be affected by severity of stuttering, temperament, avoidances, and communication models in the family. For many of us who work with individuals who stutter, effective communication is an important treatment goal. Some clients will become good communicators once the frequency and severity of their stuttering, along with their negative feelings and attitudes about speaking and stuttering, have been reduced. For other clients, guided practice and structured experiences in communication are essential. Once clients feel they can communicate easily, they often begin to seek out talking experiences, their avoidances drop away, and they become comfortable and open about any remaining stuttering that occurs. The goal of effective communication is most needed for older children and adults who have developed avoidances. Many of these clients, especially those with more severe stuttering, have been preoccupied with their stuttering and not spent much time learning to communicate effectively (Curlee, personal communication, March 3, 2004). They may still have hesitancies and a herky-jerky style of speaking that lacks the fluidity of normally fluent speech.

Create an Environment that Facilitates Fluency

This goal is paramount for working with young children who can often be treated by helping the family reduce pressures on the child's speech and increase positive aspects of the child's speaking environment to create a **fluency-facilitating environment**. For example, family members can spend one-on-one time with the child, using a slow speech rate and careful listening skills, thereby increasing the child's daily opportunities to experience fluency. The child's environment may be made more positive through praise and appreciation of his fluent speech and/or his other accomplishments. This goal of improving the child's speaking environment may also be important for school-age children. However, teachers and aides, as well as family members, need to be enlisted in facilitating the child's fluency. Older clients can make their environments facilitating to both fluency and easy stuttering by being open about their stuttering and sharing with others how listeners can be most helpful to them.

THERAPY PROCEDURES

The aim of this section is to outline the tools and strategies that clinicians can use to work on each of the treatment goals described above. By understanding which procedures are most likely to be useful in achieving each goal, clinicians can select those procedures that best suit each client and are in accord with their own beliefs. The procedures outlined here are fully described in the therapy sections on each developmental/treatment level.

My belief about stuttering treatment is that the emotions associated with stuttering must be understood and dealt with if therapy is to be successful. Therefore, I begin discussing procedures with a substantial discussion of how the clinician is involved in this process.

Procedures to Help Clients and Families Deal with Their Emotions Associated with Stuttering

In many books, this section might be called "counseling" but I prefer to describe this process as working with **emotions related to stuttering**. The clinician's attributes of empathy, warmth, and genuineness are vital to dealing with the emotions that can impede changes in stuttering and to fostering the emotional processes that can foster recovery. Although there are similarities in how the clinician responds to the parents of a child who stutters and how she helps older children and adults, there are enough differences that I describe them separately.

In working with preschoolers, working with the child's family is paramount. The family must develop faith not only in the clinician's abilities but also in her understanding and acceptance of their feelings. In the initial meetings, the family is likely to feel anxious because they have watched their child struggle, for weeks or even months, not knowing how to help him. The clinician must listen with care to how the parents (or other family members) describe the child's stuttering, his response to it, and their own responses to it. Listening to their feelings throughout the course of treatment will provide support for the family and will convey the all-important idea that they and the clinician form a team working together to help the child. As the clinician listens, she acknowledges their feelings, sometimes restating them to make sure she understands. She refrains from simple reassurance, but instead, when appropriate, shows them evidence that the child is making progress, shares information about recovery, or helps them realize all the positive things the child has going for him. This should be done, not instead of, but in addition to, acknowledgment of feelings they may express—sometimes of frustration, discouragement, and guilt, and sometimes of hope and pride. In summary, in working with young children and their families, the clinician must be aware that the family's emotions can be a part of the reason that stuttering may worsen after onset and that treatment can reverse this.

In treating clients older than preschoolers, the clinician works more with the client directly, rather than his family. The clinician's role—in helping the client deal with emotions—is to create an atmosphere in which the client feels more and more comfortable expressing feelings. These feelings may include shame and fear, and sometimes anger toward the stuttering, the clinician, and listeners. Such feelings should be accepted as normal emotions that occur when a person has stuttered for a number of years and has experienced listeners' impatience, rejection, or even teasing.

In the early stages of therapy, as the client learns more about his own stuttering, the clinician's genuine interest and curiosity about the stuttering have the potential to counteract the negative feelings the client may have—expressed or unexpressed—toward his stuttering. The goal is for the client to accept his stuttering and take responsibility for changing it. For this to happen, the clinician must show her acceptance of it. Another goal is to help the client build up tolerance to the frustration and the fear of being stuck. This must be achieved in order to reduce tension and struggle. Activities to accomplish this include stuttering openly, without avoidances, and stuttering voluntarily on nonfeared words. These activities usually cause an increase in emotion, giving the clinician an opportunity to help the client explore and accept his feelings. The clinician simply asks the client how he's feeling about doing these tasks, listens attentively, and doesn't ask the client to work on his stuttering as he talks about feelings.

The next goal is for the client to learn to stop rewarding the old struggle behaviors. This is done by progressively changing the form of stuttering from tense and rapid to loose and slow. To help the client do this, some clinicians teach what are called cancellations, pull-outs, and preparatory sets, which are explained more fully later. As this goal is being worked on, many emotions and resistances usually arise, and these are opportunities for the clinician to help the client express them, explore them, and accept them. Previously, the client may have been afraid of listeners' reactions to his stuttering; now he may be afraid of listeners' reactions (real or imagined) to his managing his speech by slowing his speech rate, using easy onsets of phonation, or prolonging stutters beyond the moment when they can be released. These are things that the client may have to do to reduce tension and struggle, but they are often hard to do with friends, family, or strangers. The clinician can help the client learn that by and large, listeners respect a person who is openly working on his challenges. And when listeners are impatient, anxious, or rejecting, it is because they have their own issues, and the client can learn to tolerate and transcend these reactions.

There is a rhythm to treatment of older children and adults who stutter. The clinician guides the client to carry out various tasks. Before, during, or after carrying them out, the client feels various emotions that are related to the stuttering and to changing it. The clinician helps the client express these emotions, and together they accept them, then move on to work on the next step together. The clinician's role in this process has been described in this way:

"(People who stutter) need a permissive figure to whom they can ventilate their anxieties and frustrations. They need a companion who can share their difficulties in communication without becoming punitive or upset. They need someone to point out a possible pathway out of communicative deviancy and who will stay with them even when they fail. They will learn all they need to about themselves by working with their stuttering. Perhaps what we are saying is that the stutterer needs a very good teacher rather than a psychiatrist." (Van Riper, 1958, p. 381)

Procedures to Reduce the Frequency of Stuttering

Operant conditioning procedures are often part of treatment approaches for achieving this goal and typically involve reinforcement for fluency and mild punishment for stuttering. Rewards may be verbal, such as the clinician's praise or approval, or tangible, such as tokens that can be redeemed for snacks, prizes, or an opportunity to take a turn in a game. Mild punishment may simply be calling attention to a stutter or requesting the individual to try the word again. Rewards for fluency and mild punishment for stuttering can be the primary tools used for beginning stuttering and are often coupled with a hierarchy based on the complexity and length of utterances. In this case, clients move from producing one or two words fluently through longer phrases to spontaneous speech. Reward and punishment may also be used as "shaping" tools for intermediate or advanced-level stuttering, in which clients begin by speaking in a way that produces instant fluency, such as speaking very slowly, and then progressing to more and more normal-sounding speech in more and more difficult situations. This approach—sometimes called "prolonged speech"—was foreshadowed in remarks by Francis Bacon in the late 1700s (Siegel, 2007). Here are Bacon's words quoted by James Boswell:

> "In all kinds of speech, either pleasant, grave, severe, or ordinary, it is convenient to speak leisurely, and rather drawlingly than hastily: because hasty speech confounds the memory, and oftentimes, besides the unseemliness, drives a man either to stammering, a non-plus, or harping on that which should follow; whereas a slow speech confirmeth the memory, addeth a conceit of wisdom to the hearers, besides a seemliness of speech and confidence." (Boswell, 1791)

The general term for treatments such as prolonged speech that focus on increasing fluency rather than decreasing the abnormality of stuttering is "fluency shaping."

Procedures to Reduce the Abnormality of Stuttering

These procedures are appropriate for clients who have developed struggle, tension, escape, and avoidance behaviors that make their stuttering stand out as abnormal to the listener and the client himself. Therapies that target the abnormality of stuttering often use reward and mild punishment to change long, tense stutters into increasingly briefer and more relaxed ones and to diminish clients' use of escape and avoidance behaviors. To meet this goal, reward and punishment are often accompanied by a systematic program for reducing negative emotions. Such programs are founded on the belief that negative emotions elicit increased tension, escape, and avoidance behaviors and that these behaviors are maintained by the fact that they are rewarded when the stutterer finally gets the word out by squeezing and pushing on it. These approaches are often referred to as "stuttering modification."

A classic stuttering modification approach is that of Van Riper (1958, 1973, 1975b), which begins first by reducing negative emotions through objective study of the stuttering, then focuses on desensitization to the frustration and embarrassment of it. Next, the clinician teaches the client to self-correct his stuttering after a stutter, then during a stutter, then before the stutter occurs. Stuttering modification and fluency shaping often result in a modified style of speaking, which contains brief disfluencies which are produced in a slightly slower than normal way of talking.

Some therapy approaches—both fluency-shaping approaches for older children and adults as well as therapy approaches for preschoolers—don't aim to reduce the abnormality of the stuttering behavior directly, but instead focus on increasing fluency with the assumption that as fluency increases, stuttering diminishes to negligible levels.

Procedures to Reduce Negative Thoughts and Attitudes about Stuttering and Speaking

There are a number of therapy procedures that can help clients become more realistic about how listeners perceive them and what this may mean to them. Cognitive therapy, for example, can be an excellent technique for helping clients think and feel more positively about their speech, listeners, and the situations that have elicited negative emotions in the past. Clients can learn to examine their thought processes and understand how what they *think* influences what they *feel* and how they *act*, particularly in regard to such maladaptive behavior as muscular tensing that leads to more stuttering. Some clinicians use **cognitive behavior therapy** as their sole treatment and others as a supplement to techniques for learning to speak fluently or to stutter in an easier way. The book, *Cognitive Therapy: Basics and Beyond* (Beck, 1995), is a good source for learning this approach, and I discuss cognitive therapy in the chapter on advanced stuttering. An excellent introduction to this approach with stuttering are two Stuttering Foundation DVDs entitled *Tools for Success: A Cognitive Behavior Therapy Taster and Implementing*

Cognitive Behavior Therapy with School-Age Children (www. stutteringhelp.org).

Procedures to Reduce Avoidance

Some clients have very little avoidance, and once they learn to speak fluently, they enter speaking situations freely without expectation of difficulty. Others, however, because of temperament, learning, or both, have a strong tendency for avoidance. Only minor avoidances may appear in beginning stuttering, but it is a problem that must almost certainly be addressed at the intermediate and advanced levels. Treatment to reduce avoidance should begin by reducing negative emotions, particularly fears of stuttering and of listeners' reactions. Fear of stuttering can be tackled by rewarding clients with praise, support, or tangible reinforcement for "catching" a stutter and holding onto it. Fear of listeners' reactions can be lessened by clients' voluntarily stuttering to acquaintances and strangers. When a stutterer can deliberately imitate his typical stuttering pattern and pretend to stutter, he finally feels in control during a stutter; this and the feeling of "stuttering" while also feeling in control is highly rewarding.

Reducing fear is not enough, however. Studies of animal behavior have shown that, even when avoidance symptoms disappear after fear is reduced, fear eventually returns and so do its symptoms—conditioned avoidance behaviors (Ayres, 1998). Thus, new responses to the old stimuli must be taught. In stuttering therapy, an example of learning a new response to an old stimulus is for a stutterer to slow his speech rate as he says a word he expects to stutter on. This is an aspect of the "preparatory set" used in many stuttering modification approaches, as well as the "downshifting" to a slower rate before attempting a difficult word, taught in fluency-shaping programs.

Avoidances are not confined to the moment just before a difficult word. Individuals who stutter may also avoid opportunities to speak by pretending to be busy when the telephone rings or by waiting for someone else to make introductions of new acquaintances. These avoidances can be treated by helping a client construct a hierarchy of easy-to-difficult speaking situations, in which he can use newly learned stuttering modification or fluency-shaping techniques. Clinicians can also motivate clients to continue seeking out new situations in which they can be open about their stuttering and can use their new strategies to manage stuttering. At meetings of the SpeakEasy Associations of Australia and the United States and conventions of the National Stuttering Association, there are always impressive testimonials by clients who have sought out public speaking opportunities, joined Toastmasters (an international organization of people who want to practice public speaking), or found other ways of increasing their approach behaviors and decreasing their tendency to avoid stuttering and speaking.

Procedures to Increase Overall Communication Abilities

For many children, adolescents, and adults, communication blossoms when fears of stuttering and listeners' reactions are reduced, and ease of speaking is increased. For others, longstanding habits of avoiding speaking situations and the accompanying lack of social experience have stunted the growth of their communication skills. For still others, concomitant problems, such as attention deficit or extreme shyness, may have prevented them from learning how to communicate well. Communication skills should be addressed in treatment whenever it appears that they are not appropriately developed. Observations of a client's communication and reports from a school-age child's teachers will indicate the areas that may need to be addressed. Specific skills that can be worked on include eye contact, turn taking, maintaining a topic, making relevant contributions to conversation, speaking intelligibly, clarifying and repairing what was said, and developing a willingness to initiate and maintain communicative interactions with others (Kent, 1993; Smith, McCauley, & Guitar, 2000). Although these skills can be worked on individually, group therapy provides excellent opportunities for clients to practice them. Direct instruction, modeling, role-playing, and video-recorded feedback with discussion can be used to teach and refine communication skills.

Procedures to Create an Environment that Facilitates Fluency

Preschool-age children, especially those on the borderline between normal disfluency and stuttering, may need only a little change in their environments for their stuttering to disappear permanently (Starkweather, Gottwald, & Halfond, 1990). Treatment focuses on parents: counseling them to reduce their anxieties, modeling for them, and continuing to support the changes they make. Parent-child interactions are usually the key element of the environment that can be changed to facilitate fluency. Video recordings and playback of these interactions in the clinic or observations at home, coupled with parent counseling, can help parents improve how they communicate with their child (Guitar, Kopff-Schaefer, Donahue-Kilburg, & Bond, 1992). Parents usually work on creating a facilitating environment during brief, one-on-one daily sessions with the child. In some families, other aspects of the environment may need to be changed, such as the home's hurried pace of life, stressful life events, and the communication styles of other family members. Older preschoolers may also benefit from a direct approach, involving contingencies for fluent speech and stuttering.

For school-age children, the creation of facilitating environments may include working with the child's family, but the school setting may be equally important, if not more so.

Clinicians often work in partnership with a child or adolescent to make school a "fluency-friendly" environment. The clinician may arrange meetings with the child and his teachers to improve the teachers' understanding of his stuttering and to open lines of communication between the child and teachers. A child's peers can be invited to treatment so that they may improve their understanding of the child's stuttering, while the process of the child's openness about his stuttering with other children is begun. Freely discussing his stuttering with other students is one of the most powerful ways for a school-age child to make his environment more fluency-friendly. For some children, a powerful boost can be given to therapy's progress if they are able, with the clinician's help and support, to make a presentation to their class about the nature of stuttering in general and their stuttering in particular.

Openness about stuttering is also a major way in which adults can create a supportive environment. By commenting on their stuttering, by showing a sense of humor about it, and by sharing what techniques they're working on, adults who stutter can create environments in which their listeners are quite comfortable with the adults' stuttering. This helps them feel free to use various fluency-enhancing techniques.

My own treatment for each age and the treatments of several other clinicians are presented in the next four chapters. Descriptions of the other clinicians' approaches include their beliefs about the nature and development of stuttering as well as rationales for their choice of goals and procedures to treat each level. Both my own approaches and those of other clinicians have been developed and refined, usually over several years' of trial and error. When possible, supporting data are provided for each treatment, but in many cases, where such data are not available, I suggest what data would be appropriate to gather.

Motor Learning Principles for Treatment

Most of our treatments involve working with the client in a relatively structured environment for a short period of time and then hoping for generalization to an unstructured environment between treatment sessions. The motor learning literature—cogently summarized by Verdolini and Lee (2004)—suggests that certain principles must be followed for generalization to take place. Table 10.1 summarizes some of their ideas and suggests how they might apply to the treatment of stuttering.

Table 10.1	Principles of Motor Learning and Their Applications to the Treatment of Stuttering
Principles of Motor Learning (Verdolini & Lee, 2004)	**Application to Stuttering Treatment**
In the first stages of motor learning, feedback is important, but then the client must evaluate his own performance for long-term change.	When teaching a technique such as easy onsets or pullouts, the clinician should let the client know when he has done well, but gradually diminish feedback and replace it with asking client to evaluate how he felt his easy onsets and pullouts were. A 1–10 scale could be used for rating them.
Rather than instructing the client, the clinician should facilitate the client's own discovery of new behaviors that work. In doing so, the clinician should utilize the client's sensory processes to discover helpful changes.	As the client is trying to change old habits of tension and struggle, he should be urged to feel, hear, or see what he is doing as he searches for ways to change. An example is Dean Williams's (2004) question to clients: "What are you doing to interfere with talking?" and his admonition to "feel what you're doing."
As new habits are acquired, old habits must be suppressed by conscious inhibition.	Prior to speaking, a client should pause and tell himself not to use an old habit (such as tensing larynx, lips, and/or jaw) and be aware of how that change feels.
In order for responses to become automatized (and therefore stable in the face of distracters), the client needs to consistently use the new behaviors in relevant stimulus situations.	Clients need to consistently use new behaviors, such as easy onsets in place of habitual tense stuttering behaviors in order to build up automaticity in their use so that they will be available under stress.
Clients should use variable practice with different stimuli and in different environments.	Clients should practice new behaviors (e.g., light contacts or slow rate) with a wide variety of words and sentences, in different types of speech tasks, and outside the clinic room as well as on the telephone in the clinic.

SUMMARY

- The clinician's attributes are a vital ingredient in treatment success.

- Empathy, genuineness, and warmth are three clinician attributes that have been considered important by Van Riper (1975a).

- An important component of best clinical practice is choosing evaluation procedures and tools that have been shown to be valid and reliable.

- Best clinical practice dictates becoming aware of evidence of effectiveness for treatment procedures that you use and adapting treatment procedures to fit clients' needs, as well as continuous assessment of improvement in attributes that have been chosen as goals for treatment.

- Continuing education is vital to keep abreast of new approaches and new evidence of effectiveness of current approaches.

- It is important for clinicians to develop an informed set of beliefs about the nature of stuttering and to fit assessment and treatment procedures to those beliefs.

- Goals for treatment and for continuing assessment should come from not only the clinician's beliefs but also from the client's (or family's) informed choices.

- Treatment procedures for meeting these goals can include methods of reducing frequency and severity of stuttering and secondary behaviors, reducing negative emotions and thoughts that interfere with fluency, increasing communication abilities, and developing environments which facilitate fluency.

STUDY QUESTIONS

1. What are the three important characteristics of a clinician described by Van Riper?

2. How might each of these characteristics facilitate progress in treatment?

3. What are the characteristics of evidence-based practice?

4. How might two clinicians' beliefs about the nature of stuttering result in two very different treatment approaches? How might these beliefs result in two similar treatment approaches?

5. Which of the treatment goals described in this chapter are appropriate for borderline stuttering?

6. Which are appropriate for beginning stuttering?

7. Which are appropriate for intermediate stuttering?

8. Which are appropriate for advanced stuttering?

9. Describe the differences between "fluency-shaping" and "stuttering-modification" approaches to treatment.

10. How might reducing negative emotion reduce stuttering frequency?

11. How might reducing stuttering frequency reduce negative emotion?

12. Which goal would you start with and why?

SUGGESTED PROJECTS

1. Video record yourself and a client during an evaluation or a treatment session. The first time you watch it, note only the things you think you do well. The second time you watch it, note two things you would like to improve. Meet with a colleague or supervisor and discuss how to improve the things you would like to and then work on those in another session and videotape yourself again. Watch this new tape for improvements in the behavior(s) you have chosen to work on.

2. Choose a test you use in your evaluation procedures, and try to find evidence of its validity and reliability.

3. Choose a treatment procedure you use, and search the literature to see if you can locate any information about its effectiveness.

4. Find a stuttering treatment approach that is described in detail and determine what the goals of treatment are, what the procedures are to reach these goals, and whether there is a description of how to measure progress on these goals. Examples of such approaches are: *Systematic Fluency Training for Young Children* by Richard Shine (Pro-Ed, Austin, TX); *Fun with Fluency-Direct Therapy with the Young Child* by Patty Walton and Mary Wallace (Imaginart International, Inc, Bisbee, AZ); *A Primer for Stuttering Therapy* by Howard Schwartz (Allyn and Bacon, Boston); and Dynamic Stuttering Therapy by Barbara Dahm (http://stutteringonlinetherapy.com/).

5. Describe in detail your own beliefs about the nature of stuttering applied to children with intermediate stuttering. Given these beliefs, what therapy goals do you have for a child with intermediate stuttering?

SUGGESTED READINGS

Bothe, A., (Ed.). (2004). *Evidence-based treatment of stuttering: Empirical bases and clinical applications.* Mahwah, NJ: Lawrence Erlbaum.

This text, available in hard copy or electronic format, contains chapters dealing with data on stuttering treatments and the scientific basis of treatment approaches.

Cordes, A., & Ingham, R., (Eds.). (1998). *Treatment efficacy for stuttering: A search for empirical bases.* San Diego, CA: Singular.

This is an excellent volume of papers by clinician-researchers who are searching for a scientific foundation for the treatment of stuttering. As the introduction makes clear, this book is the outcome of a continuing series of conferences on this topic.

Guitar, B., & Peters, T. (2003). *Stuttering: An integration of contemporary therapies.* Memphis, TN: Stuttering Foundation. (www.stutteringhelp.org)

This booklet describes in detail the two approaches mentioned in this chapter: fluency shaping and stuttering modification.

Manning, W. (2010). *Clinical decision making in fluency disorders (3rd ed.).* San Diego: Singular.

The first chapter describes many aspects of the clinician as well as of the clinical interaction in stuttering therapy. Also relevant to the material discussed earlier is Chapter 6: Facilitating the Therapeutic Process. Manning describes goals for treatment and subtleties of how and when to work toward them. Chapter 7: Counseling and People Who Stutter contains an excellent description of the therapeutic alliance and other aspects of helping the person who stutters change his behaviors, thoughts, and feelings.

Proceedings of the NINCD workshop on treatment efficacy research in stuttering, September 21–22, 1992. (1993). Special Issue of *Journal of Fluency Disorders, 18.*

This issue of the journal contains chapters by more than a dozen specialists in stuttering treatment and research. Each chapter deals with an area related to treatment efficacy. Although somewhat out of date, these chapters are good examples of the kind of literature reviews that need to be redone every two or three years.

Shapiro, D. (2011). The clinician: A paragon of change. In *Stuttering Intervention: A Collaborative Journey to Fluency Freedom.* Austin, TX: Pro-Ed.

This textbook contains two excellent chapters on clinician characteristics. One deals with the "magic" of the client-clinician relationship and touches on many of the attributes needed by effective clinicians. Another discusses the processes of students becoming qualified clinicians. The author touches on many aspects of supervision and analysis of clinical interactions.

Van Riper, C. (1958). Experiments in stuttering therapy. In Jon Eisenson (Ed.), *Stuttering: A Symposium.* New York: Harper & Row.

This chapter describes the stuttering treatments that Van Riper experimented with in his first 20 years after leaving Iowa and setting up a speech clinic at what became Western Michigan University. Of particular interest is the systematic changes he made in treatment protocols year by year to develop the most effective methods and the five-year follow-ups he made to measure long-term progress.

Van Riper, C. (1975a) The stutterer's clinician. In Jon Eisenson (Ed.), *Stuttering: A Second Symposium.* New York: Harper & Row.

This chapter is still a useful description of the attributes that may be important in clinicians who treat stutterers. It also contains excellent sections on clinicians' roles in motivating clients and discusses the subject of whether clinicians who themselves stutter should treat clients who stutter.

Zebrowski, P. (2007) Treatment factors that influence therapy outcomes of children who stutter. In E. Conture, & R. Curlee (Eds.), *Stuttering and Related Disorders of Fluency.* New York: Thieme.

This chapter has some excellent summaries of research relating to variables that can affect therapy outcome, including information about the relationship between the client and clinician.

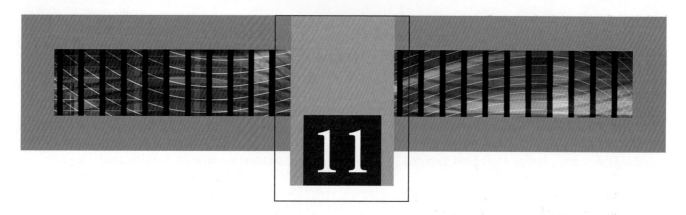

11

Treatment of Stuttering in Younger Preschool Children: Borderline Stuttering

CHAPTER OBJECTIVES

After studying this chapter, readers should be able to:
- Understand the difference between indirect and direct treatment
- Be able to plan and carry out indirect and—if needed— direct treatment of a younger preschool child
- Learn about data collection in the clinic by the clinician and at home by the parents, both of which can be used to guide treatment
- Learn the basics of treatment approaches to preschool children advocated by three other groups of authors

KEY TERMS

Younger preschool children: children between 2 and 3.5 years

Indirect treatment: therapy that involves alleviating stresses that the child might be experiencing in communication at home and in other situations

Direct treatment: therapy that works directly on the child's speech by having him speak more fluently, stutter more easily, or both

Spontaneous fluency: A child's natural fluency that occurs without work or thought on his part

Maintenance: The process of fading treatment while continuing to support the child and family so that fluency achieved in treatment does not diminish

Severity ratings (SRs): Numbers on a 1-10 scale given daily by parents to describe their child's fluency. The SR scale is shown in Figure 8.4 and described in detail in Chapter 8

One-on-one time: A period of about 15 minutes each day during which one parent is alone with the child and follows the child's lead in play and conversation. In this time, parents can practice new behaviors such as using a slower speech rate with pauses, and children can experience their parents' full attention

Percent syllables stuttered (%SS): This is one measure of stuttering frequency that is often used as data to determine how much a child is stuttering at a particular time. We suggest using %SS along with SRs as an indication of whether treatment is working

Easy stuttering: A very mild type of stuttering characterized by slow and relaxed repetitions or prolongations of sounds that are brief and relaxed. This can be a target of direct treatment, with the goal being to change stuttering into normal disfluency

Playing with stuttering: Pretending to stutter in a way that deliberately changes some aspect of the stutter, such as how many repetitions are produced. This activity is thought to decease the child's frustration and fear of stuttering and thus reduce tension and struggle

AN INTEGRATED APPROACH

In previous editions of this book I have described the stuttering in **younger preschool children** (2 years–3.5 years) to be at the "borderline" level with loose and relaxed repetitions. Treatment for them should be **indirect**, aimed at changing the environment. However, a few children this young are more advanced in their stuttering; they are starting to add tension to their stuttering and may be aware of and frustrated by it. But I would refrain from **direct treatment** aimed at having them learn to change their speech. Almost all of these children between 2 and 3.5 years have been stuttering for less than a year, and many have a likelihood of natural recovery. Therefore, everything must be done to avoid interfering with

natural recovery and instead to facilitate it. It is also important to realize that most children between 2.5 and 3 years aren't cognitively ready to learn from direct treatment how to change their stuttering (Fig. 11.1).

Most treatment of stuttering at this age is indirect because it involves working with the family environment to decrease stress and to increase fluency, rather than working directly on the child's speech. The initial focus is decreasing the family's concern, trying to understand their feelings, and helping them change selected aspects of the family-child interactions. If a child's family can discover ways to facilitate the child's fluency, they become confident in their ability to effect change and are able to assume long-term responsibility for the child's fluency. If this is not effective, then direct work on the child's speech by the clinician with some help from the family is appropriate.

In this chapter, I will use the terms "family" and "parent" or "parents" interchangeably to indicate the important adults with whom the child commonly interacts. Cultures and families differ in who should be involved in the child's treatment. When I imply that one parent is the major player in the interaction patterns I describe, the reader should freely adapt the treatment to suit each situation—one parent or two, older children or cousins, nannies or grandparents.

I will illustrate our approach to treatment with the case example of Ashley, the 2.5-year-old preschool child whom we introduced in Chapter 1.

Author's Beliefs

Nature of Stuttering

As I described in Chapter 7, stuttering at onset usually occurs as a result of the interplay between a child's constitutional predispositions and the stresses resulting from developmental demands and the environment. Treatment for stuttering in younger preschool children is based on the assumption that when stresses on the child and his speech can be decreased, his stuttering will taper off, and he will become normally fluent. I believe that the plasticity of normal neural maturation allows most of these children to compensate for constitutional predispositions toward stuttering. For such flexibility in development to blossom into normal fluency, however, the clinician and family must provide an environment that fosters fluency and diminishes negative experiences with speaking. And this must be done promptly. If too much time passes, the child may become negatively aware of his stuttering and become frustrated by it. When this happens, frustration combined with concern about negative listener reactions may motivate the child to develop escape and even avoidance reactions. These more advanced forms of stuttering are usually more resistant to treatment.

With the borderline stuttering of younger preschoolers, I seldom treat the child directly, at least not at first. Instead,

An Integrated Approach

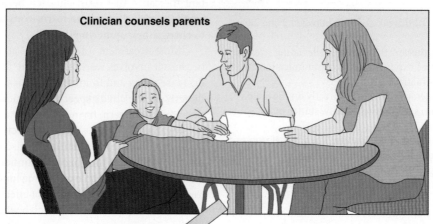

Clinician counsels parents

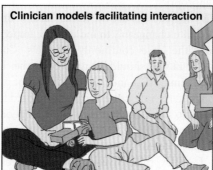

Clinician models facilitating interaction

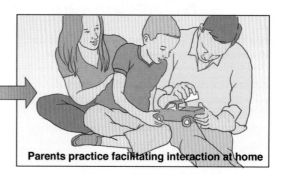

Parents practice facilitating interaction at home

Conture's Approach

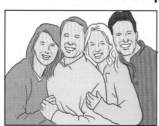 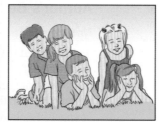

Palin Centre Approach

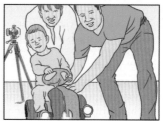

Stuttering Foundation Approach

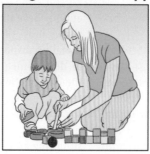

Figure 11.1 Treatments for younger preschool children who stutter.

I work with the child's family to help them reduce environmental stresses. Stress is normal in the life of every child, but the child with borderline stuttering may simply be more vulnerable to fluency breakdown under normal stresses. As you will see in my description of clinical procedures, I usually begin by informing and educating family members about ways they can reduce stresses and foster fluency. I demonstrate a facilitating style of communicative interaction as a model for the family and meet with them once a week to support and guide their efforts in finding ways to help their child.

If indirect therapy is not effective in reducing stuttering after six weeks, or if the child's stuttering proves to be more advanced than initially thought, I add more direct procedures. My direct approach for stuttering in younger preschoolers consists of a hierarchy of activities that focus on playing with stuttering and changing it to a milder form.

Speech Behaviors Targeted for Therapy

Because I don't treat the child's speech directly, none of the child's speech behaviors are specifically targeted for direct change. Instead, the family's interaction styles, including both speech and nonspeech behaviors, are the focus of treatment. For example, I help family members learn to speak in a slow and relaxed manner, and I support their efforts to make other aspects of their interactions with the child who stutters as nonstressful as possible. In those rare instances when this approach doesn't soon decrease stuttering, the child's repetitions and prolongations are targeted for change.

Fluency Goals

I believe that children who stutter at the borderline level who have no serious concomitant problems can achieve **spontaneous fluency**. With effective early intervention, this goal is readily achievable because the child's maturing nervous system gradually increases his capacity for fluent speech.

Feelings and Attitudes

The main focus of treatment is on the behaviors of family members and others who interact frequently with the child. Consequently, the child's feelings and attitudes are not dealt with directly. However, as the family and I monitor the child's fluency, we try to ensure that he is not developing negative attitudes about speaking or about his disfluencies. If the child's stuttering persists and shows periodic worsening, he may become more frustrated by it when it is at its worst and may soon acquire the escape behaviors (like increased tension in stutters) seen in more advanced stuttering. In these cases, the addition of more direct intervention is used to deal with such feelings.

Maintenance Procedures

Many younger preschool children achieve fluent speech soon after their families have made some environmental modifications, and most maintain fluency without further treatment.

However, it is important to keep in contact with the family even after formal treatment has stopped to prevent their reverting to old, more stressful interaction patterns. This **maintenance**, through telephone calls or e-mail, is gradually faded.

Clinical Methods

Working with stuttering at this level involves a variety of therapy procedures. I educate families by providing them with DVDs and reading material (such as that from the Stuttering Foundation [(SF)]) to help them understand the nature of stuttering and the ways in which they can help the child become more fluent. I counsel families by listening to their concerns and trying to understand their hopes, desires, fears, and frustrations. I brainstorm and problem solve with families when I help them choose aspects of their interaction patterns to modify. I collect data on the child's speech and on the family's perceptions of his stuttering and fluency. And finally, I provide support as the child's stuttering decreases and the family strives to maintain their new styles of interaction.

Clinical Procedures: Indirect Treatment

This section describes the stages of indirect treatment, including continuing assessment of the child's speech at home and in the clinic, introduction of a slower speech rate with pauses, and introduction of other changes that the clinician and the family choose.

Severity Ratings

As I explained in Chapter 9 on assessment, during the closing interview the family is given a copy of the **Severity Rating (SR) Scale** (Fig. 8.4), and its use is explained to them. Although the scale was originally designed for use with the Lidcombe Program, it is excellent for use with families of younger children who will be receiving indirect treatment. As you will remember, it is a 10-point scale that the family completes at the end of every day. Ratings range from 1 = no stuttering, 2 = extremely mild stuttering, all the way to 10 = extremely severe stuttering (which may never be seen in a particular child). At each clinic session, after a baseline of the child's speech is collected in the first 10 minutes, the clinician and parent compare their SRs for the child's speech during the baseline measure. Agreement is defined as the parent and clinician's SR for that sample not differing by more than one point. If the difference between the ratings is greater than a single point, the clinician's rating is assumed to be accurate, and she discusses her rating with the parent to help the parent better understand the rating system and become "calibrated." The parent uses the scale to make a daily rating of the child's speech at the end of every day and brings or e-mails the week's SR chart to the clinician for discussion in each clinic meeting.

Case Example

Ashley

Ashley's stuttering, as you will remember from the video clip and Chapter 1, was characterized by multiple part-word and single-syllable whole-word repetitions. Ashley gave little indication that she was aware of her stuttering. Because her stuttering was quite frequent and gradually worsening, Ashley underwent treatment despite her young age. Indirect treatment was carried out via once-weekly home visits by a clinician with experience in stuttering. The clinician began by playing with Ashley on the floor with a variety of toys including dolls and a dollhouse. The clinician used a slow rate of speech with many pauses, as we describe in this chapter. She did not ask Ashley to change her own rate, but only modeled the rate for Ashley and her mother, who observed. Gradually, the mother took a greater and greater part, but the clinician continued to be part of the play so she could observe the mother's own use of slower speech rate with more pauses. After each session, the clinician and mother talked about how the mother was doing. The clinician was careful to praise the mother for what she was doing well before suggesting ways she could improve. In addition to slowing her speech rate and pausing more frequently, Ashley's mother also learned to turn most of her questions into comments. The clinician took data on the child's stuttering in each session.

This play therapy continued for about eight weeks. Ashley's stuttering in the sessions disappeared, and her mother reported that she was more and more fluent in situations outside of the sessions. Recently, we video recorded an interview with Ashley at age 8, completely fluent and having no recollection of ever having stuttered.

Baseline Speech Measures

At the beginning of each clinic visit, the clinician video records and observes the first 10 to 15 minutes of parent-child play. Attending to both the child's speech and the parent's interaction style, the clinician's first task is to determine an SR for the child's speech in this parent-child play period. As noted, this will be compared with the parent's SR for the same sample. The clinician also notes aspects of the parent-child interaction, especially those on which the parent has been asked to work.

Family Interaction Patterns

As described in the section on assessment of the younger preschool child in Chapter 9, my approach to treatment involves study of and experimental change in parent-child interaction patterns. The change is described as experimental because not every change will have positive effects on the child's fluency; therefore, a change may be tried and discarded if the result of the "experiment" isn't positive. Here is a list of some conversational interaction patterns observed in some families that may be changed to facilitate the child's fluency.

1. High rates of speech
2. Rapid-fire conversational pace (lack of pauses or too-short pauses between speakers)
3. Interruptions
4. Frequent open-ended questions or questions that demand an answer
5. Many critical or corrective comments
6. Inadequate or inconsistent listening to what the child says
7. Vocabulary far above the child's level
8. Advanced levels of syntax

Table 11.1 gives some detailed suggestions for evaluating these parent-child conversational variables. Table 11.2 provides ideas for changes parents can make to facilitate their child's fluency. Rather than give them this list and ask them to change several things at the same time, I am presenting the list to let the reader know about major areas of communicative interaction to consider with each family.

Although other clinicians may begin treatment focusing on other family-child interaction variables, my own preference in most cases is to begin by helping families reduce their speech rate and increase their pausing. Supporting data on the effectiveness of parents slowing their speech rates and pausing more often is provided at the end of this section. In the next few pages, I will describe how to help parents slow speech rate and increase pause time.

Slower Speech Rate with Pauses

For most families, the clinician starts by helping the parents reduce their speech rate and increase their pause time when talking with their child. The evidence reviewed in Chapters 2 and 3 suggests that individuals who stutter have constitutional deficits that make it challenging for them to produce speech at rapid rates. If parents provide a model of slower speech with plentiful pauses, this model alone will probably influence children to speak more slowly (Guitar & Marchinkowski, 2001). More importantly, a model of slower speech with adequate pauses has been shown to reduce children's stuttering (e.g., Guitar, Kopff-Schaefer, Donahue-Kilburg, & Bond, 1992; Stephanson-Opsal & Bernstein Ratner, 1988; Zebrowski, Weiss, Savelkoul, & Hammer, 1996). The clinician emphasizes that parents should not

Table 11.1	Suggestions for Quantifying Family-Child Interaction Patterns

1. **High rates of speech.** Count the number of syllables spoken by each family member interacting with the child. Next, using a stopwatch, measure the amount of time each individual speaks. Be sure to stop timing whenever they stop speaking or pause for more than 2 s. Resume timing as soon as the speaking continues. Then, calculate the time in minutes to hundredths of a minute (e.g., 1 min and 13 s would be 1.22 min). Divide the total number of syllables spoken by the time in minutes to obtain the number of syllables per minute (SPM). For example, if a family member speaks 366 syllables in 1.22 min, their rate of speech is 300 SPM. Normal adult speaking rates are 165 to 230 SPM (Andrews & Ingham, 1971). Thus, this is a fast rate of speech.

2. **Rapid-fire conversational pace (lack of pauses between speakers).** Using a stopwatch, measure intervals from when the child stops speaking and when another family member begins. If these intervals average less than 1 s, the pace of conversation is rapid.

3. **Interruptions.** Count the number of sentences or sentence-like utterances the child speaks during the sample and the number of times a family member interrupts the child. Divide the number of interruptions by the total number of sentences. If more than 10 percent of the sentences contain interruptions, the child may feel pressure to speak quickly.

4. **Frequent questions.** Count the number of sentences spoken by family members to the child and the number of sentences that are questions. Divide the number of questions by the total number of sentences. If more than 25 percent of the utterances are questions, the child may feel pressure from having to answer questions.

5. **Many critical or directive comments.** Each sentence of family members should be characterized as being either "critical/directive" or "accepting/nondirective." Sentences characterized as critical/directive would be (1) those that convey that the speaker does not unconditionally accept the child, his actions, or his words; (2) those that pressure the child to speak or direct the child's activity; and (3) those spoken with a tone of voice that is stern or incredulous. The number of sentences that are critical should be divided by the total number of sentences. If the percentage of critical/directive comments is higher than 50 percent, the child may feel stress from high standards in the family.

6. **Inadequate or inconsistent listening to what the child says.** Assess the content of family members' sentences during each speaking turn. Note whether family members are responding to the content of the child's utterances. If more than 50 percent of family members' utterances ignore the topic the child has been speaking about, the child may feel he is not being heard.

7. **Vocabulary far above child's level.** Compare the vocabulary level of family members' speech with that of the child. If more than only a small amount of the family members' vocabulary exceeds the child's receptive level, the child may feel pressure when trying to understand family members' vocabulary.

8. **Advanced levels of syntax.** Assess the syntax used by family members when speaking to the child. If more than only a small amount is considerably above the child's current receptive level, the child may feel pressure not only to understand family members but also to use syntax that he has yet to master.

tell the child to slow his speech rate; such direct instruction tends to be ineffective and to annoy the child. Simply speaking in the style of television's Mr. Rogers will have the desired effect. Parents and clinicians can refresh their memory of this speaking style by watching YouTube videos of Mr. Rogers, including his acceptance speech at the 1997 Emmys.

Teaching Slower Speaking Rate with Pauses

After rehearsing a slower speech rate with pauses, you can meet with the parents, model this style of speaking, and ask them to try it. Sometimes beginning with a reading passage is easier than conversation. Most parents find it slightly embarrassing to speak this way at first, but your modeling this style will make it easier for them. Strongly reinforce them for the things they are doing well. Once they have a pretty good style, if you can video or audio record their speech and play

it back to them, their experience of hearing and watching themselves speak this way will help them remember it. If you have a laptop with a camera, you can record a clip of them speaking this way and e-mail it to them so they will have it at home to refresh their memories from time to time.

Trying Slower Rate with Pauses in the Clinic

After the parents feel comfortable using the new speaking style, the clinician and a parent can carry out some play interaction with the child and use the slower rate with pauses (Fig. 11.2). If the child asks the parent why he or she is talking in a funny, slow way, the clinician or parent may explain to the child that the parent talks too fast and needs to learn to slow down. With some children, we enlist them to remind the parent to slow down if they think the parent is talking too quickly. Children delight in correcting adults, especially their parents.

Table 11.2	Things Families Can Do to Help the Younger Preschool Child Who Stutters

1. **Listening time.** All children benefit from feeling that what they have to say is important. This is especially true for the child who is beginning to stutter. Set aside some time each day as "listening time" with your child. Make it 15 to 20 min at about the same time each day, so your child can depend on it. During that time, refrain from making suggestions or giving instructions. Merely "be there" for the child, listening attentively to what he or she says or quietly playing alongside the child if he or she chooses not to talk.
2. **Slow rate.** Family members may reduce their conversational rate of speech to a slow, soothing style. Speech should sound relaxed and calm, with comfortable pauses throughout. Fred Rogers on the television show "Mr. Rogers's Neighborhood" is a good model.
3. **Pauses.** The pace of conversation can be kept appropriately slow if the speaker pauses 1 to 2 s before starting to talk. This also helps to keep the speaker from interrupting another speaker.
4. **Positive comments.** Make many positive and accepting comments about what your child is saying and doing. Limit corrections or criticisms to important issues. Changes for the better usually happen more quickly when someone feels he is OK as he is. The child who feels good about himself will be better able to use "listening time," "slow rate," and "pauses" to gain more fluency.
5. **Fewer questions.** It is natural to ask a child many questions in order to encourage him to learn new things and to display that knowledge. However, this makes some children feel "under the gun." So it may be a good idea to decrease demanding questions and instructions. If you are worried that your child won't learn enough if you are too laid back, keep in mind that learning comes naturally to children. They learn best from your interest in things, especially from your interest and positive comments about the things they do and say.

Using the Slower Rate with Pauses at Home

If the clinician is not satisfied with the parents' ability to speak with the child using this new speaking style, home practice should be delayed until the parents have mastered it. However, most parents pick up the new style quickly and they can begin using it at home immediately. One parent should try to spend 15 minutes a day playing alone with the child and using the new speaking style. The best time is in the morning because it may influence the child for the rest of the day. Many families are too busy at this time, feeding and dressing their children and themselves; for them, one-on-one slow speech practice in the morning may be possible only on weekends. In this case, any 15 minutes per day of **one-on-one time** with the child is acceptable. Most important is that the parents do it every day. If one parent does most of the one-on-one play with slow speech, the other parent should also use the slower speech rate when talking with the child whenever he or she can.

Monitoring Parents' Practice of Slower Rate with Pauses

Most parents benefit from consistent support for any changes they are making in their interactions with their child. I often keep in touch with them between clinic visits via e-mail or telephone, but I always ask them to keep a journal of their experience with the new speaking style by making notes on the SR chart they are completing every evening. When parents are willing and able to video record themselves at home using the new speaking style during their 15-minute daily interactions, it is a fine motivation for them to practice and a good way for me to monitor their progress. In any case, the interaction they have with the child at the beginning of each session allows me to be sure they are using an effective speaking style as well as allows me to collect data on the child's **percent syllables stuttered** during this interaction. When I'm observing this, I can also read the SR chart with the parents' notes about their daily work between clinic visits. In the discussion that follows the parent-child interaction, I am careful to reinforce the parents for everything they are doing well. In all discussions, the clinician's role is first and

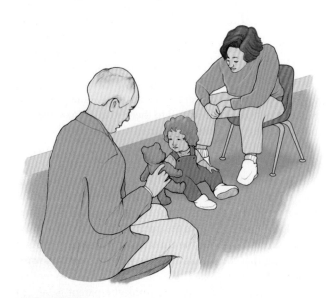

| Figure 11.2 | Clinician models interaction patterns while the mother observes. |

foremost to be an empathetic listener, allowing the parents to take the lead in assessing their progress and formulating plans to work on change.

Working with Other Aspects of the Parent-Child Interaction

As the clinician works with the parents or other family members on their speech rate and pausing, she continues to assess the child's progress toward normal fluency, as indicated by percent syllables stuttered (%SS) in the clinic, SRs at home, and discussions with the family. If these indicators of fluency do not indicate a steady downward progression of stuttering in the first three or four weeks of treatment, the clinician and family should consider other aspects of the parent-child interaction that may be putting pressure on the child's fluency. Consider items 3 to 8 in Table 11.1.

Remember that most of the interaction patterns in families of children who stutter are not abnormal or particularly negative. They usually are quite typical of the culture in which the child is being raised. However, a child sensitive to communicative pressure may benefit from some modification of family communication patterns in ways that facilitate his fluency. It is vital that the clinician help the family understand that they are not causing the child to stutter because of inappropriate communication patterns. Instead their communication is normal, but they can help their child by changing a few aspects of their communication to facilitate fluency.

One of the first things I do if I sense some aspect of the family communicative style might need a little modification, is to have the parents watch the video recording of their interaction with their child with me. As we watch together, I praise many things that the parent is doing well. Praise is vital to develop the parents' confidence and to encourage them to keep doing things they are doing well. As I praise the parents, I listen acceptingly to their comments even if they are self-critical. We watch together for things that a parent and I both feel might be putting pressure on the child. The best situation is when a parent notices something to change—something that I also feel may be pressuring the child's fluency. We then together plan to change that aspect of the interaction and observe the results.

For example, in the third week of treatment, a parent was doing a great job using a slower speech rate with pauses. However, the child's fluency—which had increased somewhat—had now plateaued. The parent and I watched the most recent video recording, and as we watched, I praised her slow speech with pauses. After a few minutes, the parent commented that she was surprised to see that she asked her child so many questions, rat-tat-tat, one right after the other. I agreed with her and we discussed alternatives, such as making comments instead of asking questions, and she tried this out during the week. The following week, the child's SRs showed further increases in fluency, and the parent's interaction at the beginning of the session revealed an impressive

decrease in questions. This change, accompanied by the slower speech rate with pausing, was enough to increase the child's fluency to normal levels, which was maintained long term.

Changes in Family Routine

In addition to changing conversational interaction patterns, a family may identify other stresses on the child that need to be changed, such as the amount of individual attention the child receives and the "busyness" of the family's schedule. My main function in helping families work on such stresses is to give them information about areas of changes that others have found helpful and to be a sounding board for their plans for changing. I encourage them to assess, informally, the effects of these changes on the child's fluency and his overall adjustment. Although my praise and appreciation may help, a significant change in the child's stuttering is the real motivator. Notes the parent makes on the chart of daily SRs will help you identify factors that may facilitate fluency or cause upward spikes in a child's stuttering. A parent, for example, noted on her SR chart that her child's stuttering flared up if she left the room while he was playing. She alleviated this stress by being careful to let the child know ahead of time if she were about to leave the room and that she would be right back.

This example is a reminder of the importance of parents' attention for a child's self-esteem. When a child senses that his mother or father understands him and genuinely cares about him (cares about what he likes to do, what he thinks about things, and how he feels), the child feels more comfortable with himself, is less anxious, and is better able to speak easily. For many younger preschool children who stutter, a little more one-on-one time spent with a parent each day, preferably in the morning, can boost fluency tremendously. Although the morning can be the most difficult time for parents who work outside the home, one-on-one fluency time in the morning can have a positive effect on the child's speech for the rest of the day. If mornings are too difficult, some one-on-one time in the afternoon can also be very helpful. The time does not need to be long, just 15 to 20 minutes, but the parent needs to be with the child in a place where they won't be interrupted.

The child should choose what to play or talk about, and the parent should follow the child's lead, participating as the child directs. As a parent becomes more and more comfortable with this nondirective play, he or she may want to explore ways of helping the child feel really understood. One of the parents we worked with, for example, learned to "mirror" her child's momentary emotions as they built a tower of blocks together. When the child placed a block on the tower and it fell off, she would quietly murmur a sound of disappointment, echoing the child's facial expression. This child made impressive gains in fluency in only a few weeks, and I believe that this parent's deep attention to the child may have contributed significantly to this change. Although not every parent could be expected to achieve the level of empathetic response that this mother did, increased caring attention is probably a realistic goal for most families.

Attentive play can become child-directed conversations as a child grows older, and such conversations can continue the process of helping the child develop a sense of being loved, understood, and appreciated. In his article *Making Time for Your Child*, the child psychiatrist Stanley Greenspan suggests "In spontaneous, unstructured talk or play, try to follow your child's lead. The goal is to 'march to your child's drummer' and to tune in to the child at his level" (Greenspan, 1993, p. 111).

The Course of Treatment

Sometimes families report that their attempts to make changes have been fairly successful. For example, they may have been able to slow their speaking rates and to simplify their language and may have seen improvement in their child. I let them know that their changes have been key factors in the child's improvement and stress the importance of continuing them. It is easy to resume old patterns after some improvement occurs, whether it's the challenge of losing weight or helping a child become more fluent.

Each child and each family is unique in how they respond to treatment, but it is possible to note some common trends. For example, some children become much more fluent soon after the family makes one or two changes in their environment. Occasionally, a child may become fluent immediately after an initial session, possibly because the family is less anxious about his disfluencies after sharing their concerns with a professional. Whatever the cause, early and immediate fluency gains should be viewed with cautious optimism. I share the family's pleasure at such dramatic change but suggest that their child's fluency may be fragile and will need to be nurtured by our continued efforts to create a facilitative environment.

Sometimes the path toward fluency is rough and irregular. The child may make little or no progress or may improve for a while and then return to his old pattern of disfluency. When this happens and the family or clinician feels frustrated by slow progress, further exploration of the family's feelings about the child's stuttering is called for. Many times family members worry about the child's future, afraid that stuttering will be a serious handicap for him. Sometimes there is lingering guilt about having caused his stuttering. Often it is hard for parents to accept the blemish they feel that stuttering creates on the family image.

Whatever the source of a family's anxieties, their concern about stuttering may easily radiate to the child in their reactions to his stutters. Unwittingly, family members may show their anxiety or disappointment through facial expressions or body language, which may make the child "hesitate to hesitate" and thus stutter more severely. Open and frank discussions with the family about their feelings and concerns are likely to be more helpful at this point than trying to change their reactions. In such discussions, the clinician's role is to make it easier for the family to talk about their concerns, so I listen carefully, try my best to understand them, and convey my understanding with acceptance and respect. When family members feel understood and accepted, it is easier for them to share their feelings and accept them. When this occurs, some feelings may change, and in turn, the child's stuttering may decrease, possibly because his stuttering no longer seems so terrible to the family.

Another barrier to changing a family's interaction patterns is the fact that some styles of interaction reflect important cultural values. For example, in the urban eastern United States, family members sometimes finish each other's sentences, conveying a closeness and solidarity within the family that is highly valued. If they are asked to speak more slowly and pause between speakers' turn takings, such changes would conflict with one of the family's implicit cultural values. Another example might be parents who frequently teach, correct, and criticize their children's behavior. This "instructional" mode of interaction may reflect the importance that the family's culture places on education.

I believe it is important to explore how the family feels about changes they are considering. In some cases, they can find ways to change other variables that will be as effective, thereby leaving unchanged those interactions that are of value to the family. Several years ago, I worked with a parent who spoke very rapidly to her child who was showing some borderline stuttering. She resisted changing her speech rate because "it isn't the way we talk." In addition, she was frequently critical of her child's behavior. Consequently, I encouraged her to use positive reinforcement for fluency, as described in the treatment of beginning stuttering in Chapter 12, which I adapted from Onslow, Andrews, and Lincoln (1994), and asked her to let her child know with upbeat statements of praise that she liked his smooth fluency. The child's stuttering diminished almost immediately, and she was delighted with her ability to help her child.

Sometimes a family may resist change and doesn't fully participate in treatment. There may be psychological issues that need to be resolved through referral to a family counselor, or the family may have other, more serious problems with which to cope. In such cases, I talk with the family directly about my concerns. This usually leads to an open discussion of their situation, a referral to a family counselor, or in rare cases, their decision to withdraw the child from stuttering therapy for the time being. If this happens, I let the family know that I remain available to them, and I try to stay in contact by occasional phone calls or e-mails to make it easier for them to resume the child's therapy if they wish to.

Maintenance

Indirect treatment of a younger preschool child is often effective within five or six sessions, over a period of one or two months. The child's speech becomes markedly less disfluent. Part-word repetitions become whole-word or phrase repetitions, which are more like typical children's disfluencies, and the family's concerns about the child's speech diminish. When this happens, I review the changes the family has made with them and the changes in their child's stuttering that reflect his improvement. Using this information, I help the family develop a plan to deal with periods of increased stress that may prompt stuttering to reappear. Most families feel that they have a handle on how to reduce stress on their child at this stage of therapy, and their experiences in observing and changing their behaviors have given them confidence. If their child's stuttering suddenly increases, they know how to examine their speech rates or attentiveness when talking to the child and how to examine other aspects of their interactions and implement needed changes.

Effective maintenance for stuttering in younger preschool children is the result of two things: (1) helping the family to view the child's stuttering more objectively with less anxiety, guilt, or panic, and (2) building the family's confidence in their own ability to implement problem-solving skills they've learned to use when the child's disfluencies increase. Sometimes, however, despite a family's best efforts to respond constructively, stuttering returns. This may occur after an increase in stress from some trauma or from normal life events, such as moving to a new house, or it may accompany a growth spurt in the child's language. On the other hand, it may be unexplainable. Whatever the cause, the family should feel comfortable getting back in contact with the clinician. I let each family know at the end of therapy that relapse is possible, not abnormal, and that I would look forward to seeing the child again if help is needed.

Supporting Data

Many years ago, my colleagues and I published a study that evaluated the effect of changing parent-child interactions with a 5-year-old child who stuttered (Guitar, 1978; Guitar et al., 1992). Although this child was an older preschooler, the principles of working with the family on their interaction style were similar to those described for the younger preschool child. Our approach to treatment was to video record parent-child interactions over five treatment sessions and then view the videos with each parent. When viewing the videos, we let the parent decide what to work on in the intervening week and then recorded a new parent-child interaction after a week of work on changing the behavior they had selected. After six sessions, the child's stuttering had diminished to the level of normal disfluency; we followed the child for 10 years, and the stuttering never reappeared. In an analysis of the parents' behavior and the child's stuttering, we

discovered that the changes in parent behavior most related to the child's improvement in stuttering were the mother's reduction in her speech rate and her becoming more accepting in her comments.

A variety of other studies have shown that changes in parent's communicative interactions affect their children's stuttering. Stephenson-Opsal and Bernstein Ratner (1988) demonstrated that when the mothers of stuttering children slowed their speech rates, the children's stuttering decreased. Starkweather, Gottwald, and Halfond (1990) reported on 29 children they treated for an average of 12 sessions (some required as many as 40 sessions), all of whom completely recovered. Their approach involved primarily modification of the parents' behavior, including reduction of speech rate, having special speech time, matching parent language to child language, and reducing parents' negative reactions to stuttering. Zebrowski and colleagues (1996) showed that decreases in mother's speaking rate and pause time were associated with decreases in stuttering in some children.

Further supporting data on this approach are presented in the outcome measures of the Michael Palin Centre's treatment of preschool children later in this chapter. Moreover, a report by Franken, Kielstra-van der Schalk, and Boelens (2005) provides evidence of the effectiveness of parent-child interaction therapy. In the next chapter on treatment of older preschoolers, the treatment approach described by Gottwald (2010) uses a great deal of indirect treatment, but supplements it with direct treatment when needed. She reports that 26 of 27 children were speaking normally a year or more after treatment ended.

Clinical Procedures: Direct Treatment

My approaches to therapy evolve as I learn more about children who stutter and treatment options. Recently my choice of a direct treatment approach for those borderline stutterers who have not responded to indirect treatment has been the Lidcombe Program, which I describe in detail in Chapter 12. The material in this section on direct treatment has been helpful for younger preschool children who need something more than indirect treatment, and I would recommend it to those clinicians who do not choose to use the Lidcombe Program or who have not yet been trained in it.

I don't use direct treatment with every child who is a borderline stutterer, but it is a powerful alternative when indirect treatment does not decrease the child's stuttering after six weeks. The causes of failure with an indirect approach are often unknown. Sometimes, a family seems unable to modify the child's environment as planned, or they do, but the child's stuttering persists unchanged or increases. In these few cases, if the child's disfluency remains at the borderline (rather than beginning) level, I try a slightly more direct approach, as described in the next section.

Direct Treatment for Mild Borderline Stuttering

Most younger preschool children with borderline stuttering are only slightly aware of their disfluencies. Their repetitions appear relaxed, and they show no signs of extra effort or attempts to "fight" their stutters. They also are normally fluent a great deal of the time, and I think they have the capacity to develop entirely normal fluency. Consequently, when I use direct treatment for mild borderline stuttering, I focus on the child's fluency, assuming that he will easily be able to increase the amount of fluency he has and "outgrow" his stuttering with our help. I follow much of the behavioral management strategies used by the Lidcombe Program, which is described in Chapter 12. I train parents to respond to fluency with praise, and unlike the Lidcombe Program, I ask them to ignore stuttering unless the child is momentarily distressed by a stutter, in which case, I suggest the parents comment acceptingly on it. Thus, it is not, strictly speaking, a Lidcombe approach.

I usually begin by training one of the child's parents to use praise for fluency during the daily one-on-one time with the child. The parent might say, "Gee, that was really smooth talking" or "I like the way you said that." The clinician and parent should decide how frequently to use positive reinforcement, but most children are annoyed by praise if the parent gives it too often. A good ratio to begin with is one praise for about every fifth fluent utterance. These fluent utterances do not need to be consecutive. A few children are annoyed by any praise at all given by the parent. In this case, the parent and the clinician can talk with the child about using something besides typical praise. Some children prefer their own phrase. One child wanted his parent to say "That was good monkey talk!" Another child asked for a gesture (thumbs up) instead of words.

As in parent-child interaction therapy, parents keep daily logs of the child's overall fluency for each day, using the 1-to-10 SRs described earlier. When the child has made substantial progress in decreasing severity, the clinician guides the parent in gradually replacing praise for fluency in the daily one-on-one sessions with praise used occasionally during other activities during the day. While the parent is carrying out this direct therapy, it is critical for him or her to attend weekly meetings with the clinician to demonstrate using the procedure, to share SRs, and to discuss progress and problems. It is also important for the family to continue one-on-one sessions with the child and to continue the changes made in their interactions and family lifestyle.

Direct Treatment for More Severe Borderline Stuttering

Some children with borderline stuttering are beginning to have negative feelings about their disfluencies but are not showing the full-blown signs of physical tension or escape behaviors that characterize beginning stuttering. Still, they may occasionally express real frustration with their stuttering.

Typically, I work with children having more severe borderline stuttering for about 45 minutes each week. I also continue to provide encouragement and support to the family in helping them make the child's environment as facilitating to fluency as possible. Our direct treatment activities are presented in a hierarchy that the clinician and child ascend as far as is necessary to bring the child's disfluencies into the range of normal. Progressive steps are taken when the clinician senses that a child is feeling competent at the current step. Thus, progress may be rapid or slow or sudden or gradual, depending on the child's feeling of comfort and mastery with the tasks at hand. There is no need to hurry this process. It should take place within the context of games and activities that make the focus on stuttering casual. The clinician needs to remain alert to the child's immediate sense of confidence and self-esteem in selecting the moment to move the child to the next step in the treatment hierarchy.

Modeling Easy Stutters

I begin direct treatment rather indirectly by providing models of **easy stuttering** in my speech. If the child's repetitions are fast and abrupt, my models are slow with gradual endings. If the child has many repetitions or long prolongations, I repeat or prolong sounds briefly. These models are done casually during play with the child. I don't produce them immediately after the child stutters but insert them randomly, about once every two or three sentences, as if I were stuttering as I talked.

Once the child has become acclimated to the models of easy stuttering after 10 or 15 minutes of play, I begin to make accepting comments about them. I might say, for example, "Hmmmm, I used slidey speech on that word, didn't I?" or "That word stuck a little, but that's OK, I slid right out of it." Most children appear to be shyly interested in what I am talking about, and direct therapy can continue to develop. A few, however, may react negatively and say such things as, "Don't do that!" or "I don't like it when you do that." For them, direct therapy needs to proceed slowly to allow my acceptance and support during play activities to gradually counteract the child's anxiety.

If the child has begun to experience the first pangs of frustration from stuttering, which can be inferred from his questions or complaints about getting stuck on words, I will try to help the child express this. Even though I am making comments that show acceptance of my own stuttering, I occasionally may produce a longer than usual stutter and say, "Sometimes they go on for a long time. That feels weird." I continue to try to sense what the child is feeling and to empathize as naturally as possible. I use this empathic focus not only when I am modeling easy stutters, but throughout direct treatment.

For children who evidence periods of acute frustration with their stuttering, parents should be coached on how to make empathetic statements in a calm, soothing, slow style when the child is going through a difficult time. As I do direct therapy, I try to involve the parents in appropriate activities both at home and in the clinic. If their indirect treatment has not been effective, I need to be sure they do not feel pushed aside by my direct therapy.

The Child Begins Active Participation: "Catch Me"

When I sense that a child is comfortable with my easy stuttering models, I see if the child will take part. I may say, for example, "Can you help me? Sometimes when I get stuck on a word, it goes on and on. Then I try to make my stuck words real slow and loose, and it helps me get unstuck. But sometimes I forget. If you hear me go on and on like thi-thi-thi-thi-thi-thi-this, just say, 'There's one,' and I'll try to make it slow and loose with slidey speech." When the child catches me, I will change a fast, tight repetition to a slow, loose one. As I model stuck words, I choose a style of stuttering similar to the child's.

Praise should flow liberally when the child catches one of my modeled stutters. This provides the child with an initial sense of competence that is associated with something he previously felt to be out of control. For many children, tangible rewards, such as small snacks or turns at a game, are important motivators and should be used along with praise to establish the child's ability to catch the clinician's stutters.

The Child Begins Active Participation: Play

This stage can either follow or precede "Catch Me." It depends on the clinician's judgment about which activity would be more comfortable for the child. Sometimes you may start one of these stages but find the child is not ready and you switch to the other. The **playing with stuttering** stage engages a child in following the clinician's lead in playfully imitating disfluencies that are similar to his own, such as repeated or prolonged sounds. The purpose is to desensitize the child to the frustration that sometimes arises in borderline stuttering. It is a process that may take place because play can give a child a sense of mastery without the risk of failure. The concept of play is quite interesting. Scientists speculate that children's play is an opportunity for them to practice and master skills that are needed in adulthood. Playing with stuttering may take advantage of children's natural tendency to play and provide them with the pleasure of mastery and control over something that has been frustrating and sometimes even frightening.

Take, for example, the child who stutters primarily in a repetitive fashion. The clinician might say, "Let's play a game of saying some sounds over and over and see how many times we can say them. I bet I can say a sound five times! Watch this. Ba-ba-ba-ba-ba! Can you do it five times?" Or it can begin by making sounds for animals, puppets, or other toys: "Hey, this is a zebragella! It goes 'lllllla! lllllla!' (using prolongations). Then it jumps around like this (clinician jumps around) and chews carpet (clinician pretends to chew the carpet)."

The clinician and child can keep incorporating such play into their routine as long as the child finds it fun and the clinician can free herself to enjoy uninhibited play. From playing with repeated or prolonged sounds, the clinician can build a bridge to playing with repeated or prolonged sounds in conversation and in time, to the child's actual stutters.

The Child Produces Intentional Stutters

After the child is able to catch the clinician's stutters and appears comfortable doing it, the clinician should begin looking for opportunities to ask the child to produce a stutter intentionally. This can be done most easily by pretending to have trouble producing slow, loose stutters. For instance, the clinician might say, "I can't seem to make this one slow and loose. Can you show me how to do it?" Again, this should be done intermittently and casually mixed in with other activities that are fun for the child.

Praise and, if needed, tangible rewards are used to help the child build confidence. When the child is able to produce slow and loose stutters, the clinician can let the parents know, in the child's presence, about this accomplishment, focusing on the child's ability to teach the clinician. If the child seems proud of this accomplishment, the clinician can take advantage of this opportunity and have the child show intentional stutters to the parents. This not only desensitizes the child to stuttering with the parent, but it also desensitizes parents to the child's stuttering and models acceptance of the child's stuttering for them.

The Child Changes His Own Real Stutters

For many young children whose stuttering fluctuates between mild and severe levels, these direct therapy activities, combined with a facilitating environment provided by parents, may be enough to advance their fluency into the normal range within a few months. For those whose stuttering persists, still another stage of direct therapy may be necessary. In such cases, I look for opportunities when the child seems ready to modify his own stutters.

I begin by responding to a few of the child's real stutters with accepting comments to help the child feel comfortable with his stutters. I might say, with an accepting voice, "Oh, that one was a little bumpy on 'my-my-my car…,'" and then return to the business of playing. After further play, when the child stutters again, the clinician can model an easier and slower style of stuttering on the same word and comment positively about it. I then ask the child to imitate my easier stutter and praise him for doing so, using reinforcements and guidance to shape his stuttering to a slow, relaxed style.

I look for slightly slower and easier stutters in the child's speech and reward them. Even if the child intentionally stutters, but in an easier way than he stuttered previously, I reward him. From this point on, the clinician uses a combination of modeling and reinforcement to shape the child's stuttering. It is the deliberate slowness and "easiness" with which the child produces repetitions or prolongations, along with the sense of playing with stuttering, that make it possible for the child to begin feeling a sense of control. This in turn should reduce his frustration and fear, further diminish tension, and enable him to move through stutters with minimal effort.

After the child is able to make his stutters slower and easier in the clinic, generalization may occur away from the clinic without the need for formal transfer activities. Such "spontaneous" generalization may be a result of the child's increased self-esteem from gaining mastery over behavior he previously felt uncomfortable about and felt was out of his control. Consequently, emphasis should be placed on the stutters that a child handles successfully, rather than when he loses control.

If generalization is not occurring automatically, I work with family members to make the child's ability to play with and modify stutters a point of pride at home. Initially, the child can teach parents and siblings to stutter in the clinic under the clinician's guidance. Then the clinician can work with the child at home and involve family members when appropriate, so that the parents learn to use positive reinforcement selectively to increase the child's slow and easy stutters and let him know that he is appreciated. Even though the emphasis here is on slow and easy stutters, the effects of speech and language maturation and the increasing confidence that the child feels in his speech as a result of reduced frustration should result in normal fluency.

OTHER CLINICIANS

The approaches of several other clinicians are described here. Many of these approaches are used not only for borderline stuttering in younger preschool children, but for beginning stuttering in older preschool children as well. I have selected them because they all involve the child's family, which I consider of major importance when working with preschool children. The nature of intervention ranges from monitoring the child's stuttering to helping parents change their interaction patterns to direct work on the child's way of speaking, if needed.

Even though some of these approaches present data on their effectiveness, clinicians using any approach should collect their own data on progress and outcome. As suggested in Chapter 8, baseline measures of the child's stuttering at the beginning of treatment should be made in a valid and reliable way. Because preschool children are highly variable, recordings of the child's speech should be made at home as well as in a clinical setting. The Stuttering Severity Instrument-4 (Riley, 2009) should be used to assess frequency and severity. When treatment begins, weekly measures of progress should be made; percentage of syllables stuttered in the clinic and daily SRs of speech at home made by a parent are effective and efficient. When the child has achieved fluent speech (SRs at home of 1 [normal fluency] and less than 1 %SS in the clinic), a maintenance program

should be started, involving continued measurement at home and during gradually faded clinic visits. Children with borderline stuttering can be expected to achieve stable, normally fluent speech within six months. Clinicians should assess how long a child is in treatment before fluency is achieved and how well the child maintained that fluency a year after treatment ends.

Edward Conture and Colleagues

Conture's indirect therapy for preschool-age children (Conture, 2001; Conture & Melnick, 1999; Richels & Conture, 2007) is carried out in parent and child groups that meet separately each session and then as a combined group. The parent group observes portions of the children's therapy and is provided information, suggestions, and opportunities to help them facilitate their child's fluency outside the clinic setting. The parents and clinician also discuss child-rearing issues that directly affect the child's ability to receive maximal benefit from treatment. The children's group helps the child learn the skills of effective communication.

During the initial phase of treatment, the groups meet once per week to establish the child's fluency. When the child's stuttering in the clinic is below 5 percent for four consecutive weeks (which usually takes about 12 weeks of treatment, but for some longer), the family then meets less frequently—but still regularly—with the clinician so that the parents can continue new behaviors more independently, and the child's increased fluency can be transferred to home and beyond. This is followed by a maintenance phase, to be described.

Conture and his colleagues stress the importance of data to guide treatment. Richels and Conture (2010) describe their evaluation procedures and the important relationships between pretreatment information and the outcomes of treatment, for example, understanding that a slow-to-warm-up child may require a longer period of treatment before becoming successful. They typically collect measures of the child's stuttering frequency at the beginning of every clinic visit and are beginning to use a rating scale on a monthly basis to examine parents' perceptions of their children's disfluencies and children's responses to stuttering beyond the clinic to determine how well treatment effects are generalizing and to guide dismissal.

Specifics of Treatment
Children's Group

The children's group begins with conversation led by the clinician. Samples of 100 words of conversation are obtained from each child to provide disfluency data for each session. Activities in the children's group then begin with rules that foster good communication, which include listening when someone else is talking, taking turns in conversations, and not interrupting.

These rules are described to the child verbally and augmented by brightly colored pictures depicting each of the three rules. Children are reinforced for using the rules appropriately. After rules are reviewed, the clinician engages the children in "story time," during which reading of an age-appropriate story is intermingled with questions of the children that match each child's language and fluency abilities (e.g., "forced-choice" questions are asked of a child who is fluent only at this level of linguistic demand, while open-ended questions are asked of a child who is ready for that level of demand). Story time is followed by a craft or game activity that blends turn taking and verbal responses consistent with each child's abilities. The clinician models the interaction strategies with which the parents are being familiarized in their group (see below).

Parents' Group

Many of the parents' group activities are focused on improved communicative interactions that dovetail with the turn-taking rules and adaptation of linguistic demand based on a child's demonstrated fluency, so that parent-child conversations at home increasingly facilitate the child's development of fluency, related speech and language behaviors, and ease of communication. The parents learn the following strategies over the course of treatment:

- Speaking more slowly (but still normally) to the child
- Adjusting the length and complexity of utterances to meet requirements of the communicative situation—generally talking to the child using shorter, simpler sentences when appropriate.
- Pausing for a second after the child speaks to give the child plenty of time to finish speaking and to slow the overall pace of conversation.
- Decreasing the number of interruptions and questions when conversing with the child
- Decreasing the number of corrections of the child's speech, language, and related communicative behaviors

Parents in the group are asked first to observe their speaking behaviors with their child, as well as the child's speaking behaviors, and then encouraged to discuss their observations with the group. Subsequently, parents learn how to make changes in these behaviors and practice them in a single setting, once a day for about five to 15 minutes (depending on the situation and the parents' comfort level with new strategies). This helps them experience and learn these changes in a relatively controlled setting, such as nightly bedtime rituals, before trying them in more spontaneous situations, such as during conversations at the dinner table. The first new behavior parents are asked to practice is to speak more slowly but normally to the child and to pause for one second after the child finishes speaking before they start speaking. This change is thought to create a speaking environment that facilitates the child's fluency and overall conversational turn taking. This approach also attempts to

produce a communicative environment in which the child is more likely to feel that he doesn't have to hurry to speak and helps to reduce how often parents are interrupting their child. The parents' pause after their child talks will also reduce the extent to which parental communicative behavior may encroach on the time during which the child may be planning and producing spoken language. Another important change for parents is to learn to use shorter and simpler sentences, not continually, but when appropriate. Parents' modeling of this behavior encourages children to decrease the speed of initiating and maintaining speech as well as more easily adjust the length and complexity of their utterances to communicative requirements, enhancing their fluency. Similarly, parents learn to adjust the level of demand of their inquiries of their child according to their observations of the child's fluency in particular situations (e.g., keeping it simple, forced-choice questions when children are more disfluent, and using more open-ended inquiries when children are more fluent).

Parents discuss and practice other new behaviors on the list and are encouraged to use the group to support each other in planning situations in which they can try out these changes and then share the results of their efforts. Parents are most successful when they don't try to change all of their behaviors in all situations but work on only one or two at a time in such specific situations as talking with their child while playing a simple board game or playing alongside the child (e.g., building with blocks, playing with Play Doh, dressing a doll, etc.) or reading a bedtime story. It is stressed to the parents that smaller periods of practice, almost every day, are more effective than longer periods of practice once or twice a week.

Throughout treatment, parents are provided with graphic descriptions of how their child is doing (Figs. 11.3 to 11.5). These "therapy graphs" depict three pieces of information: (1) total disfluencies per 100 words, (2) total stuttered disfluencies per 100 words, and (3) total nonstuttered disfluencies per 100 words. These graphs are used during therapy sessions as well as during parent-clinician counseling sessions to help parents understand expected variations in disfluencies and their child's progress over time, as well as to help the clinician plan short-term and long-term goals for each child.

Dismissal

Conture stresses the importance of the fact that once a child is ready for dismissal, treatment is not abruptly terminated but gradually faded. First, the child's treatment changes from once a week to once every other week, then to once a month, once every three months, and finally, every six months for a year. If stuttering reappears at any time during this period, the child can be brought back into treatment until he regains fluency. Although this schedule of fading is the best approach, the time of a child's dismissal

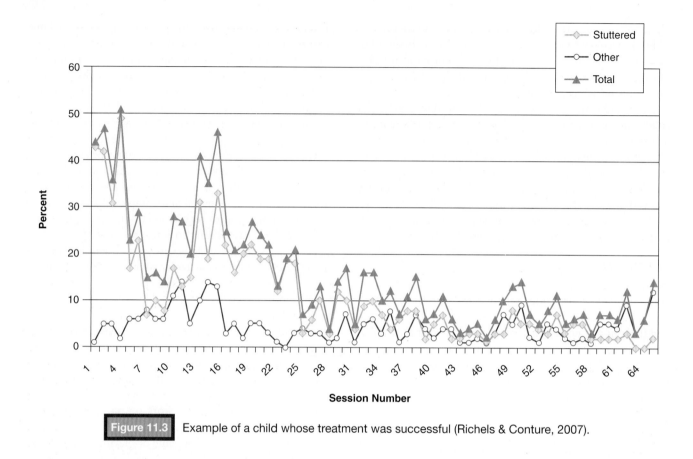

Figure 11.3 Example of a child whose treatment was successful (Richels & Conture, 2007).

is sometimes negotiated with the parents. Some parents want to continue with regular treatment longer than may be necessary, which is only allowed if it is believed to be in the child's best long-term interest (typically as a means of helping the parent(s) to prepare for independence). Other parents want to discontinue treatment after the child has become fluent but before gradual fading of treatment has been completed. In these cases, parents' wishes are granted, and the door is left open for them to return if necessary.

Based on his experience, Conture rejects a one-size-fits-all approach to determining the length of treatment and criterion for termination. Instead, he considers the individual needs of each child, the nature of his problem, the child's learning history, the parents' concerns, perceptions of their child's progress, and the extent of their involvement in therapy, in determining each child's pace in moving from skill acquisition to maintenance to dismissal (i.e., establishment of normal disfluency).

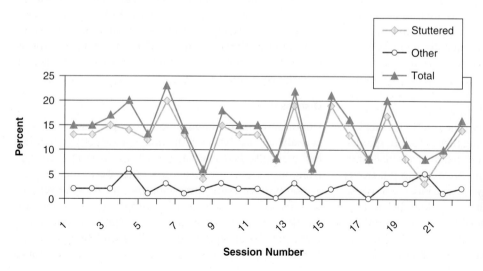

Figure 11.4 Example of a child with highly variable performance during treatment (Richels & Conture, 2007).

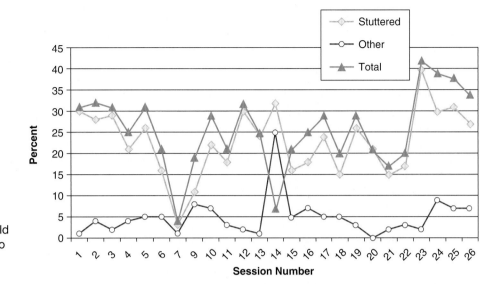

Figure 11.5 Example of a child not responding to group treatment (Richels & Conture, 2007).

Supporting Data

Richels and Conture (2007) reported on 32 children (ages 2–9 to 6–0) who stuttered on an average of 10 words per 100 (stuttering-like disfluencies), averaged 21.3 on the SSI-3 (moderate), and whose time since onset of stuttering averaged 15.5 months. All of the children had received at least 12 treatment sessions—enough time to have shown some response to therapy, according to their experience. Results indicated that on average, these children decreased their stuttering-like disfluencies by 31 percent in 12 sessions.

Palin Centre Parent-Child Interaction

Treatment

The team at the Michael Palin Centre for Stammering Children have developed a treatment for preschoolers who stutter based on the therapy of Lena Rustin (1991). This approach rests on the premise that the vulnerabilities that underlie the breakdown in children's fluency also make it harder for them to cope with typical adult-child interactions (Miles & Bernstein Ratner, 2001). Therapy uses video feedback to help parents identify interaction styles that support their children's fluency and then develop these styles in structured practice sessions at home. While the research indicates that changes in interaction style can be associated with increased fluency (Millard, Nicholas, & Cook, 2008; Guitar, 1978; Guitar et al., 1992; Kasprisin-Burrelli, Egolf, & Shames, 1972; Stephenson-Opsal & Bernstein Ratner, 1988), parent-child interaction styles are not considered to be causing the breakdown in fluency. Indeed some studies have found that interaction styles alter after the child has started to stutter (Meyers & Freeman, 1985a, 1985b; Kloth, Janssen, Kraaimaat, & Brutten, 1998).

A detailed description of the Palin Parent-Child Interaction therapy program has been published in Kelman and Nicholas (2008), and illustrative video clips can be found in Botterill and Kelman (2010). The approach begins with a thorough evaluation of a child's strengths and needs. The child's receptive and expressive language, articulation, speech rate, social communication skills, and sensitivity are evaluated. This gives an indication of any vulnerabilities which may be contributing to the stuttering. A video recording is made of the parents and child in a play situation, and this is analyzed later to establish which interaction styles are likely to be facilitating fluency and which styles need to be developed further. A detailed parent interview elicits information about the child and his fluency in the context of the family, and the parents' ideas are sought about what facilitates the child's fluency. The parents may have observed, for example, that the child is more fluent when she has had plenty of rest but less fluent when she is competing for speaking time, such as at the dinner table. The parents' ideas are valued and incorporated into treatment.

The assessment findings are presented to the parents in terms of the child's strengths and needs in a formulation, summarizing which factors may be contributing to the stuttering as well as those that are helpful for fluency development and suggesting therapy options. The clinician stresses to the parents that nothing they have done has *caused* their child's stuttering but that their participation in treatment is vital in helping the child.

Parent-child interaction therapy involves both parents with the child attending once weekly for six weeks. In the session, the clinician views a video of the interaction with the parents, inviting them to comment on the helpful things they are already doing, such as speaking more slowly or pausing for a few seconds when the child finishes a speaking turn rather than talking immediately. If the parents observe that they are talking too fast, the clinician finds examples on the video of when they are talking slower, at a more facilitating rate. The overarching principle behind changing parents' interaction behaviors is to find ways of giving the child more time to plan and execute speech. Together, the parents and the clinician decide on a target, such as increasing the parents' pause time after the child speaks. The parents work on the new target daily in five-minute practice sessions at home with the child.

In subsequent sessions during the initial six weeks of treatment, the clinician reviews the parents' homework and then records each parent interacting separately with the child. The clinician then reviews the two videos with both parents together. While watching his or her own videotape, each parent picks out several interactions with which he or she is pleased and one behavior that they might develop. The rationale for this is discussed, exploring how an interaction style can affect the child's fluency. Although much of the emphasis is on their communication interactions, the parents also learn to use praise of other skills to build up the child's confidence. The book *How to Talk So Kids Will Listen and How to Listen So Kids Will Talk* by Faber and Mazlish (1999) is used for teaching parents to praise their child once each day for something specific the child did. Other "family strategies" are also introduced, such as turn taking and managing sensitivity or perfectionism.

After six weeks of meeting with the clinician, the parents work on their own at home for a second six-week period of "consolidation" of their new behaviors. Parents send homework record sheets to the clinician each week and continue the daily five-minute interaction times that each parent has with the child. The clinician responds via e-mail, phone, or regular mail. At the end of this six-week consolidation period, the family meets with the clinician for a review of progress. If the child's fluency is significantly better and continuing to improve, the parents are asked to continue working on the changes they are making, and another review is scheduled six weeks later. If the child's fluency is not improving, more direct treatment is introduced, such as "child strategies," based on the approach of Fosnot and Woodford (1992) or the Lidcombe Program described in Chapter 12. The child's fluency is monitored for the minimum of one year.

Supporting Data

Data have been published for 13 children, showing short-term (Matthews, Williams, & Pring, 1997), medium-term (Millard, Edwards, & Cook, 2009), and long-term (Millard, Nicholas & Cook, 2008) efficacy. Using experimental single-subject methodologies, the clinician-researchers at the Michael Palin Centre have demonstrated that the indirect components of this approach (interaction and family strategies) can be effective in reducing the frequency of stuttering in children (Matthews, Williams, & Pring, 1997; Millard, Nicholas, & Cook, 2008; Millard, Edwards, & Cook, 2009). In addition, there is evidence that the approach can reduce the impact of stuttering for both the children and the parents and increase parents' ratings of knowledge and confidence in managing the stuttering (Millard, Edwards, & Cook, 2009).

By including only children who had been stuttering for more than 12 months, collecting data over a baseline phase prior to therapy, and using statistical analysis that compared change against variability in the baseline phase, the researchers concluded that improvements were attributable to the therapy.

Stuttering Foundation Approach

The Stuttering Foundation (formerly the Stuttering Foundation of America) has advocated a general approach to children who are beginning to stutter—a treatment that can be carried out by parents, ideally with guidance from a trained clinician. The SF's online store on their Web site (www.stutteringhelp.org) currently has available a number of items designed for parents of preschool-age children who are beginning to stutter. Ainsworth and Fraser's booklet, *If Your Child Stutters: A Guide for Parents,* eighth edition (2010), helps families differentiate between normal disfluency and stuttering and provides guidelines to help them create fluency-facilitating environments.

Conture's *Stuttering and Your Child: Questions and Answers,* fourth edition (2010), provides families, teachers, and others with information about stuttering and how children who stutter can be helped. It covers a wide range of issues, including stuttering versus normal disfluency, the possible causes of stuttering, changing the home environment, dealing with others' responses to the child's stuttering, and treatment. Although formal aspects of treatment are left to professionals, specific advice is given in highlighted pages about how parents, babysitters, day care centers, and teachers can help children who stutter. Parents are instructed how to be good listeners, how to increase the times when the child feels he is being heard, and how to reduce both conversational and lifestyle pressures on the child. Babysitters and day care centers are advised to react as normally as possible to the child and to treat him like other children, while ensuring that he has plenty of time to say what he wants to say without feeling rushed. Teachers are encouraged to give the child support for oral recitations, allow him the same speaking opportunities as other children, and help the entire class develop good speaking and listening practices.

The SF's most popular publication on the treatment of stuttering in young children is the video, *Stuttering and Your Child: Help for Parents* (Guitar, Guitar, & Fraser, 2006). It is available free as streaming video on the SF Web site and as a DVD that can be purchased for $10. This video, in both English and Spanish, was designed to be used by families working alone, as a preliminary tool, as well as by those who are in treatment with a speech-language pathologist. The video teaches families to make changes in the child's environment, primarily in two areas: communicative interaction and family lifestyle. It also describes when to get help from a speech-language pathologist and what to expect in an evaluation and from treatment. The SF Web site quotes an American Speech-Language-Hearing Association book review that refers to this video as "perhaps the best buy in the nation for information on children and stuttering."

All of the SF's publications emphasize that families are not the cause of stuttering but that families can create an environment that facilitates the growth of fluency. The following suggestions for changes in families' conversational interactions are described in detail in both publications, and parents demonstrate them in the video.

- Talk more slowly.
- Use plenty of pauses in your speech after the child finishes talking.
- Ask the child fewer questions.
- Spend time physically close to the child, such as having him in your lap when you read to him.
- Allow silent time in conversations so that the child doesn't feel compelled to talk and isn't interrupted.
- Help the child learn to take turns talking.

The following suggestions are for families wishing to change some aspects of their lifestyle to facilitate their child's fluency:

- Try to find an opportunity each day, preferably in the morning, when special attention can be given to the child so that he is getting one-on-one time with a parent or another caregiver. During this time, the focus should be on listening to the child and letting him direct the play. The best interactions at these times are those when the parent is talking little and is primarily there for the child as he talks and plays.
- Slow the pace of life, when possible. Give the family more time to do fewer things.
- Develop regular, consistent times for meals, naps, and bedtimes.
- Use reasonable and consistent discipline.
- Make sure the child gets plenty of rest.
- Provide plenty of time for the child to transition from one thing to another. For example, getting ready to go to a birthday party after playing quietly at home may require an extra 10 or 20 minutes because the two activities are so different.

In addition to these ideas for changing a child's environment, the SF's publications suggest that parents should try to become aware of what events or situations are associated with the ups and downs of their child's fluency. Some children who stutter are more sensitive to common, everyday life stresses; things that may not bother most children may cause a child who stutters to become more disfluent. Some examples might be visits by strangers, holidays, a parent leaving for or coming home from work, or an argument between parents. If it can be predicted when more stressful events might occur, extra support can be provided to the child during such situations.

A family that is working with their child on their own are advised that if their child's stuttering does not show a gradual decrease after these changes have been in place for over a month, they should seek help from a speech-language pathologist who specializes in treating childhood stuttering.

In addition to an extensive online bookstore with many low-cost publications and video material, the SF Web site also has a page with guidelines from ASHA for seeking insurance coverage for stuttering evaluation and treatment (www.stutteringhelp.org/insurance.htm).

SUMMARY

- Borderline stuttering in young preschoolers is characterized by an excess of normal disfluencies, particularly part-word repetitions and single-syllable whole-word repetitions. Although the child may have a high frequency of disfluencies and may repeat sounds many times, he typically is not frustrated or embarrassed by the disfluencies. If these emotional reactions do occur, they are usually transitory. Onset of stuttering is relatively recent (less than a year).
- The occurrence of borderline stuttering in young preschoolers is thought to be the result of an interaction between a child's predisposition and typical developmental and environmental stresses. The family is not to blame for the stuttering but can be vital in creating a facilitating environment that increases fluency.
- Treatment is usually focused on helping families make changes in their conversational interactions and in family routines.
- Changes in the family's interaction patterns include helping family members: (1) slow their speech rates; (2) pause for two or three seconds after the child finishes talking before they begin to speak; (3) listen attentively to what the child is saying; (4) ensure appropriate turn taking by all members of the family, including the child; (5) ask fewer questions that lead to long answers; and (6) use vocabulary and sentence complexity that are close to the child's level when speaking to him.
- Changes in the family routine should include the following: Arrange a time, preferably in the morning, when one parent or caregiver can have 10 to 15 minutes of uninterrupted time with the child. During this time, the parent should be primarily there for the child, listening and paying attention to what the child is saying and doing, and appropriately reflecting the child's feelings. This can be a time in which a parent or caregiver practices the interaction patterns suggested earlier.
- The family should be encouraged to carry out the following changes in their lifestyle: (1) create structures and predictable routines to increase the child's sense of security; (2) slow the pace of family life, so that there are calm transitions from one activity to another; (3) ensure

that the child's life is not too busy or rushed; and (4) use consistent, reasonable discipline with the child to ensure that he feels his family is in control.

- If a child's stuttering does not begin to decline within a month or six weeks, more direct treatment should be undertaken. For mild borderline stuttering in young preschoolers, parents are taught to use occasional praise for fluency during one-on-one sessions with the child. For more severe stuttering in this age group, the child is taught to change harder stutters into easier ones, using modeling, playing with stuttering, voluntary stuttering, and reinforcing slow, easy stutters in his spontaneous speech.

- Other clinicians' indirect approaches to stuttering in this age group include parent counseling coupled with monitoring of children with few risk factors, group therapy, and work with families on changing communicative interaction patterns and family lifestyles.

- One other clinician's direct approach teaches children to use slow and smooth speech and to take turns in conversation. Another approach assesses the linguistic level at which a child is fluent, then moves the child through a hierarchy of longer and more complex responses while keeping him fluent for longer periods of time.

STUDY QUESTIONS

1. What are some aspects of family conversational interactions that may put pressure on the young preschool child vulnerable to stuttering?
2. What changes can a family make in their home to relieve speech and language pressures?
3. Discuss how the clinician can facilitate changes in family routines that may help the child's fluency.
4. What are some of the barriers to change that are found in some families? How can the clinician help the family overcome these barriers?
5. Compare my direct approach to a young preschooler who stutters mildly with my approach to one who stutters more severely.
6. Compare one of the other clinician's more indirect therapies with one of the more direct therapies.

SUGGESTED PROJECTS

1. Conduct an informal ABAB study of the effect of slowing your speech rate on a conversational partner who is not aware of the purpose of your study. You will need to record your conversation so that you can analyze the data afterward. In the first A condition, conduct several minutes of conversation at a normal rate; in the first B condition, conduct the same amount of conversation at a slower rate. Then repeat the two rates in two subsequent A and B conditions. Was your speaking partner affected by your speaking rate?

2. Pretend that you are the parent of a child who is beginning to stutter. Search the library and the Internet for advice about how to help your child, and determine whether there is consistency in the advice or whether conflicting information is given.

3. Examine the materials presented in this chapter from other clinicians and determine whether the approaches are designed just for stuttering in young preschoolers or whether the authors intend them for older children as well.

SUGGESTED READINGS

Ainsworth, S., & Fraser, J. (2010). *If your child stutters: A guide for parents* (8th Ed.) **Memphis: Stuttering Foundation of America.**

This inexpensive booklet gives advice to parents who think their child is beginning to stutter.

Chmela, K. (2004). *Working with preschoolers who stutter: Successful intervention strategies.* **Videotape or DVD format. Memphis: Stuttering Foundation of America.**

This is a video of a convention presentation designed to teach clinicians how to work with preschool children who stutter, using modeling of easy, relaxed speech when talking to children and counseling parents to develop a fluency-friendly environment.

Conture, E. (Ed.) (2010). *Stuttering and your child: Questions and answers.* **Memphis: Stuttering Foundation of America.**

This booklet provides answers for parents to commonly asked questions about stuttering in young children.

Gottwald, S. (2010). Stuttering prevention and early intervention: A multidimensional approach. In B. Guitar & R. McCauley (Eds.), *Treatment of Stuttering: Established and Emerging Interventions.* **Baltimore: Lippincott Williams & Wilkins.**

This is a very useful detailed description illustrated by video clips of the direct and indirect treatment for preschoolers who stutter developed by Gottwald and Starkweather over the past 25 years.

Guitar, B., Kopff-Schaefer, H. K., Donahue-Kilburg, G., & Bond, L. (1992). Parent verbal interaction and speech rate. *Journal of Speech and Hearing Research, 35,* 742–754.

This article describes therapy with parents of a young child who stutters and the analysis of parent-child interactions.

Nelson, L. (1985). Language formulation related to dysfluency and stuttering. In *Stuttering Therapy: Prevention and Intervention with Children*. Memphis: Stuttering Foundation of America.

This chapter delineates Lois Nelson's treatment strategies for preschoolers who stutter. It is a distillation of many years of experience with stuttering children.

Reville, J. (1988). *The many voices of Paws*. Princeton Junction, NJ: Speech Bin.

This is a manual for speech-language pathologists and parents to help them work with preschool children who stutter. A slow, easy style of speaking is taught with the help of a poem about a cat named Paws.

Richels, C., & Conture, E. (2007). An indirect approach for early intervention for childhood stuttering. In E. Conture & R. Curlee (Eds.), *Stuttering and Related Disorders of Fluency*. New York: Thieme Medical Publishers, Inc.

This chapter describes a data-based treatment program that uses parent and child groups to change family interaction patterns to indirectly influence a child's stuttering.

Richels, C., & Conture, E. (2010). Indirect treatment of childhood stuttering: Diagnostic predictors of treatment outcome. In B. Guitar & R. McCauley (Eds.), *Treatment of Stuttering: Established and Emerging Interventions*. Baltimore: Lippincott Williams & Wilkins.

A very thoughtful description of the use of diagnostic data to predict short- and long-term outcomes. Interestingly, successful short-term outcomes appear to be related to less severe stuttering at the beginning of treatment, but successful long-term outcomes are more related to diagnostic indicators of expressive (rather than inhibited) temperament and to lower language scores at the beginning of treatment.

Roseman, B., & Johnson, K. (1998). *Easy Does It® for fluency: Preschool/primary*. East Moline, IL: LinguiSystems.

This manual and materials book provides instruction and materials for stuttering therapy for children from ages 2 to 6 years. The focus is on teaching fluency through the establishment of "easy speech" through modeling and then progressing up a linguistic and situational hierarchy. Desensitization to fluency disruptors is included, as well as maintenance of fluency. Some suggestions for combining phonological and fluency therapy are provided.

Starkweather, C. W., Gottwald, S. R., & Halfond, M. H. (1990). *Stuttering prevention: A clinical method*. Englewood Cliffs, NJ: Prentice-Hall.

This book details a program of assessment and treatment for children who stutter and for their parents.

Walton, P., & Wallace, M. (1998). *Fun with fluency*. Bisbee, AZ: Imaginart International, Inc.

This manual provides extensive information about working with both borderline and beginning stuttering. The manual covers both indirect and direct treatment, information, and materials for working with parents and teachers and includes many activities for children aged 2 to 7.

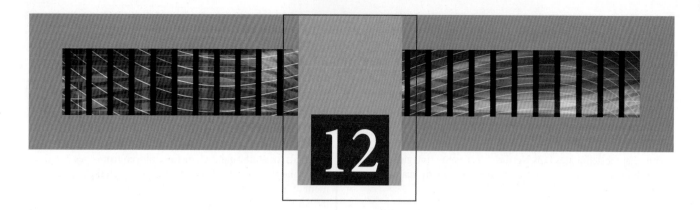

12

Treatment of Stuttering in Older Preschool Children: Beginning Stuttering

CHAPTER OBJECTIVES

After studying this chapter, readers should be able to:
- Describe the characteristics of a child who has beginning stuttering
- Describe the author's beliefs about stuttering, targets in treatment, goals for treatment, how much to involve feelings and attitudes in treatment, and maintenance procedures
- Delineate the procedures involved in the Lidcombe Program treatment, the stages of therapy, and the criteria to compete each stage
- Explain how formal training may be obtained for using the Lidcombe Program
- Outline the components of Sheryl Gottwald's "multidimensional approach"
- Describe a number of different approaches to working on stuttering and concomitant speech or language problems

KEY TERMS

Older preschool children: Children between 3.5 and 6 years of age
Lidcombe Program (LP): An operant conditioning–based approach to stuttering, delivered in the home by a parent or other caregiver and guided via weekly meetings with the clinician
Operant conditioning: A type of behavior modification that uses rewards and punishments to increase or decrease the frequency of a behavior

Verbal contingencies: Comments to the child made immediately after an event (e.g., fluent utterance; stutter) that are intended to change the frequency of that event

Stage 1 (of LP): The initial step of LP in which the child becomes normally fluent. Criteria for completing Stage 1 are three consecutive weeks in which (a) the parent's weekly SRs average below 2 with at least four 1s and (b) the clinician's SRs for entire sessions are 1s or 2s

Severity Rating Scale: A scale from 1 to 10 used daily by parent to assess child's stuttering. May be used by clinician as well during weekly clinic sessions

Stage 2 (of LP): When the child meets the fluency criteria to complete Stage 1, this maintenance stage is begun. Weekly clinic meetings are faded systematically so that the parent and child meet with the clinician in this sequence: two, two, four, four, eight, eight, and finally 16 weeks apart. The child must continue to meet fluency criteria

Demands and capacities: The perspective that the factors associated with the onset and persistence of stuttering are the demands placed on the child by her environments balanced by the child's innate capacity for fluent speech

Concomitant speech and language problems: Difficulties with articulation/phonological processing and/or difficulties with language that sometimes accompany stuttering. When this occurs in some children who stutter, it poses a problem of which disorder to work on first

AN INTEGRATED APPROACH

Children with beginning stuttering are usually between 3.5 and 6 years of age, **older preschool children**, although some children may be 7 or 8 years old. They have probably been stuttering for at least several months, and their parents may well be concerned that it is not a transient problem that will disappear on its own. What follows are some details on the core and secondary behaviors of stuttering, as well as feelings and attitudes that often mark stuttering in this age group. These children's most common core stuttering behaviors are part-word repetitions that are produced rapidly, usually with irregular rhythm. Some prolongations may also be present. Both the repetitions and prolongations may contain excessive tension, which can be heard as abrupt endings to the repetitions and as increases in vocal pitch in repetitions and prolongations. Blocks may be present but will probably not be the predominant core behavior. Secondary behaviors are typically escape devices, such as eye blinks, head nods, and increases in pitch. A few avoidance maneuvers, such as starting sentences with extra sounds like "uh" or changing words when a stutter is anticipated may be observed. Children with beginning stuttering usually feel frustrated with their difficulty in talking but have not yet developed a strong fear of stuttering or learned to be ashamed of their speech. In rare cases, if the frequency of stuttering becomes extremely high, these children may put their hands to their mouths to push words out or may momentarily avoid talking.

I will illustrate our approach with a description of Katherine's treatment. She is the 3-year-old child I introduced in Chapter 1. The course of her treatment is depicted in Figure 12.1.

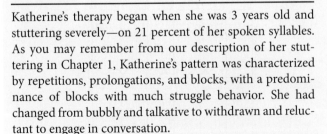

Case Example

Katherine

Katherine's therapy began when she was 3 years old and stuttering severely—on 21 percent of her spoken syllables. As you may remember from our description of her stuttering in Chapter 1, Katherine's pattern was characterized by repetitions, prolongations, and blocks, with a predominance of blocks with much struggle behavior. She had changed from bubbly and talkative to withdrawn and reluctant to engage in conversation.

At the time she came in for an evaluation, two other clinicians and I had just been trained in the Lidcombe approach—the treatment described in this chapter. Several weeks after the evaluation, we began Katherine's therapy by training her mother in using verbal contingencies (praise) for Katherine's fluent speech during daily, 15-minute structured conversations at home. We also trained her in

making daily ratings of the severity of Katherine's stuttering. During our weekly clinic meetings with Katherine and her mother, we measured the frequency of Katherine's stuttering in conversation at the beginning of each session. The rest of each session was spent on problem solving any issues that came up during the home treatment and training Katherine's mother in the next steps of treatment, in such verbal contingencies for stuttering, and then in using verbal contingencies during unstructured sessions throughout the day. After several weeks went by, we saw notable improvement in Katherine's stuttering, shown by both our weekly measures of her stuttering frequency in the clinic and her mother's daily ratings of the severity of Katherine's stuttering at home. The steady decline in Katherine's stuttering continued, interrupted by an occasional spike upward of stuttering when a momentary stressful event occurred such as a visit by relatives or a family trip. Once Katherine's

Case Example *(Continued)*

stuttering shot up for several days, and we worked with Katherine's mother to figure out the source of the problem. We discovered that Katherine's father, in his eagerness to help, began to use verbal contingencies without training when he was alone with Katherine and overdosed her with several hours of contingencies each day, instead of the recommended 12 or 15 contingencies per day. Once that was resolved and Katherine's father was trained to use contingencies judiciously, her stuttering continued to decline steadily. Katherine became fluent after about six months of treatment. Over the following year, the clinicians continued to stay in touch, but Katherine and her mother came in to the clinic less and less frequently.

Seven years after therapy had been completed, we contacted Katherine and her parents to assess her status. She had been completely fluent ever since treatment ended and today is highly verbal with only dim memories of ever having stuttered. Her parents have become a valuable resource for other parents of children who are beginning to stutter as they contemplate treatment.

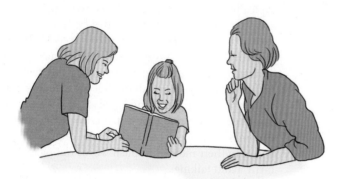

Mother and child in clinic session

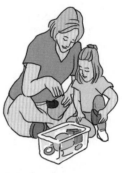

Mother and child in structured conversation at home

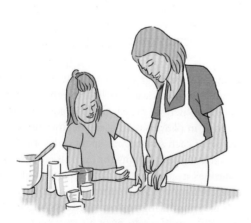

Mother and child in unstructured conversation at home

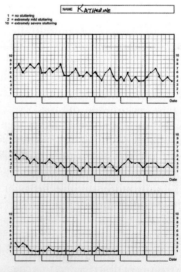

Child's Stuttering Severity Rating Chart

Figure 12.1   An overview of the treatment described in Chapter 12.

Author's Beliefs

Nature of Stuttering

I believe that beginning stuttering arises when children's basic sensory-motor difficulty interacts with their temperament and other developmental and environmental influences to produce or exacerbate repetitions, prolongations, and blocks. This is essentially the position taken by Wendell Johnson and colleagues (1959), who suggested that the problem of stuttering arises as a result of interactions among (a) the amount of the child's disfluency, (b) the reaction of his listeners to the disfluency, and (c) the child's sensitivity to his own disfluency and to listeners' reactions. I would add to Johnson's list of interacting factors any pressures that a child may feel internally (e.g., to speak quickly and in long, complex sentences) and any anxieties the child may experience as the result of moving, the birth of a sibling, or other life events.

In some children, beginning stuttering emerges gradually after they have gone through a period of borderline stuttering as younger preschool children. As these children get older and if stuttering continues, they begin to respond to negative experiences of repetitive disfluencies with increased tension.

In other children, beginning stuttering appears quickly, close to the onset of stuttering. They may be easily frustrated or highly distressed when many of their speech attempts result in repetitions or prolongations that feel out of their control. As these children attempt to cope with these core behaviors, they develop a variety of escape behaviors that are reinforced. Their eye blinks, head nods, and pitch increases are rewarded when they are associated with the release of the child's stutters. Gradually, classical conditioning influences when and where the child's stuttering occurs. Negative emotional experiences that are associated with stuttering become etched into memory and associated with various contexts, such as the telephone, impatient listeners, or particular words. As stuttering spreads and becomes more pervasive and more consistently present, these children become aware of their stuttering, although they have little shame of it and do not dread speaking situations. Because of the plasticity of the brain at this age, some beginning stutterers develop better sensory-motor control of speech, and their stuttering goes out the door it entered. Their stutters diminish in frequency and severity and disappear or become a minor nuisance. Other children, perhaps those with more widespread sensory-motor deficits, more sensitive temperament, or larger doses of other developmental and environmental stresses, continue to stutter and often develop more advanced symptoms.

Like Oliver Bloodstein (1975), I believe that if we can provide a beginning stutterer with a sufficient number of positive, fluent speaking experiences during treatment, fluency will replace stuttering. Perhaps the daily, structured practice of fluency in the approach I use reinforces the neural pathways for fluent speech so that they become more robust, more automatic, and more resistant to stress. This may happen best when treatment takes place at home, where it can be done seven days a week. It also appears effective if natural fluency is elicited in highly structured situations, systematically reinforced, and then carefully transferred to more and more real-life situations in which stuttering is occurring.

The increased fluency gained through treatment reduces the opportunities a child has to respond to any remaining disfluencies with tension, frustration, or escape and starting behaviors. It also allows time for the child's physiological system to mature and for normal fluency patterns to become stabilized.

Speech Behaviors Targeted for Therapy

Which speech behaviors are targeted for the beginning stutterer? In the major approach I advocate in this section, the **Lidcombe Program**, the clinician teaches the parent to first reinforce the child's fluent speech and then respond to stutters. The parent uses appropriate and varied verbal contingencies immediately after fluent utterances but comments gently on stutters much less frequently or gently asks the child to try the word again immediately after she stutters.

Fluency Goals

Almost all children who are treated with effective therapy for beginning stuttering will gain or regain spontaneous, normal fluency. Typically, a year or two after treatment ends, the children will have little or no recollection of having stuttered and will not have to monitor their speech or work at being fluent.

Feelings and Attitudes

As noted earlier, a child with beginning stuttering has only occasional frustration and intermittent concern about talking. She has only mild conditioned fears or avoidances of stuttering. Thus, it is unnecessary to focus directly on feelings and attitudes in therapy with a beginning stutterer.

The feelings and attitudes of these children are, however, influenced by the family. The clinician teaches the family member providing the at-home treatment to be matter-of-fact about the child's "smooth" and "bumpy" speech. The clinician and family member openly discuss the child's stuttering during their weekly meetings when the child is also present. These aspects of treatment reduce any embarrassment or shame that was associated with stuttering and foster the child's acceptance of stuttering as just a little mistake, like bumping into a table or falling off a tricycle. This is a far cry from the "conspiracy of silence" that formerly characterized the treatment of children who stutter.

Maintenance Procedures

Systematically fading contact with the child and her family is vital for maintaining fluency. In my experience, if families leave treatment after fluency is achieved without having participated in a maintenance program, stuttering is likely to return. Thus, it is important for clinicians to stress the importance of maintenance procedures at the outset of treatment. Moreover, the clinician and family should continue with careful data collection as contact is faded, so that the family can return to regular weekly meetings and discuss appropriate contingencies for fluency and stuttering if any relapse occurs.

Clinical Methods

Clinical Procedures: Lidcombe Program

For the last 14 years, I have been using the Lidcombe Program (Onslow, Costa, & Rue, 1990; Onslow, Packman, & Harrison, 2003) to treat preschool children with beginning stuttering. I was initially trained in using this program in a workshop led by Rosalee Shenker. Subsequently, I developed more expertise through consultation and mentoring from Rosalee and my colleagues, Julie Reville, Melissa Bruce, and Danra Kazenski. Follow-up training with Elisabeth Harrison further sharpened my skills. For readers interested in using this approach, I urge you to obtain formal training at one of the many workshops offered around the world by the Lidcombe

Consortium. More information on the Lidcombe Program is available at http://sydney.edu.au/health_sciences/asrc/clinic/parents/lidcombe.shtml.

Overview

The Lidcombe Program uses **operant conditioning** procedures, which are administered by a parent in the home during conversations each day and guided by weekly meetings with the clinician. Treatment begins in structured conversations designed to elicit a maximum of fluent speech by the child so that the child receives mostly positive reinforcement. Approximately every fifth fluent utterance is followed by *praise* (e.g., "That was really good, smooth talking!"); *acknowledgment of fluency* (e.g., a very low-key "That was smooth."); or *request for self-evaluation* (e.g., "Was that smooth?"), which is used only when the child has been fluent. When the child stutters, the parent provides an occasional *acknowledgment of the stutter* ("That was a little bumpy.") or *a gentle request for self-correction* (e.g., "Can you say 'truck' again?"). Table 12.1 lists verbal contingencies for fluency and stuttering.

The ratio of **verbal contingencies** for fluency to verbal contingencies for stuttering is kept very high (about 5:1) to make the program a positive experience for the child. As

Table 12.1	Verbal Contingencies for Fluent Speech
Examples of Verbal Contingencies for Fluent Speech	

- Comments should be specific to speech (i.e., "nice" or "very good" are too general).
- Always give at least five praises before doing a pick-up.
- At the end of each day, the child will have approximately 30 praises:
  - *"That was smooth."*
  - *"Great, your words are smooth!"*
  - *"Nice smooth talking!"*
  - *"No bumps there, excellent."*
  - *"I didn't hear any bumps."*
  - *"Wow, that whole story was totally smooth."*
  - *"Was that smooth?" (The answer should always be "yes" and followed up with another praise.)*
- Also praise for spontaneous self-evaluation (i.e., if the child says "I was really smooth today," or remarks on his own smooth or bumpy talking).

Examples of Verbal Contingencies for Unambiguous Stuttering

- Use low-key delivery and move quickly to a praise.
- Use one pick-up after every five praises (approximately six pick-ups a day).
- Some children become so smooth during a session they do not need any pick-ups. This is OK because the goal is practicing stutter-free speech.
  - *"Oops, I heard a little bump."*
  - *"That was a little bumpy."*
  - *"There was a bump."*
  - *"You got a little stuck there."*
  - *"You only need to say _____ once."*
  - *"Say _____ again." (Use if child is comfortable with repeating stuttered word.)*
- Remember only to praise or use pick-ups on unambiguous stutters or smooth speech; it's important not to praise bumps!

the child's stuttering decreases, structured conversations are faded and gradually replaced by unstructured conversations each day. Verbal contingencies on fluency and stuttering continue, but in more casual situations, such as when the parent is talking with the child in the car, in the kitchen, or at a store. Once the child is fluent in all situations, treatment is gradually faded in a systematic fashion. Throughout the program, the clinician and parent regularly assess the child's stuttering and use those measures to make treatment decisions.

Stage 1: The First Clinic Visit

Stage 1 of the Lidcombe Program begins with the first clinic visit when the clinician meets with the parent (or other caregiver) and child to accomplish three goals: (1) to assess the child's stuttering, (2) to explain severity ratings (SRs) to the parent, and (3) to teach the parent to conduct daily treatment conversations. Stage 1 clinic visits are typically one hour in duration.

The clinician assesses the child's stuttering using a measure of syllables stuttered during conversation between the child, the parent, and the clinician during an activity that the child enjoys. For a valid sample, approximately 300 syllables of the child's speech should be assessed, which usually takes about 10 minutes. Because the clinician will want to let the parent know what the child's frequency of stuttering is, measuring percent syllables stuttered is best done online as the child is talking, rather than from a video, using either a stopwatch and calculator (as described in Chapter 8) or a TrueTalk® handheld counting device (www.truetalk.com.au). I make no attempt to hide the fact that I am assessing the child's speech; if the child asks about it, I usually say something like, "I'm just counting how many smooth words you say." Once I assess the sample, I let the parent know the child's score, and we discuss how it compares to the child's speech in other situations.

Each day the parent uses the **Severity Rating Scale** (see Chapter 8) to assess the child's stuttering at home. The SR Scale is a 10-point scale that the parent completes at the end of every day, reflecting his or her judgment of the child's stuttering severity that day. A 1 on the scale represents no stuttering, a 2 represents extremely mild stuttering, and a 10 represents extremely severe stuttering. After discussing the scale with the parent, I ask her to tell me what rating she would give the child's speech in the clinic that day, which I compare with my own rating. It is usually possible with only a little discussion to ensure that the parent is using the scale appropriately. On the rare occasion that the parent's rating differs from mine by more than one point, I explain how I came up with my rating and then try to determine if the parent seems to understand my rationale and is likely to be accurate in her future ratings. If I have doubts, I use video clips of the child's speech to help teach the parent how to use the scale. I typically ask the parents to make videos of the child's speech at home during the first few weeks of treatment so that I can continue to "calibrate" the parent's ratings. Once I'm sure the parent understands the scale, I ask him or her to rate the child's speech at the end of every day and to bring the ratings to our weekly meetings. The standard Lidcombe procedure has the parent bring in a chart that displays each day's SRs of the child. I encourage the parents to add comments to the chart if the child has gone through a period of increased stuttering, sickness, or other event that the parent feels may have an impact on severity or the child's response to treatment.

The final thing I accomplish in the first clinic visit is to show the parent how to conduct the daily structured treatment conversations. It is most important to create situations that not only are fun but also stimulate a lot of fluent speech in the child. This enables the parent to begin treatment using a great deal of positive verbal contingencies for fluency. To demonstrate for the parent, I begin by using a picture book or picture cards with the child to elicit short, fluent words. To keep the child's interest, I talk with a lot of enthusiasm and move through the pictures quickly. I usually name a picture or two myself as a model for the child and then ask her to name some pictures. After the fifth fluent utterance, I praise her fluency immediately by saying something specifically about her speech, such as, "That was really smooth talking!" or "You said that really smoothly!" It is important to make the praise directly relevant to the child's fluency, rather than general praise. After modeling for the parent, I ask him or her to work with the child, and I coach the parent if necessary.

With children who have more severe stuttering, I may need to begin with single-syllable words or have the child repeat the word after me. Children who have milder stuttering can progress quickly from single words to carrier phrases and words to short sentences of three or four words. Figure 12.2 shows a linguistic hierarchy that most children can quickly climb on the way to natural conversations in the beginning of Stage 1.

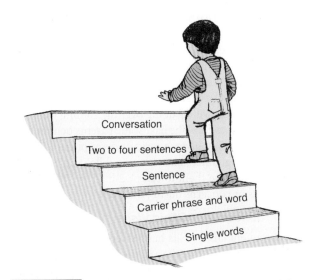

Figure 12.2 Linguistic hierarchy used for structured conversations at the beginning of Stage I.

Table 12.2	Suggested Games and Activities for Structured Treatment Conversations

- Grab bag. The parent puts interesting items into a large cloth bag or pillowcase, and the child guesses what each is by reaching into the bag and feeling the item.
- Picture naming. Using picture books or picture cards, the child names each picture. At the one-word level, the child only names the pictured object. As longer utterances are permitted, the child can use a carrier phrase such as "That's a _____," or she can name the item and its color, such as "red rabbit."
- Reading a story. Parent and child look at a familiar book while the parent reads or tells the story. To elicit a word or phrase, the parent asks the child to complete a sentence, such as "Then Goldilocks said, 'Somebody's been sleeping in my _____.'"
- Rhyme closing. Parent makes up a rhyme and leaves the last word blank, like "There was a boy who lived in Kalamazoo. He liked to climb mountains so he could get a good _____."

One of the mistakes parents often make when they first begin is to use positive verbal contingencies for fluent speech that are too general. They might say, for example, "That's good," or "You're doing well." In this case, I simply restate the need for specific praise and observe the parents doing it. Another common error is for parents to let the child make longer responses than are appropriate, thereby allowing more stuttered than fluent utterances to occur. Fortunately, a little discussion and lots of modeling will usually clear this up. For those children who need to start at the one- or two-word utterance stage, specifically praising their use of one or two words will help keep them at this level until it is appropriate for them to move to longer utterances.

As I mentioned earlier, it is crucial that the parent make the structured conversations fun for the child. It may be helpful to suggest games and activities for the sessions. Table 12.2 lists some of the activities that parents can use with the child in these structured conversations.

At the end of the first clinic visit, I review the activities and tasks the parent will be doing over the coming week and respond to any questions she has. Some parents benefit from taking notes or being given a written description of things they will be doing; others like to have a follow-up e-mail. In all cases, I encourage them to call or e-mail me if they have any questions or concerns during the week.

Stage 1: Subsequent Clinic Visits

Most subsequent clinic visits have three goals: (1) to assess the child's stuttering, (2) to discuss the current progress, and (3) to introduce new procedures when appropriate. Each session begins with the clinician and parent assessing the child's stuttering using the SRs. This assessment is made

from the child's conversational speech when talking with the parent and the clinician until a representative sample of the child's speech has been obtained (about 300 syllables or 10 minutes). The clinician gives the child's speech a rating on the SR Scale and asks the parent for her rating of that sample. If the parent and clinician ratings differ by more than one point, a discussion ensues that helps the parent align her ratings with those of the clinician. Accurate parent SRs are essential to the integrity of the treatment program. These ratings, along with the clinician's ratings, determine whether treatment is progressing successfully and signal when to fade structured treatment conversations and transition to treatment in unstructured conversations. They also indicate when to move from Stage 1 to Stage 2 of the Lidcombe Program.

After the clinician and parent complete their ratings of the child's speech, they discuss the week's SRs and the progress of the home treatment. As they talk, the child usually plays by herself in the same room, with some interaction and encouragement from the parent and the clinician. The openness with which discussions of the week's progress take place is a hallmark of the Lidcombe Program. There is no attempt to keep the child from overhearing the parent and clinician discussion of the child's stuttering. The matter-of-fact manner in which the clinician and parent discuss the child's speech seems to me to make it more likely that both the parent and child will feel less anxious about the child's stuttering and may reduce any shame the child might feel about her difficulty. During the parent and clinician's discussion, some children often make noise to call attention to themselves. In my experience, this is not because the child objects to the discussion of her stuttering but is only an attempt to get the focus back on herself. At such times, it may be helpful if the clinician simply asks the child, "Can I talk to your mommy for just a minute, and then we'll play again?" or she may take a minute to play with the child.

As the clinician looks over the parent's weekly SRs, the clinician may ask about the days in which ratings are higher or lower than average, or the clinician and parent may brainstorm solutions to problems that may be indicated by lack of change in the ratings. This is often a time when videos of the treatment conversations from home are useful, so that the clinician can assess how they are being conducted. It is also helpful to have the parent demonstrate during each clinic visit how he or she is conducting the treatment at home by doing a few minutes of structured conversation with the child using the verbal contingencies (Fig. 12.3).

When adequate progress is being made and home SRs and clinic assessments indicate that the child is becoming more fluent, new treatment procedures can be introduced.

Once a parent is appropriately reinforcing fluency, he or she may be taught to use verbal contingencies for stuttering. The mildest is verbally acknowledging the occurrence of an unambiguous stutter. Only unambiguous stutters should

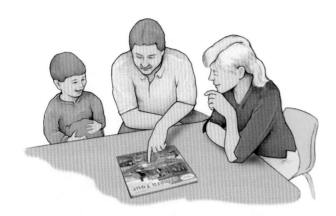

Figure 12.3 Clinician observing parent demonstrating structured conversation with child.

be acknowledged because normal disfluencies should not be treated as stutters. The descriptions of normal disfluencies and stuttered disfluencies in Chapter 7 clarify this difference. I typically model an acknowledgment of stuttering for the parent, which is given after about five instances of contingencies for fluent utterances. It is important that the parent learn to use contingencies for fluency several times before using a verbal contingency on stuttered speech. When I demonstrate acknowledgment of stuttering, I use comments like "a little bumpy one there" or "that one was a little bumpy." I make the statement quietly, immediately after the stutter and without any negative inflection in my voice. After I have modeled acknowledging stutters, I ask the parent to try it but only after he or she has praised several of the child's fluent utterances. Most children hardly seem to notice the acknowledgment, although some may stop momentarily and look at the parent when it is given. Typically, I ask parents to continue using contingencies for fluency and begin using acknowledgment of stuttering for a week before introducing further verbal contingencies for stuttering.

In the following weekly meeting, I introduce requests for self-correction of unambiguous stuttering. This verbal contingency asks the child to say the stuttered word again with a phrase like (if the child has stuttered on "I") "Can you say 'I' again?" Such requests are made in a positive, supportive manner, and it is important that the parent practice this contingency after the clinician demonstrates it. Some parents may be hesitant to request a self-correction and may convey their concern to the child. Others may inadvertently use a slightly negative or impatient tone when asking for a correction. However, a patient clinician's modeling and subsequent coaching can do wonders to shape parents' responses into helpful, supportive requests.

After the child has repeated the word fluently, the parent should praise the self-correction with comments like, "Nice job of making that word smooth." If a child ignores a parent's request for self-correction or refuses to self-correct, the

parent just moves on. If the child says the word again but stutters again, the parent may say something supportive like, "That's OK; sometimes those words are hard."

In the subsequent weeks, the clinician monitors the child's progress and ensures that the parent is delivering verbal contingencies effectively. The clinician also checks to see that the child is enjoying the structured treatment conversations and is responding well to the contingencies for both fluency and stuttering. Every child and every family are different, so the program must be individualized in each case. For example, some children may indicate they are uncomfortable with such praise as "That was really smooth talking." In this case, the parent can ask the child what she would like the parent to say when she is talking smoothly. Alternatively, the parent can use one of the other verbal contingencies for fluency. Some children who don't react well to praise will happily respond to requests to self-evaluate their fluency. One child I worked with preferred that the parent put a penny in a jar, which made a nice "plink" sound, rather than verbally praise her fluency. Another child who loved the Boston Red Sox asked his mother to say "That's Red Sox talking!" after fluent speech. You can guess what the child asked the parent to say after the child stuttered. It had to do with a New York team.

Stage 1: Introducing Unstructured Treatment Conversations

When treatment has progressed well for two or three weeks, and SRs indicate improvement, a gradual transition can be made from structured to unstructured treatment conversations. Thus, verbal contingencies of praise, acknowledgment of stutters, and requests for correction can now be given in typical daily conversations, such as during meals, riding in the car, shopping, and playing. When treatment is first introduced in unstructured conversations, structured treatment usually continues for a time to make the transition easy. When unstructured treatment has been going well for a week or two and stuttering continues to decrease, structured sessions can be faded gradually. For example, each week one or two structured conversations may be dropped until they have all been discontinued and replaced with unstructured treatment.

There are several reasons why structured treatment may subsequently be reinstated. One is if stuttering increases for a day or more; in this situation, structured treatment may be conducted until the child's fluency has returned to earlier levels. Another reason for continuing or reinstating structured treatment is if the child asks to have these conversations. Most children enjoy one-on-one time with a parent, and many ask for a structured conversation occasionally after the conversations have been discontinued. A third reason for continuing structured conversations for a period of time as the transition to unstructured sessions is made is if the parent requests it. Sometimes parents feel that things are going so well in structured sessions that they believe the transition to unstructured sessions should be made slowly.

Several issues may warrant consideration when unstructured treatment is just getting underway. Parents may wish to begin with just praise for fluent utterances and then add acknowledgment for fluency and for stuttering, requests for self-evaluation, and finally, requests for self-correction of stuttering. If problems appear in response to any of these verbal contingencies, they can be solved immediately. It is also important that verbal contingencies not be given relentlessly throughout each day but are used selectively at first, so that the parent can judge how the child is responding. If the child reacts well, which is usually the case, the parent can begin using verbal contingencies in more and more conversations, but at the same time, the parent should make sure that the child is not overwhelmed by too-frequent attention to her speech. The child needs to experience the normal flow of conversation for its own sake, rather than feel that everything she says is being evaluated. This is essential for sensitive children.

Another issue that may arise relative to unstructured treatment is who is giving the verbal contingencies. Although only one parent may have been conducting the structured treatment, both parents, and even other family members, may be involved in the unstructured treatment. When this is done, it must be done very carefully and be individualized for each family. Other adults in the home or older siblings may be appropriate in some cases, whereas a sibling close to the child's age may not be. If a child is responsive to the contingencies given by one parent in unstructured conversations, I usually try adding another family member and evaluate the child's response. I recommend that the clinician meet with any family members who are giving verbal contingencies to ensure that they understand how crucial it is that much more praise for fluency be given than requests for self-correction of stuttering and that requests for self-correction be done in a supportive manner.

Unstructured treatment at home and weekly meetings in the clinic continue until the child is essentially fluent and can move to Stage 2. This point is reached when two criteria are met: (1) the parent's SRs for three weeks in a row are all 1s and 2s, with at least four of the ratings being 1, and (2) the clinician's SRs *for the entire clinic visit* are 1s or 2s for these same three weeks. Meeting these criteria is vital if the child is to remain fluent after treatment. If the clinician has any doubts about the reliability and validity of the parent's SRs, she should request that the parent bring an audio or video recording of the child's speech at home to confirm that the criteria are met.

Stage 2: Maintenance

One of the most important components of the Lidcombe Program is its maintenance procedure. Because relapse is common in stuttering treatment, parents are cautioned when they begin Stage 1 of the Lidcombe Program that it is essential that they continue to work with the clinician through the end of **Stage 2**. They are reminded of this throughout Stage 1 so that the procedures of the second stage are expected. Stage 2 consists of 30-minute clinic visits that are scheduled at gradually greater intervals. Typically, there are two visits at two-week intervals, then two visits at four-week intervals, then two visits at eight-week intervals, and finally, one visit 16 weeks later. During this period, parents continue to provide verbal contingencies for fluency and stuttering just as they did during Stage 1 and continue to record SRs, but the clinician guides the parents in gradually decreasing their child's verbal contingencies until they are completely discontinued.

To progress through this schedule of visits, the child must maintain the same level of fluency achieved to begin Stage 2 (clinician SRs of 1 or 2 for the entire clinic visit and parent SRs beyond the clinic of 1s and 2s, with at least four ratings of 1 during any given week). When the parent and child come in for a scheduled clinic visit, they have a discussion of how the child's speech has been since the previous visit. This discussion, as always, is facilitated by the parent's SRs and reports of how the child is responding to verbal contingencies. At each visit, the clinician and parent decide whether to continue decreasing the frequency of clinic visits or to make some changes, such as keeping to the current frequency of visits, resuming unstructured treatment conversations, or reinstating both structured and unstructured treatment. It is also possible that some aspect of the verbal contingencies may need to be adjusted. For example, sometimes a child becomes so fluent that when stutters do occur, parents or other family members apply contingencies to stuttering without concurrently giving the appropriate number of contingencies for fluency. Sometimes making this adjustment will solve a problem of returning stuttering. In other cases, stuttering reappears because of momentary stress. In this case, reinstating weekly visits may help the parent and clinician get the child back on track.

Stage 2 takes about a year to complete for most children. Although minor relapses may occur, parents are usually able to accurately assess what changes need to be made to bring the child back to essentially fluent speech.

Problem Solving

Generally, the Lidcombe Program runs smoothly without much difficulty if clinicians follow the program carefully. However, it is common for minor problems to arise during Stages 1 and 2. This section describes some common problems that may occur and their possible solutions. For more detailed descriptions of troubleshooting and special cases, see *The Lidcombe Program of Early Stuttering Intervention—A Clinician's Guide* (Onslow, Packman, & Harrison, 2003).

Sometimes, progress toward fluent speech is stalled for several weeks, or previous gains are momentarily lost. If so, I usually begin by talking to the parent about what he or she thinks might be occurring. Parents are often able to pinpoint something they have changed about the way they are doing treatment. Or it may be that a parent misunderstands some aspect of treatment. Thus, it helps to have parents demonstrate how they conduct treatment, and it may be even more helpful to have them bring in a video of treatment at home. Examples of things that may go wrong include the following: (1) parents are less attentive to praising fluent speech regularly so that fewer positive reinforcements are made than requests for corrections; (2) parents become lax about the consistency of structured treatment conversations so that many days are missed; (3) other family members, while trying to be helpful, make mistakes in providing verbal contingencies because they have not been trained; (4) the child is overly sensitive to verbal contingencies and asks parents to stop using them; and (5) some children who stutter severely at the beginning of treatment have trouble generating adequate fluency in structured sessions. The problems that arise from misunderstanding the parameters of treatment can usually be resolved by supportive feedback and guidance of the parent and modeling of appropriate behavior. Other issues, such as conducting treatment inconsistently, may require brainstorming with the parent about how treatment can be conducted more regularly. If a child isn't enjoying conversations, progress will be stalled. But it is not difficult to coach parents in delivering treatment in ways that are enjoyable, effective, and fun for both parent and child. Clinicians who have worked with preschool-age children have usually learned how to keep a child interested and achieve therapy goals at the same time. It may be appropriate for other family members to become involved in unstructured treatment conversations, but they should be trained by the clinician to deliver contingencies effectively. Structured treatment may be shared by both parents and other caregivers, but the clinician should ensure that whoever is delivering treatment is doing so accurately, and direct training is the best way to achieve this.

If a child objects to the parent's verbal contingencies after treatment has gone on for some months, it is usually helpful to ask the child what he or she would prefer when fluent and when stuttering. Some sensitive children prefer nonverbal contingencies such as a wink or a "thumbs up" after several fluent utterances and just a quick eye contact after a stutter.

With children who have moderate or severe stuttering, it is critical to structure their treatment conversations so that the child is largely fluent and only stutters occasionally. This can be done by creating a linguistic hierarchy in which the child begins using short utterances and then moves to longer ones when the child is consistently fluent; ascending this hierarchy may take several days. Some parents need specific instructions on how to achieve this. The clinician can model conversations for the parent using pictures for single-word naming, differentially reinforcing briefer utterances, and requesting the child to say just one word. In treatment conversations at home, the parent can then model for the child what is expected and continue to use differential reinforcement to control the child's output.

The Lidcombe Program is an effective treatment approach but should be used only after attending a training workshop conducted by the Lidcombe Program Trainers Consortium. Information about workshops, research articles on treatment outcome, and a treatment manual are available on the Australian Stuttering Research Centre website (www.fhs.usyd.edu.au/ASRC). After training, the clinician can join the Lidcombe discussion group, which provides a wealth of information about various challenges that may arise in treatment.

Outcome Data

A number of studies have reported that the Lidcombe Program is effective in eliminating stuttering in most preschoolers. A long-term outcome study of 42 children treated with the program showed that their stuttering was at near-zero levels four to seven years after treatment (Lincoln & Onslow, 1997). Other research reported that the mean number of clinic visits needed to complete Stage 1 treatment in a sample of 29 children was 18 clinic visits (median = 16) (Rousseau, Packman, Onslow, Harrison, & Jones, 2007). In response to concerns expressed by critics that the Lidcombe Program might produce negative psychological effects, Woods, Shearsby, Onslow, and Burnham (2002) compared pre- and post-treatment measures of the *Child Behavior Checklist* (Achenbach, 1988) and the *Attachment Q-Set* (Waters, 1995) and found no ill effects of treatment on the children's psychological health. In fact, the *Child Behavior Checklist* showed improvement in the children's behavior. A randomized control trial has shown significantly ($p = 0.003$) greater improvement in Lidcombe treatment ($n = 29$) versus control ($n = 25$). Effect size was 2.3 %SS (Jones, Onslow, Packman, Williams, & Ormond, 2005). This means that the difference between the treated group and the control group was very large; in fact, the authors indicate that it was more than twice the minimally clinically significant difference stated in their treatment protocol before the study was done. While the majority of research on the Lidcombe Program has been done in Australia, publications from researchers in the United Kingdom, Canada, and other countries have appeared. For example, Miller and Guitar (2009) showed that Lidcombe can be very successful when implemented by supervised graduate students with excellent outcomes for 15 preschool children. Duration of treatment (number of sessions required to reach the end of Stage 1) was predicted by scores on the Stuttering Severity Instrument; children who stuttered more severely before treatment took longer to become fluent. This is important information for clinicians so they can let parents of children with more severe stuttering know that treatment may take 20 sessions or more.

| ANOTHER CLINICIAN

Sheryl Gottwald

I present Sheryl Gottwald's approach to working with stuttering in preschool children because it has good outcome data to indicate that it is effective. In addition, it is different

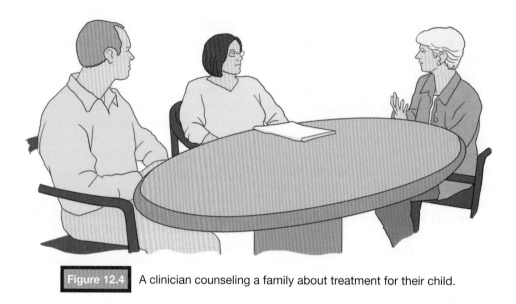

Figure 12.4 A clinician counseling a family about treatment for their child.

from the Lidcombe Program because both the child and his environment are treated, whereas on the face of it, the Lidcombe Program focuses treatment only on the child.

Gottwald (2010) has refined an approach first developed at Temple University by Starkweather, Gottwald, and Halfond (1990) and extended by Gottwald and Starkweather (1999). This treatment popularized their concept of "**demands and capacities**," described in Chapter 6, that ascribed stuttering to a combination of the demands placed on a child by her environments (internal and external) interacting with her innate capacity for fluent speech. Because there are many factors maintaining the child's stuttering, Gottwald terms her approach "multidimensional." Among the dimensions are treatment focused on the parents to reduce stresses in the child's environments and treatment focused on the child to strengthen the child's fluency.

Modifying the Environment

The initial component of treatment—individual parent counseling—provides parents with information about the nature of stuttering. For example, the clinician informs them that stuttering is highly variable and that many factors may influence its ups and downs, including factors that they may be able to change. The family is also introduced to the etiological model of stuttering, which explains it as emerging from interactions between the child's capacities and the demands placed on the child. The clinician also helps the family find ways of talking about stuttering with their child. They learn to support the child by commenting sensitively when she has difficulty getting a word out. Open acknowledgment of stuttering is intended to reduce the child's and the family's negative feelings about stuttering. For example, a parent might say to a child who has just stuttered and appears frustrated or ashamed, "Sometimes those words really get stuck. It's OK. I'm here to listen," and then the parent would show the child

nonverbally that the parent has the time and is focused on listening patiently (Fig. 12.4).

During individual counseling, families are also taught to change other aspects of their behavior that may be affecting their child's fluency. For example, family members may learn to respond to the child's stuttering without interrupting, looking away, or otherwise conveying impatience. To decrease pressure from the family's speech and language environment on the child, family members may be taught to slow their speech rates, pause more frequently, and simplify their language when talking with the child. To increase the child's self-esteem, families may be urged to create times each day when the child has a parent's full attention. Sometimes, family members may be bombarding the child with questions or otherwise pressing him to speak. As a remedy, they are shown how to talk about what they are thinking and doing as they play with the child, thereby modeling the behavior they want to encourage. Table 12.3 lists some of the things that family members can do to facilitate fluency.

In addition to changing behavior directly related to speech, families are also counseled about other stresses in the home. For example, Starkweather, Gottwald, and

Table 12.3	Modifying the Speech and Language of Family Members

1. Use a speech rate that more closely matches the child's.
2. Pause between conversation turns.
3. Eliminate questions requiring long, complex answers.
4. Respond to the content of the child's message regardless of fluency.
5. Acknowledge struggled stutters using meaningful words.

Halfond (1990) have noted that a hectic family lifestyle can exacerbate a child's stuttering. Once parents understand that a too-busy family schedule may be a factor in their child's stuttering, they are often able to reduce the hustle and bustle in the home and are gratified when their child's stuttering subsequently diminishes. In addition, a slower pace and lifestyle can often provide increased satisfaction for all family members.

Gottwald sometimes supplements individual family counseling with group therapy when that can be arranged. This gives families an opportunity to share experiences and ideas and to support one another. As members of a group, parents receive support from one another and can share ideas for helping their children. The clinician's role is to help the group members develop a sense of mutual trust by modeling concern, acceptance, and respect for all group members and their ideas and feelings. Generally, the group talks about topics they select, although the clinician may also suggest topics that are often concerns of most members, such as regression during treatment and termination of treatment.

Modifying the Child's Speech

The other major component of Gottwald's therapy—besides working with the parents or caregivers to change the child's environment—is modification of the child's speech. This involves parent and clinician modeling and reinforcement, as well as the clinician's instruction when needed. Instruction in changing stuttering with older preschool-age children is a natural outgrowth of the parents and clinician talking openly about stuttering with the child. The procedures that the authors use to modify a child's speech are as follows.

Children Who Stutter with Minimal Struggle

First the clinician talks and plays games with the child in a very fluency-enhancing setting. This situation includes the clinician talking slowly in a relaxed way with plenty of pauses and silences. Then the clinician teaches the child to talk in a slow, relaxed way. This is done with very little linguistic demand on the child; for example, a game they play may require only simple short sentences. Gradually, as the child is more and more fluent in this situation, demands are gradually increased. This may entail games and conversation involving longer and more complex utterances, or the clinician may speed up her speech rate. For those children who continue to stutter in this low-pressure situation, Gottwald teaches them to stutter using "easy bounces" at the beginning of an utterance, li-like this.

Children Who Stutter with Moderate to Severe Struggle

For those children who stutter with noticeable tension and struggle, Gottwald begins therapy by talking with them about stuttering, so that they will recognize what they are doing when they stutter and thereby increase their acceptance of it. By playing games that reward stuttering, the child changes her feelings about her stuttering and may even begin to stutter on purpose. This then leads to changing the stutters so they become gradually looser and looser. Gottwald encourages these children to use bouncy speech (re-repeating sounds easily and loosely) or stretchy speech (lllllllllike this) in which easy, loose prolongations take the place of struggled stutters. As she works on helping the children change their stutters, Gottwald also works to help them express their feelings as a way of leading to improved attitudes and cognitions.

Termination

Individual and group parent counseling and modification of the child's speech continue until the family environment and the child's speech have met the following two criteria. First, the environment has changed enough so that major stresses have diminished and the family seems to understand the dynamics that may exist between environmental stresses and the child's stuttering. Second, the child's stuttering has decreased to the point at which she is normally disfluent, with an occasional mild instance of stuttering.

Supporting Data

Starkweather, Gottwald, and Halfond (1990) reported that most of the children they have treated have regained normal fluency. Of 39 children who they treated using this approach, seven dropped out, and of the remaining 32 children, 29 recovered completely, and three were still in treatment at the time of the report. The average child requires about 12 sessions of therapy using this approach, although some children require much more before therapy can be terminated.

Gottwald and Starkweather (1999) treated an additional 15 families with their approach. Although one family dropped out, the children of the remaining 14 families achieved normal fluency and reported maintaining it a year after the children were dismissed from treatment. Further data on her approach were provided by Gottwald (2010) involving the children of 27 families. Again, one family dropped out, but 26 families reported their children had normal fluency one year or more following dismissal from treatment.

TREATMENT OF CONCOMITANT SPEECH AND LANGUAGE PROBLEMS

One of the clinical issues that should be considered, especially with beginning stuttering in older preschoolers, is the management of **concomitant speech and language problems**. Research has indicated that some children who stutter are delayed in their speech and language development, especially in their articulation or phonological development (Bloodstein & Ratner, 2008). Let me begin this section by describing how clinicians using Lidcombe deal with concomitant problems. When using the Lidcombe Program, it is imperative that only stuttering be treated during Stage 1, when the parent and child are highly involved in working on fluency. Typically, the Lidcombe Program up to the end of Stage 1 is conducted first, and then any other speech or language problem would be treated. In some cases, however, when another problem is particularly severe, treatment can be focused on that problem first until appropriate improvement is made. Then Stage 1 of Lidcombe can be implemented, and treatment of the other problem(s) can be resumed when Stage 1 is finished. During treatment of the Lidcombe Program, it is crucial that parents understand that the focus is only on fluency so that their SRs are not affected by the other disorder(s). Placing the priority on the treatment of stuttering is recommended because of its greater likelihood of chronicity and exacerbation as children grow older. This contrasts with most other developmental problems that tend to improve a little or at least not worsen appreciably if treatment for them is delayed.

A number of clinicians not using the Lidcombe Program have recommended a variety of ways of responding to other concomitant speech and language problems in beginning stutterers.

One approach is to work on phonological problems at the same time as they work on fluency, if they are severe enough to warrant intervention. When doing this, Conture, Louko, and Edwards (1993) use an indirect articulation treatment. Avoiding the traditional "corrective" type of therapy, they provide the child with plenty of models of target phonemes through extensive auditory stimulation and opportunities for improved production. This is done in an accepting environment rather than correcting the child when he is wrong and asking him to try again with more attention and effort. Diane Hill (2003) begins with receptive training and then follows with a sequence of working on phonemic change, sound play, sound approximation, and rehearsal of correct sound production in a few target sounds. If language is an issue, the clinician again begins with receptive training, followed by integrating practice with proper syntactic forms into the fluency hierarchy of more and more complex language. For example, the clinician provides appropriate instructions and materials and has the child practice a specific syntactic structure while using easy, relaxed speech.

Wall and Myers (1995) recommend that concomitant problems be treated after fluency has been stabilized if the child's disability is mild and not interfering with speech intelligibility. However, if the disability is interfering with intelligibility, the problem should be dealt with immediately because it may be adding considerable stress to the child's communicative attempts. If treatment of a phonological or articulation disorder is begun, Wall and Myers recommend that the phoneme or phoneme group selected for treatment be one that is the easiest for the child to produce. Words and syntactic structures

selected for practice material should be ones with which the child can easily cope. Work on speech sound production can be integrated with work on fluency. For example, practice of a new sound in a word can be integrated with practice of easy speech.

Finally, the "cycles" model alternates fluency treatment with language or phonology therapy over the course of the year (Hodson & Paden, 1991; described in Bernstein Ratner, 1995). Bernstein Ratner points out that this provides children with initial periods of concentrated learning of new skills (for a specified amount of time irrespective of whether or not the client meets criteria for finishing the treatment) followed by opportunities for spontaneous generalization of these skills to other settings while the other treatment is cycled in. This alternation continues until one of the problems is resolved so that all attention can then be given to the remaining issue.

SUMMARY

- The author believes that beginning stuttering arises from an interaction between children's constitutional predispositions interacting with developmental and environmental influences to produce primarily repetitive disfluencies with increased tension. Escape behaviors are also an important component of the disorder as children experience increasing frustration with their inability to complete a word.

- Children with beginning stuttering usually have a large amount of fluency that can be reinforced and generalized to situations that previously elicited stuttering.

- The Lidcombe Program is a parent-delivered, operant conditioning program for preschoolers in which the parent is guided to conduct daily treatment conversations and apply verbal contingencies to fluency and stuttering. Treatment begins in structured conversations and quickly moves to unstructured conversations throughout the day, so that treatment is conducted in the child's natural speaking environment, necessitating little work on generalization. Once the child is fluent in all situations, the clinician manages a phased withdrawal of clinic contact with careful monitoring of progress so that the family can respond to any relapses by reinstating needed features of treatment and then return to the fading process.

- Another clinician, Sheryl Gottwald, uses an approach based on the "demands and capacities" concept and treats both the family and the child.

- In the Lidcombe Program, work on other communication disorders precedes or more typically follows Stage 1 of treatment. In other treatment approaches, clinicians often integrate work on fluency with other concomitant speech or language problems. Several approaches to the challenges of treating stuttering and concomitant disorders offer different ideas.

STUDY QUESTIONS

1. Describe Stage 1 and Stage 2 of the Lidcombe Program for the beginning stutterer. What is the goal of each phase?
2. Describe structured and unstructured treatment conversations in the Lidcombe Program.
3. Describe the two major ways of collecting data on the child's progress in the Lidcombe Program.
4. Describe how data are used to guide the child's progress in the Lidcombe Program.
5. Compare the Lidcombe Program with Gottwald's approach. In what ways are they similar, and in what ways are they different?
6. Describe how the treatment of beginning stuttering and other speech and language disorders can be managed.

SUGGESTED PROJECTS

1. Develop a hierarchy based on length and complexity of utterances that could be used by a clinician who is working with beginning stuttering and wants to move from single words to conversational speech.
2. Develop a hierarchy, based on increasing social complexity, for a child with beginning stuttering. Design it for use by a typical, two-parent family with older and younger siblings and grandparents who visit frequently.
3. Interview the family of a child with beginning stuttering who was treated successfully. Find out what they perceived to be the most helpful aspects of treatment and what advice they would give to other families just beginning treatment.

SUGGESTED READINGS

Bernstein Ratner, N. (1995). Treating the child who stutters with concomitant language and phonological impairment. *Language, Speech, and Hearing Services in Schools, 26,* 180–186.

In this insightful overview of the treatment of children with concomitant disorders, Bernstein Ratner identifies several models that have evolved.

Conture, E., & Curlee, R. F. (2007). *Stuttering and related disorders of fluency.* **New York: Thieme.**

Chapter 4 gives a description of the Lidcombe Program including case studies. Chapter 5 presents a group approach to treating stuttering in preschool children and parents.

Conture, E., Louko, L., & Edwards, M. L. (1993). Simultaneously treating stuttering and disordered phonology in children: Experimental therapy, preliminary findings. *American Journal of Speech-Language Pathology, 2,* 72–81.

This article details how to use indirect articulation therapy with children at both beginning and intermediate levels of stuttering.

Guitar, B., & McCauley, R. (2010). *Treatment of stuttering: Established and emerging interventions.* **Baltimore: Lippincott Williams & Wilkins.**

Several interventions described in this book are applicable to older preschool children, and each is accompanied by video clips illustrating treatment.

Onslow, M., Packman, A., & Harrison, E. (2003). *The Lidcombe Program of early stuttering intervention: A clinician's guide.* **Austin, TX: Pro-Ed.**

This is a complete guide for both new and experienced clinicians who have been trained to use the Lidcombe Program. It is very clear and filled with clinical wisdom.

Ramig, P., & Dodge, D. (2005). *The child and adolescent stuttering therapy and activity resource guide.* **Clifton Park, NY: Thompson Delmar Learning.**

There are a vast array of activities and techniques in this book for use by clinicians using almost any approach to treatment. The book also covers evaluation, treatment planning, and report writing.

Shapiro, D. (2011). *Stuttering intervention: A collaborative journey to fluency freedom (2nd ed.).* **Austin, TX: Pro-Ed.**

The section on direct intervention in the chapter on intervention with preschool children has many excellent suggestions for treatment, including ideas for building up resistance to fluency disruptors and encouraging expression of emotion.

Zebrowski, P. M., & Kelly, E. (2002). *Manual of stuttering intervention.* **Clifton Park, NY: Singular.**

The chapter on treatment of the preschool child, particularly treatment of those children who are likely to persist in stuttering, contains many excellent ideas for direct work on stuttering. Many case examples are given.

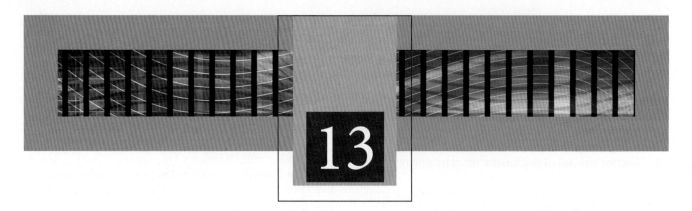

13

Treatment of School-Age Children: Intermediate Stuttering

CHAPTER OBJECTIVES

After studying this chapter, readers should be able to:

- Describe the characteristics of a child who has intermediate stuttering
- Describe the author's beliefs about stuttering, targets in treatment, goals for treatment, how much to involve feelings and attitudes in treatment, and maintenance procedures
- Explain the key concepts for working with children of this age
- Outline the goals and activities of these components of treatment: exploring, learning and generalizing fluency skills, reducing fear and avoidance, coping with teasing, being open about stuttering, and maintaining improvement
- Describe important aspects of working with parents and working with teachers to help the school-age child who stutters
- Describe the treatment procedures of (a) Yaruss, Pelczarski, and Quesal; (b) Harrison, Bruce, Shenker, Koushik, and Kazenski; and (c) Walton

KEY TERMS

School-age children: Children between 6 and 14 years old

Superfluency: A style of speaking that incorporates fluency-shaping components such as slow speech rate and gentle onset of phonation

Fluency skills: The elements of superfluency, such as slow rate and easy onset of phonation

Controlled stuttering: Using techniques to modify stutters so that they are brief and relaxed

Voluntary stuttering: Deliberately stuttering so that one loses some of the fear of stuttering

Acceptable stuttering: Stuttering that is mild enough that it doesn't bother either the speaker or the listener and doesn't interfere with communication

Cognitive behavioral therapy: Working with thoughts and beliefs that may give rise to the negative emotions associated with stuttering

Desensitization: Helping the individual become less sensitive to negative experiences such as stuttering or negative listener reactions

Proprioception: Using sensory feedback from speech movement (such as the feeling of the jaw and tongue moving) to guide speech in place of auditory feedback that may be faulty in stutterers

Fluency disrupters: Stimuli that put pressure on someone's speech so that he or she stutters. Examples are interruptions and fast-talking conversational partners

AN INTEGRATED APPROACH

The **school-age child** with intermediate stuttering is usually an elementary or junior high school student between 6 and 13 years of age who has been stuttering for several years. I use the word "child" or "student" to refer to the client, but I am aware that when a youngster is 10 years or older, in many ways he is more like an adolescent than like a child. The typical intermediate stutterer exhibits tense part-word and monosyllabic whole-word repetitions, as well as tense prolongations; however, blocks with tension and struggle are the most evident sign of stuttering. This child may use escape devices, such as body movements or brief verbalizations (e.g., "uh"), to break free of stutters. He may also use various avoidance strategies such as starters, word substitutions, circumlocutions, and evasion of difficult speaking situations. He experiences more frustration and embarrassment than beginning stutterers do and has distinct anticipation of stuttering on specific sounds, words, and many speaking situations. His major fear is the moment of stuttering itself, and he has a definite concept of himself as a stutterer.

My approach to intermediate stuttering is markedly different from the fluency shaping I use with beginning stuttering. I typically begin treatment with a stuttering modification approach—exploring stuttering—which focuses on decreasing the child's fear and increasing his understanding of stuttering. After that, treatment progresses to teaching the child to use "**superfluency**," which is a style of speaking that incorporates fluency-shaping components such as slow speech rate and gentle onset of phonation. After that, I help the child replace anticipated or actual stutters by "turning on" superfluency in more and more real-world situations. Then I return to aspects of stuttering modification that help the child keep the fear of stuttering reduced and that help maintain fluency (Fig. 13.1).

I will illustrate our approach to treatment with the case example of David, the 6-year-old elementary school student whom we introduced in Chapter 1.

Author's Beliefs

Nature of Stuttering

I believe that in intermediate levels of stuttering, neurophysiological factors combined with a vulnerable temperament interact with developmental and environmental factors to prevent natural recovery and produce or exacerbate the core behaviors of repetitions, prolongations, and mild blocks. Children respond to these disfluencies with increased tension that in turn increases the frequency and duration of repetitions, prolongations, and blocks. As school-age children who stutter experience more and more of these increasingly severe core behaviors, they become frustrated because parts of their bodies are out of control and they can't stop it. In desperation, they blink their eyes or nod their heads to break out of a stutter. They feel embarrassed as their stuttering becomes more bizarre and they realize they are the only kids doing it, unlike their peers or anyone else they know.

The more they stutter when talking to family and friends, the more these children dread it happening again. These moments of dread or anticipatory fear spread via classical conditioning—that is, through the repeated pairing of negative stuttering experiences with various sounds, words,

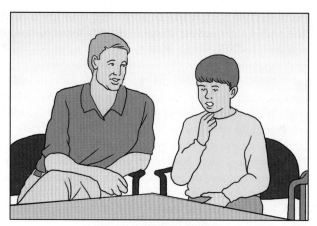

**Student Explores
His Stuttering**

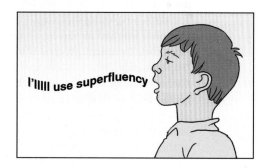

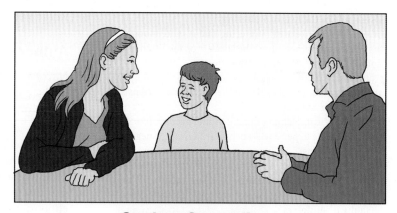

**Student Generalizes
His Fluency Skills
to New Listener**

Figure 13.1   Overview of the chapter.

Case Example

David

When David was 6, he began weekly treatment with me (and a graduate student), when I was using an early version of the treatment described in this chapter. In those days, I used primarily stuttering modification, but the modified stuttering became a fluency skill for David. In other words, he used his modified stutters on both stuttered words and some fluent words as well.

In the first months of treatment, David was extremely sensitive about his stuttering and unwilling to work directly on it during the exploration stage of treatment. In fact, he wouldn't even discuss his stuttering and would often wander out of the therapy room when I brought it up. My response was to pepper my speech with easy stutters (slightly drawn out onsets of words llllliiike this). I'd occasionally probe whether he was willing to talk about his stuttering (he wasn't). Our activities were confined to shooting hoops with a basketball net attached to the back of the door and bowling with plastic pins and balls as I kept up a steady flow of easy stutters. I would sometimes comment that I needed to use easy stutters to control my stuttering (David later said he never believed I really stuttered, but was just pretending). One day, David spotted a jar of candies on my desk and asked if he could have one. I traded him one in exchange for him trying an easy stutter. Thus began a steadily effective therapy strategy. Over the next year, he increasingly warmed to the idea of changing his stuttering from hard blocks to easy "slide-outs" (as he called them) while earning candies. The candies always went home in a bag that his mother put away in a drawer and then surreptitiously returned to me for recycling as rewards for easy stutters.

David learned other **fluency skills** such as slowing and proprioception, but always favored slide-outs. We practiced them with many listeners in many different situations. At some point, David decided on his own to keep a score sheet of the number of slide-outs he used in the therapy room and outside. Perhaps because he received a reward for each slide-out, at first, David began to put in slide-outs even on words he wasn't stuttering on. Slide-outs became a fluency skill for him. Soon, David would give himself a check mark for each slide-out without my having to tell him; I intermittently praised him after he used a slide-out and reinforced himself. I think this self-reinforcement was an important part of his therapy that he invented himself.

In addition to working on the ease and fluency of his speech, David improved his attitudes about speaking, largely through talking with his class about his stuttering. Always a bit of a ham, David was happy to make presentations to his classes in second, third, and fourth grades. He showed posters and video clips he had made, answered questions, and had other students come up and "learn how to stutter." During his elementary school years, the course of therapy was full of bumps and detours, as well as great gains in fluency. Once when his family sold their house and built a new one in a different neighborhood, he was thrown for a loss and started to stutter more severely again. During this time he was also teased by another student who was having his own problems at home and school. A few months' work with David, his parents, his teachers, and his friends, as well as the child who teased him, brought him through this relapse stronger than ever, and he continued to gain confidence in his speech throughout junior high and high school without further therapy. When he graduated he was essentially fluent with a few minor repetitions and prolongations.

I should add to this account that David's parents were a major help to his therapy. They were always willing to come to our clinic and talk over his progress (even in the early days when he wasn't making any), as well as promoting therapy activities at home (such as buying him a punching bag to release his frustrations during a relapse). At my suggestion, they tried to reinforce his fluency at home, particularly at the dinner table. This lasted all of two weeks and came to a screeching halt when David declared he just wanted to talk and not be doing therapy at home as well as at the clinic. What he wanted was just his parents' general support of him, which they gave unstintingly.

David's sister and brother were very sympathetic to him when he was going through a bad patch, and David was surprisingly open to talking with them about his stuttering. David was also open with many others about his stutter, including my class and a local television show. I think another key aspect of his recovery was his participation as a mentor when he was in high school in group therapy for younger school-age children. He was a much-loved "older brother" to the group and helped them immensely by modeling his slide-outs as well as leading them into situations outside the clinic. He even threw in some voluntary stutters to give them courage to try it too.

and speaking situations. As more of their talking is infected with stuttering, they try to cope by avoiding—dodging feared words and difficult situations, saying "I don't know" when asked a question, or throwing in extra sounds to get a stuck word going. Avoidance behaviors are reinforced when these tricks are intermittently successful in preventing stuttering. Because longer and more abnormal stutters lead to more negative listener reactions, children with intermediate stuttering develop the belief that stuttering is bad, and therefore they are bad when they stutter. Shame about their speech becomes a feature of their daily life.

Because the tension response, escape and avoidance behaviors, and negative feelings and attitudes are all learned, I believe they can be modified by new learning. The context for this change must be an accepting, supportive environment that focuses on the child as a person, rather than just on his stuttering. Many intermediate stutterers feel that they have failed in previous therapy and thus have disappointed their parents and teachers by not becoming fluent. Thus, I must help these children feel accepted with their current level of stuttering as well as help them experience mastery and success with their speech *and* with their communication.

If treatment can provide an intermediate stutterer with a sufficient number of emotionally positive speaking experiences in therapy, such as experiences in which he feels "in control" of his speech, the increased fluency and positive feelings associated with speaking will generalize to other environments. The clinician can use operant and classical conditioning principles to achieve this, rewarding beneficial changes in stuttering and associating speaking with pleasure. Furthermore, because predisposing neurophysiological factors may contribute to the core behaviors in the speech of many intermediate stutterers, it is also important to help students at this age cope effectively with any remaining disruptions in their speech. These twin goals of coping with the remaining stuttering and positive speaking experiences can be achieved using a combination of stuttering modification and fluency shaping. In implementing these goals with a school-age child, I find that the child's age and maturity influence the selection of clinical procedures.

Finally, it is important to reduce developmental and environmental influences that may be contributing to the child's stuttering. I can do this by working with the child's parents and classroom teachers, helping them create an environment that accepts the child regardless of his progress with speech, thus helping him feel free to work on his speech with the further outcome of facilitating change. In addition, I help the child communicate directly with his parents and teachers about how they can best help him deal with his stuttering.

Speech Behaviors Targeted for Therapy

The speech behaviors targeted for intermediate stuttering therapy are both stuttered and fluent speech. Unlike treatment of beginning stuttering, this therapy begins with a focus on stuttering behaviors that are first explored and then changed. Subsequently, fluent speech becomes the target for therapy and is shaped using various tools, such as easy onsets and light contacts.

Fluency Goals

Which fluency goals are realistic for school-age children? Some intermediate school-age stutterers may become normal or spontaneously fluent speakers, which is more likely for younger than for older school-age children. Those who don't become completely fluent without having to think about their speech will need to use controlled fluency to sound like typical speakers. This is often a difficult task for a youngster (or indeed any speaker) to do on a consistent basis. Although he may use controlled fluency in some situations, a child this age often may not have the motivation or self-discipline to control fluency throughout his daily talking. Thus an alternate fluency goal is **controlled stuttering**. This is achieved by helping the child use easy, **voluntary stutters** (sometimes called "slides"), or he can hang onto stutters and ease out of them ("pullouts"). Both of these strategies will give the child a sense of control over his speech and will thus inhibit the tension response, escape, and avoidance behaviors. Essentially we are asking him to stutter in an honest, straightforward way without the ducking and dodging that so often interfere with communication. As you can imagine, this approach will involve techniques such as those used in cognitive behavioral therapy to help him stop trying to hide or avoid his stuttering. In short, a realistic fluency goal for many intermediate school-age stutterers is **acceptable stuttering**, fluency mixed with mild or very mild stuttering.

Feelings and Attitudes

How much attention should be given to an intermediate stutterer's feelings and attitudes about his speech? Whenever a child is experiencing frustration and embarrassment and is beginning to experience some fear related to speech (which is usually the case for intermediate school-age children who stutter), I believe it is important to reduce these negative feelings. Furthermore, because these children are beginning to avoid certain words and speaking situations, it is important to eliminate or reduce these avoidances. All of this necessitates the child feeling the clinician's acceptance of him *as he is now*. This acceptance is conveyed, especially at the beginning of therapy, by the clinician's accepting curiosity about what the child is doing when he stutters, why he does it, and whether that helps him. It is also conveyed by the clinician's genuine interest in the child, even apart from his stuttering and fluency.

Maintenance Procedures

The typical intermediate stutterer usually needs more hours of treatment than a beginning stutterer. And after formal treatment has ended, it is likely that he will need continued contact to maintain improvements in his fluency. A systematic, planned program of gradual fading of treatment contact is recommended. In addition, if he can become a mentor to younger children who stutter, it will help him maintain fluency as well as bolster his self-esteem.

Clinical Methods

My approach to intermediate stuttering is to use a combination of stuttering modification and fluency-shaping strategies for the child. Soon after I begin therapy with the student, I also work with his parents and the teachers to create "stuttering-friendly" environments that increase the student's comfort using the techniques we learn together in treatment. The measures I use to assess progress are described in the section titled "Progress and Outcome Measures."

Clinical Procedures: Working with a Child

My clinical methods for intermediate stuttering have been influenced by many people, but Charles Van Riper has been my prime inspiration. Many of the techniques and much of the philosophy in my approach come straight from a chapter in Van Riper's treatment book entitled *The Young Confirmed Stutterer* (Van Riper, 1973). I am also indebted to Richard Boemhler for my understanding of how to replace stuttering with controlled normal fluency and to Julie Reville, who shared her intuitive clinical approaches with this age group. Many activities that she and I developed for treating children with intermediate stuttering are presented in our workbook, *Easy Talker* (Guitar & Reville, 1997). More recently I have been influenced by Danra Kazenski, who has a fine understanding of stuttering and of school-age children. Her clinical approaches include the Lidcombe Program (LP) adapted for school-age children and the use of **cognitive behavioral therapy** for this age group and for their parents.

Key Concepts

Van Riper (1973) cited fear, avoidance, struggle, and shame as four major characteristics of the young confirmed stutterer. I will begin with a brief snapshot of these factors and how they can be dealt with in treatment.

1. *Fear and avoidance are major factors in intermediate stuttering.* Fear produces tension, making it difficult for youngsters to change their old, struggled patterns to more relaxed, forward-moving ways of saying words. Treatment, then, must reduce fear. These children have had too many experiences when their articulators are jammed up and they unable to make a sound. They have learned to cope by avoiding words and situations and using starters and postponements. To counteract this, therapy must tip the balance toward an "approach" attitude by helping children explore their stuttering, learn about it, and learn new responses to old cues. Both stuttering modification and fluency shaping can achieve this.

2. *Struggle must be reduced to approximate normal speech.* Struggle arises when a child desperately wants to get a word out and to finish the communication but has contracted his muscles so tightly that the word can't come out. You can better understand a stutterer's experience if you imagine yourself stuck and in a hurry to get unstuck—for example, being stuck in bumper-to-bumper traffic when you are late for an important meeting or trying to open a stuck front door when a taxi is waiting. When a child is trying to talk and a sound is stuck, he feels helpless, out of control, and frustrated. He pushes harder and harder, tension spills out to muscles throughout his face, and finally the sound spurts out. Relief! The word is finished, communication is completed, *but the struggle is rewarded.* Therapy to deal with this cycle of struggle and reward must use a two-pronged approach: (1) reducing the negative emotions and rewarding the easier speech that results, and (2) teaching the child to use controlled fluency (which I call "superfluency") instead of stuttering. Often just the practice of voluntary stuttering reduces negative emotions, and just the practice of using superfluency over and over makes spontaneous fluency possible.

3. *Reduce shame by openness.* Bill Murphy has spoken and written in some detail about the shame associated with stuttering. His Stuttering Foundation video, *The School-Age Child Who Stutters: Dealing Effectively with Guilt and Shame* (1999) is an excellent resource for clinicians. Murphy notes that, whereas guilt is associated with something you have done, shame is related to the way you are. Thus, the intermediate stutterer has begun to feel that stuttering is a part of him; he thinks of himself as unable to talk right, and it is the way he is. Shame can often be reduced by being more open about shaming experiences. For example, individuals who were sexually abused as children are sometimes ashamed because of it; however, they discover that when they talk about their experiences to counselors or very close friends, they feel relief from the shame. This occurs with stuttering as well. When a child can talk to an accepting clinician about his stuttering experiences, especially negative listener reactions, his shame decreases. When he can talk to his parents about his stuttering and they can listen and accept his feelings, his shame decreases more. When he can talk to his peers, maybe even his whole class, his shame may almost disappear.

There are two more key concepts to keep in mind when working with intermediate stuttering. I have learned them through my own experience and by watching colleagues work with children who stutter.

4. *Therapy must be fun.* Rewards and games take the sting out of stuttering and reduce the anxiety associated with having to work on something shameful and difficult. Children in school settings are often reluctant to come to therapy as so vividly portrayed by David Sedaris in *Me*

Talk Pretty One Day (Sedaris, 2000). To draw them in, clinicians need to make therapy exciting, interesting, and above all, emotionally safe. When I worked in a junior high school in Washington, D.C., kids thought it was cool to go to the "speech room," where there were always interesting games on tap, including poker. After we started the poker, even the principal wanted to come for a visit.

Many times, when a school-age child is reluctant to come to therapy or work on his speech, all that may be needed is an effective reward system. I have had success with a child's favorite candies and engaging activities. Every child will have his own favorites, and parents can be consulted about what is OK with them. With youngsters who are transferring new skills to outside situations, I have used a point system so they can time playing an exciting game back at the clinic. In the session before a child and I go to the mall, we plan what we do and how many points each assignment will bring. When I am working in the treatment room, I have an array of games and activities as reinforcers and a "prize cart" hidden away in a special room where they can cash in tokens for their choice of a small gift. Snack reinforcers are highly effective for children in a therapy group, too. In our school kids' group, I use healthy snacks to reward new behaviors, such as easy voluntary stutters.

5. *Clinicians should first perform any tasks they ask children to perform.* Van Riper (1973) uses the term "identification" in a variety of ways. It is not only a term for getting to know one's stuttering, but it also describes the bond between the clinician and client. For the youngster with intermediate stuttering, a major factor in treatment is that the child identifies with the clinician and therefore wishes to please and emulate her. On the clinician's part, this means that she must be accepting of the child, be interested in him as a person, and must also model the behaviors that she wants the child to learn. Whether she's teaching easy stuttering or gentle onsets, the clinician must show the child what the new skill looks and sounds like. When she wants him to use easy stuttering on the phone, she should make the first phone call. When first putting pretend stutters in her speech, the clinician can let the child know that she doesn't really stutter (unless she does) but that she has practiced stuttering so that she can feel what the child feels. Most children are delighted to help the clinician improve her pretend stuttering so that having the student coach the clinician in stuttering boosts the student's sense of mastery.

Beginning Therapy

In this first phase of treatment, I have a number of objectives. First, I help a child explore his stuttering; in part, this means that we talk about the moments of stuttering when they happen. As the child explores his stuttering, I try to help him understand what is happening when he stutters. Also, I help him identify easy stutters in his speech and suggest that

those forms of easy talking are one of our goals for therapy. When he learns how to use easy stutters whenever he wants to replace hard stuttering, we'll call it his "superfluency." This intensifying of the goal takes us into the realm of children's dreams and sets the stage for future accomplishments. Exploring, understanding, and setting our target for therapy are three objectives that are all interwoven into the fabric of our first phase of therapy.

When I meet a student for the first time, I let him know that I'm here to help him with his stuttering, but first I want to know more about him. I ask about what he likes to do after school and on the weekends, as well as about his family, his likes, and his dislikes. I want him to see that I'm a good listener and hope this emerges naturally out of my real interest in his world. His daily life, his favorite activities, and his experiences provide the metaphors and analogies that we will use as we work together on his stuttering. As we talk, I convey my comfort with his stuttering by my relaxed attention during his moments of stuttering. At first, I just watch and listen carefully to learn what he does when he stutters; eventually, when he seems to be ready, I help him explore his stutters, as described in the following paragraphs.

Exploring

Exploring is the opposite of avoiding; it is an "approach" behavior that can reduce negative emotions. When I proposed a theoretical background for persistent stuttering in Chapter 6, I speculated that the temperament of many children who have developed intermediate-level stuttering may be biased toward avoidance and withdrawal from threatening stimuli. This idea is put into practice by engaging such youngsters in activities that counteract their natural tendency to avoid.

Exploring the Goals of Therapy

It is important for a student to know where he's going in therapy and to know that the clinician has a map to guide him on his trip through sometimes difficult territory. Depending on his age, I will ask him about past therapy, what he learned, and what he'd like to get out of therapy. Most school-age children will probably answer that they would like their stuttering to be totally gone. I might respond that we can work toward that goal, but then I would ask him if it would be OK if he had a little stuttering sometimes when he's excited or in a hurry. I let him know that at first, he and I will be working to get to know his stuttering and what makes it happen. Then we'll work on helping him change his talking so that it will be easier. I might tell him this at the very beginning of therapy or after several sessions. It's often helpful to draw some pictures or diagrams to make the activities and sequence of therapy easier to grasp. Figure 13.2 shows the sequence of therapy for our approach. It may help the student you are working with if you and the student redraw the sequence as you explain what the student will be doing in each stage.

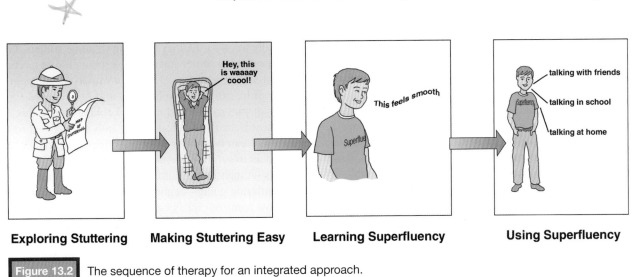

Exploring Stuttering   **Making Stuttering Easy**   **Learning Superfluency**   **Using Superfluency**

Figure 13.2   The sequence of therapy for an integrated approach.

Exploring Beliefs about Stuttering

I think it is important for an intermediate stutterer to be given some explanation for his stuttering. He knows he stutters and has been stuttering probably for a number of years, and he needs to have an explanation for why he talks differently than his friends. So, what do I say to this youngster?

Choosing words that are appropriate for the child's age and comprehension level, I let him know that stuttering is not his fault and that much of it is learned and can be unlearned. I let him know that he must already be a good learner to have learned all the things he does when he stutters. This means he will be good at learning some new, easier ways of handling his stutters. To help him realize that stuttering is not his fault, I may say that just like some kids have trouble drawing pictures of things or other kids find it hard to play a musical instrument, he has a little more trouble getting words out smoothly if he is talking fast and has lots of ideas to get out. I let him know about famous people who also have the same problem, like the movie actors Bruce Willis, James Earl Jones (Darth Vader in "Star Wars"), Samuel L. Jackson, and Nicholas Brendon (star of the TV show "Buffy the Vampire Slayer"). Many sports stars also stutter (or used to), such as Shaquille O'Neill and Tiger Woods. Lots of famous people stutter, but they have learned to change their stuttering so it is hardly noticeable, and so can he.

I go on to explain that any inborn tendency to stutter accounts only for the fact that sometimes when he talks fast or is excited or tired, he finds that he stumbles over words. This is the part I call natural stuttering. Other parts, the most bothersome parts, like getting really tight when he stutters or putting in extra sounds or eye blinks, are learned. If they are learned, he can change them. One tool I sometimes use to help teach intermediate stutterers about stuttering is the video, *Stuttering: For Kids by Kids*, which is available from the Stuttering Foundation (Scott & Guitar, 2004). This DVD has great examples of kids who stutter talking about the difficulties they face and how they have worked on their speech.

In helping a child to better understand his stuttering, I think it is beneficial for him to know that a lot of children stutter and that he is not the only person in the world who stutters. Often a child may not know any other child who stutters and may believe that he is one of only a very few who have this problem. So, I tell him that about one in 100 kids stutter and that there are over 2 million people in the United States and millions more around the world who stutter. I believe this sort of information helps a child to feel less alone because of his stuttering.

Exploring the Core Behaviors of Stuttering

I guide a child to approach and explore the core behaviors of his stuttering using three principles taken from research on phobias in animals and humans (Mineka, 1985). These principles adapted for stuttering are (1) the clinician must be unafraid of stuttering; (2) the child must explore and study his stuttering; and (3) the longer the child is able to remain in contact with moments of stuttering, the more his fear will be reduced.

The Clinician Must Be Unafraid of Stuttering

The clinician can demonstrate her lack of fear of stuttering by her curiosity about the child's stuttering by having the child teach her to imitate his stuttering and by taking the lead in practicing in all situations (unless the child wants to take the lead). The clinician should cultivate and renew her own lack of fear of stuttering. She should be able to pseudo-stutter comfortably when talking with the child alone as well as in public to acquaintances and strangers.

The Child Must Explore His Stuttering

The second principle, that the child must explore his stuttering, is the basis of much of the activity in this first phase of treatment. After I get to know a child and he feels at ease with me, I bring up the topic of stuttering with him. My aim is to help him become interested in his stuttering rather than denying it and hoping it will go away. Because talking about stuttering is often uncomfortable for a child, I begin our discussions when we are drawing pictures, playing a game, or doing something else the child enjoys. Thus, I can alternate between helping the child explore his stuttering and moving back to an activity that is fun. To begin, I simply comment on the child's stuttering in an accepting manner. For instance, I may say something like "Hey, you really eased out of that one pretty well," or "That was a tough one, huh?" I take note of how he responds and whether he appears uncomfortable or whether he acknowledges his stuttering even subtly and non-verbally when I comment on it. This first approach to stuttering may go quite easily if I have won the child's trust and he is not excessively embarrassed by his stuttering. Those who are very sensitive can be helped to face their stuttering by proceeding slowly.

For a particularly sensitive child, I begin by providing him with a feeling of mastery over something else, such as a board game, drawing, or "shooting hoops" in the therapy room. I then alternate between exploring his stuttering and giving him relief through other activities of his choice. As I explore a child's stuttering with him, I not only comment on it but also ask him to describe what he's doing when he stutters. For example, I might say, "OK, there was an interesting one. What did you do when you stuttered on that word?" Then, I help him feel and identify what he actually does when he stutters. For many children, this focus on stuttering behavior—especially if they are rewarded for it—creates an openness about stuttering that can change their emotions from shame and helpless confusion to a more hopeful and objective outlook.

At some point during early exploration of a child's stuttering, I teach him about "speech helpers," which are the lungs, larynx, and articulators, and their involvement in speech production. A cardboard or plywood cutout of a head, neck, and chest with speech helpers drawn on it may help. For examples, see Exercise 1-1 in *Easy Talker*, our workbook that is listed in Suggested Readings at the end of the chapter; also watch the "Exploring Talking and Stuttering" part of *Stuttering: Basic Clinical Skills*, a DVD available from Stuttering Foundation (Guitar & Fraser, 2007) This part of the video includes having the child getting to know his stuttering (and therefore being less afraid) as well as learning to change it.

For a more sensitive child, I start with instructions about how speech helpers work during fluent speech and later explore what the child does with his speech helpers when he stutters. For children who are less emotional about their stuttering, I might incorporate instruction about speech helpers into our exploration of what they are doing when they stutter. In this part of treatment, the child learns the parts of his speech mechanism, what he does when he talks, and what he does when he stutters. The child is also learning that stuttering is not a scary monster that attacks him, but simply things he does as he tries not to stutter.

As the student and I talk about his speech helpers and what he may be doing with them when he stutters, I ask him to actually feel what he may be doing when he stutters. I ask him to pretend to stutter and make the pretend stutter as tight as a real stutter would be. This is an important moment in therapy. If he can stutter voluntarily and be rewarded for it, his fear of stuttering will diminish. Looking ahead, this is a step toward changing a real stutter into a loose, voluntary stutter that can be easily released. Anticipating this, I coach the student to get the pretend stutter tight, then feel what he's doing as he stays in the stutter, then—while keeping the pretend stuttering going—begin to loosen it and let the sound or airflow come out freely before ending it slowly. Voluntary stuttering can be used throughout therapy. It is a rehearsal for the different ways the student will handle real stutters. Some students find that voluntary stutters turn into real stutters; when this happens, it provides an opportunity for the student to learn to tolerate the real stutter and gradually turn it into a voluntary, loose stutter. Occasionally students balk at voluntary stuttering and refuse to put pretend stutters in their speech. I accept this and move on to other therapy techniques.

Once a child is able to tolerate discussing his stuttering and even modifying pretend stutters, I move on to activities that focus more consistently on stuttering. I begin by having the child try to "catch me" stuttering. I throw in a few pretend easy stutters and ask him to let me know by signaling whenever he notices a stutter in my speech. Easy stutters can be repetitions, prolongations, or blocks, but they are produced slowly and without much tension. I reward him when he successfully catches my easy stutters, and I sometimes talk about what I did when I pretended to get stuck. This lets him know that I am not afraid of stuttering and in turn provides a model of talking objectively about stuttering. Most clinicians can do this legitimately even though they don't stutter. Most children know that the clinician's stutters are voluntary and are OK with it. After several minutes of putting easy stutters in my speech, I might ask the child to signal me when *he* stutters. If he misses many of them, I make sure I'm really rewarding those that he catches and then comment on a few that he has missed. I am careful to find some easier stutters in his speech and compare them with harder ones. I discuss with the child, as I have earlier, that this is one of our goals for therapy: to replace his hard stuttering with the easier talking that I call "superfluency." He has more control over his speech than he thinks.

An important goal at this stage is to continue making stuttering something that we can talk about. This openness decreases some of the fear, frustration, and shame associated with stuttering. I can judge progress on this goal by noticing how a child reacts when I put stuttering in my speech and when I ask him to explore his stuttering. I continue to question the child about his stutters while I maintain an interested, enthusiastic, and accepting style of inquiry. What did he do when he stuttered? Where was it tight? Could he show me again what it sounded like? Again, I continually assess how much confrontation a child can tolerate and intersperse it with activities the child enjoys. An important focus of this phase of therapy is easy stuttering. Therefore, as the youngster and I explore his stuttering together, I help him identify relatively easy and relaxed stutters in his current speech. Because I have filled my own speech with models of these, the child is usually familiar with these targets. It will help, however, if I audio or video record his speech and play back those segments in which there are only good examples of easy stuttering. With an initial emphasis on these mild stutters, we can then move to longer and tenser stutters that the child can readily identify in his own speech. Audio or video playback works quite well if the child can be put in charge of recording and playback. Some students will get a kick out of learning to edit their videos so they look and sound pretty good.

The Longer the Child Is Able to Remain in Contact with Moments of Stuttering, the More His Fear Will Be Reduced

The third principle taken from the phobia literature suggests that extended amounts of time in contact with stuttering will help reduce fear of it. The idea of being "in contact" with stuttering behavior may have an important meaning in the context of speech motor control. A child who has been stuttering persistently for several years may have lost easy access to proprioceptive awareness of his speech or may never have had it to an appropriate degree. This may make it difficult for him to use proprioceptive information to coordinate speech movements. Therefore, as a child explores his stuttering, I help him increase his awareness of what he's doing when he stutters, particularly for more severe moments of stuttering. If I can guide him to stay in the moment of stuttering beyond the time when he can release the block, he can feel what he's doing and then will realize that he can control the tension and movement of his speech structures. *The shift that he will feel as he holds on to stutters for an extended period of time will seem like a change from being out of control to being in control.* It may indeed result from a change in the activity of brain areas that control speech movements, such as a shift from a motor area of the brain that is not well supplied with sensory feedback to a motor area with better sensory information (Guitar, Guitar, Neilson, O'Dwyer, & Andrews, 1988).

Several years ago, a graduate student and I were helping a 10-year-old girl learn to stop fighting her stutters and learn to handle them with grace and ease. One of the steps in her exploring her stutters was to get to know her stutters and "make friends with them." The graduate student, Charles Barasch, wrote a poem for the girl to help her accomplish this:

Getting Unstuck
  for a young stutterer
When breath hides in your stomach
like a fish under stone,
and when it's hooked thrashes
and teases, dive down and follow,

let it think it's pulled you in
while you swim past swaying weeds,
through the shadow and light
inside yourself. And when it thinks
it owns you, sing to it like a mermaid,
it will fall in love with you
and do whatever you want.
It will follow you home
and be your liveliest companion,
it will dance for you
and do tricks for your friends,
you will think you've never met anyone
so intelligent or funny.
The house you set up together
will be happy until the end of your days.

Exploring Secondary Behaviors

The aim of the exploration phase of therapy is not to identify every aspect of a child's stuttering in great detail but to develop an "approach" attitude, to decrease fear, and to learn the rudiments of easier stuttering and easier talking. However, most school-age children who stutter have some avoidance behaviors, and if we can help these children become aware of them, avoidances are likely to diminish. I usually begin by mentioning some examples of starters, postponements, and other avoidance behaviors that I have seen in other children. For instance, I may tell the child about other kids I know who use "well" or "um" before difficult words, who don't talk in class because they're afraid they might stutter, or who substitute easy words for hard ones. I make it clear that these avoidances are very understandable and nothing to be ashamed of, but they also get in the way of being able to talk easily. By sharing such examples with the child and asking him if he has tried any of them, I make it easier for him to be open about the secondary behaviors he uses or at least those he is aware of using. If a child has difficulty identifying or discussing secondary behaviors, I put it aside for the moment. He may be better able to explore these behaviors after he has learned some coping skills.

Exploring Feelings

In addition to identifying the strategies that a child uses to hide or avoid his stuttering, I also explore the feelings underlying his need to use them. Many children are unwilling or perhaps unable to discuss in much detail their feelings of embarrassment or fear associated with stuttering. I do not push a child on this point, but let him know that these sorts of feelings are understandable and natural. I encourage his expression of such feelings, reinforce any of his comments about them, and continue to show my acceptance. I use several approaches to help a child express and thereby diminish feelings about stuttering. I often comment on the experiences and feelings that other children have when they stutter, such as the angry and sad feelings that result from being teased, being told by adults to slow down, having words finished for them, and being interrupted. Kristin Chmela and Nina Reardon have produced an excellent workbook to help children express and manage their feelings about their stuttering and about themselves (Chmela & Reardon, 2001).

I find that some children express their feelings more freely through drawings. Thus, I often ask them to draw pictures of what stuttering is like. I begin by telling the child that some stutters are like a stuck door (or whatever is most relevant to his type of stutters), and I draw something that represents the feeling. I usually make jagged lines to represent frustration and talk to the child about how stutters like that might feel. Then, I ask the child to draw a picture showing how it feels when he gets stuck on a word. In explaining his drawing, the child is often able to express how he feels. Therefore, I use drawing throughout therapy to help the child deal with old feelings of hurt and new feelings that are encountered during various stages of therapy. My experience has been that children's feelings often affect their fluency. The more practice they get in expressing their feelings, the less those feelings interfere with talking.

Another way in which drawings can be used to explore feelings is by using a metaphor proposed by Joseph Sheehan (1970) called "The Iceberg of Stuttering." Clinicians from the Michael Palin Centre make great use of the iceberg analogy by having children draw their own icebergs showing their stuttering behaviors as the small top part of the iceberg and their feelings in the large underwater portion. A good depiction of this can be seen in the video mentioned earlier, *Stuttering: Basic Clinical Skills* (Guitar & Fraser, 2007).

By now, the child has shared with me his moments of stuttering and the strategies he uses to hide them. Moreover, he has found me to be an understanding and accepting listener. Some deconditioning of speech fears has already occurred, and the child has also learned some of the terms I will be using in the remaining phases of therapy. Thus, some basic groundwork has been laid for the following phases of treatment.

Teaching Fluency Skills

In *Treatment of the Young Confirmed Stutterer*, Van Riper advocates building up the child's fluency: "We always try to increase the amount of fluency in these children, and we want them to feel it and recognize it when it does occur rather than to focus their attention only on the stuttering" (Van Riper, 1973, p. 434). Following Van Riper's lead, I teach these children to increase their fluent speech by using a variety of skills. Once a child has learned these skills, he can use them to replace stuttering with superfluency. I find that this work on fluency goes best if I have first given the child some of what Van Riper calls "**desensitization**." Some desensitization occurs in the preceding phase of exploration when the child learns to feel what he's doing when he stutters, hold onto the stutter, and reduce his physical tension.

This has set the stage for a focus on fluency by reducing the child's emotional response to stuttering. He may then be calm enough in speaking situations outside the clinic to use his fluency skills to move through the feared word(s) slowly, carefully, and smoothly. For most children, progress in this area is slow. One day they can use fluency skills in real-world situations, and a week later they can't. As the clinician gains experience, she is able to discern whether to keep practicing fluency skills, return to desensitization activities, or both.

There are some intermediate-level stutterers who are more like beginning stutterers in their relative lack of fear toward stuttering. These youngsters may need only a small amount of desensitization, and they begin therapy by learning fluency skills to replace stuttering. Other children may indeed fear stuttering but be unable to make progress in desensitization until they have increased their fluency and thus may benefit from *starting therapy* with fluency skills training and then work on desensitization.

Specific Fluency Skills

The skills described in this section are also described in the workbook, *Easy Talker* (Guitar & Reville, 1997), which includes reproducible worksheets for each skill. There is no magic to the order in which these skills should be taught. In this section, I will begin by describing what skills I think are the easiest before going on to those that are a little harder or more abstract. They may be taught in any order or all at once; with the latter option, the clinician models fluency with flexible rate, easy onsets, light contacts, and proprioception, and then shapes the child's responses.

Flexible Rate

Flexible rate is simply slowing down the production of a word, especially the first syllable (Boehmler, personal communication, 2003). Slowing is thought to be effective in reducing stuttering by allowing more time for language planning and motor execution (see "Fluency-Inducing Conditions" in Chapter 1). This skill is called "flexible rate" rather than "slow rate" to emphasize that only those syllables on which stuttering is expected are slowed, not the surrounding speech. I also think that "flexible rate" is more acceptable to school-age children who may be tired of hearing people tell them to "slow down."

Flexible rate is taught first by having the clinician model production of words in which the first syllable and the transition to the second syllable are said in a way that slows all of the sounds equally. Vowels, fricatives, nasals, sibilants, and glides are lengthened, and plosives and affricates are produced to sound more like fricatives without stopping the sound or airflow. After the clinician's model, the child produces the word with flexible rate, and successive approximations of the target (i.e., improvements) are reinforced. Practice should include all the sounds of the language; you can use a search engine to find interesting word or phrase lists, such as animals and the sounds they make (http://www.abcteach.com/free/l/list_animal_sounds.pdf). Younger children may be helped to learn flexible rate by running an obstacle course of chairs and tables in which they have to slow down as they move around obstacles but can speed up in parts of the course without obstacles. As you and the child run the obstacle course, you can tell a joke or a story and slow down both your speech and your movements as you negotiate the obstacles. Older children can get the idea by using analogies from their areas of interest. For example, some video games have race cars that can be slowed down on curves and sped up on straightaways.

Pausing

Winston Churchill, who stuttered, gave many fine speeches and most are notable for their pauses. Listen to his "Their Finest Hour" speech, especially the end. You will hear that although Churchill used pauses to reduce his stuttering, he also achieved great dramatic effect with them. The school-age child who stutters—as well as the adult—can use pausing to reduce muscle tension and allow the brain to stay at a processing speed that is comfortable.

I use pausing when I use flexible rate to downshift in preparing to say a feared word a little more slowly. You can teach it to children by having them act out a pause in running an obstacle course as mentioned in the preceding section. Then they can transfer pausing to appropriate places in their conversational speech. One of the youngsters I work with recently told me he pauses after being called on in class before he begins his answer to a teacher's question to take charge of the pace of speaking.

Easy Onsets

These are labeled as "Ee-Oo's" in our *Easy Talker* workbook (Guitar & Reville, 1997); they refer to an easy or gentle onset of voicing. My perception of my own stuttering is that if I begin a "feared" sound with a rapid onset of voicing (i.e., a hard glottal attack), I get myself into a "stuck" posture that feels like I can't move it. But if I start my vocal folds vibrating gently at first, I can usually get voicing going without stuttering. For me and probably for many others who stutter (but not all), vowels in word-initial positions are easier to use with an easy onset than are consonants. Vowels following a word-initial voiceless consonant, however, are fairly difficult for me. For example, I might prolong the "s" in "sun" and may block on the "u" unless I consciously employ a gentle onset on the /u/.

Again, teaching easy onsets is like teaching flexible rate. You model the target behavior on lots of different sounds and then have the child imitate your models and reinforce his successive approximations. Some children, particularly younger ones, may be helped to get the concept by performing an action, such as bringing their hands together slowly, as they produce an easy onset.

Light Contacts

Light contacts means producing a stop consonant by just brushing the articulators together, keeping airflow going as the stop is produced.

Just as a hard glottal attack can trigger stuttering, hard articulatory contacts can also bring it on. When someone who stutters anticipates difficulty with a sound, he'll often "preset" his articulators into a stuck position before starting a word, or he may even rehearse the stuttering behavior (Van Riper, 1936). Producing consonants with light contacts prevents the stoppage of airflow and/or voicing that can trigger stuttering. Light contacts are taught by modeling a style of producing consonants with relaxed articulators and continuous flow of air or voice, depending on the consonant. Plosives and affricates should be slightly distorted so that they sound like fricatives but are still intelligible. For example, when I produce the /b/ in "Barry" using a light contact, I slow down the movement into and out of the lip "closure." Instead of stopping the airflow and voicing by closing my lips, I let my lips loosely vibrate and allow the /b/ sound semi-closure continue for a little longer than normal. For a /p/, my lips barely touch and air flows out of my not-quite-closed lips, creating a slight turbulence so that it sounds a little like an /f/. For those readers who are phonetically minded, I'm actually producing fricative cognates for the /p/ and /b/ sounds. Because these sounds aren't used contrastively in English, my listeners don't notice, but my stuttering does!

Teaching a child to use light contacts is accomplished by modeling a variety of words with initial consonants and reinforcing the child's successive approximations of the target. To make the concept more interesting and perhaps clearer, you can use a variety of games to demonstrate light contact. For example, you might try catching soap bubbles or throwing and catching water balloons or raw eggs. You can also use games that build towers or require you to gently pick up an object (like jackstraws, also called pickup sticks) without disturbing other objects. These activities enable the child to use a light, gentle touch in a vivid way. Once a child gets the basic idea of using light contacts in speech, you can combine flexible rate, easy onsets, and light contacts together in practice on multisyllable words, while using these skills on the first syllable and transition to the second syllable and finishing the word at a normal rate.

Proprioception

In the present context, **proprioception** refers to sensory feedback from mechanoreceptors in muscles of the lips, jaw, and tongue (Abbs, 1996). This feedback may be crucial in controlling speech movements, and its use as a concept in stuttering therapy may have originated from Van Riper, who suggested that "…some of the stutterer's difficulties seem to originate in the auditory processing system. (Therefore,) if we can get him to concentrate upon proprioceptive feedback rather than auditory feedback, we can bypass these difficulties"

(Van Riper, 1973, p. 211). Recent brain imaging studies reviewed in Chapters 2 and 3 support Van Riper's contention that the auditory systems of people who stutter may be dysfunctional (e.g., Ingham, 2003; Stager, Jeffries, & Braun, 2003), but there is also evidence that other sensory systems may not be functioning normally either (e.g., De Nil & Abbs, 1991). The work of Cykowski, Fox, Ingham, Ingham, and Robin (2010) suggesting that stutterers may have inadequate density in left-hemisphere fiber tracts that connect sensory integration areas and motor planning areas is another sliver of evidence suggesting problems in sensory processing. The effectiveness of teaching proprioception may be that it promotes conscious attention to sensory information from the articulators, perhaps bypassing inefficient automatic sensory monitoring systems and thereby normalizing sensory-motor control.

Children can be taught to use proprioception in a number of ways. One of my former students, David Stuller, has taught proprioception by having a child first hold a raisin in his mouth and report on its taste, shape, size, and other attributes. This activity tunes the child into sensations from his mouth before introducing speech, which may have negative associations for more severe or more sensitive intermediate stutterers. Children can also learn proprioception by picking a word from a list and then closing their eyes and silently moving their articulators for this word and being rewarded when the clinician guesses the word. During this game, children can be coached to feel the movements of their lips, tongue, and jaw as they say a word. Proprioceptive awareness can also be enhanced by using masking noise or delayed auditory feedback to interfere with self-hearing. Although it is not always easy to judge accurately whether or not a child is using proprioception, I look for slightly exaggerated, slow movements to verify that a child is trying to feel the movements of his articulators.

Once a child seems to have acquired proprioception skills, they can be combined with flexible rate, easy onsets, and light contacts as described in the next section. I call using the combination of all these skills "superfluency."

Replacing Stuttering with Superfluency

The use of superfluency to replace stuttering begins with practice on fluent speech. I start with three-word sentences like, "I am great!" and have the child practice putting superfluency on the first syllable and the transition to the second. Using multiple letters to represent superfluency, I would depict its production like this: "IIIIaam great." By first modeling the production and then listening and watching the child imitate it, the clinician shapes the child's superfluency skills. Clear and enthusiastic feedback to the child will help him learn; a reward system will make learning fun.

At first, it is important to ensure that all the elements (flexible rate, easy onset, light contacts, and proprioception) are present. Later on, when a child has learned to use superfluency

successfully, he may develop his own version that may use only those elements necessary for him to be fluent. Some children become quite fluent and may need to use superfluency only rarely because, for them, having a tool that replaces stuttering with fluency gives them confidence and replaces anticipation of stuttering with anticipation of fluency. Thus, they appear to no longer put their articulators in anticipatory postures or have anticipatory tension that triggers stuttering.

After starting with a simple three-word sentence, the clinician continues having the student practice superfluency using both long and short sentences with a variety of initial sounds and with superfluency used in a variety of positions. At first, she has the child imitate her model but then fades the strength of that cue. The more successful the child is in learning good quality superfluency, the less the clinician needs to model the sentences. For those sentences not imitated after the clinician's model, the child can read the sentence from a list using superfluency on words that are circled. Here are a few sentences to use: "Just do it!" "Show me the money," "Yes, we have no bananas," and "Step away from the car." Video or audio playback of the child's successful utterances can be helpful in creating an auditory target in the child's mind to guide him.

After a youngster has mastered the use of superfluency on fluent utterances at the one-word level, the focus should be on conversation. At first, the clinician should model superfluency on many of her utterances, both on sentence-initial words and on initial sounds of other words in sentences. The child should be rewarded for superfluency during the time he is working to master it in conversation, but systematic fading of his rewards should be used to make the skill independent of the clinician's feedback. In any case, the activity must be fun for the child, especially if he is taken out of class for therapy. I often use rewards that release frustration toward past stuttering, such as shooting a ping-pong ball gun or throwing a stuffed rat at cans and bottles that have pictures of "stutters" taped to them. A burp gun that shoots ping-pong balls is available from www.HammacherSchlemmer.com.

Some children respond well to concrete representations of new skills they are trying to learn. To help them get the idea of shifting into superfluency from normal speech as they attempt a difficult word, I use the idea of "downshifting" a car or truck. In Vermont, it's easy to have kids imagine they are driving a four-wheel drive truck and need to downshift when they see deep snow ahead. In other areas, downshifting may be needed before driving through deep mud or up a steep hill. Downshifting can be acted out by the clinician and child by talking and changing into superfluency as they talk when encountering pretend snow, mud, or a hill while walking around the therapy room. Some children may have trouble perceiving when they might stutter on an upcoming word. These children can often be helped in two ways. First, they may be given a little training on the side, using reinforcement for stopping after a stutter, then during a stutter, and finally before a potential stutter. Second, they may benefit from massed practice of superfluency on fluent words, letting them shift into superfluency before an anticipated stutter becomes automatic.

During the conversation, because superfluency on fluent utterances is being rewarded, the child will probably get into a mindset that will make it easy for him to use superfluency with words on which he expects difficulty. Sometimes you can tell when a child uses superfluency on an expected stutter rather than an expected fluent word, and sometimes you can't. However, the child can often tell you when he is actually using it on an expected stutter, and you should give him an extra reward for these times. There is no harm done when the child uses superfluency on an "expected" stutter that was really just a fluent word. The more practice the better. When the child has replaced stutters with superfluency in the therapy room and superfluency is comfortable for him to use, he can begin using it in structured situations.

Transferring Superfluency to Structured Situations

This section describes not only the specifics of transferring fluency skills, but also additional elements, such as being open about stuttering, which will help make transfer successful and aid in maintenance.

Transfer of superfluency to replace stuttering with other listeners and in other situations begins by setting up a hierarchy with the child of easy-to-difficult situations, in which the child and I can use voluntary downshifts to superfluency together. I use the word "voluntary" here to mean that superfluency is used on nonfeared words—that is, words on which the child doesn't expect to stutter. In the context of using voluntary superfluency, anticipated stutters will eventually occur, and the child will be primed to replace them with superfluency. We begin each session by working together to plan a hierarchy and determine the number of reward points for each accomplishment. At this time, I am getting information from the parents about the child's progress at home.

At an appropriate level of difficulty in the hierarchy, I bring the parents into therapy and have the child teach them about downshifting into superfluency and then develop a plan to have the child use both voluntary and real (when stuttering is expected) downshifts at home. One or both parents, depending on the child's preference, should help him keep a log of the number of downshifts he makes each day. However, involving parents as therapy helpers is not effective for some children. They prefer not to have their parents function in this way but merely want their parents to be supportive listeners. In such cases, I sometimes telephone the child at home and have him record himself talking to me with superfluency from his home. If he's motivated, he can listen to the recording on his own.

By now, the child may be speaking with little difficulty in many situations, but some situations are probably still giving him problems. As I continue the transfer process, I turn more attention to those situations in which the child is having trouble using superfluency successfully to replace his stuttering.

Desensitizing the Child to Fluency Disrupters

Most children at intermediate levels of stuttering have an "Achilles heel," and sometimes, they seem to have one on each foot. For example, some find it hard to maintain fluency when they are talking in a group where children are interrupting each other. Others have more difficulty when telling a story or joke to a friend or when talking in a noisy environment like an industrial arts (shop) class. When a child is vulnerable to particular situations, I begin by role-playing the situations in the safety of the treatment room, and then I gradually move the child into more life-like approximations of the situations. If the child has difficulty using superfluency when he's being interrupted, we plan some role plays. I let the child interrupt me so that I can model using superfluency with all its bells and whistles to retain a calm, smooth utterance despite the interruptions. We then switch roles, and I interrupt him. When we have done that and he seems to be confident in using superfluency to deal with interruptions when talking to me, we enlist other children or adults to help out in the role playing. By doing this many times over many sessions, the child usually learns to handle this type of difficult situation.

Scaffolding

I have found it useful with some children to "scaffold" their use of superfluency by letting the listener(s) know that we are working on our speech and sometimes by coaching the child in that fluency-friendly environment. I am always careful to plan this beforehand with the child and ensure that he is comfortable with it. For example, I may tell a stranger in a mall that the child and I are working on our speech and we'd like to ask him some questions. Depending on the child's readiness, I may ask the first question or the child may. If the situation has been difficult in the past, I may coach the child in his use of superfluency as he speaks by giving him subtle signals that we have worked out beforehand.

Transfer on the telephone lends itself to a great deal of scaffolding, which can be faded as the child is more and more successful. For example, the clinician and child may plan a variety of gestures or signs that can provide support as the child makes telephone calls to practice superfluency. If we are practicing voluntary superfluency, which is always a good thing to do, I'll make the first phone call and have the child signal me to put in superfluency whenever he wants. Then we will reverse roles. Sometimes, physical contact helps focus a child on his speech even in the face of some fear. If you and the child are comfortable with it, you could place your hand on the child's arm and squeeze it to let him know you notice that he has shifted to superfluency or to remind him to do so.

Reducing Fear and Avoidance

Some children take a little longer than others to transfer their superfluency skills. They may have learned fears and avoidances that will require a concerted effort to overcome. It helps many children in this situation to deal with their fears if the right analogies or comparisons can be found. I get them to think about other fears they have overcome or about people they know, such as family members, who are afraid of such things as the dark, bugs, snakes, or swimming in deep water, and I enlist the child's help in listing ways they might overcome their fears. I also look for examples in pop culture, like Harry Potter or Spiderman. By analyzing how people get over their fears and describing the rewards of facing fears and conquering them, I am often able to motivate children to tackle their fears of difficult words and situations.

Sometimes we forget that fears are very natural and perhaps some fears—like a fear of crocodiles—are important to help us survive. Let the child know that it's natural to be worried about words or situations that have given him trouble in the past. But he should also know that the fear of these things itself causes him to tense up and stutter. Here are some steps for him to reduce his fears: (a) be OK with having some fear; (b) study the words or situations so he can learn about them; (c) practice his superfluency over and over before saying a difficult word or talking in a difficult situation; and (d) get rewarded for going ahead and trying something despite his fear, even if he's not completely fluent. In fact, if the child can just shoot for making his stuttering gradually easier and easier—gradually more and more like superfluency—it will be an easier target to hit, and he will succeed more and more.

Making a Hierarchy

In preparing to help a child plan a hierarchy to overcome fear and avoidance, I make up a hypothetical situation. For example, I might talk about overcoming fear of jumping off the high diving board at the local swimming pool (Fig. 13.3) and suggest if the child wanted to overcome his fear of the high board, it would be best for him to start by jumping off the side of the pool. When he could imagine being comfortable with this, he could imagine jumping off the low board. After becoming comfortable with diving off the low board, he would be ready to take on the medium-high board. Eventually, he would reach the high diving board. After jumping off the high diving board a number of times, he would find himself no longer afraid of it. Therefore, there would be no reason for him to avoid the high diving board any more. I then explain to the child that I will use this same

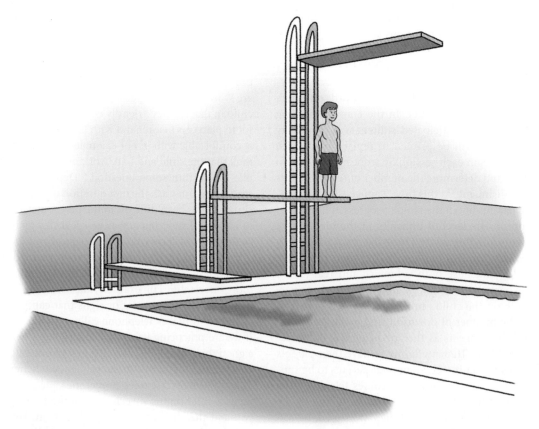

Figure 13.3   Using an easy-to-hard hierarchy to overcome fear and avoidance.

easy-to-hard strategy, or hierarchies, to help him overcome his speech fears and avoidances.

Reducing Word Fears

It is usually easier to help a child overcome his fear and avoidance of particular words than of particular situations. This is because I can provide the child with more support in confronting word fears in the therapy room than I can provide when he confronts his situational fears in daily life. I can also use feared words over and over again within the therapy situation. For example, I worked with a young school-age stutterer who consistently substituted "me" for "I." This was not because of a language disorder, and his parents reported that he had used "I" appropriately for a number of years before he began using this substitution. With this child, I began to practice saying "I" in unison with him, while we both used superfluency saying the word and strongly reinforced his efforts. Next, we used "I" many, many times in carrier phrases while playing games, with both of us using superfluency when saying "I." Gradually, the child regained his confidence in saying "I." Within a week or two, his avoidance of "I" was eliminated in therapy, and his parents reported that he was again using this pronoun appropriately at home.

Reducing Situation Fears

Now, let's consider the situation of a student being afraid to speak aloud in the classroom. In this case, I would invite with the child's consent one or two of his classmates into therapy. I would play the role of the classroom teacher and have this small group of two or three children ask and answer questions. When the child began to feel comfortable doing this, I would expand the group to three or four classmates. Next, it might be helpful for the child and the rest of us to go to his classroom during the noon hour or at recess. After explaining our goal and therapy procedures to the classroom teacher, I would have the child sit at his desk and have the teacher ask questions about his lessons. These activities are about as far as I can go in simulating a child's fear of this situation. The child needs to take the last step of these therapy procedures by himself. He has been successful in a series of situations that successively approximate his feared situation, and his classroom teacher is now sensitized to his problem and understands his therapy. The chances are that after some initial ambivalence, he will overcome his reluctance to talk in class.

Developing an Approach Attitude

In working on his fears and avoidances, the child must understand (as we've suggested before) that he doesn't have to be completely successful in using superfluency in all situations all of the time. In fact, as he first tackles feared words and situations, he may stutter in his old way many times. Even so, he should be rewarded for trying. The "approach attitude," which I sometimes refer to as "seeking out" (Guitar & Reville, 1997), may reduce fear and tension so that superfluency is

more obtainable. Repeated exposure to the feared objects when supported by the clinician will make a big difference in transfer of new skills to feared words and situations.

Coping with Teasing

It is important to minimize any teasing that a child is receiving because of his stuttering. The clinician can deal with it at any time, but it may be helpful to address teasing after the child has mastered some fluency skills and is transferring them. I address this issue in more detail when I discuss counseling parents and classroom teachers. Regardless of how hard parents, teachers, clinicians, and friends may try to eliminate teasing, I doubt that it is possible to eliminate all of it. Thus, I try to give a child some defenses against the teasing that he is likely to receive.

I agree with Van Riper (1973) that the best defense against teasing is acceptance if a child is emotionally mature enough to feel and express acceptance. For example, if a child can say, "I know I stutter, but I'm working on it," or some similar statement, this will disarm most teasers. Nobody likes to tease someone who does not appear to be bothered. Running away, on the other hand, just reinforces teasing. Nevertheless, I have found that it is difficult for a school-age child to calmly accept and admit his stuttering when he talks to his tormentors. When I have been successful, I have done the following things.

First, I discuss the importance of calmly and openly admitting stuttering to teasers, rather than saying nothing. I explain how this type of response usually discourages teasers. I then explore with the child the sorts of statements he can imagine himself making. The words he uses must be words with which he feels comfortable. Next, I initiate role playing with the child. As I play the role of the teaser, the child's task is to respond calmly to my heckling. He practices saying the types of statements he has chosen to use to counteract the teasing. I role play this many times until the child feels comfortable with his response and can see himself doing this in a real-life situation. Finally, the day comes when he tries out this new behavior. I hope it works, but if it does not, I am there to give the child support and encouragement.

I have also found that if I have two or more children who stutter or if I can form a group of several children who have speech or language problems, we can write and perform a play together about a child who stutters who triumphs over teasing.

Some children are especially sensitive to teasing and need patience and understanding as they work to develop effective responses. These children may have more inhibited temperaments, and their first reaction to a threatening situation is to withdraw or avoid. Hence, these children need practice in asserting themselves. In our role playing, I experiment with a variety of ways in which the child can feel that he confronted the teaser. For some children, it might be teasing back; for others, it might be reporting the teaser to a teacher or the principal. A tactic taught by Bill Murphy, an experienced speech pathologist who also stutters, is to have children say "So?" back to the teaser after every taunt. Because it's a short utterance, children who stutter can often say it fluently and with gusto. Other excellent advice is contained in a publication by Murphy and others titled, *Bullying and Teasing: Helping Children Who Stutter* (Yaruss, Murphy, Quesal, Reardon-Reeves, & Flores, 2004). A good list of information about teasing of children who stutter can be found at http://www.mnsu.edu/comdis/kuster/infoabout-stuttering.html#teasing.

Being Open about Stuttering

One of the best ways to combat fear, embarrassment, and the physical tension that these emotions often elicit is for the child to be open about his stuttering, to talk about it casually with friends, to refer to it in humorous ways when it happens, and to educate people about it. Children differ widely in their readiness to be open about their stuttering. However, once most of them feel some sense of mastery over what has made them feel helpless in the past, they are much more able to let people know about it. If a child stutters in class, I rehearse casual comments that he can make about his stuttering when he is giving an oral report or answering a question in class. He might say, for example, "My report is about how maple syrup is produced. Before I begin, I just want to say that I'll probably stutter sometimes while I'm talking, but don't let it bother you. I'm dealing with it." Or he might say, "It makes it easier for me if you can keep pretty good eye contact with me when I get stuttery." Basically, it is not so much the content that is important as the fact that the child acknowledges his stuttering and that he's working on it. He feels good that he has acknowledged it, and his audience is more comfortable than if he stutters and tries to hide it.

A child may also benefit from developing a repertoire of casual comments to make about his stuttering if he gets particularly hung up on a word while talking to friends, relatives, or strangers. He might learn to say, "Wow! I really got hung up there," or "I'm really running into a lot of blocks; I'd better slow down a bit." In my experience, the most effective comments are those that the child comes up with spontaneously when he feels comfortable with his stuttering. These are unforced, often funny remarks that put the child and his listeners at ease.

Teaching other children and his teachers about stuttering can be a powerful tool in combating the shame and embarrassment that often accompany a school-age child's stuttering. Although this can be done with small groups of students brought into the therapy room or in meetings with the child and his teachers, our experience has been that eventually sharing information about stuttering in front of the entire class is extremely effective for many children. When and if a child is ready to do this, we work together to prepare, rehearse, and then give a presentation that informs the class about stuttering in general and the child's own stuttering in particular. A question-and-answer period is a crucial part of the presentation because it gives the child's classmates a chance to express their curiosity about stuttering. It also gives the child an opportunity to become an expert in the very behavior that previously made him feel so helpless.

Here is an example of how this can work. A second grader who was very sensitive about his stuttering was also rather proud of a brief segment on a local television station that showed him working on his stuttering. He was willing to show a video of this segment in class and answer questions about his stuttering. The following year, I accompanied him to class for a full-scale presentation about stuttering. This presentation included posters he had made, demonstrations of therapy techniques, and a question-and-answer segment. A year after this program, the child had a particularly rocky beginning to the school year because his stuttering had returned full-force after his family moved to a new house in a new neighborhood. However, he was still willing to do another presentation with me. This time he used more video clips of himself talking, because he was more reluctant to talk at length and talked to the class about some of the "ups and downs" in his progress with stuttering.

Maintaining Improvement

By this point in therapy, a child is usually speaking well in most situations. He is having a great deal of natural fluency in many situations and either superfluency or acceptable stuttering in others. His speech fears and avoidances have been eliminated or significantly reduced. I do not dismiss the child from therapy at this point but gradually phase him out of therapy. I see him for therapy on a weekly basis for a month or so, then on a twice-monthly basis for another month or so. If all continues to go well, I see him for a series of "checkups" over the next two years, first monthly, then bimonthly, and finally once a semester.

During these checkups, I obtain samples of the child's speech and oral reading and discuss with him how he has been talking in everyday speaking situations. I also interview his parents and classroom teacher about his speech at home and school. If I find that the child's fluency has regressed or that he has begun to use avoidance behaviors again, I re-enroll him in therapy. My experience is that a number of children may have one or two mild regressions before their fluency stabilizes. Such regressions are often associated with the beginning of a school year or with transfers from one school to another or with other disrupting factors.

When I return a child to therapy, it is usually for only a month or two. During these "booster" sessions, he may need to have his fluency-enhancing or stuttering modification skills "tuned up." He may need a brief refresher course on the importance of not avoiding, or he may just need an opportunity to talk to an understanding listener about his stuttering. In time, these regressions and our reevaluations become further apart until finally the day arrives when the child, his family, and I decide to dismiss him from treatment.

My hope is that even though "dismissal" sounds rather final, the child realizes that he has an ally in me and in other SLPs who know about stuttering. That attitude could help him return to treatment if he thinks he needs some additional help—in a month, a year, or a decade.

Clinical Procedures: Working with Parents

I have five goals in mind when counseling parents of an intermediate stutterer: (1) explaining the treatment program and the parents' role in it; (2) discussing the possible causes of stuttering; (3) identifying and reducing fluency disrupters; (4) identifying and increasing fluency-enhancing situations; and (5) eliminating teasing. I will discuss each of these goals in turn.

Explaining the Treatment Program and the Parents' Role in It

First, I discuss the stages of our therapy program with the child's parents, letting them know how I hope to take the mystery out of stuttering for the child by exploring with him what he does when he stutters. I also tell them about our goal of teaching the child to use superfluency to replace stuttering and how it is a gradual process. At times, it may even sound like their child is stuttering in slow motion when he uses superfluency. Second, I tell them that therapy may take time, perhaps one to three years and in some cases even longer. Third, I inform them that communicating with their child about his stuttering is important and that they should express their acceptance of his stuttering and acknowledge their understanding that it is often difficult for him to work on it.

Explaining the Possible Causes of Stuttering

I believe it is important for the parents of a school-age stutterer to be given an explanation of the possible causes of stuttering. I explain current thinking about the nature of stuttering. In some cases, parents have no information about the causes of stuttering. Since I want them to participate in their child's treatment, they need to understand the rationale for our treatment program. Many parents feel guilty about their child's stuttering because of some outdated or inaccurate information they may have. They may have been exposed to an explanation that is no longer valid, or they may have been given some erroneous information by a well-meaning but misinformed friend or relative. Such parents then blame themselves for some supposed misdeed on their part. They need good, current information about the nature of stuttering. Often, just supplying this information relieves them of their guilt. The following materials have been helpful supplements to parent counseling:

1. On the "Stuttering Home Page" website (http://www.mnsu.edu/comdis/kuster/), there is a link titled "Information about Stuttering," which leads to another link for parents of children who stutter. Articles, essays, books, and other materials for parents are provided directly there or are described so that parents can find them elsewhere.
2. On the National Stuttering Association website (http://www.westutter.org/whoWeHelp/NSA-Family-Programs/parents/School-Age.htm), there is a wealth of information for parents of school-age children who stutter.
3. On the Stuttering Foundation website (http://www.stutteringhelp.org/), a link titled "If You Think Your Child is Stuttering: 7 Ways to Help" provides useful information to parents. The Foundation also has two videos, *Stuttering: Straight Talk for Teens* and *Stuttering: Straight Talk for Teachers*, that are also helpful for parents.

Using language that is appropriate to the parents' level of understanding, I provide the type of information that I presented in the early chapters of this book. I describe how developmental and environmental influences may interact with predisposing physiological and constitutional factors to produce or exacerbate a child's initial repetitions and prolongations. The child responds to these disfluencies with increased tension in his effort to inhibit them. In time, the child also learns a variety of escape and possibly starting behaviors to cope with his repetitions and prolongations. I go on to suggest that predisposing physiological factors are most likely neurological in nature and are related to a child's deficits in speech production. I suggest that the child may have problems in timing the fine motor movements required for fluent speech. I add that children who stutter may also have a more sensitive temperament, and that could compound the stuttering by making the child more likely to have learned emotional reactions to his speech difficulties. I also note that in many cases, the predisposing physiological factors may be genetic in origin. Thus, there are many possible sources for his speech difficulty. I also suggest that because of the way the brain may be organized, the child may have special talents in the areas of drawing, music, engineering and other visual and creative endeavors.

I explore, with the parents' assistance, the developmental and environmental influences that may be interacting with the child's predisposing factors to affect his stuttering. These are reviewed in Chapters 4 and 5. In some cases, I may not identify any developmental or environmental factors that seem to be contributing to the problem; however, when I do identify one or more possible factors, I attempt to lessen their influence. My experience suggests that in most cases, the solution to reducing the impact of developmental and environmental influences is fairly straightforward. In a few cases, when it may be more difficult, I have suggested that counseling by a family therapist may be helpful.

I also talk with parents of a school-age child who stutters about avoidance behaviors. I describe these behaviors to them and explain how the child's word and situation avoidances are behaviors he has learned to use in coping with the embarrassment and fear of talking. I also explain how in therapy, I will be helping the child eliminate his use of these avoidance behaviors. I will also point out that avoidance learning is unfortunately a rather tenacious form of learning so that they will need to model patience as the child "unlearns" avoidances.

Some parents feel responsible for their child's stuttering and may feel they need to find a cure for it. While I'm discussing the possible causes of stuttering and after I've mentioned the possible neurological differences in children who stutter, I often bring up the possibility that their child will always stutter but that it needn't interfere with his life. Because this can be such an important issue for parents, I try to judge whether this moment is the right time to discuss it. For example, if this is an initial phone conversation, I might not bring it up at that time. But if this is a face-to-face meeting and we have some time to talk about their concerns, I find it helpful to let parents know that a child who is still stuttering after age 9 or 10 years will probably continue to have at least a little stuttering throughout his life. In saying this, I am sure to indicate that most individuals who stutter into adulthood don't let their stuttering get in the way of their goals, and I will cite some examples of famous people who have achieved success even though they stuttered. At this point, I am careful to let them respond to this information. Parents sometimes envision difficulties in academic, social, and career areas for their child who stutters, and it is important for them to express these concerns and for me to listen deeply to them.

Identifying and Reducing Fluency Disrupters

As I explain in later chapters, environmental influences are often critical factors for managing beginning and borderline levels of stuttering in preschool children. Intermediate-level stuttering in school-age children is more complex and requires direct treatment of a child's behaviors and attitudes, but environmental factors are important for this level of stuttering as well. The home environment of a school-age child who stutters may involve stresses and **fluency disrupters** that can be substantially alleviated if the clinician can join forces with an interested, motivated family. I begin by asking family members to observe when the child stutters most and when he stutters least. With this information, I brainstorm with them various ways to reduce potential stresses and to observe the effects on the child's stuttering. For example, some children stutter a lot when there is competition for attention at the dinner table or when several children arrive home from school at the same time, all wanting to talk to their parents. In other cases, changes in a family routine may spark an increase in a child's stuttering. Whatever the sources of stress, I encourage the parents and other family members to take the lead in identifying them and in planning ways of reducing such stress. Even in cases in which stress may result from relatively abstract sources, such as a family's attitude that stuttering is shameful, the family is unlikely to

change unless they feel that they and their points of view are respected and understood by the clinician. In an accepting environment, a trusting relationship can be developed, and a family may be open to seeing the child and his stuttering in new ways.

Increasing Fluency-Enhancing Situations

During the process of identifying the times when a child stutters more frequently, families also discover there are times when a child is extremely fluent. These may be specific situations or just days or weeks when the child is particularly fluent. Whatever the case, families can find ways of increasing factors that promote fluency and giving a child plenty of opportunities to talk when he is fluent. For example, a child may be especially fluent when he is talking to a parent at bedtime, when he is sleepy and relaxed. This provides a parent an opportunity to comment on the child's "smooth speech" and to let the child know that they can imagine how good it must feel to talk easily. Help parents find ways of increasing fluency-enhancing situations and of reinforcing their child's fluency without implying that the times when he stutters are bad. Encourage the family to empathize with the child that fluency is great but that stuttering just can't be helped sometimes.

For those children who are willing to work on their fluency with members of their family, a program of home therapy can be developed cooperatively by the child, parent(s), and clinician. Regular contact between the clinician and family members is important to facilitate and guide this component of treatment. Face-to-face meetings are ideal, but phone calls, journals, or e-mail will also suffice. A typical home program would include severity ratings made by both parents of the child's speech at home and by the child of his speech at home and at school. The specific behaviors to be rated and an effective reward system are negotiated by the child, parents, and clinician.

Eliminating Teasing at Home

If any of an intermediate stutterer's siblings are teasing him about his stuttering, his parents need to stop it. I have found the best way to do this is to have parents have a serious talk with the teaser. They need to explain that teasing makes stuttering worse and must be discontinued. Usually, this is sufficient. If it is not, I have found it effective for me as the child's clinician to talk to the sibling about the importance of not teasing his or her brother or sister. Having an adult other than a parent talk seriously about this matter sometimes carries more weight with teasers.

Another important issue for parents is their reactions to teasing by other children at school. Although this is a serious matter, parents may do more harm than good if they are overly upset by teasing. The child who is teased will take his cue from his parents. If parents are anxious or distraught about their child's being teased, the child will be more deeply affected by it. If parents let the school take care of the incident and convey to the child that they have faith in his ability to handle it but are also empathetic to his concerns, they will help the child maintain a good perspective on it.

Clinical Procedures: Working with Classroom Teachers

I believe it is very important to have an intermediate stutterer's classroom teacher involved in the student's treatment program (Fig. 13.4). After all, the child spends as much, if not more, time with the teacher than any other adult. I have four goals in mind when I am working with a classroom teacher: (1) to explain the treatment program and the teacher's role in it; (2) to facilitate the teacher talking with the student about his stuttering; (3) to help the student and teacher work out the child's class participation; and (4) to help the teacher eliminate teasing.

Explaining the Treatment Program and the Teacher's Role in It

Involving the student's classroom teacher(s) in treatment works best if the student gives his permission for this to take place. Even the most reluctant students usually agree to let me make a contact with the teacher. If the student has several teachers, I always ask which teacher(s) the student would like me to talk to. Sometimes, a meeting with several teachers at once is efficient. When I worked as a speech-language pathologist in

junior high and elementary schools, I gave in-services about stuttering to teachers at the beginning of the school year. If such in-services can be arranged, the Stuttering Foundation DVD *Stuttering: Straight Talk for Teachers* (Trautman & Guitar, 2005) makes a powerful addition to a presentation on the problems faced by school children who stutter and how teachers can help them. Or consider showing another of the Foundation's DVDs: *Stuttering: For Kids, by Kids* (Scott & Guitar, 2004).

It is beneficial for classroom teachers to have an overview of the student's treatment program, so I discuss how I am helping the student increase his fluency, eliminate his avoidance behaviors, and improve his overall communication ability. I want the teacher to understand the rationale behind these procedures. Therefore, I am careful to answer any questions the teacher may have, believing that helping the teacher understand our goals will have at least two benefits: (1) the teacher will have a better understanding of how to interact with the student and (2) the teacher will be better able to give me feedback regarding the student's fluency in the classroom. I use the Teacher's Assessment of Students' Communicative Competence (TASCC) (Smith, McCauley, & Guitar, 2000) described in Chapter 8 to measure the student's baseline levels and progress. I also explain the teacher's role in the student's therapy and discuss why and how I would like the teacher to implement the three goals of how to talk with the student about his stuttering, how to help him cope with oral participation, and how to eliminate any teasing he may be receiving. I discuss each of these in the following paragraphs.

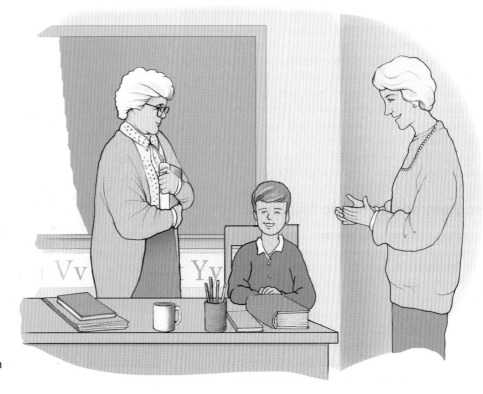

Figure 13.4 It is important to have the classroom teacher involved in the child's treatment.

Talking with the Child about His Stuttering

A friend of mine recalled going all the way through school from kindergarten through high school without any teacher ever mentioning his stuttering. He stuttered severely year after year, and everyone knew he stuttered, but nobody ever acknowledged it. This silence, he said, was very painful. I believe that it is better for a classroom teacher to sit down with a student who stutters and talk calmly with him about his stuttering, letting him know that she is aware of his stuttering and would like to help him in any way possible. The teacher should tell the student that she will not interrupt or hurry him when he is talking. Just this sort of acknowledgment and acceptance of the student's stuttering by a teacher will make the child feel more comfortable in the classroom.

Coping with Oral Participation

The teacher should also talk with the student about his oral participation in class. I believe it is important for a school-age child who stutters to participate orally in class. It is also important for him to feel comfortable participating, and the teacher should seek the student's input on this matter. Possibly some classroom procedure, such as calling on students in alphabetical order, is creating apprehension for the student who stutters and could be modified. For example, the student may prefer to be called on early, before his apprehension builds up. With an understanding of the student's feelings and flexibility in procedures, most teachers can help a student who stutters become much more comfortable in his oral classroom participation.

Eliminating Teasing

It is not unusual for stutterers in elementary or junior high school to be teased about stuttering at school. If a classroom teacher becomes aware of teasing, she should attempt to stop it. As I indicated during my previous discussion of teasing in the home, I believe the best way to do this is to have a serious talk with the teaser. The teacher needs to explain that the child's teasing is making the stutterer's speech worse and that he needs to discontinue it immediately. The teacher should make it clear that this behavior will not be tolerated. Some teasers are themselves troubled children and will need help from the school counselor to change their behaviors.

Progress and Outcome Measures

Measures of progress and outcome, as described in Chapter 8, need to be taken to assess the effectiveness of treatment. Data on stuttering and fluency (%SS, Stuttering Severity Instrument [SSI-4], measures of attitudes [CAT and A-19], and assessment of communicative competence [TASCC]) can be used to measure progress during treatment and outcome after maintenance.

This concludes the description of my approach to treatment of a school-age child with intermediate stuttering. I now describe the clinical procedures of some other clinicians.

OTHER CLINICIANS

Scott Yaruss, Kristin Pelczarski, and Bob Quesal: Treating the Entire Disorder

This intervention is described in detail and illustrated with a 20-minute DVD in Yaruss, Pelczarski, and Quesal (2010). The goal is to help the child become the most effective communicator he can be. Subgoals include (a) increasing the child's fluency and reducing his stuttering, (b) reducing the child's and the environment's reactions to the child's stuttering, and (c) helping the child increase participation in social and academic activities (Fig. 13.5).

Minimizing the Impairment (Increasing Fluency and Decreasing Stuttering)

The clinician begins by working directly on the child's fluency, helping him learn to reduce speaking rate and increase pause time. This is done in such a way that the changes in the child's speech are enough to promote fluency but not so much that the style of speaking sounds abnormal. As the clinician helps the child make changes in his speaking rate and pausing, she also teaches the child to reduce physical tension in his speech mechanism. For this purpose, light contacts and easy starts are incorporated into the child's speech, especially at the beginnings of utterances.

This more fluent style of speaking is taught in easy-to-more-difficult hierarchies. First the child uses this style of speaking while reading and then progresses to more and more natural conversations in the treatment room. Then the child practices this speaking style in gradually more challenging real-life situations, using a progression that the child and clinician design together.

Minimizing Negative Personal Reactions

To help the child decrease his negative reactions to his stuttering, the clinician helps the child use voluntary

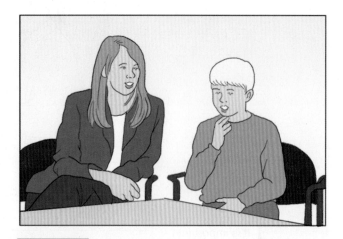

Figure 13.5 A clinician like Kristin Pelczarski helping a student feel what he is doing when he stutters.

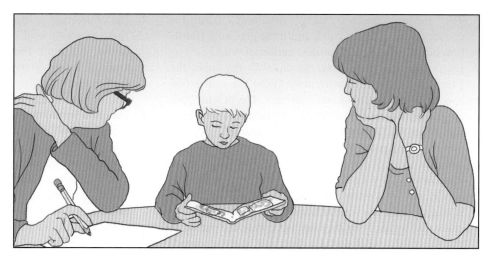

Figure 13.6 A clinician like Rosalee Shenker working with a student and his mother using the Lidcombe Program for school-age children who stutter.

stuttering in easy-to-more-difficult situations. The clinician also uses "cognitive restructuring" (e.g., Rapee, Wignall, Psych, Hudson, & Schniering, 2000) to help the child change his thoughts about his stuttering and his imagined listener reactions to it. This is assisted by role playing situations to explore what really might happen in various situations and what are realistic and unrealistic expectations. The clinician both accepts the child's fears and helps the child rethink imagined reactions.

The clinician can also help the child find groups of other kids who stutter, either online or by arranging such a group.

Minimizing Negative Environmental Reactions

To reduce negative reactions from parents, teachers, and peers, the clinician helps the child educate these groups about stuttering and what they are doing in treatment. Helping the child reduce his negative emotional reactions to his stuttering will also help the child respond to bullying, teasing, or other hurtful responses from peers by making matter-of-fact responses to provocations. Class presentations by the child and the clinician can also be used to educate peers and create a more stuttering-friendly environment.

Helping the Child Participate More Fully in Social and Academic Situations

To achieve this goal, the hierarchies that the child and clinician constructed while working on speaking strategies are adapted to help the child participate in more and more social and academic situations. The authors advocate a "generalization scavenger hunt" to organize and motivate this part of treatment. In a nutshell, the child and clinician develop a list of important speaking situations that the child may face during a typical day. These usually include conversations with family, classmates, and friends outside of school. The hierarchy is arranged in an easy-to-harder matrix with a list of strategies to enhance fluency and reduce stuttering to choose from for each situation. As the child goes through a typical

day and enters a planned situation, he picks which strategy he'll use in that situation. This whole procedure, practiced as frequently as possible, enables the child and clinician to track progress and decrease the amount of limitation and restriction that stuttering puts on the child's life.

Assessment of Progress and Outcome

Because this treatment is aimed at the overall effect that stuttering may have on a child's life, a major assessment tool is the *Overall Assessment of the Speaker's Experience of Stuttering* (Yaruss & Quesal, 2006; Yaruss, Coleman, & Quesal, 2007a, 2007b). Changes in the child's stuttering frequency and severity can be tracked by use of the SSI-4 (Riley, 2009), and the child's attitudes toward speaking can be assessed using the Communication Attitude Test (Brutten & Vanryckeghem, 2006). Yaruss, Pelczarski, and Quesal (2010) encourage collection of data on the effectiveness and efficacy of this approach using these measures.

Harrison, Bruce, Shenker, Koushik, and Kazenski: Lidcombe Program for School-Age Children

I have taken most of this description of the LP for school-age children from a chapter by Harrison, Bruce, Shenker, and Koushik (2010). The LP for preschool children described in detail in Chapter 12 forms the basis of LP for school-age children. The principal elements are:

1. The treatment has two stages: Stage 1, in which a stable level fluency is established in the clinic and beyond, and Stage 2, in which fluency is maintained, but clinic visits are systemically faded in duration and frequency.
2. The treatment is parent-delivered; in Stage 1 the parent and child meet with the clinician once a week for an hour, during which time the parent is trained, and progress is assessed (Fig. 13.6).

3. The parent conducts daily structured treatment conversations with the child, and these gradually transition into unstructured treatment conversations.
4. During the treatment conversations with the child, the parent gives verbal contingencies (VCs) for stutter-free speech and for unambiguous stuttering. The VCs for both are the same as those in Table 12.1 in the previous chapter describing the LP for older preschool children.
5. Severity Ratings (SRs) are used by the parent and the clinician to track the child's progress. This is a 1-to-10 scale in which 1 = no stuttering, 2 = extremely mild stuttering, and 10 = extremely severe stuttering. The parent is taught to use the scale at home for daily ratings and is calibrated regularly by the clinician asking the parent to rate the child's speech during a clinic visit, and the parent's and the clinician's ratings are compared. The parent's rating must not differ from the clinician's by more than one point. If it does, the parent must be trained further in the use of the scale. In addition to the parent's daily SRs, the clinician also assigns an SR to the child, rating the child's speech over the entire clinic visit.
6. Criteria for moving from Stage 1 to Stage 2 are three consecutive clinic visits in which the clinician's ratings of the child for the entire visit is a 1 or a 2, and the parent's ratings of the child's speech over the past week are 1s and 2s with at least four 1s.
7. Stage 2 is completed when the child maintains criteria-level fluency during the gradually faded clinic visits, spaced in this progression: two, two, four, four, eight, eight, and 16 weeks apart.

Some *adaptations for the school-age child* include the following, although these adaptations are optional:

1. The child may be taught to collect his own daily SRs. These may be useful because they may reflect the child's fluency in school. The child may enjoy charting his own progress, using a diary or a graph to keep track. However, the parent's SRs, along with the clinician's SRs, remain the primary measure of progress.
2. The child should be encouraged to discuss with his parent the types of VCs he would prefer. Anything goes, as long as the VCs for stutter-free speech are reinforcing to the child and the VCs for unambiguous stutters call attention to the stuttering without rewarding it.
3. Some school-age children may prefer tangible rewards in addition to VCs. They may be used for progress in reducing SRs or just for participating in the program. Tangible rewards for fluent speech in many different situations will speed generalization.

My colleague Danra Kazenski, who has worked with school-age children using the LP for more than 5 years, has these additional suggestions:

1. Develop VCs and tangible reward systems that take advantage of the child's interest (Fig. 13.7). For example, use a coin jar decorated with the child's favorite sports teams. Use code words that make the child feel really good about his fluency, such as "Now you're talking like LeBron James!"
2. Encourage and reward self-corrections. Ask the child after he's been fluent "Was that smooth?" Give the child bonus points if he fixes a stutter without the parent having commented on it, or if he identifies his fluent speech without prompting.
3. The more independence you can give the child, the better, as long as the parameters of the LP are respected.

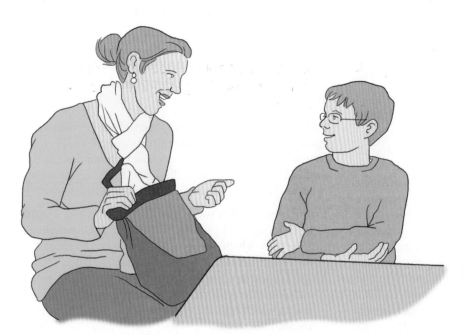

Figure 13.7   A clinician like Danra Kazenski using a mystery bag of toys as she reinforces a student in the Lidcombe Program for school-age children who stutter.

Patty Walton: Fun with Fluency for the School-Age Child

Patty Walton makes a statement near the beginning of her book that shows that she knows what treatment of school-age children who stutter is really like. She says "The greatest challenge clinicians face in treating school-age children who stutter is finding a balance between getting them to speak more easily and letting them stutter sometimes" (Walton, 2012). Walton is very realistic about the likelihood that most of these children will still have some residual stuttering even with the best treatment. She also realizes that the clinician must not be punitive toward any remaining stuttering, or she will lose the child's trust.

Walton's well-organized approach begins with a careful assessment that includes measures of stuttering severity, analysis of the child's stuttering pattern, assessment of the child's reaction to his stuttering, and his attitudes and emotions. She also assesses the parent's attitudes and behaviors toward their child's stuttering.

Her treatment plan will vary with each child, but the following components are the core of her approach:

1. Fluency-shaping techniques, beginning with "stretching" out the first sound of phrases, and including—only if necessary—easy onsets, light contacts, and other tools to increase fluency.
2. Stuttering modification techniques, to be used if the child is reacting negatively to his stuttering: voluntary stuttering, pull-outs, and other ways of making the child feel more in control of his stuttering.
3. Working with the child's attitudes and emotions, if the child perceives his stuttering to be negative or if he's being teased. In this area, Walton encourages the child to express his feelings about his speech, empowers him to take control of his stuttering, and helps him realize that success needn't be complete fluency, but may be stuttering in a way that feels in control.
4. Parent counseling, which involves educating parents about stuttering and about treatment, teaching strategies that the parents can be involved in to help the child at home, openness about stuttering at home so that stuttering is OK to talk about, helping parents have realistic expectations about treatment, and encouraging them to reduce criticism of the child and his speech.
5. Working with teachers, including finding out from teachers about the child's speech in the classroom, educating teachers about stuttering (particularly this child's), and enlisting teachers' support to facilitate transfer of therapy techniques into the classroom.

Walton emphasizes the importance, throughout therapy, of listening to the child—no matter whether the child is stuttering or not—to validate what he says, what he thinks, and how he feels.

SUMMARY

- My integrated approach to stuttering in school-age children begins with an exploration of stuttering to decrease some of the negative emotions associated with it and then teaches "superfluency," incorporating flexible rate, pausing, gentle onsets, light contacts, and proprioception to enhance fluency and manage stuttering. The young client then works on reducing his fear and avoidance by being open about stuttering, becoming desensitized to fluency disrupters, and learning to deal with teasing.

- The other clinicians, whose therapies are described in this chapter, use many of these same techniques. Some reinforce fluency in a hierarchy from words to sentences to conversation in the clinic and then to everyday situations outside the clinic. Most of them foster a change in attitudes about speech and stuttering, not only to provide positive expectations for fluency but also to help clients accept any residual stuttering so that they will deal with it rather than avoid it. Many also prepare the child to deal with teasing. Thus, the core of these programs is similar, but each clinician adds innovations. I've included several different approaches to help readers see how they too may consider adding different elements to their treatment.

STUDY QUESTIONS

1. What is the "approach" attitude that is recommended for school-age children who stutter? What are some reasons why an "approach" attitude might help a child with intermediate stuttering?
2. Many clinicians, including the Lidcombe group, believe that direct work on a child's attitude about speaking is not necessary because operant conditioning can change the child's speaking behaviors, which will automatically change his attitude. Do you agree? Give your rationale.
3. What is a "stuttering-friendly" environment, and how could you create one in a child's home and school?
4. Describe what the "exploration" phase of my treatment approach is designed to accomplish and how it meets that goal.
5. Suggest three ways in which you might assess to what extent the goals of the exploration phase of treatment have been met with a particular child.
6. Given what you learned about the nature of stuttering, explain why slowing speech rate (as in "flexible rate") might reduce stuttering.
7. When you are working on a transfer hierarchy and the child seems unable to transfer superfluency to a particular situation, such as giving a book report, what do you do to achieve success on this step?

SUGGESTED PROJECTS

1. Avoidance reduction is an important component of the major treatment described in this chapter. Experiment with your own fears and avoidances to see if you can decrease them by using a "seeking out" attitude. For example, if you dislike making phone calls, devote a week to making extra phone calls and seeking out opportunities to make phone calls you usually wouldn't make. After the week is over, assess whether this experience decreased your dislike of making phone calls.
2. Watch the Stuttering Foundation video *Stuttering: Straight Talk for Teens,* and plan how you might use various clips from it to help a child explore his own and others' stuttering.
3. Draw a "roadmap" with pictures that you could use to help a school-age child at the beginning of therapy learn about what he will be doing over the course of therapy.
4. Develop new ways, new metaphors, and new activities to help a child learn each of the components of "superfluency."

SUGGESTED READINGS

Craig, A., Hancock, K., Chang, E., McCready, C., Shepley, A., McCaul, A., Costello, D., Harding, S., Kehren, R., Masel, C., & Reilly, K. (1996). **A controlled clinical trial for stuttering in persons aged 9 to 14 Years.** *Journal of Speech and Hearing Research, 39,* 808–826.

This article describes three different treatment approaches for intermediate stuttering and assesses the effectiveness of each.

Dell, C. (2000). *Treating the school-age stutterer: A guide for clinicians* (6th ed.). **Memphis: Stuttering Foundation of America.**

This bargain-priced booklet contains a wealth of clinical information about stuttering modification with the school-age child, as well as helpful advice on working with parents and teachers.

Guitar, B., & Reville, J. (1997). *Easy talker: A fluency workbook for school-age children.* **Austin, TX: Pro-Ed Publishers.**

This is a workbook for elementary school children that tells the story of several children at a camp working on their stuttering. Along with the story, sequenced concepts and techniques are presented, with workbook activities for children to complete. This book integrates stuttering modification and fluency shaping.

Harrison, E., Bruce, M., Shenker, R., & Koushik, S. (2010). **The Lidcombe Program for school-age children who stutter.** In B. Guitar & R. McCauley (Eds.), *Treatment of Stuttering: Established and Emerging Interventions* (pp. 150–166). **Baltimore: Lippincott Williams & Wilkins.**

A detailed description (with video) of how the Lidcombe Program, originally designed for preschool children, can be adapted for school-age children.

Manning, W. (2009). *Clinical decision making in fluency disorders.* **New York: Delmar Publishers.**

The chapter called "Treatment of Young Children," contains excellent information on both fluency-shaping and stuttering modification approaches with children between 2 and 12 years old.

Ramig, P., & Dodge, D. (2005). *The child and adolescent stuttering treatment and activity resource Guide.* **Clifton Park, NY: Thomson Delmar Learning.**

Goals of treatment, ideas for IEPs, steps in treatment, activities to teach elements of therapy, tips for involving parents and teachers, and a multitude of handouts (in Spanish and English) are some of the valuable contents of this book. Cluttering evaluation and treatment are also covered.

Van Riper, C. (1973). **Treatment of the young confirmed stutterer.** In *The Treatment of Stuttering* (pp. 426–451). **Englewood Cliffs, NJ: Prentice-Hall.**

In this chapter, Van Riper provides a comprehensive discussion of a classic stuttering modification approach to the treatment of the intermediate stutterer.

Walton, P. (2012). *Fun with Fluency: For the school-age child.* **Austin, TX: Pro-Ed.**

This is a well-organized approach that combines stuttering modification and fluency shaping for the school-age child who stutters. This book provides a great deal of material that can be copied and used for each individual child.

Yaruss, J. S. (Ed.) (2003). **Facing the challenge of treating stuttering in the schools. Part 2: Selecting goals and strategies for success.** *Seminars in Speech and Language, 24,* February issue.

This journal issue is full of relevant and practical ideas for working with intermediate stuttering in a school setting.

Yaruss, J. S., Murphy, B., Quesal, R., Reardon-Reeves, N., & Flores, T. (2004). *Bullying and teasing: Helping children who stutter.* **New York: National Stuttering Association.**

The philosophy behind this book is to empower children who stutter to take charge of teasing situations themselves. However, it also provides excellent suggestions for parents, teachers, SLPs, and school administrators.

Yaruss, J. S., Pelczarski, K., & Quesal, R. (2010). **Comprehensive treatment for school-age children who stutter: Treating the entire disorder.** In *Treatment of Stuttering: Established and Emerging Interventions* (pp. 215–244). **Baltimore: Lippincott Williams & Wilkins.**

This chapter and accompanying video provide an excellent illustration of a broad-spectrum approach to treatment that targets affective, behavior, and cognitive aspects of stuttering.

Zebrowski, P., & Kelly, E. (2002). *Manual of stuttering intervention.* **Clifton Park, NY: Singular Publishing Group.**

Chapter 5 of this book ("Therapy for the Elementary School-Age Child") describes an approach similar to that described in this text with many fresh ideas. In addition, a section is devoted to group therapy with this age group.

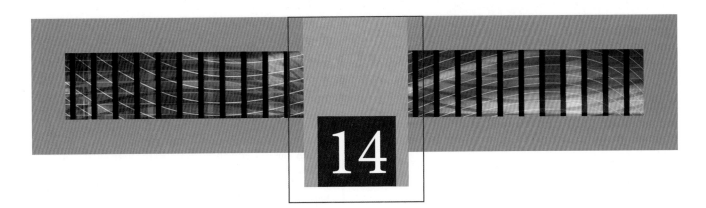

14

Treatment of Stuttering in Adolescents and Adults: Advanced Stuttering

CHAPTER OBJECTIVES

After studying this chapter, readers should be able to:

- Describe some of the behavioral, cognitive, and emotional characteristics of stuttering in adolescents and adults
- Explain what components of advanced stuttering may be learned, thus making them candidates for unlearning
- Describe three fluency goals that are appropriate for adolescents and adults who stutter
- Explain how classical conditioning principles can be used to help individuals unlearn old responses that account for many stuttering behaviors and attitudes
- Explain why fears and other emotions must be dealt with in treatment, along with changing how the individual speaks
- Explain what is accomplished in the first stage of treatment, "exploring stuttering"
- Describe how the clinician can help the client deal with feelings associated with stuttering
- Describe and demonstrate the five components of controlled fluency
- Delineate some of the important principles that must be followed to transfer a new behavior from the therapy room to outside situations
- Explain how voluntary stuttering may help a person who stutters

- Give several examples of how a person who stutters can be open about his stuttering
- Indicate some of the things the client must do to maintain fluency gains after treatment

KEY TERMS

Controlled fluency: A highly conscious style of speaking that induces fluency by modifying certain elements of speech

Spontaneous fluency: Speech without stuttering that doesn't require thinking about it

Acceptable stuttering: A mild form of stuttering that neither interferes with communication nor bothers the speaker or listener

Counterconditioning: A way of decreasing a response such as fear of stuttering by pairing the previously feared stimulus (stuttering) with a positive stimulus (praise)

Deconditioning: Similar to counterconditioning except that instead of a positive stimulus the previously feared stimulus (stuttering) is paired with a neutral stimulus (no negative consequence)

Exploring stuttering: Activities that help the client get in contact with the experience of stuttering without the negative emotions usually associated with stuttering. It is a type of approach behavior that can achieve deconditioning thereby decreasing fear

Holding onto stutters: With the clinician's encouragement and guidance, staying in the moment of stuttering by, for example, prolonging the posture and tension that characterize the stutter without trying to escape from the moment of stuttering

Reducing physical tension while holding onto stutters: The client may automatically reduce tension when she is able to stay in the stutter without feeling an urgent need to push out of it. However, it helps to have the client learn to consciously reduce tension in the moment of stuttering (before releasing it) to transfer that skill to conversational speech in daily situations

Proprioception: Attending to the movement of one's articulators, with the aim of using that sensory information to replace auditory input from one's own speech (which may be faulty)

Flexible rate: Slowing the beginning of a word, especially when stuttering is expected

Pausing: Inserting pauses while speaking at appropriate linguistic locations, with the aim of gaining control of one's speaking and processing speed

Easy onsets: Beginning phonation by gently bringing the vocal folds together instead of bringing them together quickly and with force

Light contacts: Touching the articulators together lightly while speaking so as to avoid "setting off" a stutter by pushing too strongly

Voluntary stuttering: Stuttering on purpose or at least producing speech in a way that mimics stuttering, with the aim of reducing fear of stuttering

Approach behavior: Consciously going toward something that was previously feared (or still is feared). Part of the reason that stuttering persists is that the individual avoids stuttering and saying feared words and entering feared situations, causing the fear to continue. By deliberately approaching feared words and situations again and again, fear diminishes and so does stuttering

Becoming your own clinician: Near the termination of therapy, the client becomes more and more able to give themselves assignments to maintain the fluency they achieved working with their clinician

AN INTEGRATED APPROACH

Individuals with advanced stuttering are usually older adolescents or adults who have been stuttering for many years. Their patterns, which are well entrenched, consist of blocks, repetitions, and prolongations that are usually accompanied by tension and struggle, as well as escape and avoidance behaviors. Typically, these individuals have developed negative anticipations about speaking situations and listener reactions. Sometimes, their stuttering has been such an important factor in their lives that they have chosen occupations beneath their abilities (Van Riper, for example, worked as a farmhand digging potatoes after he earned his Master's degree in English literature). Adults with advanced stuttering sometimes turn down promotions if more speaking is required than in their present positions and will often not participate fully in group discussions, team meetings, and conversations. On the other hand, some seek out therapy in an effort to become more fluent to meet the speaking demands of a higher position available to them. In rare instances, some adult stutterers hide their stuttering by avoiding words or situations so completely that don't show the usual signs of stuttering. They are sometimes referred to as "interiorized" stutterers.

Because the complex patterns of advanced stuttering involve behaviors, emotions, and cognitions, treatment is most effective if it targets all of these areas. These patterns are so deeply etched into the brain that treatment is best if it is intense, long-lasting, and provides long-term maintenance. My approach to treatment is a brew blended from many sources. I have tried to integrate these procedures so that clients reduce their negative emotions and avoidances and learn to respond differently with more fluent speech to old cues that have always triggered stuttering (Fig. 14.1).

Our integrated approach to stuttering in adolescents and adults is illustrated below, using an example of a highly motivated young adult. If any of the terminology used in this description is not clear, it will become clear upon reading about the treatment process later in the chapter.

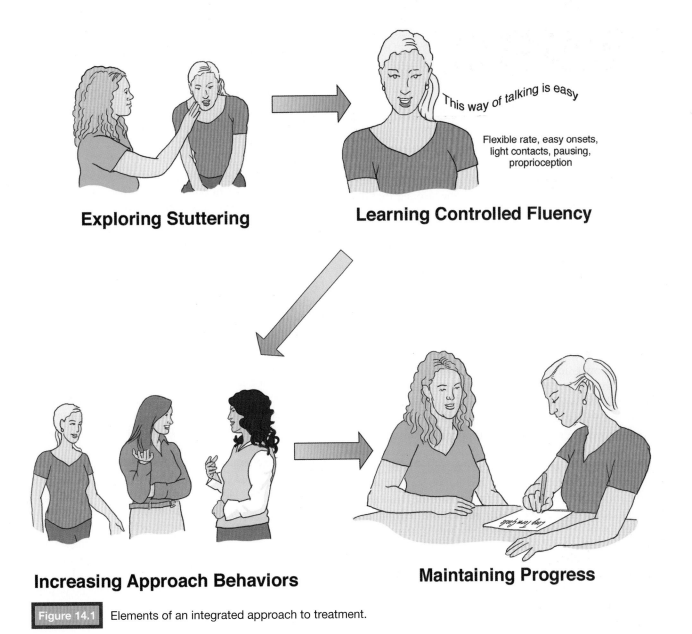

Exploring Stuttering

Learning Controlled Fluency

This way of talking is easy

Flexible rate, easy onsets,
light contacts, pausing,
proprioception

Increasing Approach Behaviors

Maintaining Progress

Figure 14.1 Elements of an integrated approach to treatment.

Author's Beliefs

The assertions that follow are not facts, but rather my inferences about advanced stuttering and its treatment. The reader should keep in mind that it is filtered through my own experiences as a person who has stuttered since age 3, who received therapy at age 21 from Charles Van Riper, and who has had both successes and failures over the 45 years I have worked as a stuttering therapist.

Nature of Stuttering

As I described in Chapter 7, I believe that the origins of advanced stuttering arise from a physiological predisposition for inefficient neural activation patterns for speech and a vulnerable temperament interacting with environmental

influences to produce and exacerbate core behaviors of repetitions, prolongations, and blocks. In the early stages, a child responds to these early core behaviors or disfluencies with tension and hurry. As the child continues to experience and react to core behaviors, she copes by using a variety of escape behaviors, which are reinforced through operant conditioning. During this same period, negative feelings, such as frustration, shame, and fear, become associated with stuttering. These feelings generalize through classical conditioning to more and more words and situations. Finally, the young stutterer begins to avoid feared words and situations, which is perpetuated through intermittent reinforcement. If these underlying processes continue until an individual reaches adolescence or young adulthood, the client will become an advanced stutterer.

Case Example

Malisa

In September of 2011, a young woman who teaches elementary school in Vermont came to us for treatment of her stuttering. She reported having difficulty talking to the parents of her students, introducing herself to new people, and making telephone calls. She also felt that her stuttering was keeping her from reading her poetry aloud at public gatherings. Malisa had a family history of stuttering and in fact had no memory of speaking without stuttering, even as a child. Our initial evaluation measures showed that her frequency of stuttering in conversation was 7.4 percent syllables stuttered, and her rating on the SSI-4 was severe. The Overall Assessment of Speakers Experience of Stuttering (OASES, a measure of how much impact stuttering has on the individual's daily life) was moderate.

Two of my graduate students and I worked with Malisa during the fall and spring academic semesters last year. We began by helping her explore her stuttering and her feelings about it, through having her feel what she was doing when she stuttered, watching herself stuttering in the mirror, and discussing stuttering experiences and accompanying feelings, both in the past and present. After several weeks, we progressed to having Malisa stay in the moment of stuttering—learning to tolerate the frustration of being stuck—then gradually reduce the tension and slowly finish the word on which she was stuttering. She practiced these "pullouts" while watching herself in the mirror with us in the clinic, on video playback, and also in the nearby student center. When our work involved speaking to strangers in public, we would do the task first, using voluntary stuttering, as we stopped people on the sidewalk or in a building and asked questions using pullouts. Then Malisa would gamely choose someone, approach them, and try to employ a pullout on her real stutters. There were plenty of failures as well as successes, but Malisa was quick to learn from our suggestions and worked diligently, both in her sessions with us and her assignments to practice at home.

The first five or six sessions focused not only on stuttering behaviors, but also on feelings associated with stuttering. Malisa's fear of stuttering diminished as she learned more about her stuttering, explored past experiences and feelings, and repeatedly sought out opportunities to practice. Once Malisa was making changes in her overlearned stuttering patterns as well as in her feelings and attitudes, we introduced some elements of "controlled fluency"—easy onsets, proprioception, flexible rate, and pausing. After practice on using these in her fluent speech, we helped Malisa employ them to deal with anticipated stutters. Again, Malisa was a quick learner and was successful turning some of her stutters into easier, briefer stutters so that they felt comfortably in control. Malisa also worked on voluntary stuttering and letting listeners know that she stuttered.

By the end of the spring semester, she was doing well, but still had some challenges when the stress was high or when she was caught by surprise. By May, 2012, after a total of 21 sessions, Malisa's percent syllables stuttered in conversation had decreased (from 7.4) to 1.4. Her SSI-4 score had decreased from severe to very mild, and her OASES score was "mild/moderate" (having been moderate). The percent syllables stuttered and SSI-4 scores may well have been influenced by the fact that we were now a familiar audience. In an eloquent letter of thanks to the clinic, Malisa wrote, "The last two semesters of work with you and (the two graduate students) have been pivotal in changing my outlook and stuttering behavior. … To be confident in 'voice' is a life skill with far-reaching effects." She added that she had just published a poem in a literary journal and was able to read it in public, not with complete fluency, but in a way that made her proud.

Malisa will continue treatment as this book is published. In consultation with her and keeping in mind her personal goals, it is likely that she will want to keep working on being able to say what she wants to say when she wants to say it.

Because increased tension, speeding up of speech rate, secondary behaviors, and feelings and attitudes are largely learned, they can be modified. Operant and classical conditioning principles are used to make these changes. However, because predisposing physiological factors contribute to these behaviors and because many years of learning have reorganized the brain in advanced stutterers, *complete* unlearning may not be possible. Thus, it is crucial to help advanced stutterers learn how to cope with residual disruptions in speech if they are going to maintain improvements in fluency.

Speech Behaviors Targeted for Therapy

In this section, I include both *new* behaviors, which should be learned, and *old* behaviors, which must be reduced or eliminated. In most advanced stutterers, well-learned tension and speeding-up responses are cued by anticipated and actual stuttering, which is typically accompanied by a considerable overlay of other learned secondary behaviors. To cope with these learned behaviors and to speak more fluently, advanced stutterers must decrease their fear of stuttering and eliminate their escape and avoidance behaviors. Then they must learn to respond to anticipated stuttering by speaking slowly and mindfully (but fluently) for several syllables. In the chapter on treatment of intermediate stuttering, I referred to this style of speaking as "superfluency." In this chapter, I call it "**controlled fluency.**" It often works best, however, if clients decide for themselves how to refer to what they do when they use a controlled, mindful form of fluency to replace stuttering. A single word that they can repeat in their heads as a reminder and label for successful implementation may work best.

Another target of therapy is actual rather than anticipated moments of stuttering. Individuals with advanced stuttering have learned, through many years of stuttering, to respond to moments of stuttering by tensing muscles, especially in the mouth and larynx areas. Thus, some residual stuttering will occur unexpectedly, but it can be diminished if an individual develops a reliable coping response. This response is to loosen muscle tension and slow down speaking rate during stutters so that fluent speech and the feeling of control can be regained soon after. An example that comes to mind is from my own experience as a stutterer. After several years of greatly improved fluency, I tried to shout to a friend who was walking down a hallway, headed away from me, which is usually a tough situation for someone who stutters. When I tried to yell "Paul," I found myself jammed in an old, habitual, tense block without any sound coming out. Once I realized what I was doing, I actually laughed at the return of my old habit, then relaxed my tense posture almost automatically and got speech going again, slowly but fluently.

Fluency Goals

The ultimate goal that most advanced stutterers have in mind when they start therapy is spontaneous "fluency" in all situations, or in other words, normal speech. In my experience, most advanced stutterers do not reach this level of fluency. After treatment, clients may have periods of **spontaneous fluency,** lasting from a few hours to a month or more, but usually some stuttering returns, especially in stressful situations. At these times, I would like clients to have three options available.

First, when they feel it is important to be fluent, I want them to be able to apply fluency skills successfully to achieve controlled fluency, which I will describe in detail later. Second, when they feel it is important to be fluent but are unable to achieve controlled fluency, I want them to be able to apply and feel comfortable using skills to produce easy, mild forms of stuttering. Third, when they feel it is not as important to sound fluent and do not want to put the effort

into doing so, I would like them to be comfortable having mild, **acceptable stuttering** so that they stay relaxed when they stutter, continue to talk, and communicate well. These fluency goals seem realistic to me. However, in the final analysis, it will be the clients who choose which of these options they will use.

Feelings and Attitudes

I believe that adolescents and adults with advanced stuttering often have negative feelings and attitudes toward their stuttering and themselves. These emotions and cognitions need to receive considerable attention in therapy. These individuals also need to eliminate or drastically reduce avoidances. Although this is technically part of behavior change, avoidance reduction is intimately tied to fear reduction. Individuals will never reduce their fear of words and speaking situations that they continue to avoid. Reducing this fear is critical if clients are going to be successful in using either controlled fluency or mild, acceptable stuttering. Otherwise, their fears will create excessive muscular tension and speeding up, and they may be unable to alter their speech production toward fluency under conditions of high fear. I also believe that avoidances and speech fears need to be substantially reduced to enable clients to maintain their improvement over the long run. If negative feelings and attitudes are not significantly diminished, they will become the seeds for relapse, which is prevalent among advanced stutterers.

It is important for clinicians to understand classical conditioning principles when attempting to eliminate clients' avoidance behaviors or to reduce their negative feelings and attitudes. Increased muscle tension, for example, may become classically conditioned when stuttering produces strong negative emotion, which in turn triggers an automatic "tension response" (see Chapter 6). Sounds, words, or situations that are associated with this experience eventually become the triggers for increased muscle tension. One strategy for changing classically conditioned responses is **counterconditioning,** which takes place when words and situations that elicit fear (the conditioned stimuli) are experienced over and over again in the presence of positive feelings. For example, when stutterers confront and explore their stuttering in the presence of an accepting and understanding clinician, counterconditioning occurs. The clinician's positive regard and reinforcement of such exploration decrease the client's fears and negative feelings. Another approach, **deconditioning,** occurs when words and situations that elicit relatively low levels of fear are experienced over and over, in the absence of the feared consequences, until clients' fears are dissipated or extinguished. This is why hierarchies of least-to-most fearful stimuli are helpful for reducing negative emotions. By beginning with clients' least fearful words or situations and gradually working our way up the hierarchy, their fears become systematically reduced. This requires repeated experiences confronting fearful words and situations at each rung of the hierarchy ladder. Examples of these strategies are discussed in the section on clinical procedures.

Maintenance Procedures

Effective maintenance depends on clients becoming their own clinicians, which should begin early in therapy. Clients learn to evaluate their own performance in mastering stuttering modification and fluency-shaping techniques and to monitor their speech fears and avoidances. I gradually shift more and more of the responsibility for therapy to clients as they improve, and it is important for them to have a realistic understanding of what they should expect in terms of their long-term fluency. Thus, clients need to understand the concepts of spontaneous fluency, controlled fluency, and acceptable stuttering in setting their own fluency goals. It is also important that they appreciate the relationship between conscientious practice of what they have learned in therapy and the attainment of their fluency goals.

Clinical Methods

Like the approach described for intermediate stuttering with school-age children, my management for advanced stuttering in adolescents and adults begins with stuttering modification activities (specifically exploring the behaviors, cognitions, and emotions) to decrease negative emotion associated with stuttering. Subsequently, I teach fluency skills similar to the superfluency used with the school-age client. Then I help the individual transfer and stabilize those skills with stuttering modification activities such as using a hierarchy of more and more challenging situations, voluntary stuttering, and seeking out feared words and feared situations. The measures I use to assess progress are described shortly.

Clinical Procedures

Procedures described here for working with advanced stuttering in adolescents and adults borrow liberally from many clinicians. Three individuals who have had a particularly strong influence on my approach are Gavin Andrews (Andrews & Ingham, 1971), Richard Boehmler (1994), and Charles Van Riper (1973). I am also indebted to numerous colleagues in the field, as well as to my students and clients who have generously shared their ideas.

Key Concepts

1. *Treatment of adolescents and adults usually takes a long time, demands considerable motivation, and must maintain a focus on many fronts.* As you may remember from Chapters 11 and 12, treatment of preschool children can be as brief as a few months. But the older individual has been stuttering for many years, and much maladaptive learning has taken place. Therefore, as you will see, my approach has many stages, each subsequent stage building on the former and requiring continuing hard work on

changing behaviors and emotions. There are exceptions; some clients are so ready to change and so emotionally robust that treatment feels like sailing with the wind at your back.

2. *Treatment should be tailored to each client's needs.* Although it would be easier if one sequence of treatment fits all clients, stuttering therapy is not so simple. Each person's biological makeup and life experiences differ; therefore, individuals require different therapy ingredients in the overall recipe for their success. Of the procedures presented in this section, *controlled fluency* is the heart, because all clients will benefit from this. But in order for it to work, the client must not be hampered by fear of stuttering and fear of listener reaction. To deal with these fears, most clients will need to follow the procedures at the beginning of treatment that are concerned with confronting, accepting, and exploring stuttering. However, mild stutterers who are not uncomfortable with their stuttering and who talk freely and easily with all types of listeners may not need parts of exploring stuttering. Moreover, they may not need to work on using voluntary stuttering or feared words and entering feared situations, which is described in the section on increasing approach behaviors. The last section, which deals with maintenance, is probably crucial for every client; it is the foundation for long-term success.

   A clinician just learning how to carry out stuttering therapy may want to go through each step of treatment just as I have described them. An experienced clinician may want to reorder the steps to suit the client or may omit steps she believes the client doesn't need or add new steps of her own.

3. *Successful outcome of treatment requires focused attention to speaking, especially when stuttering is anticipated.* Brain imaging studies of the effects of treatment (e.g., Boberg, Yeudall, Schopflocher, & Bo-Lassen, 1983; Kroll, De Nil, Kapur, & Houle, 1997; Neumann et al., 2003; Neumann, Priesbuch, Euler, Wolff von Gudenberg, & Lanfermann et al., 2005) suggest that successfully treated stutterers have increased left-hemisphere activation after treatment compared to before treatment. These researchers interpreted their results as reflecting greater self-monitoring and attention to sequencing and timing of speech (e.g., De Nil, Kroll, Lafaille, & Houle, 2003; Neumann et al., 2003). It is probable, given the nature of the treatments used in these studies (fluency-shaping), that the increased left-hemisphere activity was the product of stutterers using skills taught in the treatment, like those of controlled fluency. These skills include slowed speech rate, pausing, easy onset of phonation, light articulatory contact, and proprioception. They are used when stuttering is anticipated but are practiced in fluent speech.

4. *Successful outcome of treatment depends, in part, on increasing approach behaviors and reducing avoidance.*

Evidence from treatment outcome research suggests that successful long-term outcome is associated with positive communication attitudes and low levels of avoidance (e.g., Guitar, 1976; Guitar & Bass, 1978). Work on attitudes, negative emotions, and avoidances takes two forms in an integrated approach to therapy. First, use of controlled fluency, described earlier, will positively affect attitudes and emotions through repeated experiences of fluency in situations where stuttering previously prevailed. Second, direct work on decreasing fear and avoidance can be effective in reducing stuttering (Van Riper, 1958). Neurophysiologically, the emphasis on approach activities may "kindle" emotional regulation by the left hemisphere, which, in turn, may "dampen" the avoidance and fear responses regulated by the right hemisphere (Davidson, 1984; Kinsbourne, 1989; Kinsbourne & Bemporad, 1984). Thus, work on controlled fluency and attention to approach behaviors both may be associated with increased left-hemisphere activity.

5. *Adults who stutter may continue to have speech-processing deficits after treatment and may need to continue to compensate for them.* Brain imaging research suggests that even after successful treatment, adults who stutter are likely to continue to show abnormally low activity in left-brain regions that are active for speech processing in nonstutterers (Neumann et al., 2003). Thus, the treatment program described in the following pages includes provisions for dealing with residual stuttering through long-term work on controlled fluency as well as work on new responses to residual stuttering in a way that is comfortable for both the speaker and listener and thus doesn't interfere with communication.

6. *Measurement of progress and outcome are important.* I use two principal measures of behavioral change in treatment. As I noted in Chapter 8, "Preliminaries to Assessment," percentage of syllables stuttered (%SS) provides a useful measure of the frequency of stuttering for snapshots of progress during treatment. Frequency of stuttering is particularly handy for assessing audio-recorded samples of speech made outside of the therapy setting. At crucial times in treatment, such as after the "Understanding and Exploring Stuttering" stage of treatment, after "Learning and Generalization of Controlled Fluency," and at the termination of formal treatment and later, I use the SSI-4 to assess overall severity of stuttering.

To assess a client's progress and outcome in terms of her feelings and attitudes about communication, I use the Modified Erickson Scale of Communication Attitudes (S-24), which was also described in Chapter 8. This measure has been adapted for repeated use and has been shown to be predictive of treatment outcomes (Andrews & Cutler, 1974; Andrews & Craig, 1988; Guitar & Bass, 1978). I use this measure before beginning the "Maintaining Improvement" stage of treatment so that

I can assess the extent to which a client has generalized positive feelings and attitudes about communication situations. If a client shows more negative attitudes than the average normal speaker, it is a cue to continue working on approach behaviors and ensure that she has mastered the use of controlled fluency in all situations. Evidence for the validity and reliability of these measures can be found in Chapter 8.

Beginning Therapy

There are several issues I deal with in the first therapy sessions. The first is to understand what treatment goals the client has. Frequently, we have discussed this in a preliminary way during the evaluation, but once treatment actually gets underway, it is important to revisit this topic and to clarify for both the client and clinician what they are working toward. During this discussion, I bring up the options of spontaneous fluency, controlled fluency, and acceptable stuttering. The client and I will discuss various situations in her life that are likely to be affected by stuttering, and we explore what level of fluency is important in each of them. We look for situations in which the client is satisfied with her fluency and discuss what her speech is like at such times. We try to find levels of stuttering or fluency that would be good targets to shoot for.

A second issue the client and I deal with early on is to make a map of a possible course of treatment. Mindful of what the client's goals are, I provide brief descriptions of the stages of treatment we can go through, matching treatment to the client's present situation and her desires for improvement. The general plan I would describe is first for the client to get to know what she does when she stutters, including her behaviors, thoughts, and feelings about her stuttering, and her listeners' possible reactions. After that, she would learn to increase overall fluency and deal with anticipated stuttering by employing various controlled fluency skills to reduce tension, slow her speech rate, and monitor her speech. Gradually, working more independently, she would seek out formerly feared words and situations and replace her old avoidance behaviors with a more assertive attitude, more fluency, and a more confident, more relaxed approach to those stutters that remain. Finally, in the later stages of treatment, I would help her work out a plan to use her new fluency in more and more situations and to gradually become her own clinician so that she can diagnose and repair her speech if stuttering creeps back in.

Exploring Stuttering

The aim of this first phase of treatment is to help the client become more objective about her stuttering and to lift the clouds of dread and mystery that surround stuttering. Objectivity is fostered through step-by-step procedures of the client learning about her pattern of stuttering behaviors, as well as through the overall feeling of acceptance she gains from the clinician's support and encouragement. As this

Table 14.1	Steps in Exploring Stuttering—The First Stage of Therapy	
Step	Activities	Goals
Understanding stuttering	Provide handout and discuss the elements of the client's stuttering with her	To objectify what has been mysterious and scary; beginning of desensitization
Approaching and exploring stuttering in the treatment room	Client and clinician catch and hold stutters. Client learns to feel what she's doing physically when she stutters. Client learns to reduce tension during stutters	Continuing desensitization. Beginning of learning to modify stutters
Approaching and exploring stuttering outside of the treatment room	Client and clinician observe stuttering and client's reactions to it outside the clinic. As the stuttering is studied, client tries to catch and hold stutters outside of the treatment room. Continuing discussion of how client feels about her stuttering. Audio recording by client of her stuttering in various situations followed by discussions with clinicians	Continuing desensitization. Client learns that she can tolerate her stuttering with more and more listeners. Client learns to stay in stutter until she can reduce tension and finish the word with a feeling of control

process goes on, the client becomes more optimistic about changing her stuttering. She realizes that stuttering consists of behaviors that she can control and feels supported by the clinician's belief in her ability to change.

Steps in the exploration process are outlined in Table 14.1.

Understanding Stuttering

The goals of this step are for clients to understand the rationale for exploring their stuttering and to become partners in planning therapy. I begin by giving clients a handout on Understanding Your Stuttering (see tan box below). As we discuss it, I find out from a client about other domains that she's worked on previously and improved, like skiing, painting, golf, or photography. We discuss how emotions and attitudes can get in the way of new learning and may perpetuate old behaviors. I draw an analogy between the skills

that the client has worked on and the tasks before us, which is to learn to increase fluency and modify stuttering. We discuss the idea that if she can learn what she's doing when she stutters, then she may feel more objective and optimistic about her stuttering and be able to change what she's doing and become more fluent. I try to convey the idea, which will be repeated in many forms, that she has learned to speak in an inefficient way that is at least in part influenced by her desire not to stutter. However, despite years of stuttering, she can now learn to replace it with a controlled form of fluency. This process begins by her **exploring stuttering** and getting to know it and decreasing her understandable tendency to avoid or escape from it. I also discuss the fact that, as with learning other skills, she will need to practice new techniques until they are second nature to her and even after that.

UNDERSTANDING YOUR STUTTERING

We want to better understand your stuttering, and we want you to do the same. You may not really know what you do or how you feel when you stutter. Because it's unpleasant, you have probably attempted to hide it from yourself as well as from others. Let's begin to explore your stuttering by discussing the following components of the problem. Once you explore and better understand your stuttering, it will lose its mystery, and you will be less uncomfortable with it.

Core Behaviors

These are the repetitions, prolongations, and blocks (getting completely blocked on a word) that you have; they are

the core or heart of the problem. Core behaviors were the first stuttering behaviors you had as a child.

Why do you have these core behaviors? Research suggests that people who stutter may have "timing" problems related to their control of the speech mechanism. For fluent speech to occur, muscle movements involved in breathing, voice production (voice box), and articulation (tongue, lips, jaw) must all be well coordinated. Evidence suggests that people who stutter experience a lack of coordination among these muscle groups during speech. Furthermore, research implies that these physical timing problems are so slight that they often show up as stuttering when feelings and emotions are strong enough to cause a breakdown in the coordination of the

(Continued)

speech mechanism. In therapy, we will teach you techniques to assist you in coping more effectively with these core behaviors.

Secondary Behaviors

Secondary behaviors are tricks or crutches you use to avoid stuttering or to help you get a word out. They are behaviors you have learned over the years to help you cope with the core behaviors, and they can be unlearned. These behaviors occur more quickly and less consciously than the development of superstitious behaviors, but they are not unrelated (e.g., wearing a lucky shirt). There are different types of secondary behaviors. Which of the following do you use?

Avoidance Behaviors

The category of avoidance behaviors covers all the things you might do to keep from stuttering. Word and situation avoidances include substituting words, rephrasing sentences, not entering feared speaking situations, and pretending not to know answers. You might also use "postponements," such as pausing before a difficult word or repeating another word or phrase over and over before trying to say a word on which you expect to stutter. Another avoidance trick some stutterers use is called a "starter." This is when you might say a sound or word quickly just before a difficult word, as in saying "umwould you like to go to a movie?" Hand or body movements might be used in the same way.

Escape Behaviors

These behaviors are things a stutterer does to get out of a word once she is stuttering, such as a head nod, jaw jerk, or eye blink. You may have developed escape behaviors that are so subtle that you don't notice them anymore. Some of them might be called "disguise behaviors" because they are attempts to hide your stuttering as it is happening. These include covering your mouth with your hand or turning your head when you stutter.

Feelings and Attitudes

When you began to stutter as a child, you were probably unaware of your stuttering. Because you have been stuttering for many years, however, you may have experienced many frustrating and embarrassing speaking situations. Consequently, if you're like most stutterers, you have probably acquired some negative feelings and attitudes about your speech. You may feel embarrassed, guilty, fearful, or even angry. Fear is the most common feeling. Stutterers typically fear certain speaking situations and certain sounds or words. What feelings and attitudes do you have regarding your stuttering? As part of your therapy, we will help you reduce these unpleasant feelings and attitudes.

With my help, you will explore and describe the various components of your stuttering problem. Before you can change something, you need to understand what you are changing. And if you can break it down into manageable chunks, you can change it more easily.

Approaching and Exploring Stuttering in the Treatment Room

The goal is for the client to make the first steps toward approaching her stuttering, rather than backing away from it. As we begin studying her stuttering, I often use an illustration or model of the speech mechanism to show the client the structures associated with speaking and how they work in fluency and in stuttering. The client needs to learn about the core, escape, and avoidance components of her stuttering and to some degree, why they occur. The client should also feel that the clinician is genuinely interested in her and in her speech. Because approach behaviors are thought to be regulated by the left hemisphere, they may dampen negative emotions that are right hemisphere-based (Davidson, 1984; Kinsbourne, 1989; Kinsbourne & Bemporad, 1984). Hence these approach activities are meant, in part, to decrease the client's fear of stuttering.

The activities associated with this step involve examining moments of stuttering as they occur in the treatment room. I explain to a client that to begin our work on her stuttering we will work together to understand it and

explore what she is doing when she stutters. One of the aims of our work is to reduce the client's fear of stuttering. For years, she has been feeling "trapped" in the stuckness of stutters, helpless and struggling, with little or no reliable way to escape. If she is like most people who stutter, the very act of struggling to escape from stutters increases her muscle tension and consequently the feeling of being stuck. But being able to stop struggling and tolerate her experience of being trapped reduces her tension and perhaps provides more positive sensory feedback to the brain, allowing her to move forward in speech. I usually try to have the client feel tension at first and then gradually lower the tension while holding the posture and then finishing the word.[1] Progress on this step can be assessed by the client's movement up the hierarchy for this activity. The hierarchy goes from her controlling my pseudo-stuttering

---

[1]Staying in a stutter but gradually reducing the tension before finishing the word is essentially what Van Riper called a "pullout." At first, emphasis is on staying in the stutter; then once that is mastered, the client can learn to deliberately reduce tension and finish the word.

with her hand signal, all the way to her **holding onto a stutter** for several seconds in a conversation with a friend or stranger while maintaining good eye contact and staying relaxed.

I use the handout in the tan box below on "Holding onto the Stutter" to provide the client the rationale for the activities associated with this step. Or I may just verbally convey the same information.

HOLDING ONTO THE STUTTER

The experience of being caught in a moment of stuttering (repetition, prolongation, or block) can be frustrating and scary. When your mouth doesn't do what you want it to, you feel out of control. If it goes on for several seconds or your listener is upset or impatient, you may feel devastated. As unpleasant as these core behaviors are, you need to increase your tolerance for them to learn that you can experience them without panicking. Instead of avoiding them or hurrying to get out of them, you need to learn to experience them and remain calm so you can change them.

So, how do you learn to remain calm while you're jammed (blocked) in a moment of stuttering? We'll use a technique called "holding onto the stutter" or "staying in the stutter." When you are stuttering and I signal you, you are to hold onto that moment of stuttering until I signal you to come out of it. If you are repeating a syllable, you are to continue repeating it; if you are prolonging a sound, you are to continue prolonging it; and if you are having a block, you are to maintain that phonatory arrest or articulatory posture. By experiencing these core behaviors of repetition, prolongation, and block over and over again while remaining relatively calm or becoming calmer as the freezing continues, you will find your tolerance for them increasing. You will no longer become fearful at the thought of getting stuck on a word, and you will find the core behaviors becoming more relaxed; that is the key to change.

We will begin by reversing roles—in other words, you will signal me to hold onto a pseudo-stutter for several seconds when I voluntarily stutter. Then I will have you hold onto one of your real stutters for only a brief period of time, possibly one or two seconds. That is, when you get caught in a stutter, I will signal you to hold onto that stutter and keep it going until I signal you to complete the word slowly. While holding onto a repetition, prolongation, or block, you are to try to stay as calm as possible. Just experience the stutter and be as calm and relaxed as you possibly can. As your tolerance increases, I will gradually increase the length of time you are to hold onto your stutters. Eventually, you will hold onto your stutters until the tension and struggle have dissipated and you can end them easily and slowly. This will involve you signaling yourself and me when you begin a stutter and when you will come out of the stutter. I will also have you watch yourself in a mirror as you are holding onto your stutters. Again, just experience your stuttering and try to remain as calm as possible. Remember that after you feel the tension ebb away, finish the word slowly and deliberately.

By experiencing these moments of stuttering over and over again in this manner, you will gradually lose much of your fear of them. You will find yourself feeling more comfortable when you are talking, and you will be talking more fluently.

When I think the client understands the task, I talk about something of interest, such as our self-help group or the overall course of stuttering therapy. I put in some really obvious voluntary stutters that would be easy for me to hold onto, such as voiced continuant consonants like /l/ or /r/. If she doesn't immediately signal me to hold onto the stutter, I explain again how she should do that. Then I get back into stuttering, and when she signals, I prolong the sound and continue to maintain the tension I have while staying calm and relaxed. I emphatically praise her catching my stutters because even someone else's voluntary stutters may be hard for a sensitive client to bear. As we go along and discuss my stutters and what I'm doing physically when I stutter, I use a large array of different sounds and I try to stutter in the manner that she does. Then we reverse roles.

After I get the client's OK to interrupt her, I ask her to talk about her hobbies, her work, or her school—anything

easy for her to talk about. As she talks, I watch for one of her more severe stutters and then signal her to hold onto it. This may take some coaching and practice because people who are not trained in our field may not understand how to hold onto the exact sound that is being stuttered. Particularly hard are plosives, and the client may need extra coaching to stay right in a /b/ or /p/ that is stuttered (by producing it as the fricative counterpart to those stops), without going on to the next vowel sound.

I show genuine interest in her stuttering and make observations about it such as, "I noticed on that one it looked like you squeezed your lips together trying to get the word out." I also ask questions like, "Is that how you usually stutter on words that start with 'B?'" As we explore stuttering together, I use my interest and acceptance to begin the process of *desensitization*. During this activity, I teach clients about different components of stuttering, including core, escape, and

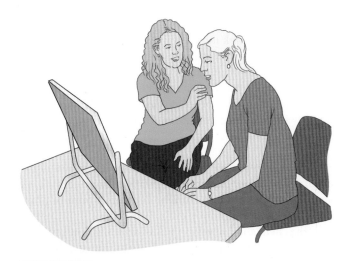

Figure 14.2 Exploring stuttering with the help of a mirror.

avoidance behaviors, particularly as they apply to the client's stuttering. This activity continues at a pace suited to a client's comfort talking about her stuttering. When the client is relatively comfortable examining her stuttering, I may use a mirror to help her explore and confront her stuttering, as depicted in Figure 14.2.

Note that while we work on approaching stuttering and exploring it, I find ways to express a matter-of-fact acceptance of the client's stuttering. For example, I try to use vocal intonation to express approval and curiosity—just about the fact that she can look at and talk about her stuttering. I am especially pleased when she can follow my instructions to "stay in the stutter"—meaning keep the moment of stuttering going deliberately even though she would like to finish the word.[2] When the client stays in the stutters, she learns that when she can tolerate the "stuckness," she can **reduce her physical tension while holding onto the stutter**. This is a key experience. It is the discovery that she herself has the power to control what happens when she stutters.

As indicated earlier, an important sequel of learning to catch and hold onto stutters is to reduce physical tension to the point (and beyond) where the stutter can be released and the word finished. As I mentioned in the last chapter, some clients call this "catch and release." Note that the release must be done only after the tension is reduced to normal speech levels. This process involves powerful learning (operant conditioning). The relief felt by the client when she can release

and finish the word reinforces the reduction of tension to normal levels. Thus it will usually happen automatically if the client works on it. Soon, for many clients, the reduction of tension occurs *before* they start saying the word. Van Riper's term for this, when it is done deliberately, is "preparatory set."

Approaching and Exploring Stuttering Outside the Treatment Room

After the client has many experiences in the therapy room "catching" her stutters, holding onto them, feeling what she's doing physically, and describing what she feels she's doing, we make plans to transfer this learning to real-world situations. At first, we just work on observing the stuttering—like scientists observing and taking notes on a new species of frog. We don't worry about her trying to be more fluent outside the treatment room yet, but it would not be surprising if she feels more in control of speech because she reduces the tension before finishing the word as a by-product of not having to panic while in a stutter. The client and I build a hierarchy of situations in which the client can just observe her stuttering objectively rather than running from it or trying to hide it. We also begin to observe listener reactions as well. In the beginning, the clinician provides as much support as possible. For example, I often begin by making a phone call to a store to ask what their hours are. I put in a handful of voluntary stutters, similar to the client's. We discuss my pseudo-stutters as well as the listener reactions. This works really well if I can do it on a speakerphone so the client can hear how the listener responds. When she's ready, the client makes a phone call, and we discuss her stutters and the listeners' reactions. Many listeners, of course, are patient and even encouraging. A few, who may be confused or anxious, may answer abruptly or even hang up. These sorts of activities desensitize the client to her own stuttering and to listener reactions. We discuss the listener reactions, and I encourage her to vent feelings if a listener responds rudely.

The expressing of feelings is a vital part of therapy. As I work with an adolescent or an adult, I try to attend to the client's emotions so that therapy can keep moving forward. (Perhaps I should better say "lurching forward in fits and starts." *Therapy is rarely simple and predictable, and experienced clinicians know they must tolerate a messy process.*) I discussed dealing with emotions in Chapter 10, and some points are worth repeating. Wherever change is going on, emotions bubble up; stuttering therapy is no exception. The clinician should expect emotions and even try to elicit them so that he can listen and accept, just as he accepts the person who stutters and her stuttering. Feelings of frustration, anger toward the self and toward the clinician, and hostility toward listeners are all common. When the client talks about her feelings, sometimes stuttering worsens, but the clinician should just accept whatever stuttering accompanies the expression of feelings, rather than "doing therapy" on the stuttering. Not every clinician is a natural in dealing with feelings. It may

---

[2]When I ask a client to "stay in the stutter" I am borrowing a technique from the late Dean Williams, who was a master stuttering clinician at the University of Iowa. Dean was able to work temporary miracles by having a client stay in a moment of stuttering, feel what they were doing, and reduce the tension. When a client did this, she often became suddenly very fluent.

take consistent reviewing of recordings of therapy sessions for most clinicians to recognize when a client is expressing feelings and to become alert enough to encourage the client to discuss them further. Sometimes emotions come in the disguise of resistance—refusing to work on stuttering outside the therapy room, doing assignments half-heartedly, and other signs of holding back. Resistance is often a sign that, as Van Riper has pointed out, "the basic disorder is being affected" (Van Riper, 1958). This term is borrowed from psychoanalysis and indicates a client is resisting the effects of therapy because change is threatening. At least in stuttering therapy, if not in all therapy, resistance can be seen as a hopeful sign, but the clinician must discuss resistance with the client, and elicit the feelings beneath. As we'll see, as treatment moves outside the therapy room, resistance becomes more likely.

When we go into situations outside the clinic together, I use a small audio recorder to record our work for further discussion. I usually do the assignment first, modeling the sort of conversational interaction that we'll use in our sample. If we are walking outside on a sidewalk, I'll ask someone passing by what time it is or where a certain building or store is. I put in a few voluntary stutters and maintain a calm demeanor with good eye contact. Then the client and I discuss the stutters and the listener reactions. At this point if the client is game, we plan a speaking opportunity for her. If she's not, then I ask her to pick a situation for me to do more stuttering in, and I carry out more voluntary stuttering while she listens and watches. Even if she's only observing, the client usually gains a lot by seeing my calm demeanor even while having severe (voluntary) stutters and by noticing that most listeners are very patient. If the client continues to resist approaching strangers and difficult situations, her feelings about this should be explored back in the therapy room. When the client is ready—either in this session or a later one—she goes into a planned situation and uses her typical speech, fluent or not. Most often there will be some natural stutters that we can discuss immediately on the sidewalk or in a store. We also record her stutters and listen to them again, back in the clinic. As we listen to the recording, we discuss not only what the client was doing but also how she was feeling. If this goes well, I then ask the client to take the recorder home and record some samples of her stuttering at home or at work and write down her observations about her stuttering when she later listens to it and finally shares it with me.

In the next session, when she brings a recording back I respond enthusiastically. Remember that one goal of treatment is to activate "approach" behaviors and lessen avoidance behaviors; recording stutters at home or at the office is indeed an approach behavior. If a client has been unable to carry out this task, she and I do the task together and record her stuttering in a situation outside the room or on the telephone.

During the sessions in which the client and I analyze her typical stuttering, I also look for stutters that are mild, brief,

and forward-moving and call the client's attention to them. I ask the client to look for them in her samples collected outside and in her stuttering in the therapy room. As we attend to these, I let the client know that these are models of how she can learn to handle her stutters. In fact, she can make them more like fluent speech, so that neither she nor her listeners will hear them as stutters. They will, in fact, become similar to the way persons who don't stutter would handle disruptions in their speech (Boehmler, personal communication, 2004). Another thing to watch for and praise is the client finishing her stutters with greatly reduced tension. In some clients, it happens naturally; in others it must be practiced and reinforced.

The client and I develop transfer activities that continue to strengthen her approach attitudes and behaviors but that are not beyond her present capacity. She continues to record her stuttering in situations outside the clinic and take notes on listener reactions. It is important to ensure that the client is engaged in therapy activities on days when she is not attending treatment, and it helps if she and I keep in telephone or e-mail contact between treatment sessions.

Teaching the Client to Evaluate and Reinforce Her Behavior

An important component of treatment is helping the client learn to observe, evaluate, and reward (when appropriate) her own behavior. This is vital for generalizing the changes the client is making to her everyday environment, and it should start early in treatment. A chapter by Finn (2007) provides an introduction to this process. Finn describes the process as comprised of several steps:

1. Training the client to observe her behavior. In this stage of treatment, it is recording the stuttering and making notes on listener reactions. The clinician can work with the client in outside situations (with debriefing in the treatment room) to teach her how to carry out this assignment. They can decide together how many times the client should do this between sessions.

2. Training the client to self-evaluate her work. The client and clinician can together evaluate the frequency and quality of the client's recordings and observations of listener reactions.

3. Training the client to reinforce herself when she achieves a targeted goal. For example, she may want to reward herself each time she records her stuttering and take notes on listener responses. The client knows best what would truly be reinforcing, so deciding what to use for reinforcement should be a discussion led by the client. Finn suggests, as many have, that effective rewards are often things that the client is likely to do. Examples are drinking a favorite beverage, eating a favorite food, and reading a magazine or book. The client might want to give herself an instant reward such as a point or token that is counted toward

a total that must be achieved before a tangible reward is collected.

Positive reinforcers can be coupled with mild punishments to be most effective. The chapter by Finn (2007) and the references he provides are a rich source of ideas about how to incorporate self-management into treatment. Self-management can be used in each stage of treatment, and this will prepare the client to become her own clinician when treatment is finished.

Learning and Generalizing Controlled Fluency

Learning Controlled Fluency

The next goal is to have clients learn a controlled type of fluency to replace their stuttering. Some clinicians prefer to delay working on this goal until negative emotions have been reduced further through voluntary stuttering. I find that teaching fluency skills at this point increases motivation and makes the confrontation of stuttering more tolerable for most clients. Progress toward confronting stuttering and reducing negative emotion has been started in the previous work on understanding and exploring stuttering. Further work on reducing negative emotions will be done after controlled fluency is learned. In fact, however, negative emotions are usually diminished as work on increased fluency is successful.

As a client works on controlled fluency, progress is assessed in the clinic by the clinician's judgment of whether the client can successfully produce speech with each of the components described in the following sections and whether she can use the components together in conversational speech that sounds natural.

The fluency skills learned in this step are the same as those used with intermediate-level stuttering, but for the sake of review, I have outlined them in Table 14.2.

Once a client seems to have acquired the necessary **proprioception** skill, it can be combined with **flexible rate, pausing, easy onsets**, and **light contacts** into an overall style of speaking sometimes called "prolonged speech" or "smooth speech." I refer to this combination as "controlled fluency," which means the same as the term "superfluency," which I used in the chapter on treatment of intermediate stuttering. The clinician should feel free to use whichever term seems appropriate for the client. When the client is first using this style of speaking, it requires concentration, which may activate left-hemisphere speech centers (De Nil et al., 2003).

Transferring Controlled Fluency into Fluent Speech

The goal of this step is for clients to learn to use controlled fluency in their normally fluent speech to "put money in the bank," as Van Riper used to say. Thus, if a client can use the careful, deliberate style of speech that I call controlled fluency in her normally fluent utterances, she will benefit greatly from the practice. This will improve the chances that when she anticipates stuttering, she can call upon controlled

Table 14.2	Fluency Skills
Skills that the client can use all together to produce more fluent speech. The client can also use only some of them depending on what suits her.	
Fluency Skill	**Description**
Flexible rate	Flexible rate is simply slowing down productions of a syllable, most commonly the first and second phonemes of a word (Boehmler, personal communication, 2003). Slowing is thought to be effective in reducing stuttering by allowing more time for language planning and motor execution to occur.
Pausing	Inserting brief pauses at grammatical junctures or before an important word or phrase. Pauses may reduce physical tension and allow more time for linguistic processing. Good examples can be heard in the audio recording of Winston Churchill's "Their Finest Hour" speech (http://www.youtube.com/watch?v=G4BVzYGeF0M).
Easy onsets	Easy or gentle onset of voicing. This seems to prevent stuttering by not allowing the speaker to close her vocal folds tightly before trying to start airflow through the glottis, as stutterers often do.
Light contacts	Producing sounds by making articulatory contacts very gently or not fully making the contact. For example, a /k/ would be produced as a continuant rather than as a plosive by not completely constricting airflow. This may reduce the likelihood of a stutter because the speaker is not able to tightly squeeze one articulator against another.
Proprioception	Conscious attention to the movements of the articulators. May be taught by first having the client block out the auditory system using masking or talking at a normal speed while under delayed auditory feedback.[3] Then the client can learn to attend to proprioception without using any external stimulus.

[3]You can turn your iPad or iPhone into a delayed auditory feedback (DAF) device by buying an app for just under $20 from speech4good.com. Teach proprioception by having the client speak under DAF and try to "beat" the delay by attempting to talk at a normal rate, ignoring auditory feedback and just attending to the feeling of movement from her articulators (proprioception).

fluency, and it will work for her. She may not always turn a stutter into a fluent utterance, but she may be able to produce the stutter with a feeling of being in control. This requires a well-learned and available behavior (controlled fluency) that can be called upon even under stress. To make the behavior available under stress, the client must practice it over and over until it is second nature to her.

Once clients have mastered controlled fluency, they don't need to use it for the entire sentence. Using controlled fluency on the first word of a sentence or on a word within a sentence can be another way to keep this tool sharp. Some of my clients call these single-word uses of controlled fluency "slide-outs." Other clients and my graduate students refer to them as "slides," a term coined by Vivian Sheehan (*personal communication*, November 1999). Clients should be encouraged to develop their own names for the techniques they find helpful.

Assessing success on this step is a matter of designing a hierarchy of speaking contexts in which controlled fluency can be used to replace normal speech and measuring a client's progress ascending the hierarchy. When I use the term "normally fluent" speech, I am not referring to perfect speech, which is not the goal of treatment, but to speech like that of nonstutterers, which contains its share of normal disfluencies (e.g., whole-word and phrase repetitions) that the speaker handles easily.

To begin, the client and I design a hierarchy of speaking contexts that progresses from using controlled fluency on single syllables at the beginnings of sentences to using controlled fluency on various syllables in other sentence positions. It is important to remember that this is done only on words on which the client expects to be fluent. We start with conversations between ourselves in the treatment room and progress to outside speaking situations in which the client expects to be fluent. These may include simple telephone conversations in which the client asks what time a store closes, asking questions of store clerks, and stopping unfamiliar people on the street and asking them questions. The client and I then jointly design more transfer activities for a variety of natural situations in her life. At least some of these speaking opportunities should be audio recorded so that we can evaluate the quality of her controlled fluency outside the treatment situation.

One way to help the client practice controlled fluency on words in her normal speech is to help her set up a quota to meet by noon of every day. She should develop a tallying system, such as using a wrist counter like those used by golfers to tally strokes, or carrying a box of 20 Tic-Tacs and eating one for each word produced with controlled fluency on the first syllable. For my own self-therapy, I prefer to use a golf stroke counter because its noticeable presence on my wrist reminds me to practice controlled fluency on the initial syllables of many sentences throughout the day. Alternatively, I can set the alarm on my wrist watch (or iPhone, if I had one) to chime once an hour to remind me.

Replacing Stuttering with Controlled Fluency in the Treatment Room

In this step, the goal is for clients to learn to use controlled fluency in response to old stimuli that were followed by stuttering. This means that the client needs to learn to use controlled fluency when she anticipates stuttering and before she finds herself stuck in a block. With lots of practice and success in many situations, she will develop confidence in her ability to speak with controlled fluency instead of stuttering. In time, she will learn to do it in such a way that her controlled fluency becomes more or less indistinguishable from normal fluency for both listeners and the speaker. Progress is assessed by measuring the frequency of stuttering in various situations.

I begin by having a client replace stuttering with controlled fluency during conversation in the treatment room. If she has practiced using controlled fluency in her natural speech, she knows what it feels and sounds like and has started to "groove" it. As a client begins to use controlled fluency to replace stuttering, she may benefit by looking in a mirror as she converses with me, watching for upcoming stutters, and focusing on what she is doing as she starts to respond. Then, as she works to use controlled fluency to replace anticipated stutters, the mirror helps her to monitor her speech in a more focused way. If a client has trouble "downshifting" to controlled fluency before stutters, I have her signal me when she anticipates a stutter and then plan her controlled fluency response. I sometimes use Van Riper's (1973) technique of having a client pantomime her target response before she begins it. Enthusiastic but gradually faded praise is helpful. I also use video recording and replaying samples of her *successes* to help her learn. Early in this process, I ask the client to evaluate her response, sometimes providing feedback and sometimes not as I foster the goal of self-evaluation.

As a client is learning controlled fluency, I introduce "cancellations" (Van Riper, 1973) as a way of having her mildly punish herself when she fails to downshift into controlled fluency and stutters instead. Cancellations, which are taught by modeling, involve pausing for several seconds after a stutter (the pause functions as a "time out"), having the speaker mentally prepare to use controlled fluency during the pause, and then using controlled fluency on the word just stuttered and continuing to talk. The opportunity to continue talking is a positive reinforcer for the controlled fluency. I am diligent in rewarding cancellations with verbal praise because they are one of the most powerful tools available for self-therapy. I gradually fade my praise and help the client to develop her own reward system. When used regularly throughout acquisition, transfer, and maintenance stages, cancellations can make controlled fluency a durable replacement for stuttering.

I would like to highlight the point just made because it is important. Cancellations are an operant conditioning procedure. The pause after stutters is a "punishment" that decreases the frequency of stuttering, and the opportunity to continue speaking is a reward that will increase the use of controlled fluency. Cancellations are especially effective because they are self-administered operant procedures that a client eventually uses herself as she takes charge of her own treatment. A good description of cancellations by a fan of this technique can be found on pages 84 through 90 of the book *Forty Years after Therapy* by George Helliesen (2002), which is listed in the suggested readings for Chapter 1.

Transferring Controlled Fluency to Anticipated Stuttering

When a client seems confident in her responses during conversations with me in the treatment room, she and I design a hierarchy of increasingly difficult contexts in which to practice. Typical hierarchies involve (1) inside the clinic with me, (2) on the telephone while I'm with her in the clinic, (3) outside the clinic with me, (4) everyday speaking situations.

The first hierarchy of inside the clinic with me varies the physical location and social complexity of therapy sessions in the clinic, which means conducting therapy in other locations in the clinic and bringing other people into therapy sessions. The size of the audience can be increased, and people from the client's world, such as family and friends, can also be brought into therapy. The client and I rank such situations from easiest to most difficult, and then she goes through these situations in sequence, using controlled fluency, both in her natural speech and when she expects to stutter, and cancellations if she does stutter. Usually, we work out a point system generating self-rewards to increase her motivation.

I have found that most advanced stutterers need a separate hierarchy for the telephone. The same strategies or principles used in implementing the hierarchies discussed earlier are applied here as well. Thus, telephone calls, at first in the clinic with the clinician present, are arranged in a hierarchical order. The client practices using controlled fluency in fluent speech and on anticipated stutters or uses cancellations, if needed, during these calls until she meets the criterion for success, and the clinician continues to support and reinforce her during these activities. Soon, the client will report successes in her daily use of the telephone outside of the therapy room.

Once a client has completed the in-clinic telephone hierarchy using controlled fluency, it is time to move on to non-telephone speaking outside the clinic in which I can accompany the client. We jointly select and sequence hierarchy situations and activities for this. Examples of these situations are asking directions from strangers or obtaining information from store clerks (Fig. 14.3). For some part of this hierarchy, a survey about stuttering given to strangers (Do you know what stuttering is? Do you know anyone who stutters? How do you think you should respond to someone who is stuttering?) can be a powerful device to practice replacing anticipated stuttering with controlled fluency. It has the side benefit of discovering what attitudes about stuttering really are.

For any given situation, the criterion for success is that both the client and clinician agree that the client used these

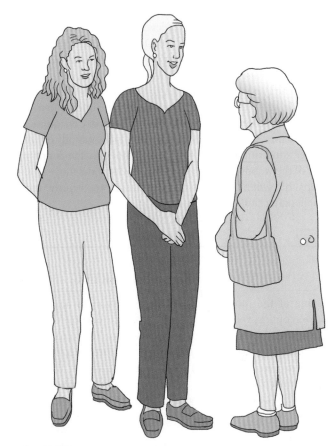

Figure 14.3 Transferring controlled fluency in conversation with a stranger.

skills as well as she did in the clinic. This means that the controlled fluency she used to replace stutters and in fluent speech feels and sounds as good as it did when she used them in the clinic. Some instances of cancellation are acceptable in achieving success, but most stutters should be replaced by controlled fluency on the first try. This is a subjective evaluation, but realistically, it is the type of evaluation the client will use on her own in the future. It is also important that the client experience success in using controlled fluency in fluent speech. Then she must learn to replace anticipated stuttering in each situation a number of times so that she gains confidence in her ability to use controlled fluency. After gaining skill and confidence in using controlled fluency in outside situations with the clinician present, it is time for the client to move on to the next, more difficult hierarchy.

The everyday speaking situation hierarchy consists of situations from the client's environment and requires her to complete them on her own. Clients usually rank a dozen or more speaking situations that they encounter in a typical month, from least to most difficult. As a general rule, the client should feel that she has successfully used her transfer skills a number of times in the immediately preceding, easier situation before moving to a more difficult step or situation on the hierarchy. This is important in developing her skills and confidence in using these techniques. During regular therapy sessions, the clinician monitors the client's progress through this hierarchy, praises her when she is successful, encourages her when she is not, and makes suggestions when she has problems. In time, the client will report to the clinician that her speech is becoming much better in her everyday encounters.

By now, the client will be speaking more fluently or with easier stuttering in most situations. Although she is not yet out of the woods, she is well on her way. We now move to the steps that will help clients transfer fluency to even the most challenging situations.

Increasing Approach Behaviors
Using Voluntary Stuttering

Voluntary stuttering can be a very potent procedure for reducing tension and avoidance and thereby facilitating the use of controlled fluency to replace stuttering. By using voluntary stuttering, the client is performing an **approach behavior**, which is intended to decrease fear and tension. This makes it more likely that the client will be able to use controlled fluency successfully. Every clinician should be familiar with voluntary stuttering. The handout (tan box below), which I give to clients in this stage of therapy, explains the whys and wherefores of voluntary stuttering.

USING VOLUNTARY STUTTERING

One of the most important goals for you to achieve in overcoming your stuttering is to reduce negative feelings associated with it, such as embarrassment, fear, and shame. The more embarrassed you are by your stuttering, the more fearful you are of getting jammed up in a stutter; the more ashamed you are of your stuttering, the more you will try to hide it. The more you try to hide your stuttering, the more tense you will become, and the less you will be able to use controlled fluency. This process needs to be reversed.

One way to reduce these feelings is to stutter voluntarily. If you are afraid of something and run away from it, you will always be afraid of it. The way to overcome fear is to confront it and discover that it's not as bad as you thought. By confronting your fear, you will learn that you are tougher than you think. By stuttering on purpose, first in easy situations and later in more difficult situations, you will learn that you can stutter without fear and shame.

You will begin using voluntary stuttering in the clinic, and I will help you start by putting easy repetitions and prolongations in your speech on nonfeared words. Don't be alarmed if you stutter on some of the words on which you use voluntarily stuttering. This is a common experience. Just keep on stuttering voluntarily until you can finish the word comfortably and without struggling. Ideally, you will voluntarily stutter with your usual amount of abnormal physical tension, but then you should consciously reduce the tension so that it is at a normal level when you finish the word. We will continue to practice this until you are able to remain calm while voluntarily stuttering here in the clinic.

The next step will involve you going with me into the real world to do voluntary stuttering together. Again, you will use easy repetitions or prolongations while talking with strangers on nonfeared words. You may be surprised that most people are accepting of stuttering and will wait for you to say what you want to say. A few may frown or try to finish your sentence for you, but these will be trophies to collect, listeners we can discuss together later. While testing reality in this way, you will learn to tolerate your stuttering and any listener's reactions and to stay cool.

You will also need to use voluntary stuttering in your own environment to reduce your old fears. Old feelings die slowly! However, if you conscientiously do voluntary stuttering sufficiently often over a long period of time, you will find your old fears decreasing. You will no longer be hiding your stuttering, you will be able to use controlled fluency to replace stuttering, and you will be talking more comfortably and fluently. When you are ready to do voluntary stuttering on your own in your everyday speaking situations, we will work together to help you prepare assignments.

When I first introduce voluntary stuttering to clients, many think I am crazy. After all, they came to therapy to rid themselves of stuttering, not to do more of it. At this point, I explain the rationale behind voluntary stuttering: stuttering is perpetuated by fear of stuttering, and reducing this fear will reduce the stuttering. An analogy often helps. For instance, suppose a person wanted to overcome a fear of dogs. This could not be done by running away from them. Instead, the person would have to begin seeking out contact with dogs with knowledge of how to approach them. The best way to do this would be to have the guidance of someone who was an expert on dogs and was not afraid of them and who would guide the person's contact with dogs in a series of small steps.

For example, the first step might involve only looking at puppies in a pet store; the next step might be talking to a clerk about the puppies. Then, the person might briefly pet a puppy and then perhaps pick up the puppy and hold it for a short period. This process would need to be repeated over and over again with gradually larger and larger dogs. Eventually, the person would learn how to approach a dog in a friendly way. As the person learned how to approach and make friends with dogs, her fear would gradually decrease.

This same process can be followed with stuttering. With my guidance, the client begins to stutter on purpose and learn that she has nothing to fear. She'll learn that voluntary stuttering frees her from the need to be perfectly fluent and enables her to use controlled fluency because she is less tense and no longer feels a need to "hold back." The success of this process depends a great deal on a clinician who is comfortable with stuttering. Thus, clinicians need to desensitize themselves to stuttering by practicing voluntary stuttering until the experience of stuttering and the experience of negative listener reactions do not bother them.

After explaining the rationale behind voluntary stuttering, I teach clients how to stutter voluntarily. First, I model brief, easy repetitions or prolongations while remaining calm and relaxed, and I follow this voluntary stuttering with controlled fluency. Then I encourage the client to attempt some voluntary stuttering followed by tension reduction and controlled fluency and enthusiastically reinforce her efforts. If she finds this too difficult, however, I do it with her and have her shadow my voluntary stuttering, tension reduction, and controlled fluency. With appropriate modeling and support, most stutterers are able to do some voluntary stuttering within just one session. I continue giving the client lots of praise for her courage in doing something she may find difficult and am careful to point out that what had been so fearful at first no longer seems so scary.

After the client becomes comfortable using voluntary stuttering followed by tension reduction and controlled fluency in the clinic, it is time for her to move out into the world. First, the client and I establish a hierarchy of situations in which she can use voluntary stuttering. The clinician should always go into situations with the client and use voluntary stuttering during the beginning steps of the hierarchy. I ask her to rate my listeners on a scale that reflects a range of qualities. For example, a "1" might be someone who laughs or looks away, and a "10" might be someone who is attentive and listens patiently. The client may want to continue using this rating system when it is her turn to practice voluntarily stuttering as well because it can countercondition old emotions of feeling victimized and helpless.

I voluntarily stutter in such situations as asking directions from strangers or getting information from store clerks, and I remain calm as I do it. If all of my listeners are patient and understanding, I ask the client to choose listeners whom she feels might be more difficult. After I've completed several of these, it is the client's turn to stutter voluntarily with strangers. We then continue to take alternate turns, which provides additional counterconditioning as the client and I compare our ratings of listeners and take turns choosing

listeners for each other. In time, a stutterer's feelings of assertiveness and exploration usually increase, which diminishes feelings of fear and avoidance.

I am careful not to allow a client to get in "over her head" with listeners who may be too difficult. I also lavish praise on each of the client's attempts, acknowledging how difficult it can be and try to be sensitive to how much she wants to discuss each event. After a good workout with store clerks, for example, I may suggest that we take a break for coffee or a soda at a restaurant, where we can practice voluntary stuttering with the waitress and enjoy the counterconditioning effects of drinking and eating while doing something that was previously unpleasant.

The client and I continue working together on voluntary stuttering until she feels comfortable. Then she works her way through the rest of the situations in her hierarchy on her own. She has to continue putting voluntary stuttering into her speech in each situation until her fear subsides before going on to the next situation. I check clients' progress during therapy sessions, commending them when they are successful while supporting, encouraging, and counseling them when they run into problems. Voluntary stuttering is a procedure that clients will continue to use throughout active treatment and maintenance and is not an activity that will soon be discontinued.

A recent written booklet that is focused on voluntary stuttering may be of some inspiration to clients, especially those who are skeptical of this technique. It is titled "The Greatest Moment My Life: One Man's Story of Beating Stuttering and Becoming a Public Speaker" (Stewart, 2012). It is described more fully at the end of this chapter under *Suggested Readings*.

Reducing Fear of Listener Reactions

The goal of this step is for the client to continue to reduce avoidance, self-consciousness, and shame about her stuttering through further "approach" activities, such as being open about her stuttering. Until recently I had clients work on being open about their stuttering much earlier in therapy, but I have found that this is often a difficult step. It has been easier for clients to do this after they have made considerable progress increasing fluency and reducing the severity of their stuttering. The success of these activities can be assessed in terms of reductions in stuttering severity, increases in her speaking in situations that she previously avoided, and reports of greater comfort in talking despite stuttering. This step and the next can be the most difficult part of treatment for many clients, who often require encouragement and support from the clinician. It may help to remind them of where they are in the progression of treatment and to review the rationale for confronting fears associated with their stuttering.

The major activity of this step involves the client talking to others about her stuttering, which I initiate by giving her a handout (see tan box) on being open about her stuttering.

DISCUSSING STUTTERING OPENLY

One way to become more comfortable with your stuttering is to discuss it openly with your family, friends, and acquaintances. When you get to the point of being open about your stuttering, you will lose much of your fear of it and be more relaxed. In most cases, your listeners know you stutter, you know you stutter, but nobody ever says anything about it. It's like having a giraffe in the room and nobody mentioning it. You would feel much more comfortable about your stuttering if you could talk about it openly. Your listener would also be more comfortable if you were open and more accepting of your stuttering. Your listener often takes his cue from you regarding how to respond. If you look uncomfortable, he will probably feel uncomfortable, but if you are open and comfortable with your stuttering, your listener will probably feel at ease.

How can you be more open about your stuttering? Tell family and friends that you are in therapy and explain what you are doing and why you are doing it. After you have talked about it, encourage them to ask you questions about it. Create an opportunity to let them know how you would like them to respond to your stuttering. For example, some of your family and friends may finish words for you when you stutter. If you can, let them know at the appropriate moment that you would rather they wait until you're finished. Or some of your listeners may look away when you stutter. They may think this helps you. If this makes you uncomfortable, as it does most people who stutter, let your listeners know that it is helpful if they will maintain eye contact when you stutter.

Another good practice is to make comments about your stuttering. If you feel like it, you can make a funny comment about your stuttering to put yourself and your listeners at ease. For example, if you have to introduce yourself and you think you will stutter on your name, you can say, "Make yourself comfortable, it may take me a few minutes to say my name." One of my friends who stutters says to a listener after he has stuttered when introducing himself, "If I stutter on my name, it's only because the witness protection program just changed it." Or just comment casually on a hard block you've had by saying, "Whew, that was a hard one." The more you do this, the less panicked you will feel when you stutter. Another opportunity for being open about your stuttering is when you are faced with making a speech or presentation to a group. Just before you begin speaking, let the audience know that you stutter. They'll find out anyway, but saying it upfront will put everyone, including yourself, much more at ease.

A few advanced stutterers will find these assignments easy, but most will not. I make sure that a client feels she and I are working as a team and that I am supportive and empathetic. I usually help her make lists of the situations in which she will begin to be open about her stuttering and then model an example for her. For example, if commenting on stuttering during a telephone call is on her list, I would call a store, pretend to stutter, and immediately make a comment, such as, "Wow, looks like I'm really stuttering more than usual today." Recently, when working with a young man who was quite sensitive and reluctant to talk openly about his stuttering, I had him video record me as I interviewed three different people on a busy shopping street. After getting permission to video record, I asked them a variety of questions about stuttering and found that each gave positive, supportive answers. The young man seemed impressed that the public was, after all, not uptight about stuttering. He then asked to do the next interview. Exercises such as this can help clients test reality and find out that much of their anxiety and disapproval about stuttering is in their minds rather than in those of the listeners. However, I prepare clients for the possibility that there will be a negative listener reaction (although this is rare) by expressing the hope that at least one listener will be impatient or rejecting so that we can see if we can retain our calm under stress.

Usually, by using a hierarchy of situations, stress can be increased slowly. A client and I plan a hierarchy of tasks in which a client is open about her stuttering. We might go, for example, from a casual comment she might make to a store clerk about having a stuttery day all the way up to telling a group of people that she stutters and is working on it. In psychological terms, reductions in negative emotions that are associated with less stressful tasks will generalize to more stressful tasks. Consequently, when a client gets to the more stressful tasks, they will no longer be as difficult.

After the client completes the assignments on her hierarchy, she discusses the outcomes with me. I diligently give her a great deal of praise for confronting her fears and discussing her stuttering openly. At times, I may need to encourage or even push her to move on to the next step; however, I need to be sensitive to the intensity of her feelings so that I don't expect too much too soon. The client needs to feel she is in control of the amount of stress under which she puts herself.

The client will probably never completely finish with this activity because discussing her stuttering openly will always be an important strategy for her, not only during therapy but possibly throughout her lifetime. It can help her maintain her improved fluency long after therapy has ended. Thus, I get the client started on her hierarchy, then move on to the next technique, and she will continue to work on discussing her stuttering openly in outside assignments while also working on other techniques or procedures. I encourage the client to keep a written record of her progress up this hierarchy so that she may refer to it if, after termination of therapy, she begins to hide her stuttering and old fears creep back in. Using her old records and seeing her old victories may motivate her to try anew to stutter openly, comment on

her stutters, and reestablish her freedom to work on her stuttering in difficult situations.

Using Feared Words and Entering Feared Situations

Using feared words and entering feared situations are important approach behaviors that help clients continue their progress in replacing stuttering with controlled fluency. Some clients will have accomplished a great deal in this area during the transfer of controlled fluency to replace stuttering. However, most will benefit from practice in seeking out remaining fears. I use the following handout (see tan box below) to begin teaching this step and supplement it with examples and discussion.

USING FEARED WORDS AND ENTERING FEARED SITUATIONS

An important goal for you to achieve in overcoming your stuttering is to reduce your avoidance of feared words and feared situations. In the past, you have probably changed words that you were sure you would stutter on and have also shied away from people and places that were very difficult for you. The problem in doing this is that avoidance perpetuates stuttering. It also perpetuates further avoidance, reducing your opportunities to communicate. To make real progress in therapy, you will need to change your avoidance mindset to one of approach and begin to seek out words you have stuttered on and situations you have found difficult in the past. These will be opportunities for you to make your controlled fluency stronger and more resistant to stress.

If you have not already developed this habit, you should now begin to approach words and situations that you previously avoided. It may help to use some voluntary or easy stutters on words you don't fear in difficult situations. Even though you may still stutter, the fact that you have an approach attitude will keep you from tensing and holding back as much as you usually do, and you will sometimes be surprised to find that you don't stutter as much as you expected.

This is hard work and very challenging for most people. It is certainly hard for most nonstuttering people who avoid some speaking situations, like talking on the telephone. But try to set yourself reachable goals and reward yourself when you accomplish each one. Try to stop substituting easier words for harder ones, rephrasing sentences to get around feared words, and pretending you don't know the answer to questions when you really do. Instead of using these sorts of tricks, try to say exactly what you want to say, even if you stutter. If you are afraid you will stutter on a word you are about to say, commit yourself to saying that word, even if you stutter. Even better of course would be to use some aspect of controlled fluency, like flexible rate or proprioception as you start the feared word. But you can't always do that. It's better to say what you want to say, even if you stutter. In time, you

will find your old fears decreasing, and with this decrease in word fears, you will find your word and sound avoidances decreasing and your fluency increasing as well.

From today on, you should try not to avoid talking while in the clinic. In fact, talk as much as you possibly can. If you want to talk about a topic or ask a question, do it. If you think you are going to stutter on a word, go ahead and stutter. In the long run, this is much better than avoiding or postponing. You will learn that you can tolerate your stuttering, will be more comfortable with it, and will gradually become more fluent.

Eliminate your avoidance of feared situations by talking in all of those situations that you avoided in the past. For example, introduce yourself to strangers, start using the telephone more than you usually would, and look for opportunities to speak in groups. If you are aware of any fear of a speaking situation, take that as a sign to approach and enter that situation. Your willingness to speak in these situations will make things much easier for you in the long run. You will find your situation fears decreasing and your wanting to avoid these situations also decreasing; a by-product of this decreased fear will be increased fluency.

In addition to not avoiding speaking in the clinic, you should begin today to eliminate the use of word and situation avoidances in the real world. You will need to develop an approach set in your own speaking environment, and I will help you set up a series of outside speaking assignments from least to most fearful to help you overcome your use of avoidances. Now and then, old speech fears will be too strong, and you will use avoidances, but give it a try again the next day. In time, you will find the old fears decreasing and your tolerance for stuttering increasing. You will also be more comfortable with yourself as a speaker and speak more fluently. However, you will need to keep working on this approach attitude for a long time because it is very important that you conquer your avoidances and keep them vanquished.

After the client has read the handout, I answer any questions she may have. I then encourage her to try to not use any postponements or word avoidances when in therapy from then on. If she does, I have her use a cancellation by redoing the sentence while using controlled fluency on the word(s). When I think she deliberately uses a word that she appeared to want to avoid, I strongly reinforce this approach behavior. I also set up activities in which the client purposefully has to say feared words that we had previously identified and uses controlled fluency when producing these words. These activities may involve her reading word lists and text that is loaded with her feared words or involve her composing sentences with these words. I warmly praise her each time she does not postpone or avoid a feared word, especially when she successfully uses controlled fluency. Sometimes she may be unable to use controlled fluency; however, I am accepting of these occasions and let her know that I understand how hard it can be. This will help her become more comfortable saying these words and will reduce her tendency to want to avoid them.

To help the client eliminate her use of avoidances outside the clinic, I assist her in setting up a hierarchy of word and situation avoidances she commonly uses in daily life. Like all hierarchies, it should be sequenced from least to most difficult for the client. By using this strategy, her fears will be kept to a minimum. A typical step in the hierarchy is the stutterer's deliberate use of certain feared words throughout the day. How often should she use these feared words? They have to be used over and over until she no longer wants to avoid them. Another step in the hierarchy has the stutterer entering situations that she usually avoids in daily life (Fig. 14.4). As before, she needs to enter these situations until she loses her motivation to avoid them. Many of the assignments can be completed as the client goes through her daily routine and will not take any extra time. For instance, she just needs to answer the telephone whenever it rings with the feared "hello" said using controlled fluency or introduce herself to a different person each day. Other assignments may have to be created, and she may need to go out of her way to perform them. For example, the client may have to shop for an item whose name contains one of her feared sounds or fabricate reasons for making telephone calls to local businesses. When I was trying to get over my fear of words beginning with the /l/ sound, I went into many stores asking about **l**uggage, **l**ocks, and **l**ampshades.

To help the client get started on an outside hierarchy, it is helpful for me to join her for some of the assignments. Thereafter, she has to complete the assignments by herself and discuss her progress and any problems with me during regular therapy sessions. I make sure that she keeps on track in completing her hierarchy and provide her with the necessary support and sometimes gentle nudging to help her do so. After the client has worked through as many situations as she and I think are sufficient, it is appropriate for her to complete the Modified Erickson Scale of Communication Attitudes.

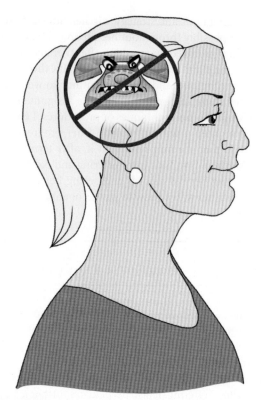

Figure 14.4   The client reduces fear and avoidance by approaching previously feared situations.

This will give me an indication of whether or not there are still situations that need to be approached and mastered.

Like discussing stuttering openly, eliminating the use of avoidances is a strategy that stutterers will need to use throughout therapy and beyond. So, once a stutterer has begun outside assignments successfully, it is time to move on to steps that will create the foundation for long-term change. Self-evaluation and self-reinforcement are crucial elements in a client's learning to decrease avoidance. As described in an earlier section, these behaviors need to be explicitly trained.

Maintaining Improvement

The goal of this last phase of therapy is to help clients generalize their improvement—that is, transferring their reduced negative feelings, attitudes, avoidances, and increased fluency to all remaining speaking situations and maintaining this improvement following termination of therapy. I introduce the following procedures during this phase: (1) **becoming your own clinician** and (2) establishing long-term fluency goals.

Becoming Your Own Clinician

If clients with advanced stuttering are going to generalize improvement to all speaking situations and maintain this improvement, I believe that they must assume responsibility for their own therapy. The literature on self-management provides helpful guidance for fostering this transition. The article "Self-Regulation and the Management of Stuttering" (Finn, 2003) is a good example. Finn points out that having clients set their own goals is a key element of success. I would also highlight the importance of teaching clients to formulate their own plans that target specific behaviors for specific changes. An article in *Time* (Riley, 2005) on surviving disasters suggests that survivors of September 11 and other catastrophes often had developed a plan of action beforehand so that they were not affected by the common human response to unexpected stress—freezing. Such plans will help clients become committed and focused in their efforts to improve their fluency.

I use the handout on "Becoming Your Own Clinician" shown in the tan box below to help clients learn how to combat avoidance and continue improving their fluency skills.

BECOMING YOUR OWN CLINICIAN

Now that we have covered all the therapy techniques you will need to meet your therapy goals, it is time for you to become your own speech clinician. Although you have improved your fluency and reduced your emotional reactions to stuttering, you will probably still encounter some situations that will give you trouble. Thus, you will need to learn how to handle these situations as well as maintain the fluency you have gained.

Handling the difficult situations that remain will require you to be honest about where you think you may still stutter and what your fears are. Fear doesn't stand still; if you ignore it, it will grow, but if you pursue it, it will die. So you must be vigilant for words and situations that continue to spark fear in you and make you feel as if you won't be able to handle your speech the way you want. For these words and situations, you must be ready to use your techniques to work on these fears, such as controlled fluency in both fluent speech and when you anticipate stuttering, openness about your stuttering, and voluntary stuttering. Up to this point, we have worked together to develop and carry out such plans, but now you will have to take more and more responsibility for them.

Working on feared words and situations is not limited to your initial course of therapy. It also involves maintaining the level of fluency you have now because adult stutterers often relapse or slip back some after they leave therapy. Relapse is not inevitable, but neither is it surprising. After all, you have had years of practice in stuttering. In fact, you are an expert. You have avoided words and situations for a long time, and your negative feelings and attitudes about your speech are well learned. Because stuttering is deeply etched into your brain, you may always have some core behaviors and will need to cope successfully with them. Therefore, you need to become your own speech clinician. You will have to keep applying—on your own and long after you leave therapy—the techniques you have learned in therapy.

So what is involved in being your own clinician? You will need to learn to give yourself assignments to overcome remaining difficult speaking situations and any new ones that crop up. If you still avoid speaking in a certain situation, you will need to design assignments that will eliminate this avoidance. If you are still fearful while talking in some situations, you will need to undertake assignments to reduce this fear. If you are still stuttering a lot in a given situation, you will need to plan assignments that will improve your fluency in this situation. At the beginning of therapy, I helped you create these assignments, but as you improved, more and more of the responsibility was turned over to you. We will continue to do this. With additional practice, you will be able to determine your therapy needs and to develop assignments to meet these needs. When you can do this, you will have become your own speech clinician.

I have found the following approach is effective in meeting this goal. Every day you need to work on reducing any remaining speech fears and eliminating any remaining avoidances. For example, if you still feel fearful while talking in a certain situation, you could give yourself a daily quota of tasks to perform in that situation, including being open about your stuttering and using controlled fluency in your fluent speech and voluntary stuttering. Every day you will also need to work on improving your fluency. If you are still doing a lot of stuttering in a given situation, you could set a daily quota of talking time in that situation during which you will use controlled fluency. These are only examples; the important thing is for you to ask yourself every day which situations are still giving you problems and to give yourself assignments designed to overcome these problems. Now, let's get started in helping you become your own speech clinician.

By this time, a client is probably getting close to completing her everyday speaking situation hierarchy. I point out to her, however, that completing this hierarchy is not enough and that she needs to pursue any other situations that are still giving her trouble. I ask her the following kinds of questions: Is she avoiding talking in any more situations? Is she still unduly afraid while talking in some situations? Is she unable to successfully use controlled fluency in fluent speech and when anticipating stuttering in some situations? Is she hesitant to use voluntary stuttering in some situations?

If she answers yes to any of these questions, she needs to target these situations in assignments.

If the client is still avoiding some situations, I remind her of the importance of using feared words and entering feared situations. I may have her reread the handout and then prepare assignments to overcome her current avoidances. I try not to assume any more responsibility than is necessary. I try to ask helpful questions but want her to figure out on her own what she needs to do. As time goes on, I will gradually have the client assuming more and more responsibility for planning her own assignments.

If the client is still unduly apprehensive about talking in some situations, I remind her of the importance of discussing stuttering openly and of using voluntary stuttering to reduce her negative feelings. I help her create assignments using techniques that will make her feel more comfortable in these situations. Here again, I don't assume any more responsibility than necessary and focus on guiding the client to becoming her own speech clinician.

If she is having difficulties using controlled fluency to replace stuttering in some situations, I explore the nature of her difficulties with her and help her determine what types of assignments she needs to work on to be successful. Maybe she needs more practice in some less difficult situations before she can reasonably expect to be successful in the more

difficult situations. Perhaps she needs to further reduce her speech rate and muscle tension in these difficult situations so that her motor control does not break down as readily. I have found that some clients strive to be as fluent as possible in all situations; however, others are happy with some residual stuttering if it doesn't interfere with their communication. I am accepting of this because I realize that clients must set their own goals. During all of our discussions, I try to keep in mind that my goal is to help the stutterer become independent. So, I gradually become less directive and gradually turn all of the responsibility for her assignments over to her. Throughout this phase of therapy, the client should be working daily on outside assignments and discussing her progress with me during therapy sessions. During this same period, I am more and more of a consultant, helping the client feel that she can go out and fly on her own.

Establishing Long-Term Fluency Goals

Before therapy ends, it is very important for a client to be aware of what she can expect in terms of fluency after termination from therapy. By having realistic goals, she can substantially decrease the possibility of becoming disappointed and frustrated with her speech and not developing feelings that may lead to relapse. To begin this topic, I share with her the handout shown in the following tan box.

ESTABLISHING LONG-TERM FLUENCY GOALS

You are at the point in your therapy when you need to consider your long-term fluency goals. Before you do this, I need to define three of the terms we will be using: "spontaneous fluency," "controlled fluency," and "acceptable stuttering." Spontaneous fluency refers to speech that contains no more than occasional disfluencies, and there is no tension or struggle. This fluency is not maintained by paying attention to or controlling your speech. Therefore, you don't use controlled fluency to be fluent. You just talk and pay attention to your ideas. It is the fluency of normal speakers.

Controlled fluency is another name for normal-sounding fluency that is under your active control. It has some or all of the characteristics you've practiced: flexible rate, pausing, easy onsets, light contacts, and proprioception. It sounds similar to spontaneous fluency except that you must attend to or control your normal-sounding speech to maintain relative fluency. You sound fluent only because you are working on your speech at the time.

Finally, acceptable stuttering refers to speech that contains noticeable but mild stuttering that feels comfortable to you. You are not avoiding words or situations, and you feel OK about yourself as someone who stutters at times. You may have acceptable stuttering when you don't care

about working on your speech. Or you may have it when you are trying to use controlled fluency but can't quite get a handle on it. It's healthy to feel OK about the occasional mild stuttering you have in either case.

Now, let's consider long-term fluency goals. A few adults who stutter become spontaneously fluent in all speaking situations on a consistent basis. They become normal speakers. In my experience, however, most adult stutterers do not reach this goal. Instead, they have situations, such as talking to close friends, in which they are spontaneously fluent. In other situations, such as speaking in groups, their stuttering tends to give them trouble. In these troublesome situations, I think it is important for these stutterers—and possibly you—to have the following options.

First, *if* it is important to you to sound fluent in a specific situation, I want you to be able to use your controlled fluency skills. I know this is possible in most situations, especially if you have been putting money in the bank by practicing controlled fluency in your fluent speech. I also know that there will be some situations in which you will not be totally successful. In such situations, I want you to feel comfortable with acceptable stuttering.

Second, if it is *not* important to you to sound fluent in a situation, and you do not want to put the effort into using

(Continued)

controlled fluency, I would like you to feel comfortable with acceptable stuttering.

These options or goals are both realistic and acceptable. In other words, you don't have to sound perfectly fluent all the time or work on your speech constantly. Indeed, attempting to sound fluent all the time by using controls can become burdensome. Where are you now with regard to these fluency goals? Are you satisfied with your present fluency? Where would you like to be in the future with regard to these goals? We should discuss these issues, and you should begin to make plans based on your answers.

I make sure that the client understands the concepts of spontaneous fluency, controlled fluency, and acceptable stuttering. When I am convinced that she understands what is meant by these terms, I explore with her the types of fluency she currently has in various, everyday speaking situations. If she is unsure, she gives herself assignments to help her find out whether or not she is satisfied with the types of fluency she has in these situations. If she is satisfied, then she has met her goals, and the end of therapy is near. She can continue working along the lines discussed in the previous section on "Becoming Your Own Clinician."

I have observed a couple of problems that frequently occur with clients' fluency expectations or goals. First, many clients experience a great deal of spontaneous fluency at this point in therapy. They expect and want this spontaneous fluency to last forever without any effort on their part. It can last, but that will require continued work. A client will need to continue giving herself assignments to keep her negative feelings and attitudes at a minimum and to extinguish her avoidance behaviors. She will also need to continue working on her controlled fluency so that she has confidence in her ability to use it when she chooses. Spontaneous fluency will be a by-product of these efforts, and I must help the client understand this. If she doesn't understand, she will be disappointed and possibly panicked when she begins to lose some of her spontaneous fluency, which could lead to relapse.

A second problem frequently involves clients with more severe advanced stuttering. These clients often fail to achieve a great deal of spontaneous fluency. If they are going to talk better, they need to use controlled fluency constantly. Even then, they often achieve only acceptable stuttering, which can be discouraging. It may be too much of a burden for them to constantly monitor and modify their speech. In time, they will become tired and give up doing anything at all, and relapse will soon follow. I need to help these clients accept and become comfortable with their acceptable stuttering. I also need to help them realize that they will need to expend substantial effort to maintain this level of fluency. Clients with severe advanced stuttering may benefit especially from the support provided by a self-help group to help them maintain the motivation needed for continued self-therapy (Yaruss, Quesal, & Reeves, 2007).

Once a client feels she is meeting her fluency goals and has become her own clinician, the frequency of her therapy contacts is systematically reduced. I typically fade contacts to once a week for a month or two, then to once a month for several months, and finally to once a semester for two years. This gradual transition provides the client with some continued support. For example, if she is doing well, I reinforce her feelings, and if she is having a few problems, I can help her find solutions. Of course, if she has relapsed completely, she can be reenrolled in therapy. Ultimately, the day comes to say "goodbye." I commend her for all her efforts and let her know that if she ever needs me again, she should feel free to contact me.

Throughout the fading process, I assess her speech using the SSI-4 for samples gathered in the clinic on video and percent syllables stuttered for the samples she brings me from outside situations. I also use such measures as the OASES, the Erickson S-24, and the Iowa Scale of Stutterer's Reactions to Speaking Situations, which are presented in Chapter 8. The process of us mutually analyzing her fluency and working on areas that need further practice helps to keep her focused on using controlled fluency. It also increases the chances that she will become largely spontaneously fluent and her controlled fluency will become more and more automatic.

OTHER APPROACHES
Comprehensive Stuttering Program

I am presenting the comprehensive stuttering program (CSP) because I am a supporter of group therapy for adults and adolescents who stutter. The CSP offers a mix of fluency-shaping and cognitive components, so that both behaviors and attitudes are addressed. A similar approach is offered by Kroll and Scott-Sulsky (2010). Follow-up studies from both treatments provide good evidence of the programs' effectiveness.

The CSP was developed by Einer Boberg and Deborah Kully (1985) as a three-week treatment program based on earlier programs that used prolonged speech to induce fluency and then used principles of conditioning to transfer and maintain fluency in clients' everyday lives (Ingham & Andrews, 1973; Webster, 1974). Over the last 20 years, Kully and Marilyn Langevin have refined their approach so that elements of stuttering management, cognitive behavioral therapy, and self-management have become crucial elements of the treatment.

The following description of the program is taken from Kully and Langevin (1999) and Langevin, Kully, Teshima, Hagler, and Prasad (2010). Clients begin by learning very slow, prolonged speech that has the following components: (1) smooth, unrushed breathing patterns with appropriate breath grouping, (2) gentle onset of voicing, (3) continuous airflow and smooth continuous movement of articulators within breath groups, and (4) light contacts of articulators. Once clients learn these skills, they gradually increase their speech rate and monitor their speech naturalness. At the same time, they learn Van Riper's (1973) techniques of cancellation and pullout to deal with stutters that may emerge as clients increase their speech rates. Clients then learn cognitive-behavioral techniques to be comfortable using their techniques in public to reduce avoidance and deal with residual stuttering. They also learn to improve their overall communication skills and attitudes, as well as skills to manage regression and relapse, if they occur.

Once clients have learned these skills and are speaking fluently in the clinic, they begin transfer activities. These are essentially hierarchies, suited to the needs of each client, in which the client uses her newly acquired skills to speak fluently with managed stuttering in gradually more difficult situations. Clients then consult with their clinicians to design individual maintenance programs to use after they terminate formal therapy. They are encouraged to join support groups and return to the clinic for follow-up treatment if needed.

Outcome data have been reported on both one-year and five-year follow-ups. Kully and Langevin (1999) found that in a group of 25 adolescent clients, mean pretreatment %SS was 14.32, and mean score for Erickson Scale of Communication Attitudes (S-24) was 16.81 (mean for nonstutterers reported by Andrews and Cutler [1974] was 9.4). One year after treatment, mean %SS was found to be 3.89, and mean S-24 scores were reduced to 11.57.

Results of a five-year longitudinal follow-up study of 18 clients (mean age = 23.8 years) revealed that the mean stuttering frequency, measured as %SS in telephone calls, decreased from 15.86 to 4.98. This difference was statistically significant and the effect size was large (1.16). Additionally, there were no significant differences among the measures obtained immediately post-treatment and the five follow-up measures, indicating that improvements in stuttering were stable for the five-year follow-up period. Regarding self-report, because the questionnaire return rate for years 3-5 were not representative of the entire group (i.e., less than 50 percent were returned), results for two-year follow-up were reported. Langevin and colleagues (2010) found that statistically and clinically significant differences in attitudes, perceptions of stuttering, and speech-associated confidence were being maintained at the two-year follow-up. In particular, the mean communication attitude score, as measured with S-24, decreased from 19.72 (SD = 3.30) to 11.10 (SD = 5.88), indicating that group attitudes were approaching

those of typically fluent speakers (9.4). In summary, 15 of 18 clients maintained "clinically meaningful" speech gains at five-year follow-up (50 percent improvement in %SS at the five-year follow-up relative to pretreatment %SS and no more than 3 percent increase in %SS measured at follow-up relative to immediately after treatment).

Camperdown

Sue O'Brian, Mark Onslow, Angela Cream, and Ann Packman (2003) developed the Camperdown program for adults. It is based on earlier prolonged speech treatments (e.g., Ingham & Andrews, 1973) but requires less treatment time and gives clients more self-reliance in the establishment, transfer, and maintenance of their controlled fluency.

The program has four stages. First are the individual teaching sessions, in which clients learn prolonged speech and practice using two 1-to-9 scales to track their progress. One is the *stuttering severity* scale (1 = no stuttering; 9 = extremely severe stuttering) and the other is the *speech naturalness* scale (1 = extremely natural speech; 9 = extremely unnatural speech). Unlike traditional methods of teaching prolonged speech via detailed instruction in slow rate, gentle onsets, light contacts, and continuous airflow, the Camperdown approach uses an exemplar video of a clinician speaking with prolonged speech at approximately 70 syllables per minute (or a 7 on the naturalness scale). Clients are coached by the clinician to imitate the model and to continue to practice using the model with the clinician's feedback until they can maintain 100 percent fluent prolonged speech in the clinic setting. This involves frequent self-evaluation of their naturalness and severity ratings during multiple monologues to achieve consistently fluent speech.

After clients can produce the monologue fluently with prolonged speech, they complete a group practice day, in which they learn to speak at gradually faster rates, fluently and naturally, and to assess their speech on the severity scale as well as a nine-point naturalness scale. Subsequently, they begin individual problem-solving sessions, consisting of weekly individual meetings with a clinician to facilitate generalizing fluent speech to everyday situations. These sessions involve the clinician mentoring clients' planning and carrying out generalization activities, as well as further practice of fluent speech. Clients' speech has to meet two criteria for three consecutive weeks at this stage. Both within-clinic and beyond-clinic conversations must show low levels of stuttering severity (ratings of 1 to 2) and normal levels of speech naturalness (ratings of 1 to 3).

The final stage of the program, performance-contingent maintenance, lasts about a year and involves repeated clinic maintenance visits by clients. During these visits, stuttering severity and speech naturalness levels are expected to be equivalent to those required previously. If these severity and naturalness criteria are met, clinic visits are scheduled at fading intervals: two weeks, two weeks, four weeks, eight weeks, and 24 weeks. If the criteria are not met at any visit, that visit is repeated, and progress is momentarily stalled until it is met.

The authors of the program indicate that this approach is an important advance over previous stuttering treatments because it requires relatively little treatment time (i.e., 20 hours to establish fluency). Because the program doesn't involve extensive teaching and measurement of prolonged speech targets, the authors believe that it can be used by generalist clinicians rather than just stuttering specialists. A more detailed description of the program is available from the treatment manual, which can be downloaded from the Australian Stuttering Research Centre website: http://sydney.edu.au/health_sciences/asrc/health_professionals/asrc_download.shtml. This can also be reached by Googling "Camperdown."

Several studies have been carried out to assess the long-term outcome of this approach. O'Brian and colleagues (2003) reported on 30 adults who reduced stuttering from a pretreatment mean of 7.9 %SS to a mean of 0.4 %SS at the end of treatment and maintained that same reduction when measured a year after treatment ended. O'Brian, Packman, and Onslow (2008) designed a telehealth model of the Camperdown program, conducted entirely by e-mail and telephone consultation, reporting a 75 percent reduction in stuttering from before treatment to six months after. Carey, O'Brian, Onslow, Block, Jones, and Packman (2010) conducted a randomized control comparison of Camperdown done via telehealth with Camperdown done face to face. The telehealth group had a mean pretreatment %SS of 6.86 and reduced it to 2.58 one year after treatment had ended; the face-to-face group had a mean pretreatment %SS of 5.44 and reduced to 2.5 one year after treatment had ended. This suggests the telehealth version is as effective as the face-to-face version.

Successful Stuttering Management Program

I have known several people who have not been helped by treatments focused on fluency alone but have found the successful stuttering management program (SSMP) to meet their needs. This program can be done intensively in a brief period of time and may be appropriate for individuals who have strong fears and avoidances and who do not have access to regular weekly treatment.

The SSMP was developed by Dorvan Breitenfeldt in 1963 and is now offered in a residential three-week treatment program at Eastern Washington University by Kim Krieger and her colleagues. There are two phases to the program: the first is reducing fear and avoidance, and the second is learning to manage stuttering and transfer improvements to outside situations. Much of the work in both phases of the program is done outside the clinic.

Phase I begins with stutterers making lists of their covert and overt symptoms, learning to maintain eye contact with listeners when they stutter and learning to "advertise" their stuttering to listeners. Starting on the very first day and continuing throughout the program, clients conduct surveys about stuttering with strangers outside the clinic, both in person and on the telephone. These surveys provide the participants an opportunity to practice skills they are learning in the clinic, such as reducing secondary behaviors, maintaining eye contact with listeners, and learning to accept their stuttering as they change it to an easier form.

Phase II accelerates the learning of easier stuttering, with clients learning to use light articulatory contacts, prolongation of the first sounds of words, pullouts, and cancellations. These techniques are then combined in "controlled normal speech," which teaches clients to begin words normally, prolong the first sound, and move through the word without stopping. This appears to be similar to Van Riper's "preparatory set." The initial practice in the clinic is followed by practice in many outside situations; at the same time, clients work on various lifestyle changes, such as organizational ability, appearance, social skills, and physical conditioning. The final step involves planning for long-term success, including learning to become one's own clinician, negative practice (deliberately stuttering in the client's old way), five-day refresher sessions, self-help groups, and networking via e-mail, Skype, and Facebook.

Pharmacological Approaches

Because the use of drugs in the treatment for stuttering has a long history but until recently has been short on scientific evidence, this section will be more of a review than a recommendation. Complaints and concerns about the lack of tightly controlled drug studies goes back at least as far as Van Riper (1973), who noted that a valid drug study would involve at least two groups of stutterers: one group would receive the drug and the other group would receive a placebo that had the same side effects. Another critically important aspect of a good study is "double-blinding;" neither the experimenter nor the participant knows whether he or she was given the drug or the placebo. A third characteristic is that the experimenter should make multiple measures of the drugs' effects on the frequency and severity of stuttering, as well as measures of how the study's stutterers perceived their speech. Van Riper pointed out that the few early studies that used placebos and were double blind had mixed results, although tranquilizers and sedatives seemed to reduce the severity of stuttering and make subjects feel better about their speech. At one time, there was some hope that an antipsychotic drug called haloperidol, which blocked receptors for the neurotransmitter dopamine, might prove to be effective.

In a later review of pharmacological approaches to stuttering, Brady (1991) reported that improved studies indicated that tranquilizers and sedatives reduced the severity of stuttering compared to placebos, and he also discussed a number of studies on haloperidol. Several authors (Prins, Mandelkorn, & Cerf, 1980; Rosenberger, 1980; Swift, Swift, & Arellano, 1975) who studied haloperidol suggested that its effectiveness might result from diminishing the uptake of dopamine, which could interfere with fluency if it were produced in excess. Although haloperidol seemed to work directly on stuttering symptoms, rather than through overall sedative or tranquilizing mechanisms, major side effects contraindicated its use. Its side effects included drowsiness, sexual dysfunction, excess movement of limbs, and the risk of a permanent, neurologically based movement disorder, tardive dyskinesia. When I worked in Australia, I participated in a haloperidol trial and found that it reduced the tension in my stuttering, allowing blocks to seemingly melt in my mouth, but the side effects were hard to bear. I was always on the verge of falling asleep, but my legs were uncontrollably wiggling.

A recent research review by Maguire, Yu, Franklin, and Riley (2004) presented the evidence that medications that reduce the uptake of dopamine can be effective in reducing stuttering. These authors recently completed a study of olanzapine, a dopamine antagonist, which doesn't have the same side effects as other drugs that reduce dopamine, such as haloperidol or its replacements risperidone and pimozide. In a double-blind study, 5 mg/d of olanzapine was reported to significantly ($p < 0.05$) reduce stuttering compared with the placebo on each of the following three measures: the SSI-3, the clinician's global impression, and the participant's self-rating of stuttering. The only side effect noted was a tendency for weight gain, but that was minimized via counseling about diet and exercise. Maguire, Riley, Franklin, and Gumusaneli (2010) described their model of the action of the neurotransmitter dopamine in the etiology of stuttering and presented an update on the effect of a new drug called pagaclone. In a separate publication, Maguire, Franklin, Vatakis, Morgenshtern, Denko, and colleagues (2010) showed that pagaclone reduced stuttering in 88 patients by 19.4 percent, whereas a placebo group of 44 patients reduced stuttering by only 5.1 percent in an eight-week trial. When this trial was over and all patients were offered pagaclone, the entire group showed a reduction of 40 percent after a year of treatment. The only significant side effect was headache, experienced by about 12 percent of the pagaclone patients.

In summary, although case studies appearing in the literature (e.g., Brady & Ali, 2000) frequently report the success of a variety of medications, large-scale double-blind studies most frequently support drugs that interfere with the uptake of dopamine, especially olanzapine and pagaclone. It appears, however, that at this time and for most individuals who stutter, medication for stuttering has not proven any more effective than traditional treatment.

Treatment and Support Groups

My description of treatment groups will largely draw on my own experience as a client in one of Van Riper's stuttering modification treatment groups (see Van Riper [1958] for a description of his group therapy) and as a clinician in fluency-shaping therapy groups (Guitar, 1976). Manning (2010) provides a good description of group stuttering therapy, in general.

Among the benefits of group therapy is the mutual support that its members experience as they face the challenges of confronting and changing their stuttering. An effective group leader will facilitate extensive interaction among group members so that they encourage each other, share hopes and fears, and provide a safe haven for trying out new behaviors. Many of us in Van Riper's group paired up to do some of our beyond-clinic assignments together. We were able to give each other helpful feedback, both in our group sessions and when we went out together to work on our speech in shopping areas and restaurants. Seeing each other's stuttering made ours more bearable, and vying with each other to bring back "trophies" of successful changes in our speech was healthy competition. The techniques we were taught and the changes we made in our behaviors, feelings, and attitudes were, I suspect, much the same as would have occurred in individual therapy, but the group made the road we had to travel less lonely. Van Riper measured the outcome of his treatment five years after the end of therapy, using the following five criteria: (1) the client's speech must be at or below 0.5 on the Iowa Scale of Severity of Stuttering (Sherman, 1952); (2) the client must not be avoiding words or situations; (3) stuttering must not be interfering with the client's social or vocational adjustment; (4) the client's word and situation fears must be close to zero; and (5) the client's stuttering must present no concern to himself or others (Van Riper, 1958). The seven members of our group have had our ups and downs, and several of us have had some additional therapy, but most of us did fairly well, but not perfectly, in terms of Van Riper's criteria.

The fluency-shaping groups I worked with in Australia (Guitar, 1976; Howie & Andrews, 1984) focused first on learning a prolonged speech pattern to replace stuttering and shaping conversational speech to sound essentially normal. Group members then generalized their fluency to their natural environments. In this approach, the group functioned primarily as a setting in which conversational speech could be practiced, with only minor attention to the support that group members provided each other. Treatment in a group promoted an efficient use of the clinician's time as well as opportunities for members to practice using fluent speech in the give-and-take of a conversation among six people. Results of treatment varied widely for individuals (Guitar, 1976), but the overall group mean of percent syllables stuttered went from 14 percent before treatment to 3.9 percent a year after treatment, with essentially normal mean speech rates (Howie & Andrews, 1984). Subsequent modifications of the program brought follow-up percentages to even lower levels (1-2 %SS) (Andrews & Craig, 1982).

Support or self-help groups differ from treatment groups because their main function is to provide an atmosphere in which members can freely share their feelings and develop a sense of connectedness to others who stutter, and they can provide an excellent opportunity for maintenance of improvement made in formal therapy. In my experience, getting together with others who stutter and sharing experiences, especially triumphs and frustrations, motivates continued work on techniques. Our group at the University of Vermont, which has been running for more than 30 years, is a mix of support and therapy. Participants share their experiences, comment supportively on each others' techniques, give themselves speech assignments, both for that meeting and for the two weeks in between meetings, and tell funny stories. There is much therapeutic humor, directed both at stuttering and at difficult listeners.

Ramig (1993) surveyed 62 self-help participants and found that 49 of them believed that their fluency had improved "at least somewhat" as a result of attending meetings regularly. The majority of respondents felt that the group experience improved their feelings about themselves, as well as their comfort in their personal and work environments. Information about the return rate of the survey was not available. Ramig did note that there is a paucity of research on the impact of self-help groups on the lives of people who stutter, and he gave 17 suggestions for designing studies on self-help groups.

An excellent review of self-help groups as a supplement to traditional therapy was presented in a chapter by Yaruss, Quesal, and Reeves (2007). This chapter lists several national self-help for stuttering organizations and provides evidence of benefit to participants gathered by self-report studies.

Assistive Devices

For hundreds of years, practitioners have offered stutterers an incredible array of devices to help them speak more fluently. These devices have included ivory forks placed under the tongue, auditory feedback-delaying devices inserted in the ear, respiration-monitoring belts snugged around the chest, and masking noise generators triggered by sensors wrapped around the throat (Van Riper, 1982). Some have been used alone, and others have been used as an adjunct to therapy. Many have helped stutterers who have not been able to find relief through traditional therapy, but too often, false hopes for a miracle cure have been raised.

Merson (2003) presented a brief overview of devices such as the Edinburgh Masker, the Fluency Master, the Case Futura delayed auditory feedback (DAF), and the SpeechEasy. He reported that he only uses such devices with clients who seem to not be helped by other therapy procedures alone, using these devices only as an adjunct to more traditional stuttering modification and fluency-shaping therapy techniques. Of the 10 patients who have used the Fluency Master (masking triggered by phonation) for 12 to 24 months, five reported that their stuttering was 100 percent reduced, two reported a 50 percent reduction, one stopped using it, and two more could not be contacted. Of the 37 patients who had used the SpeechEasy for three to five months, 55 percent reported that its effectiveness was retained, 53 percent reported less frequent stuttering, 52 percent reported less tense stuttering, and 28 percent reported that their speech was more fluent *without* the SpeechEasy. These data are not objective measures of fluency but are the subjective reports of clients who were surveyed and may be unreliable.

Another "soft" source of information about the use of assistive devices is a survey conducted by the Stuttering Foundation (Fraser, 2004; Trautman, 2003). The Foundation contacted 800 adults who had requested information about electronic devices from its website. Just over 100 individuals returned the survey, and of these, only 22 had actually bought a device. Most of those who didn't buy a device cited high costs and the absence of evidence of long-term benefit. Of those who bought devices, 12 bought a SpeechEasy, six bought a Casa Futura DAF, three bought a Fluency Master, and one bought an unspecified device. Initial reports suggested that 14 of the 22 purchasers were happy with their devices. A later follow-up survey to learn how they felt after having used their device for a year was able to reach eight of these 14 individuals. Of those eight individuals, three were still happy with their device, three were not happy, and two reported mixed reactions. Some of those who were no longer happy with their devices reported that it didn't work when their stutters were those that stop phonation; others reported that their device didn't work well in noisy environments.

Ramig reported (personal communication, March 8, 2005) that he and his private practice colleagues have evaluated over 60 stuttering patients over a two-year period, fitting over 40 of them with a SpeechEasy device. Only a few of those patients were able to receive supplemental traditional therapy. He indicates that the device helped one-third of the clients significantly, one-third were helped marginally, and one-third were not helped at all. For some of his clients, it is the only effective treatment they have experienced. Ramig further notes that for the device to be useful for most clients, the clients must be able to initiate appropriate voicing during their stuttering blocks, and they must pay attention to the auditory feedback from the device. He emphasizes that he only dispenses the device for adults, teens, and children over 11 years old, believing that younger children can be helped by other therapeutic approaches. His reluctance to fit very young children stems primarily from the thought that their auditory cortex is not yet fully developed and the fact that the effect of prolonged exposure to DAF and frequency altered pitch is unknown at this time.

Ramig, Ellis, and Pollard (2010) have written a comprehensive chapter on the SpeechEasy, including video clips of clients using it and talking about their experiences with it. It is a thorough account of his and other's experiences using the SpeechEasy with clients.

SUMMARY

- Advanced stuttering is characterized by repetitions, prolongations, and blocks, accompanied by overlearned patterns of tension, struggle, and escape and avoidance behaviors. Clients will also typically have negative attitudes, feelings, and beliefs about stuttering and about speaking.

- The author believes that because these behaviors are so well-learned, treatment must focus on teaching the stutterer new fluency and coping skills as responses to old cues that will still tend to elicit struggle and avoidance behaviors.

- Treatment begins by increasing motivation to change and decreasing fear and avoidance. Then, new controlled fluency skills are taught in the clinic and generalized to the client's daily life. These skills are practiced on non-feared words as well as when the client experiences old cues that previously triggered tension, struggle, and avoidance behaviors. For many clients, continued work is needed on increasing approach behaviors and decreasing avoidance behaviors. For all clients, the responsibility for managing their own speech is gradually transferred to them over the course of treatment.

- A variety of other treatments are available for advanced stuttering, including individual and group approaches, intensive and nonintensive treatment, medication, and assistive devices. Knowing about these options can give you a wider range of options to offer your clients, especially those who need something more or something different from the integrated approach offered in this chapter.

STUDY QUESTIONS

1. Summarize the main differences between *intermediate stuttering in school-age children* and *advanced stuttering in adolescents and adults* and the treatment approaches used for them.

2. If the aim of therapy is to learn to respond to anticipated stuttering with controlled fluency, why are actual moments of stuttering also targets of treatment?

3. Do you think it is a treatment failure if a client has mild stuttering after treatment? Explain the reasoning behind your answer.

4. Explain the difference between *counterconditioning* and *deconditioning* using examples from stuttering therapy.

5. If the purpose of treatment is to become more fluent, why do I suggest that the client ought to work on exploring her stuttering?

6. In my approach to treatment, I advocate teaching clients four separate components of "controlled fluency" before they combine them. Clinicians using the Camperdown program prefer to teach clients a variant of controlled fluency using a video model of someone speaking with all the components already combined (speaking with prolonged speech at 70 syllables per minute). What are the advantages and disadvantages of each approach?

7. Why do I advocate learning controlled fluency in fluent speech? How many reasons can you think of?

8. Many clients are reluctant to use voluntary stuttering. What are some reasons you could give them as to why it may be helpful? Are there any clients with whom you would not use it?

9. Which clients would be most suited for treatment with a pharmacological approach? Which clients would be most suited for an assistive device?

10. What do you think are the most valid measures of the benefits of a treatment approach?

SUGGESTED PROJECTS

1. Choose a behavior of yours that you would like to change, and develop a self-therapy plan to explore your present behavior, identify the change you would like to make, and develop a hierarchy to practice the new behavior. Report on your success.

2. Write out a talk that you could have with a new adult client to describe the possible course of treatment (see the section on "Beginning Therapy"). Make your talk both challenging and inspirational.

3. If you are a nonstutterer, your biggest fear in doing voluntary stuttering is probably that you will be unable to stutter convincingly, and a listener will unmask you. Confront that fear by stuttering to several listeners, and see if that decreases your fear.

4. After you have learned controlled fluency, see if you can use it on just single words ("slideouts") 20 times before noon. In trying to do this, see if you can develop a novel way to remind yourself.

5. Watch a session of the Van Riper videos (for example, the session on desensitization), and see if you can determine what made him so effective as a stuttering therapist.

SUGGESTED READINGS AND VIEWINGS

Fraser, M. (2002). *Self-therapy for the stutterer* (10th ed.). Memphis: Stuttering Foundation.

This self-help book contains a sequenced program for the adult stutterer to use, either on his own or with the help of a clinician or supportive friend. It describes many of the techniques you have been reading about in this book. In addition, it contains many personal and inspirational messages for the reader. I recommend it not only to individuals who stutter but also to clinicians so that they may get another perspective on adult stuttering therapy.

Guitar, B., & Guitar, C. (2005). *If you stutter: Advice for adults* (DVD). Memphis: Stuttering Foundation.

This video presents a broad spectrum of treatment approaches, and many of them are demonstrated by adults who have benefited from stuttering therapy.

Guitar, B., & McCauley, R. (2010). *Treatment of stuttering: Established and emerging interventions.* Baltimore: Lippincott Williams & Wilkins.

This edited book has four approaches for adults and adolescents who stutter: two behavioral treatments, one involving the SpeechEasy device, and one on pharmacological therapy. Each chapter is illustrated with a video that depicts the treatment process as well as before- and after-therapy interviews with clients.

Manning, W. (2010) *Clinical decision making in fluency disorders* (3rd ed.). Clifton Park, NY: Delmar, Cengage Learning.

An excellent and sensible book about stuttering therapy by a knowledgeable clinician.

National Stuttering Association Website: www. westutter.org.

This site contains a wealth of information for adolescents and adults who stutter, including basic information about the nature of stuttering and treatment opportunities. A DVD, *Transcending Stuttering,* about the struggle and triumph of many individuals who stutter, is among NSA's recent offerings.

Shapiro, D. (2011) *Stuttering intervention: A collaborative journey to fluency freedom.* Austin, TX: Pro-Ed.

This book is a thoughtful account of working with people who stutter, written by an experienced clinician who stutters

himself. Shapiro is particularly eloquent on the feelings that affect people who stutter.

Stewart, S.W. (2012). *The greatest moment of my life: One man's story of beating stuttering and becoming a public speaker.* Self-published. Available for about $25 from stephenstewart497@gmail.com.

This 60-page booklet is the story of a man who stuttered severely and found fluency after working hard on a program of therapy centered on voluntary stuttering. He describes the program in detail, but also explains how his life changed after that. He became a minister, gave sermons easily, and was president of his local chapter of Toastmasters International, an organization that focuses on public speaking.

Stuttering Foundation Website: www.stutteringhelp. org.

Background information on stuttering and its treatment, books, videos, and lists of clinicians who specialize in stuttering are offered on this site.

Stuttering Home Page: www.mnsu.edu/comdis/kuster/ stutter.html.

Developed by Judy Kuster at Mankato University, the Stuttering Home Page offers a wide variety of helpful pages and links. On this site, the user can connect to chat rooms and access an annual online conference and its archives, the latest research, and commentary by people who stutter. Links to stuttering sites in other countries are also provided.

Van Riper, C. (1975b). *Therapy in action (video).* Memphis: Stuttering Foundation.

This nine-part video shows a master clinician conducting stuttering modification treatment with an adult stutterer. Van Riper takes this young man from the assessment to the final treatment meeting in seven sessions. There are then one-year and 20-year follow-up interviews. Van Riper introduces each session describing what he has planned for the session and then follows the session with a commentary on what was accomplished.

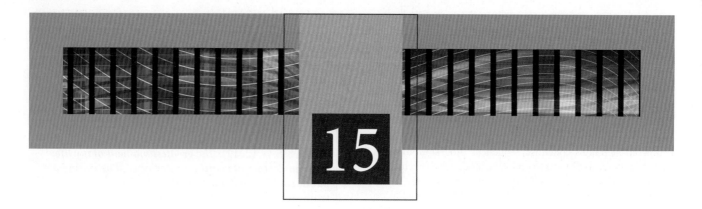

15

Related Disorders of Fluency

After studying this chapter, readers should be able to:
• Describe the multiple possible etiologies of neurogenic
  stuttering
• Describe the speech characteristics of neurogenic stuttering

• Describe evaluation and treatment of neurogenic stuttering
• Describe the conditions that may give rise to psychogenic
  stuttering, particularly in regard to information that may be
  obtained from the case history and interview
• Describe the speech characteristics of psychogenic stuttering
• Describe aspects of evaluation that can differentiate
  between psychogenic and neurogenic stuttering
• Describe trial therapy for psychogenic stuttering and how
  that may be continued beyond the initial trial
• Describe the characteristics of cluttering including concomitant problems
• Describe the evaluation of cluttering including concomitant
  problems
• Describe why motivation is a major issue in the treatment
  of cluttering
• Describe the major areas that should be focused on in
  treatment

**Stuttering associated with acquired neurological
disorders (SAAD):** A term that has been suggested to
replace the term "neurogenic stuttering"
Pacing: A treatment technique in which each individual syllable is spoken separately, sometimes accompanied by physical
movement such as tapping a finger as each syllable is spoken
Delayed auditory feedback (DAF): Hearing one's own
voice a half-second or so after speaking. This is usually done
via a computer program, with the client speaking into a
microphone and hearing himself through headphones. It
typically forces a client to speak more slowly and reduces
stuttering dramatically
Fluency-inducing or fluency-enhancing conditions:
Stimuli that usually cause a person who stutters to speak much
more fluently. Examples are speaking in a rhythmic or staccato
manner, speaking under loud masking noise so the client can't
hear his own voice, and speaking while very relaxed

Trial therapy: A brief treatment of stuttering carried out during the evaluation to determine which treatment techniques are most effective

Prolonged speech: A treatment for stuttering, which induces the client to stretch out sounds, start new words with a gentle onset of phonation, and touch the articulators lightly when producing consonants

Traumatic brain injury (TBI): An injury to the brain from an external force. This may be either an injury that penetrates the skull (such as a bullet shot into the head) or a closed-head injury (such as bomb concussion) where penetration does not occur

Posttraumatic stress disorder (PTSD): An anxiety disorder that occurs after a person has experienced a traumatic event

Central language imbalance: Difficulty organizing spoken language

Mazing: A disorder of spoken language characterized by false starts, hesitations, and revisions that make the speaker's message difficult to understand

This chapter discusses three fluency disorders that are related to the "developmental" stuttering discussed in the first 14 chapters. These disorders—neurogenic stuttering, psychogenic stuttering, and cluttering—are similar to developmental stuttering in some ways, but are distinctly different in etiology, symptoms, and treatment. Figure 15.1 gives an overview of the chapter.

NEUROGENIC ACQUIRED STUTTERING

Nature

The term "neurogenic acquired stuttering" denotes stuttering that appears to be caused or exacerbated by neurological disease or damage. It is typically acquired after childhood, and its etiology may be stroke, head trauma, tumor, disease processes such as Parkinson's, or drug toxicity. Additional though rare causes are dialysis dementia, seizure disorders, bilateral thalamotomy, or thalamic stimulation (Duffy, 2005). Recently, stuttering has been seen in active duty service members with combat-related brain injury and co-occurring posttraumatic stress disorder (PTSD).[1]

Understanding neurogenic stuttering can help us understand some aspects of typical or "developmental" stuttering. Moreover, neurogenic stuttering in patients may be an early diagnostic sign of a neurological problem. Helm-Estabrooks (1999) describes this eloquently:

---

[1]This etiology is discussed in the section on psychogenic stuttering when I talk about differential diagnosis between neurogenic and psychogenic stuttering.

"Fluent speaking is, perhaps, the most refined motor act performed by humans, requiring complex coordination of many different muscle groups. It can be sensitive, therefore, to even small changes in neurological status, which may be why stuttering occurs in a wide range of neurological disorders, from Parkinson's disease to closed head injury. If this fact is ignored, clinicians may be overlooking an important early indicator of neurological disease" (p. 265).

Some writers prefer to use the term "neurogenic disfluency," because they don't consider neurogenic stuttering to be true stuttering. Such usage may, however, blur the distinction between two different phenomena that may occur with neurological insults. One is an increase in normal types of disfluencies (e.g., whole-word and phrase repetitions, revisions, interjections, and pauses); the other is a speech disorder presenting stutter-like disfluencies (i.e., part-word repetitions, prolongations, and blocks), sometimes accompanied by tension, struggle, escape, and avoidance behaviors.

Although much of the literature on neurogenic stuttering consists of single-case studies (e.g., Bijleveld, Lebrun, & van Dongen, 1994), there have been several attempts by clinician-researchers to summarize their findings on multiple cases and thereby develop a clearer picture of the disorder. Canter (1971) wrote a seminal article that went beyond case studies to suggest a possible way of categorizing types of neurogenic stuttering. He proposed three subgroups. One is dysarthric stuttering—seen, for example, in individuals who have Parkinson's disease or have a cerebellar lesion—in which stuttering appears to emerge from the same lack of neuromotor control as the primary dysarthric disorder. The second is apraxic stuttering, in which stuttering may arise from a basic problem in motor planning. Both silent blocks and repetitions occur as the speaker struggles to sequence the appropriate speech movements. The third subgroup is dysnomic stuttering, which sometimes accompanies aphasia. Stuttering symptoms occur as an individual searches for the word he is having trouble retrieving. Canter speculated that there may be a parallel to this type of stuttering in children who have word-retrieval problems and who develop stuttering as a result of their emotional reactions to the word-retrieval difficulty.

Rosenbek (1984) made the point that neurogenic stuttering should be distinguished from other disfluent behaviors that are associated with neurological problems, such as palilalia (word and phrase repetitions produced with increasing rate and decreasing loudness). It should also be distinguished from repetitions that some patients make as they try to correct their speech motor or linguistic errors. Observations of his own patients led Rosenbek to suggest that stuttering following nervous system damage is characterized primarily by involuntary repetitions of correct sounds and syllables, not those produced in error that occur at any place in a word (initial, medial, final). He was distressed by the lack of detail in clinicians' descriptions of patients with this disorder and

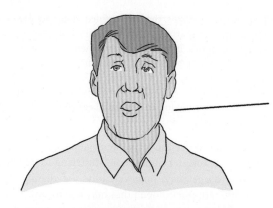

I-I recently-ly had a st-st-stroke

Neurogenic Stuttering

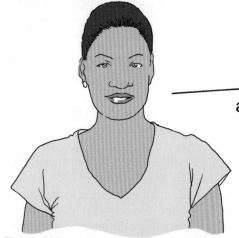

I've j....(silent block)...j ust ex-ex-ex-experienced
an e....(silent block) ..... e motionally upsetting event

Psychogenic Stuttering

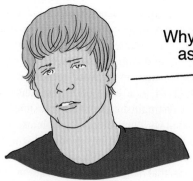

Why-why uh does everyone...you know..uh...tell me ...
ask me ..uh...to...uh...to repeat....well.... to repeat
what I've....what I've....uh....just said?

Cluttering

Figure 15.1 An overview of the material covered in Chapter 15.

called for a moratorium on the use of the term, "neurogenic stuttering," until more is known about it. Despite his call for a moratorium, case studies of "neurogenic stuttering" have continued to flow forth in the literature.

Helm-Estabrooks (1999), also unhappy with the term "neurogenic stuttering" thought it should be replaced with "**stuttering associated with acquired neurological disorders,**" which she abbreviates as **SAAD**. Part of her argument for using this new term is that this diagnostic category should include those adults whose preexisting childhood stuttering either worsened or recurred as a result of an acquired neurological disorder. Her point was that the stuttering in these cases was not initially caused by a neurological disorder. However, "neurogenic" can apply to disorders that are either caused or modified by neurological conditions (Merriam-Webster, 2004), and the term "neurogenic" is commonly used in our field and is a good deal simpler than SAAD. Thus, "neurogenic stuttering" is the term I use in this chapter.

Diagnosis and Evaluation

Helm-Estabrooks (1999) and Ringo and Dietrich (1995) provided a framework for assessing neurogenic stuttering and distinguishing it from other disorders. These authors suggested that the following procedures are important not only for evaluating individual cases but also for gathering data that may make a contribution to the literature.

1. A complete case history reflecting:
   - Onset of stuttering and its association with other neurological or psychological signs
   - The client's level of concern, anxiety, or fear about his stuttering
   - Extent to which stuttering interferes with communication
   - Changes in stuttering since onset
   - The client's history and family history of speech, language, or learning problems
   - The client's and relatives' handedness
   - Neurological and psychological health history

This information can be gathered initially through a case history and then supplemented during the interview.

2. Direct assessment of speech:
   - The Stuttering Severity Instrument should be administered, and speech should be video recorded during conversation and reading samples.
   - Stuttering in speech samples should be analyzed for:
     - Proportion of stuttering on function (grammatical) words versus content (substantive) words
     - Presence of stuttering on non-initial syllables, such as in these words "exciteme-me-ment," "cowb-b-b-oy," and "canister-er-er"
   - Absence of secondary (i.e., escape and avoidance) behaviors such as eye blinks, head nods, and use of "um" to get a word started.
     - The same short passage should be read aloud six times to determine if stuttering is reduced progressively through the repeated readings. See Chapter 1 for more information and references for this adaptation procedure.
   - Speaking in a variety of fluency-inducing conditions should be explored, especially speaking in a rhythm while swinging an arm, speaking while listening to loud masking noise, and speaking slowly under delayed auditory feedback (DAF) set at a 250-ms delay.

3. Other assessment components:
   - Helm-Estabrooks (1999) recommended using the Aphasia Diagnostic Profiles (Helm-Estabrooks, 1992) to exclude the possibility that the stuttering actually reflects language formulation problems.
   - Helm-Estabrooks (1999) also recommended that if other neurological problems are present and might interfere with treatment, neuropsychological testing would be important for assessing the client's capabilities.
   - De Nil, Jokel, and Rochon (2007) also strongly suggested testing for other disorders that may affect communication or treatment. These include dysarthria, aphasia, motor disorders, cognitive disorders, and chronic pain. These authors also provide an assessment battery that includes measures of attitudes about stuttering, including the S-24 (Andrews & Cutler, 1974) and the Locus of Control for Behavior (Craig, Franklin, & Andrews, 1984).

The information gathered from the above procedures can be used to improve our understanding of neurogenic stuttering, to differentially diagnose neurogenic stuttering (i.e., distinguish it from other fluency disorders), and to help in planning treatment. The data on the client's and relatives' handedness and history of speech, language, or learning problems are primarily used to determine if a client might have a predisposition for stuttering. Left-handedness or ambidexterity as well as a history of speech or language problems in a family may predispose an individual for stuttering (Geschwind & Galaburda, 1985). If a client began to stutter or if previous stuttering recurred or worsened in association with the occurrence of neurological problems, neurogenic stuttering should be suspected. On the other hand, stuttering that appeared in conjunction with the onset of psychological problems may be of psychogenic origin. Sometimes these etiologies are difficult to sort out and are discussed further in the section on psychogenic stuttering.

Turning now to direct assessment of speech, the following characteristics have been suggested as *more typical of neurogenic* than developmental stuttering (Canter, 1971; Helm-Estabrooks, 1999; Ringo & Dietrich, 1995; Rosenbek, 1984). These characteristics are described in Table 15.1.

Table 15.1	Characteristics More Typical of Neurogenic Stuttering
Domain	Characteristic
Locus of stuttering	In neurogenic stuttering, stuttering occurs on *function* words as well as content words. In developmental stuttering, it occurs much more frequently on content words (Bloodstein, 1995). In neurogenic stuttering, stuttering is *not restricted to initial* syllables in words, whereas it occurs primarily on initial syllables in developmental stuttering (Bloodstein, 1995).
Secondary behaviors	In neurogenic stuttering, there are relatively *few* secondary symptoms, and those that do occur are mild. In developmental stuttering—particularly in adults—there are usually escape and avoidance behaviors, which are sometimes severe.
Response to fluency-inducing conditions	In neurogenic stuttering, there is *little or no adaptation* with repeated readings of a passage. In developmental stuttering, there is a sudden decrease in frequency of stuttering in the second reading of the passage followed by further decreases that are increasingly smaller and smaller with each successive reading, so that by the fifth reading there is a 50 percent reduction on average (Bloodstein, 1995).
Emotional response	In individuals with neurogenic stuttering, there is relatively little fear and anxiety associated with the act of stuttering or speaking in general, although there may be frustration or annoyance. In developmental stuttering, most adults who stutter have fears and anxiety about stuttering and speaking (Bloodstein, 1995; Van Riper, 1982).

Summarizing the evaluation and diagnostic procedures, I think it is probably impossible to be certain that an individual has neurogenic stuttering rather than disfluencies caused by other impairments. Consequently, every effort needs to be made to rule out memory problems, language formulation problems (such as in aphasia), and emotional distress as the source of a client's disfluencies.

Considerations for Treatment

Helm-Estabrooks (1999) suggested several criteria for determining which clients have the potential to benefit from treatment. She noted that some neurogenic stuttering is quite mild and may not result in a handicap that warrants treatment. Other individuals, whose stuttering may be a serious handicap, may have other health problems which are far more serious, such as a progressive or fatal neurological disorder. A third consideration is the extent to which other neurological problems, such as dementia, may interfere with treatment. If a client does have severe and persistent stuttering, is motivated to undergo treatment, and has adequate cognitive and linguistic abilities to benefit from treatment, then several treatment options are available.

Treatment Approaches

Because individuals with neurogenic stuttering do not usually have the cognitive and emotional involvement that characterize developmental stuttering in adults, treatment is often entirely behavioral. An exception is when the neurological etiology of the stuttering is known and can be treated by surgery or drugs.

De Nil, Jokel, and Rochon (2007) noted that not all patients with neurogenic stuttering need treatment because as Helm, Butler, and Cantor (1980) have indicated, neurogenic stuttering may appear and then gradually improve without treatment.

1. Behavioral treatments. Many of the treatments (or components thereof) that are used for developmental stuttering have also been used for neurogenic stuttering with some success.
   - **Pacing**. This is essentially a technique of speaking one syllable at a time, so that each syllable is spoken separately, without the usual coarticulation across syllables. As a result, speech is produced more slowly and with a regular, staccato rhythm. This treatment was developed by Helm (1979) for patients with palilalia (i.e., rapid repetition of whole words and phrases), but has been used for neurogenic stuttering as well (Helm-Estabrooks, 1999). To facilitate pacing, especially in those patients who have difficulty slowing their speech, pacing devices can be used. One example is a pacing board (Helm-Estabrooks & Kaplan, 1989); another is a molded form that fits over the patient's finger (Rentschler, Driver, & Callaway, 1984). With either of these devices, the patient moves a finger from place to place, timing each syllable with a finger movement. Helm-Estabrooks (1999) suggested that pacing could begin with a device and progress to simply tapping rhythmically on the thigh to produce fluent speech. My own experience with developmental stutterers who have used syllable-timed speech to become fluent is that this treatment does not easily generalize to normal sounding (nonstaccato) speech.

- *Auditory masking and* **delayed auditory feedback (DAF).** Rentschler, Driver, and Callway. (1984), Marshall and Starch (1984), and Helm-Estabrooks (1999) reported that masking and DAF can be used as therapeutic tools to induce fluency in neurogenic stutterers, and in some cases, fluency can then be generalized.
- *Slow rate and easy onset.* Market, Montague, Buffalo, and Drummond (1990) conducted a survey of clinicians who had worked with acquired stuttering and found that many of them reported success with fluency-shaping tools, such as slow rate and easy onset.
- *Stuttering modification.* Only a modest percentage of the clinicians surveyed by Market and colleagues (1990) reported that they had used such stuttering modification tools as light contacts, preparatory sets, cancellations, and pull-outs.
- *Electromyographic biofeedback for tension reduction.* Reports by Helm-Estabrooks (1986) and Rubow, Rosenbek, and Schumaker (1986) suggested that training patients to relax muscles with the help of biofeedback can be effective in reducing neurogenic stuttering.

2. Neurosurgery. Sometimes when a neurological problem requires surgical intervention, the surgery resolves or improves stuttering. Cases reported by Donnan (1979) and Jones (1966) suggested that for whatever reason, surgery that resolved a neurological problem may also resolve stuttering. Andy and Bhatnagar (1992) reported on four patients who were improved by surgical implantations of electrodes to stimulate the thalamus for other neurological conditions. The implication is that some disturbance in neurological functioning can result in stuttering, and when the neurosurgery changes this neurological functioning, stuttering can be resolved. This finding is consistent with recent evidence suggesting that brain structure and function may be aberrant in developmental stuttering (e.g., Cykowski, Fox, Ingham, Ingham, & Robin, 2010; Foundas, Bollich, Corey, Hurley, & Heilman, 2001; Sommer, Koch, Paulus, Weiller, & Buchel, 2002).

3. Medications. As I described in Chapter 14, a number of drugs such as haloperidol, olanzapine, and pagoclone have been tried with varying degrees of success with developmental stuttering. These medications have not been tried, as far as I know, with neurogenic stuttering. Rather, case studies have reported that drugs for seizure disorders, schizophrenia, depression, anxiety, Parkinson's disease, and asthma can precipitate stuttering in individuals who have not stuttered previously (Baratz & Mesulam, 1981; Duffy, 2005; Elliott & Thomas, 1985; McClean & McClean, 1985; Nurnberg & Greenwald, 1981; Quader, 1977). In most of these cases, stuttering is reduced or eliminated when drug dosage is adjusted or an alternative drug is used. In other studies, drugs have been given for other symptoms and have relieved stuttering (Perino, Famularo, & Tarroni, 2000; Turgut, Utku, & Balci, 2002).

Overall, there is no clear consensus about effective treatments for neurogenic stuttering, and few studies present evidence of the long-term effectiveness of treatment. In part, this may be because the many different etiologies of neurogenic stuttering and the relative rarity of this disorder make long-term group studies of treatment of neurogenic stuttering unlikely.

Summary and Conclusions

Acquired neurogenic stuttering differs from developmental stuttering in a number of ways. Neurogenic stuttering usually has a sudden onset in adulthood, stuttering may occur with similar frequency on function and content words, stuttering is less restricted to the initial syllables of words, repeated readings of the same passage have less of an effect on neurogenic stuttering, many fluency-inducing conditions do not reduce stuttering, and often there is little fear and few secondary behaviors. Effective therapy may include surgery and drug adjustments for the underlying neurological problem as well as behavioral approaches, such as pacing or slowing speech.

Having highlighted the differences between developmental and neurogenic stuttering in this brief summary, I would also like to consider their similarities by asking this question: What does acquired neurogenic stuttering tell us about developmental stuttering? First, I will assume that both developmental and acquired neurogenic stuttering have neurological deficits at their cores. The evidence regarding acquired neurogenic stuttering suggests that insults to the brain in most regions (except for the occipital lobe and cranial nerves)—left hemisphere, right hemisphere, and subcortical areas—can result in at least temporary disfluencies (Duffy, 2005). Thus, it may be that neurological disturbances can affect fluency by interrupting speech and language information flow at many different places in the neural circuitry of these functions. In a chapter on neurogenic stuttering, De Nil, Jokel, and Rochon (2007) suggest that "…the neurological origin [of neurogenic stuttering] needs to be sought in a disruption of neural circuitry rather than a lesion in one specific brain region" (p. 330). In developmental stuttering, there may be several different inherited or congenital deficits in the neural circuitry subserving speech and language, but these different etiologies could produce mistimings or discoordinations that have a small range of possible outcomes in disturbances of fluency, such as repetitions, prolongations, and blocks, making it appear as a unitary disorder. In other words, if interruptions of the flow of information during speech processing could occur at many different sites, these interruptions may be limited in their possible effects. Perhaps only repetitions, prolongations, or blocks are the natural outcome of such interruptions—in both developmental and neurogenic stuttering.

The evidence that acquired neurogenic stuttering is often not accompanied by fear or secondary symptoms suggests that they are independent of the core symptoms, which supports the belief that these aspects of stuttering are reactions that develop as a child experiences more and more negative reactions to his difficulty by listeners and himself. Of course, there are adult developmental stutterers who lack fear and secondary symptoms, hinting at the possibility that they may be a subgroup of developmental stutterers who resemble neurogenic stutterers.

Other frequently mentioned differences from developmental stuttering are that many neurogenic stutterers stutter as much on medial as on initial consonants and sometimes stutter on final consonants. In addition, they are as likely to stutter on function words as on content words. Ringo and Dietrich (1995) pointed out that the profession, as yet, lacks adequate data to be confident of these findings. However, these data hint at the fact that neurogenic stuttering may not be influenced as much by linguistic variables as is developmental stuttering. I wonder, therefore, if the linguistic variability of developmental stuttering might be just an artifact of its onset during a critical period of language learning.

In conclusion, professionals working with clients having acquired neurogenic stuttering should be encouraged to develop systematic ways of collecting and sharing data (see Appendix B of Ringo & Dietrich, 1995) so that this infrequently occurring disorder can be better understood. As a consequence, we may better understand stuttering of all kinds.

PSYCHOGENIC ACQUIRED STUTTERING

Nature

Psychogenic stuttering, like neurogenic stuttering, is a late-onset disorder (late teens and older). Its major identifying feature is that it typically begins after a prolonged period of stress or after a traumatic event. It has sometimes been characterized as a conversion symptom (i.e., a physical or behavioral expression of a psychological conflict) (Lazare, 1981). Unlike malingering or faking, this type of stuttering is not conscious, volitional behavior by the client, but it is involuntary. Several authors (Baumgartner, 1999; Duffy, 2005; Mahr & Leith, 1992; Roth, Aronson, & Davis, 1989) have described its manifestations, diagnosis, and treatment, and this section borrows a good deal from them.

The stuttering pattern of this disorder resembles developmental stuttering in terms of core behaviors (i.e., repetitions, prolongations, and blocks), but in some cases, secondary behaviors may be unusual and occur independently of attempts to produce stuttered words (Baumgartner, 1999). Psychogenic stuttering may occur alone or together with other signs of psychological or neurological involvement. Strict definitions of psychogenic stuttering exclude cases in which childhood stuttering had been resolved but then reappeared under prolonged or sudden stress. Nonetheless, these cases may respond to treatment as readily as do many cases of true psychogenic stuttering.

When I conducted intensive group stuttering therapy in Australia, I treated a young man whose stutter had started in his late teens. He had never stuttered as a child, nor did he have a family history of stuttering. The onset of his stuttering occurred when, unable to afford graduate education in his preferred area, geology, he went into a teacher training program which included a practicum experience. During this classroom training, he began to stutter, was required to leave teacher education, and was then able to attend graduate school in geology. He came to our intensive group stuttering therapy stuttering rather severely, but quite well adjusted otherwise. After three weeks, he was completely fluent (as were the other members of the group), and he continued to maintain his fluency (unlike some of the group members) for as long as I was able to follow him, 18 months beyond the end of treatment.

I have no evidence of this, but I would speculate that for this young man, the anxiety of teaching for the first time created some initial disfluency when he spoke to his classes. Perhaps anxiety interferes with fine motor control in many people. After this initial loss of speech motor control, his natural self-consciousness, combined with a desire to find a way out of the teaching profession, somehow turned a spontaneous and momentary disfluency into a full-blown stutter. Because it had become conditioned to many stimuli associated with speaking, the stuttering persisted even though he had left teaching and returned to his first love, geology. Speculating further, his treatment may have been successful because the stuttering had begun within the past few years, and he was ripe for relearning his natural fluent speech pattern. If true, then some cases of psychogenic stuttering may resolve if they are treated promptly with an intensive speech retraining program and if the conflict which triggered the stuttering is alleviated.

Diagnosis and Evaluation

Roth, Aronson, and Davis (1989) pointed out that adult-onset stuttering can have several etiologies that need to be considered: purely neurogenic, purely psychogenic, psychogenic accompanied by psychogenically based neurologic signs, psychogenic with coexisting (but unrelated) neurologic disease or disorder. Thus, one of the first aims of an evaluation is to rule out a neurological etiology, particularly since adult-onset stuttering is sometimes the first sign of a neurologic disorder. A multidisciplinary approach, involving neurology, psychiatry, and speech-language pathology, may be best, especially if a client has neurological signs, such as headache, dizziness, or numbness of extremities.

The evaluation should include:

1. A complete case history obtained either exclusively in an interview or followed up with an interview. The case history should obtain information concerning:
   - Onset of stuttering, including circumstances surrounding onset, such as whether it occurred during prolonged or acute stress and the nature and pattern of the stuttering when it began
   - Changes in stuttering since onset and whether there have been times of complete fluency
   - Current pattern of stuttering, its situational variability, and its impact on the client's life
   - Whether the individual stuttered previously at any time and if so, its nature and pattern and the extent of recovery
   - Family history of stuttering and other speech, language, or learning problems

   If the clinician can maintain an interested, accepting attitude, the client is more likely to reveal vital information about the emotions associated with the stuttering. Baumgartner (1999) noted that clients' expression of feelings may be accompanied by increased fluency, which is a sign of psychogenic basis for the stuttering.

2. Baumgartner (1999) suggests giving adult-onset clients a motor speech exam (Duffy, 2005) to rule out such motor speech disorders as apraxia or Parkinson's disease that might underlie stuttering. He also suggests that if clients evidence signs of language or cognitive problems, these should be further tested.

3. As with neurological stuttering, clients should be asked to speak under traditional **fluency-inducing or fluency-enhancing conditions** that were listed in the evaluation procedures for suspected neurogenic stuttering. If a client stutters even more frequently or severely while speaking under these conditions, psychogenic stuttering should be suspected (Baumgartner, 1999).

4. **Trial therapy** should be carried out, and the clinician should model what is expected of the client and liberally provide praise and support to encourage him. More specific steps include the following:
   - Have the client try to stay in a moment of stuttering. The clinician first models this, then instructs the client, and may even need to use a cue to help the client "catch" a moment of stuttering and hold on to it. In this and subsequent steps, the client may stop holding onto a stutter because he has run out of breath or for other reasons. The clinician should accept this and instruct him to "get the stutter going again," even though at this point, it may be a voluntary behavior rather than a true stutter.
   - While the client is holding onto a stutter, have him touch places on his face or throat where he appears to be tensing or "holding back" the word that is being stuttered.
   - While the client is holding onto a stutter, have him change the tension, the speeding up, or other elements of the stutter, so that the sound becomes prolonged voluntarily.
   - When the client has changed the "holding back" behaviors, the clinician should then coach him to slowly finish the stuttered word, making a slow transition from the stutter into the remainder of the word.
   - Following this, the clinician should guide the client through the first four steps on his own while reading aloud or conversing.

   These steps of trial therapy could be replaced by another behavioral treatment the clinician typically uses. Another trial therapy approach is given in the section on stuttering onset as a result of stress and injuries while in the military. In any case, the point of trial therapy with psychogenic stuttering is to see if the client becomes dramatically more fluent during trial therapy—another sign of psychogenicity. Whatever approach works should be used as a complete approach to treatment, with steps for generalization.

5. Analysis of stuttering. Samples should be obtained of the client's conversational speech and reading aloud so that baseline measures of stuttering severity can be made with the SSI-4, and the patterns of stuttering can be examined. As mentioned above, unusual struggle behaviors, especially if they are independent of moments of stuttering, are signs of possible psychogenicity of stuttering.

Diagnosis of psychogenic stuttering is usually tentative. The clinician must weigh multiple factors, and even then, a conclusive diagnosis might never be reached. The most clear-cut pieces of evidence for this diagnosis are (a) adult onset during psychological stress and (b) the absence of neurological factors associated with the client's stuttering. Two other factors can help support the diagnosis—(c) dramatic improvement with trial therapy and (d) unusual or bizarre struggle behaviors.

Considerations for Treatment

Individuals who are able to decrease their stuttering in trial therapy and whose psychological adjustment is adequate are often good candidates for stuttering therapy. Even though they may need psychotherapy eventually, speech therapy may start immediately. On the other hand, clients who are unable to improve fluency during trial therapy and/or who are dysfunctional because of psychological issues may benefit from receiving psychotherapy concurrently with (or prior to) stuttering therapy. Individuals who resist the idea that their stuttering may have a stress-related basis and who do not improve with trial therapy may not be good candidates for treatment or may need extended treatment.

Treatment Approaches

Several published reports on psychogenic stuttering suggest that speech therapy can be very effective with this group of clients (Baumgartner, 1999; Duffy, 2005; Mahr & Leith, 1992; Roth, Aronson, & Davis, 1989). Baumgartner emphasized that clients benefit from an understanding that their stuttering is not the result of neurological problems and from the clinician's continuing encouragement about their progress.

Most treatments used with developmental stuttering have been reported to be effective with psychogenic stuttering (Roth, Aronson, & Davis, 1989). In my own experience, a **prolonged speech** fluency-shaping approach was very beneficial for a young adult who had developed stuttering suddenly when he did not want to pursue a career in classroom teaching but was required to do so because of the financial support he'd received for his education. Roth, Aronson, and Davis (1989) suggested that approaches such as easy onset, light contact, and easy repetitions can be effective. Baumgartner (1999) worked with clients to diminish extra motor behaviors and reduce the physical tension associated with their efforts to speak. Duffy (2005) provided a seven-step procedure in which the clinician helps the client reduce tension and changes repetitive stutters into more normal-sounding prolongations while giving support and reassurance for gradual progress. Weiner (1981) employed desensitization combined with vocal control therapy that emphasized adequate respiratory support, gentle onsets, and optimal vocal resonance. Transfer was carried out using a hierarchy of easy-to-difficult situations. Unfortunately, no long-term treatment outcomes for therapy with psychogenic stuttering have been reported.

There are still many mysteries to be solved about psychogenic stuttering. One is whether the anomalies in brain activity patterns seen in developmental stuttering (Chapters 2 and 3) are present in this disorder. Another is whether psychological stress produces mistimings and discoordinations that result in the disorder or whether psychological factors actually result in highly coordinated struggle behaviors that reflect the speaker's efforts to speak despite primitive reflexes holding back speech. It is appropriate to ask what, if anything, psychogenic stuttering teaches us about developmental stuttering. Some electromyographic studies of developmental stuttering have shown co-contraction of speech production muscles in a fashion that impedes speech flow (Freeman & Ushijima, 1975; Guitar, Guitar, Neilson, O'Dwyer, & Andrews, 1988). If the same co-contractions are evident in psychogenic stuttering, it may suggest that these muscle activities in developmental stuttering are learned "holding back" responses rather than evidence of discoordination.

Stuttering as a Result of Stress and Injuries While in the Military

This is a special section for those readers who will be working with active duty military service members or veterans whose stuttering appeared as the result of stress or injuries while in combat. The information comes from a presentation at the 2011 ASHA Convention about this topic presented by

Roth, Manning, and Duffy (2011) (https://cms.psav.com/cPaper2012/myitinerary/day.html).

Sudden-onset stuttering not infrequently appears in military personnel who have been in combat and who have sustained **traumatic brain injury (TBI)** and/or **posttraumatic stress disorder (PTSD)**. Such stuttering presents a challenge in terms of differential diagnosis (neurogenic, psychogenic stuttering, or a combination) and treatment. The combined experiences of Carole Roth, Kevin Manning, and Joe Duffy provide some guidelines for assessing and treating these clients. Their stuttering-like behaviors can include initial syllable or whole-word repetitions, prolongations, tension with facial grimaces, posturing of articulators or whispering before starting speech, hesitations, and/or blocking before initial sounds. These speech behaviors may be accompanied (and exacerbated) by attention problems, slow speed of processing, and word-retrieval problems. Other signs of PTSD may be present such as problems sleeping, nightmares, or difficulty concentrating.

Differential diagnosis is not always possible and may not be absolutely necessary. Signs of neurogenic stuttering, as indicated in the earlier section, include stuttering on both content and function words, lack of secondary symptoms such as tension and struggle, no reduction of stuttering during repeated reading of a passage, and little fear and anxiety about speech (e.g., De Nil, Jokel, & Rochon, 2007). Signs of psychogenic stuttering, as indicated, include onset during psychological stress (which may include experience of combat injury), dramatic improvement during trial therapy, and absence of verified neurological impairment.

In the evaluation (and treatment) it is important to listen carefully to the client's complaints and take them seriously. Moreover, the clinician should help the client understand why combat stress may produce stuttering. For example, the clinician can describe how all speakers may become disfluent if they are under the stress of hurry, confusion, or indecision. Combat stress can be thought of as an extreme and prolonged instance of this. A key part of the evaluation is trial therapy, which should be carried out with a very positive, confident manner. Duffy (in Roth, Manning, & Duffy, 2011) suggests the clinician put her hands on the thyrohyoid area, feel for tension, and have the speaker talk while the clinician pulls the thyroid cartilage down to a more relaxed position. The client can be told that he is maintaining excessive tension in this area; the clinician can then guide him through a hierarchy of producing vowels, single words, sentences, and conversation in a very relaxed and slow style. Psychological basis of the stuttering is supported if the client becomes very fluent in this trial treatment. The clinician should be careful to explain the client's fluency to him, relating it to the relaxation which counteracts the excess tension developed as a response to stress.

If fluency is not obtained through muscle relaxation, a fluency-shaping technique such as slow, prolonged speech should be used. Whichever technique is effective should be explained to the client and taught in subsequent sessions, with appropriate generalization to the client's everyday life. In many cases, group stuttering therapy or group psychotherapy (led by a psychologist) can be an effective adjunct to individual treatment, especially if some focus is made on other aspects of PTSD.

Summary and Conclusions

In the past 10 years, there has been an increasing acceptance of the idea that disfluencies associated with psychological trauma and stress may actually be a type of stuttering. The main diagnostic markers are (a) stuttering onset that occurs in late adolescence or adulthood; (b) stuttering onset that is associated with prolonged or acute stress; (c) unusual struggle behaviors that may not always be associated with moments of stuttering; (d) stuttering that increases in fluency-inducing conditions; and (e) dramatically improved fluency during trial treatment. Compared with neurogenic stuttering, there is relatively little known about the speech characteristics observed in psychogenic stuttering (such as the linguistic loci of stutters) nor is there consensus on the common types of core behaviors associated with this disorder.

| CLUTTERING

Nature

Many years ago, cluttering was described as "...a torrent of half-articulated words, following each other like peas running out of a spout" (Van Riper, 1954). The essence of cluttering, as this quote suggests, is rapid speaking that is difficult to understand. Words may be collapsed, syllables may be omitted, or sounds may be slurred. Cluttering is often accompanied by disfluencies that differ from those typically heard in stuttering; instead, clutterers may produce fillers, incomplete phrases, word and phrase repetitions, revisions, and hesitations—all usually without tension. A clutterer's speaking rate is not continuously rapid, however, but gives the impression of coming in sudden impulsive bursts that are filled with misarticulations and disfluencies. In contrast to stutterers, clutterers become more fluent—as well as slower and more intelligible—when they make an effort to control their disorder. This rarely happens, unfortunately, because most clutterers are often not aware they are "cluttering" unless someone brings it to their attention.

Several excellent publications on cluttering have described the disorder as manifesting the above speech characteristics but also as being characterized by, in many cases, language and learning problems (St. Louis, 1996; St. Louis, Raphael, Myers, & Bakker, 2003; St. Louis, Myers, Bakker, & Raphael, 2007; Ward & Scott, 2011). The language problems were first recognized by Weiss (1964), who described cluttering as a problem of "**central language imbalance**" that may reflect a disorganized formulation process. The person who clutters seems to be unable to put his thoughts into coherent sentences and link them together in a logical way. Such language behavior is sometimes termed "**mazing**," a metaphor for repeated false starts, hesitations, and revisions that leave listeners puzzled about a speaker's verbal destination. The concomitant problems of people with cluttering may include distractibility, hyperactivity, learning difficulties, articulation problems, and auditory processing problems. Cluttering is sometimes accompanied by stuttering.

Cluttering, then, appears to be a disorder whose core signs or symptoms are rapid and irregular speech rate that is often unintelligible and replete with nonstuttered disfluencies. Language is often disorganized and the individual often lacks awareness of his difficulty and of listener cues signaling lack of understanding. Neuropsychological problems may or may not be present. Speculation about the neurophysiological basis of the disorder suggests abnormalities in the basal ganglia (Alm, 2004; Kent, 2000).

Diagnosis and Evaluation

The process of evaluating a client for possible cluttering differs for different ages (school-age versus adult) and will vary depending on the setting in which the evaluation takes place (e.g., school versus university or hospital clinic). In many cases, especially with school-age children, a multidisciplinary approach to evaluation is important and may involve the SLP, classroom teacher, special educator, psychologist, and audiologist. In the following section, I give some general guidelines that reflect information gleaned from several sources, including Myers and St. Louis (1986; 2007); St. Louis, (1996); St. Louis and colleagues (2003); and van Zaalen, Wijnen, and Dejonckere (2011).

Case History and Interview

The case history can be filled out by a client (or parent) beforehand and used as a guideline for the interview. Among the important areas to be covered in the case history and interview are:

- The client's, parents', and/or teachers' perceptions of the problem. What aspects of the cluttering "syndrome" are the presenting problem (from the viewpoint of the person completing the form and participating in the interview)? Because the individual who clutters is himself often unaware of his own speech, an adult or adolescent may report that his problem is that people say he's sometimes hard to understand. It should be ascertained, however, how cluttering affects him. For example, does he have a hard time in school, social situations, or his job because people don't always understand him?
- How long the problem has existed. In some cases, cluttering might have begun in preschool years, but it is usually not until the school years when listeners tell him that he's mumbling or talking too fast, or that they simply can't understand him. Nonetheless, it is useful to gather information

about the individual's speech and language development—whether it was delayed, advanced, or atypical.

- When and where the problem appears. Cluttering can be variable, so it's important to understand which situations are particularly troublesome. This may depend on the listeners and the demands of the situation. Some children may do well when they are reading or giving one-word answers, but may lose intelligibility during narratives. Adults who clutter may be fluent and intelligible when speaking to close friends, but their intelligibility may suffer when speaking in more demanding situations.
- Background on the individual and his family. It is helpful in understanding a client's cluttering to view it in a larger perspective, including whether other members of the client's extended family clutter or have other communication or learning problems, whether the client has other problems, such as stuttering, that interfere with communication, and whether the client has received treatment for his communication problem(s) and how successful treatment has been.
- Reasons for seeking treatment at this time. A major determinant of success in cluttering therapy is the client's motivation. It is important to find out from the case history or interview whether the client is aware of his cluttering and whether it bothers him enough to undertake the hard work that successful therapy will require.
- Other problems. The case history and interview should determine if the client has any of the other problems that often accompany cluttering, such as receptive or expressive language difficulties, articulation problems, central auditory processing deficits, attention deficit/hyperactivity, reading problems, or learning disabilities.

Direct Assessment of Speech

The client's speech should be examined on a variety of tasks in a variety of situations. Cluttering, like stuttering, varies a great deal so it is easy to gain a false impression from a small sample of speech gathered in the clinic. The website for the International Cluttering Association (http://associations.missouristate.edu/ICA/) contains a link to software for evaluating cluttering.

Recording of Speech

The client should be digitally audio or video recorded for 15 or 20 minutes while performing a number of speaking tasks, including:

- A narrative about a topic not related to his speech, such as describing what he did on his last vacation or a favorite movie. This should be done in a way that really engages the client in talking so that a natural, unguarded sample can be obtained.
- Reading a passage appropriate for his reading level
- A conversation in which the client talks about something that really interests him

- For clients who report that their cluttering is situational, a sample should be recorded in the relevant environments.
- Van Zaalen, Wijnen, and Dejonckere (2011) also recommend that older clients should be asked to produce words that may be difficult, such as "statistical" or "chrysanthemum," as well as words with differing stress patterns such as "apply," "application," and "applicable" to assess their ability to handle complex phonological sequences and changing linguistic stress patterns. These authors also recommend retelling a story.

Analysis of Speech

After the recording has been made, the speech samples should be analyzed to assess speech rate in syllables per minute using the procedures described in Chapter 8. Many individuals who clutter can reduce their overly fast rate when they try so the narrative and reading samples may show slower rates than do conversation samples. If it is the clinician's impression during the evaluation that the client's speech rate was not slower during narrative or reading compared to conversation (as would be expected for most speakers), she should ask the client to engage in a narrative task and try to speak at a slow, normal rate. The client's ability to slow his speaking rate may be a good prognostic sign, because much of cluttering therapy is focused on slowing a client's speaking rate. The various samples can be compared to the speech rate norms for different ages that were given in Chapter 9.

Many clutterers don't speak at a consistently fast rate, but at a relatively normal rate with sudden bursts of rapid speech. Assessment, therefore, should include measures of speech rate during these bursts and how frequently they occur. A comparison may be made between the client's articulatory rate (i.e., syllables per second with pauses are excluded) during fast bursts of speech and during regular speech. The articulatory rates of typical adults in conversation are six to seven syllables per second (St. Louis et al., 2003).

Analysis of Stuttering Versus Cluttering

Analysis of speech samples should also include separate counts of normal-type disfluencies and stuttering-like disfluencies (see Chapters 7 and 9 for this distinction). The number of syllables that are normally disfluent and the number that are stuttered can be expressed as a proportion of the total number of syllables spoken in the sample. These measures will reflect the proportions of stuttering and cluttering in the client's speech. Some clients have both stuttering and cluttering in their speech, but one usually predominates. It has been suggested that when stuttering is mixed with cluttering, a client's cluttering may not be noticed until his stuttering is substantially reduced by therapy (Bakker, 2002; St. Louis et al., 2003).

Analysis of Meaningful Versus Extraneous Syllables

When I evaluate a client with cluttering, I find it useful to calculate the ratio of the number of syllables spoken that are part of the intended message if that can be reliably discerned to the number of syllables spoken that are extraneous to the message. For example, in the utterance, "Well, you see, I think, I think the, the, the sky is well is blue" (15 syllables), we can assume that the speaker meant to convey "I think the sky is blue" (six syllables). Thus, nine syllables, or 60 percent of the utterance, are extraneous which undoubtedly detracts from the speaker's communicative effectiveness. This measure may be helpful also in assessing a client's progress in therapy.

Analysis of Intelligibility

The intelligibility of a sample should be assessed by having one or more listeners unfamiliar with the client gloss (i.e., interpret) each word and each utterance. The percentage of words and of utterances that understood can be calculated, providing pretherapy measures of a client's intelligibility.

Language Assessment

The language skills of clients who clutter are likely to be affected by the disorder. In fact, Weiss (1964) described cluttering as a central language imbalance, suggesting that language deficits are its core.

Wiig (2002) suggested that many aspects of clutterers' language can be effectively tested using the Clinical Evaluation of Language Fundamentals (CELF-3) (Semel, Wiig, & Secord, 1996). Obviously this applies to the CELF-4 which is appropriate for individuals from 5 to 21 years old. This test assesses "the relationships among semantics, syntax/morphology, and pragmatics, and the interrelated domains of receptive and expressive language." Wiig suggested that it be administered in such a way that a client's responses could be timed, because under time pressure, which simulates everyday conversational situations, the clutterer's scores might well be lower.

It may also be helpful to assess a client's pragmatic behaviors in the videotaped conversational sample described above. Pragmatic skills that may be lacking include appropriate turn-taking, supplying complete information to the listener, and repairing communication when it breaks down. Other aspects of language assessment are described in van Zaalen, Wijnen, and Dejonckere (2011) and Myers and St. Louis (2007).

Assessment of Cluttering Characteristics

Clients may exhibit a variety of traits that are part of the cluttering syndrome. The clinician may find it helpful to use Daly's Predictive Cluttering Inventory (2006), available in seven languages from http://associations.missouristate.edu/ICA/Resources/Resources%20and%20Links%20pages/clinical_materials.htm. This checklist evaluates a client in four areas: pragmatics, speech-motor control, language-cognition, and motor coordination-writing problems. It can be used for assessing areas of deficit as well as for treatment planning. These ratings help the clinician determine which cluttering characteristics are most salient and are therefore most in need of treatment.

Assessment of Coexisting Disorders

In the process of gathering information about a client, the clinician may become aware of challenges that affect communication but are not the province of only the SLP. These may include auditory processing disorders, attention-deficit disorder, hyperactivity, reading difficulties, social adjustment problems, illegible handwriting, and learning disabilities (Ward & Scott, 2011). These challenges may best be assessed with the help of other specialists, such as an audiologist, psychologist, learning specialist, reading specialist, and the classroom teacher.

Considerations for Treatment

Because clients who clutter are usually not aware of their problem and are often surprised when listeners don't understand them, they rarely seek treatment. Indeed, those who do seek treatment are often referred by someone else. Some clutterers, however, can be motivated to work hard in therapy and can make good progress. Two positive prognostic signs are the ability to speak without cluttering if asked to do so and a specific reason for improving, such as keeping a job or receiving a promotion at work. Children who clutter can often be engaged in games and activities that will create motivation for their work in treatment.

Treatment Approaches

The evaluation procedures described above should suggest the areas that are particular challenges for each client. Treatment can then focus on these areas of need. Bennett Lanouette (2011), Myers (2002; 2011), and Myers and St. Louis (2007) outlined several cluttering therapy strategies that they have explored in their work with cluttering over several years. I describe them in the following section with some minor changes:

1. Increase the client's awareness of his speech rate and his ability to decrease rate.
   - Simulate various speaking rates by having the client move his arm or walk at slow, medium, and fast tempos. Then, teach the client to attend to his sensory feedback while he is doing this so that he learns the feeling of these rates.
   - Alternate between speaking and moving various body parts or walking at various rates while attending to sensory feedback.
   - Use movements and walking paced by fast and slow music.
   - With children, engage in activities in which they can get speeding tickets or give speeding tickets to the clinician for speaking too fast.
   - Teach clients to attend to various verbal and nonverbal cues from a listener that indicates they are speaking too

quickly or cannot be understood. For example, listeners may frown or show puzzlement on their faces or repeatedly ask the speaker to repeat himself.

- For readers, put symbols at periods and commas, such as red or yellow lights, to help them slow their speech rate at relevant places in a text.
- Teach phrasing and pausing in conversational speech.
- Use the concept of a speedometer for children and ask them to speak at 75 miles per hour or at 35 miles per hour.
- Teach clients to speak with strong stress patterns by reciting poetry, for example.

2. Improve linguistic skills.
- Teach clients to chunk and sequence their thoughts by having them write a story or narrative on cards, sequence them, and then tell the story aloud using the cards.
- Involve clients in skits and plays so that they learn to follow a script and use turn-taking.
- Teach them such narrative skills as turn-taking in conversation and staying on topic in conversation.
- Teach them how to use complex sentences with subordinate clauses.

3. Facilitate fluency.
- Use DAF to help clients learn to speak in a slower, more fluent manner.
- Use DAF to teach proprioception, by having clients speak at a normal rate under maximal delay (i.e., 250 ms) by ignoring auditory feedback.

4. Increase the client's knowledge and awareness of cluttering.
- Teach clients about the disorder of cluttering using Daly and Burnett-Stolnack's (1995) checklist to help the client learn which cluttering behaviors he has.
- Have the client transcribe and analyze a recording of his cluttered speech.
- Help the client become aware of his thought processes when he is talking in fast bursts of disorganized speech.

Further suggestions for treatment were presented by St. Louis and colleagues (2003), which included:

1. Rather than admonish the client to "slow down," have him match the clinician's speech rate using a computer-based program to display the clinician's and client's utterances. The Visi-Pitch® and the Computerized Speech Lab from Kay Elemetrics are examples of programs that can do this.

2. To help clients achieve their potential to use normal speech, have them imagine themselves (i.e., in their mind's eye and ear) speaking effectively and have them use positive self-talk to strengthen their visual and auditory images. It may help also for the client and clinician to video record the client's best and worst speech and play these samples back to him to remind him of the range of his options.

3. When working on intelligibility and organization, begin with short utterances that are spoken clearly, and then gradually increase length and complexity while ensuring

high quality of fluency, articulation, rate, and organization. Video recording and replaying them can help clients establish an auditory-visual image for what they are aiming.

In his chapter on treatment of cluttering, Daly (1986) provides his own guidelines for many of the treatment strategies described earlier. He believes that video feedback and analysis of audio samples are crucial for increasing a client's self-awareness. He also advocates helping clients learn to use relaxation exercises, mental imagery, and positive self-talk. His chapter has many references, which can help clinicians learn more about these activities.

There are very few studies of the treatment outcomes of cluttering therapy, and the ones that do exist consist of only one or two cases. A special edition of the *Journal of Fluency Disorders* (vol. 21, nos. 3–4, September–December 1996) on cluttering has a number of case studies. For example, data on a clutterer-stutterer treated in a three-week intensive smooth speech program indicated that the client's stuttering and speech rate were reduced to near-normal limits and that the gains appeared to be retained 10 months after treatment.

Summary and Conclusions

Cluttering is a disorder with a probable neurological etiology. It is characterized by an excess of disfluencies, rapid rates of speech that often occur in momentary bursts, and lack of intelligibility, especially in bursts of increased rate. Although there is relatively little research on the nature and treatment of cluttering, there is some consensus that it isn't viewed as a problem until a child has reached school age. Evaluation procedures include (a) obtaining background information to determine, among other things, whether or not the client is aware of the problem and is motivated to undergo therapy, (b) direct assessment of speech on several different tasks to measure: (i) frequency and type of disfluencies, (ii) speech rate and intelligibility overall as well as during fast bursts of speech, (c) language testing, particularly pragmatics and other aspects of expressive language, and (d) assessment of other, possible concomitant disorders. Treatment should address the interdependent qualities of speech rate, fluency, intelligibility, and expressive language. Although many clinicians report success with motivated clients, there are essentially no outcome data on a particular treatment approach for cluttering.

Because cluttering most often co-occurs with stuttering, the disorders appear to be related in some as yet undetermined way. Given the strong effect of slow speaking on stuttering and cluttering alike, it is possible that subgroups of stutterers and clutterers have difficulty maintaining a slow enough rate to match their capacity to synchronize the elements of language and speech output. Perhaps each disorder has a particular level of processing at which such dyssynchrony occurs.

Table 15.2	Comparative Characteristics of Developmental, Neurogenic, and Psychogenic Stuttering and Cluttering			
	Developmental Stuttering	Neurogenic Stuttering	Psychogenic Stuttering	Cluttering
Etiology	Probably neurophysiological (anomalies in left hemisphere) exacerbated by temperament and environment	Stroke, head trauma, tumor, disease process, drug toxicity, dialysis dementia, seizure disorder, bilateral thalamotomy, thalamic stimulation	Prolonged stress, psychological conflict, psychologically traumatic event; emotional arousal or emotional conflict appears to interfere with speech production.	Probably neurological, possibly related to dysfunction in basal ganglia
Typical onset	Usually ages 2–5, with some onsets in school years	Usually after childhood, following a neurological event. However, in rare cases, stuttering could be the first sign of a neurological problem.	Usually after childhood, following prolonged stress or after a psychologically traumatic event. Sometimes occurs in conjunction with apparent neurological problems.	May be present in preschool years, but often not diagnosed until problem interferes with school performance
Speech characteristics	Single-syllable whole-word repetitions, part-word repetitions, prolongations, and blocks. Frequency is usually more than 3 percent syllables stuttered. Secondary behaviors (escape and avoidance) common. Pattern varies somewhat.	Stuttering appears on function as well as content words; stuttering not restricted to word-initial syllables; absence of secondary behaviors; little adaptation in repeated readings; stuttering not markedly reduced in fluency-inducing conditions.	Stuttering remains constant or increases while speaking under fluency-inducing conditions; may have unusual struggle behaviors; stuttering may show stereotyped pattern; client may show dramatic improvement with trial therapy.	Excess of normal disfluencies, lack of intelligibility, especially during rapid bursts of speech. May slur syllables and leave out others entirely.
Client's level of concern	Client typically shows frustration and embarrassment about stuttering, as well as fear of speaking.	Client may be annoyed or frustrated, but not fearful or anxious about stuttering.	Variable, from indifferent to concerned.	Frequently unaware of problem, except when listeners tell him they can't understand what he's said.
Other diagnostic information	Frequency and severity are often variable from day to day and situation to situation.	Need to rule out possibility that disfluencies are from memory or language formulation problems or from emotional distress about neurological problem.	Absence of neurological problems which could cause stuttering; client may benefit from psychotherapy as well as stuttering therapy if inclined.	Often accompanied by stuttering, as well as language, attention, auditory processing, writing, and reading problems, and other learning disabilities.
Treatment	School-age children and adults benefit from integration of behavioral, affective, and cognitive focus of stuttering therapy.	Pacing, masking, delayed auditory feedback, slow rate, and easy onset	Fluency shaping or tension reduction.	Increase awareness of cluttering, particularly fast speech rate. Help client self-regulate speech rate and fluency. Improve expressive language skills.

SUMMARY

Table 15.2 summarizes the characteristics of neurogenic stuttering, psychogenic stuttering, and cluttering and compares these characteristics with those of typical developmental stuttering.

STUDY QUESTIONS

1. If you had only one activity you could do with a client to differentiate neurogenic from psychogenic stuttering, which activity would you choose and why?

2. After reading about neurogenic stuttering, do you think that Canter's three categories of neurogenic stuttering are adequate? Why or why not?

3. Name four characteristics of stuttering behavior that appear to distinguish neurogenic stuttering from developmental stuttering.

4. What are contraindications (if any) for treatment of neurogenic stuttering?

5. If an adult-onset client had evidence of a neurological disorder, would you rule out psychogenic stuttering? Why or why not?

6. Compare the reported treatment success of psychogenic stuttering and neurogenic stuttering.

7. What are the contraindications (if any) for treatment of psychogenic stuttering?

8. What are the two most salient problems in cluttering?

9. Why might language and learning problems be related to the speech problems of cluttering?

10. What are the contraindications (if any) for treatment of cluttering?

| SUGGESTED READINGS

Neurogenic Stuttering
De Nil, L., Jokel, R., & Rochon, E. (2007). Etiology, symptomatology, and treatment of neurogenic stuttering. In E. Conture & R.F. Curlee (Eds.), *Stuttering and Related Disorders of Fluency* (2nd ed.) (pp. 326–343). New York: Thieme Medical Publishers.

This chapter covers prevalence and incidence of neurogenic stuttering in detail not seen elsewhere. The authors also present a critical review of the reported speech characteristics of neurogenic stuttering and indicate how different etiologies (e.g., stroke versus head wound) may produce different speech characteristics.

Duffy, J. (2005). *Motor speech disorders* (2nd ed.). St. Louis: Elsevier, Mosby.

Chapters 13, 14, 19, and 20 provide excellent coverage of the nature of neurogenic and psychogenic stuttering as well as their management. Duffy is particularly good at describing etiologies of these disorders and the other conditions with which they may be associated. His sections on management reflect his extensive clinical experience.

Ringo, C. C., & Dietrich, S. (1995). Neurogenic stuttering: An analysis and critique. *Journal of Medical Speech-Language Pathology*, 3, 111–122.

This article is particularly useful in that it critically examines characteristics of neurogenic stuttering that have been proposed by various authors since Canter's (1971) seminal publication about differential diagnosis of neurogenic stuttering. Each of seven characteristics is examined in light of evidence that it is present in neurogenic stuttering in a way that is different from its manifestation in developmental stuttering. Suggestions are made to standardize the data to be collected and reported on individual cases.

Psychogenic Stuttering
Baumgartner, J. (1999). Acquired psychogenic stuttering. In Curlee, R.F. (Ed.), *Stuttering and Related Disorders of Fluency* (2nd ed.) (pp. 269–288). New York: Thieme Medical Publishers.

This chapter is an excellent starting place for anyone interested in learning about psychogenic stuttering. Baumgartner has been writing about this topic for several years and has firsthand clinical experience with individuals who have psychogenic stuttering, thus making the chapter a solid source for information.

Roth, C. R., Aronson, A. E., & Davis, L. J. (1989). Clinical studies in psychogenic stuttering of adult onset. *Journal of Speech and Hearing Disorders*, 54, 634–646.

This journal article examines the records of 12 patients who were evaluated and treated for psychogenic stuttering. Because the subjects were patients at the Mayo Clinic, they were examined thoroughly for psychological/psychiatric and neurological functioning in a standardized way, providing substantial evidence of the psychogenic nature of the stuttering. A case study is given to illustrate how stuttering can appear as a conversion reaction to emotional conflict. Clinical recommendations are given.

Cluttering
Kuster, J. Online resources on cluttering: The other fluency disorder. http://www.mnsu.edu/comdis/kuster/cluttering.html.

This webpage is a treasure trove of useful resources on cluttering. Among them are videos, assessment techniques, computer-assisted cluttering instruments, treatment suggestions, links to support groups, and an extensive section on research.

Myers, F. L., & St. Louis, K. O. (2007). *Cluttering* [DVD]. Memphis: Stuttering Foundation of America.

This video provides excellent examples of cluttering in several young adults, as well as clear guidelines for evaluation and treatment.

St. Louis, K. O., Raphael, L. J., Myers, F. L., & Bakker, K. (2003, Nov 18). Cluttering updated. *The ASHA Leader*, 4-5, 20–22.

This article, which is available online at www.asha.org, provides a clear synopsis of how to identify and evaluate cluttering, as well as specific suggestions for treating the core behaviors. For those who know little about cluttering, this publication is an excellent place to begin.

Myers, F. L., & St. Louis, K. O. (Eds.) (1986). *Cluttering: A clinical perspective*. San Diego, CA: Singular Publishing Group, Inc.

This book, with an interesting forward by Charles Van Riper, is the first text on cluttering since the classic text on cluttering by Deso Weiss (1964). Chapters by the authors and other clinicians working with cluttering provide an overview of the disorder as well as practical suggestions for evaluation and treatment.

St. Louis, K. O. (Ed.) (1996). Research and opinion on cluttering. *Special Issue of Journal of Fluency Disorders, 21.*

This special issue of JFD is rich with case studies of evaluations and treatments of individuals who clutter. It is therefore one of the few sources with data on treatment outcome, although the heterogeneity of the cases and the manner in which they are studied highlight the fact that research on cluttering is in its infancy. The cases studies are bracketed by overviews of the disorder at the beginning and critical reviews at the end that summarize the case studies and call attention to the poverty of credible data. A chapter by Myers is particularly valuable for its annotated list of publications on cluttering between 1964 and 1996.

Ward, D., & Scaler Scott, K. (Eds.) (2011). *Cluttering: A handbook of research, intervention and education*. Hove, UK: Psychology Press.

This is a rich compendium of international authors discussing the nature of cluttering, as well as assessment and treatment. The two chapters on treatment have excellent overall organization as well as many ideas for specific activities. There are several chapters that describe clients with cluttering who also have other disorders such as Down syndrome, learning disabilities, and autism spectrum disorders.

REFERENCES

Abbs, J. H. (1996). Mechanisms of speech motor execution and control. In N. Lass (Ed.), *Principles of experimental phonetics* (pp. 93–111). St. Louis, MO: Mosby.

Achenbach, T. M. (1988). *Child behavior checklist for ages 2-3.* Burlington, VT: University of Vermont.

Adams, M. (1977). A clinical strategy for differentiating the nonfluent child and the incipient stutterer. *Journal of Fluency Disorders, 2*, 141–148.

Adams, M. (1990). The demands and capacities model I: Theoretical elaborations. *Journal of Fluency Disorders, 15*, 135–141.

Adams, M., & Hayden, P. (1976). The ability of stutterers and nonstutterers to initiate and terminate phonation during production of an isolated vowel. *Journal of Speech and Hearing Research, 19*, 290–296.

Adams, M., & Runyan, C. M. (1981). Stuttering and fluency: Exclusive events or points on a continuum? *Journal of Fluency Disorders, 6*, 197–218.

Ainsworth, S., & Fraser, J. (2010). *If your child stutters: A guide for parents* (8th ed.). Memphis, TN: Stuttering Foundation.

Ahern, G. L., & Schwartz, G. E. (1985). Differential lateralization for positive and negative emotion in the human brain: EEG spectral analysis. *Neuropsychologia, 23*(6), 745–755.

Alfonso, P. J., Story, R. S., & Watson, B. C. (1987). The organization of supralaryngeal articulation in stutterers' fluent speech production: A second report. *Annual Bulletin Research Institute of Logopedics and Phoniatrics, 21*, 117–129.

Allen, S. (1988). *Durations of segments in repetitive disfluencies in stuttering and nonstuttering children.* Unpublished manuscript. E.M. Luse Center, University of Vermont, Burlington.

Allen, G. D., & Hawkins, S. (1980). Phonological rhythm, definition, and development. *Child Phonology, 1*, 227–256.

Allman, J. M., Hakeem, A., Erwin, J. M., Nimchinsky, E., & Hof, P. (2001). The anterior cingulate cortex: The evolution of an interface between emotion and cognition. *Annals of the New York Academy of Sciences, 935*, 107–117.

Alm, P. A. (2004). Stuttering and the basal ganglia circuits: A critical review of possible relations. *Journal of Communication Disorders, 37*, 325–396.

Alm, P. A., & Risberg, J. (2007). Stuttering in adults: The acoustic startle response, temperamental traits, and biological factors. *Journal of Communication Disorders, 40*, 1–41.

Ambrose, N. G., & Yairi, E. (1995). The role of repetition units in the differential diagnosis of early childhood incipient stuttering. *American Journal of Speech-Language Pathology, 4*, 82–88.

Ambrose, N. G., Cox, N. J., & Yairi, E. (1997). The genetic basis of persistence and recovery in stuttering. *Journal of Speech, Language, and Hearing Research, 40*, 567–580.

Ambrose, N. G., Yairi, E., & Cox, N. (1993). Genetic aspects of early childhood stuttering. *Journal of Speech and Hearing Research, 36*, 701–706.

American Speech-Language-Hearing Association. (1995). Guidelines for practice in stuttering treatment. *American Speech-Language-Hearing Association, 37*(Suppl. 14), 26–35.

Anderson, J., & Conture, E. (2000). Language abilities of children who stutter: A preliminary study. *Journal of Fluency Disorders, 25*(4), 283–304.

Anderson, J., Pellowski, M., & Conture, E. (2001, November). Temperament characteristics of children who stutter. Paper presented at the Annual meeting of the American Speech-Language-Hearing Association, New Orleans, LA.

Anderson, J., Pellowski, M., Conture, E., & Kelly, E. (2003). Temperamental characteristics of young children who stutter. *Journal of Speech, Language and Hearing Research, 46*, 1221–1233.

Andrews, G., & Craig, A. (1982). Stuttering: Overt and covert measurement of the speech of treated subjects. *Journal of Speech and Hearing Disorders, 47*, 96–99.

Andrews, G., & Craig, A. (1988). Prediction of outcome after treatment for stuttering. *British Journal of Disorders of Psychiatry, 153*, 236–240.

Andrews, G., & Cutler, J. (1974). Stuttering therapy: The relation between changes in symptom level and attitudes. *Journal of Speech and Hearing Disorders, 39*, 312–319.

Andrews, G., & Harris, M. (1964). *The syndrome of stuttering.* London: Spastics Society Medical Education and Information Unit in association with W. Heinemann Medical Books.

Andrews, G., & Ingham, R. (1971). Stuttering: Considerations in the evaluation of treatment. *British Journal of Communication Disorders, 6*, 129–138.

Andrews, G., & Tanner, S. (1982). Stuttering treatment: An attempt to replicate the regulated-breathing method. *Journal of Speech and Hearing Disorders, 47*, 138–140.

Andrews, G., Hoddinott, S., Craig, A., Howie, P. M., Feyer, A.-M., & Neilson, M. D. (1983). Stuttering: A review of research findings and theories circa 1982. *Journal of Speech and Hearing Disorders, 48*, 226–246.

Andrews, G., Howie, P. M., Dozsa, M., & Guitar, B. (1982). Stuttering: Speech pattern characteristics under fluency-inducing conditions. *Journal of Speech and Hearing Research, 25*, 208–216.

Andrews, G., Morris-Yates, A., Howie, P. M., & Martin, N. G. (1990). The genetic nature of stuttering. *Archives of General Psychiatry, 48*(11), 1034–1035.

Andy, O. J., & Bhatnager, S. C. (1992). Stuttering acquired from subcortical pathologies and its alleviation from thalamic perturbation. *Brain & Language, 42*(4), 385–401.

Arndt, J., & Healey, E. C. (2001). Concomitant disorders in school-age children who stutter. *Language, Speech, and Hearing Services in Schools, 32*, 68–78.

Arthur, G. (1952). *Arthur adaptation of the Leiter international performance test.* Los Angeles: Western Psychological Services.

Ayres, J. J. B. (1998). Fear conditioning and avoidance. In W. O'Donohue (Ed.), *Learning and behavior therapy.* Boston: Allyn & Bacon.

Azrin, N. H., & Nunn, R. G. (1974). A rapid method of eliminating stuttering by a regulated breathing approach. *Behavior Research and Therapy, 12*, 279–286.

Baer, D. (1990). The critical issue in treatment efficacy is knowing why treatment was applied. In L. B. Olswand, C. K. Thompson, S. F. Warren, & N. J. Minghetti (Eds.), *Treatment efficacy research in communication disorders* (pp. 31–39). Rockville, MD: ASHA.

Baker, D. J. (1967). The amount of information in the oral identification of forms by normal speakers and selected speech-deficient groups. In J. F. Bosma (Ed.), *Symposium of oral sensation and perception* (pp. 287–293). Springfield, IL: Thomas.

Bakker, K. (2002). Putting cluttering on the map: Looking back/looking ahead. Paper presented at the annual meeting of the American Speech-Language-Hearing Association, Atlanta, GA.

Barasch, C. T., Guitar, B., McCauley, R. J., & Absher, R. G. (2000). Disfluency and time perception. *Journal of Speech, Language and Hearing Research, 43,* 1429–1440.

Baratz, R., & Mesulam, M. (1981). Adult-onset stuttering treated with anticonvulsants. *Archives of Neurology, 38,* 132–133.

Baumgartner, J. M. (1999). Acquired psychogenic stuttering. In R. Curlee (Ed.), *Stuttering and related disorders of fluency* (2nd ed., pp. 269–288). New York: Thieme.

Beal, D. S., Gracco, V. L., Lafaille, S. J., & De Nil, L. F. (2007). Voxel-based morphometry of auditory and speech-related cortex in stutterers. *Neuroreport, 18*(12), 1257–1260.

Beck, J. S. (1995). *Cognitive therapy: Basics and beyond.* New York: Guilford Press.

Beitchman, J., Nair, R., Clegg, M., & Patel, P. G. (1986). Prevalence of speech and language in 5-year-old kindergarten children in Ottawa-Carleton region. *Journal of Speech and Hearing Disorders, 51,* 98–110.

Bennett Lanouette, E. (2011). Intervention strategies for cluttering disorders. In D. Ward, & K. S. Scott (Eds.), *Cluttering: A handbook of research, intervention and education* (pp. 175–197). Hove, UK: Psychology Press.

Berk, L. E. (1991). *Child development* (2nd ed.). Boston: Allyn & Bacon.

Bernstein Ratner, N. (1981). Are there constraints on childhood disfluency? *Journal of Fluency Disorders, 6,* 341–350.

Bernstein Ratner, N. (1995). Treating the child who stutters with concomitant language and phonological impairment. *Language, Speech, and Hearing in Schools, 26*(2), 180–186.

Bernstein Ratner, N. (1997). Stuttering: A psycholinguistic perspective. In R. Curlee and G. Siegel (Eds.), *Nature and Treatment of Stuttering: New Directions (2nd ed.).* Needham, MA: Allyn & Bacon, 99-127.

Bernstein Ratner, N., & Sih, C. C. (1987). Effects of gradual increases in sentence length and complexity on children's dysfluency. *Journal of Speech and Hearing Disorders, 52,* 278–287.

Bernstein Ratner, N., & Silverman, S. (2000). Parental perceptions of children's communicative development at stuttering onset. *Journal of Speech, Language and Hearing Research, 43,* 1252–1263.

Bernthal, J., Bankson, N., & Flipson, P. (2009). *Articulation and phonology disorders: Speech sound disorders in children* (6th ed.). Boston: Pearson/Allyn & Bacon.

Berry, M. F. (1938). Developmental history of stuttering children. *Journal of Pediatrics, 12,* 209–217.

Berry, R. C., & Silverman, F. H. (1972). Equality of intervals on the Lewis-Sherman scale of stuttering severity. *Journal of Speech and Hearing Research, 15,* 185–188.

Biederman, J., Rosenbaum, J. F., Chaloff, J., & Kagan, J. (1995). Behavioral inhibition as a risk factor for anxiety disorders. In J. Bierderman, J. F. Rosenbaum, J. Chaloff, & J. Kagan (Eds.), *Anxiety disorders in children and adolescents* (pp. 61–81). New York: Guildford Press.

Bijleveld, H., Lebrun, Y., & van Dongen, H. (1994). A case of acquired stuttering. *Folia Phoniatrica et Logopedica, 46,* 250–253.

Black, J. W. (1951). The effect of delayed side-tone upon vocal rate and intensity. *Journal of Speech Disorders, 16*(1), 56–60.

Bloch, E. L., & Goodstein, L. D. (1971). Functional speech disorders and personality: A decade of research. *Journal of Speech and Hearing Disorders, 36,* 295–314.

Blood, G. W. (1985). Laterality differences in child stutterers: Heterogeneity, severity levels, and statistical treatments. *Journal of Speech and Hearing Disorders, 50,* 66–72.

Blood, G. W., & Blood, I. M. (1989). Multiple data analysis of dichotic listening advantages of stutterers. *Journal of Fluency Disorders, 14,* 97–107.

Blood, G. W., Blood, I. M., Tellis, G. M., & Gabel, R. M. (2001). Communication apprehension and self-perceived communication competence in adolescents who stutter. *Journal of Fluency Disorders, 26,* 161-178.

Bloodstein, O. (1944). Studies in the psychology of stuttering: XIX. The relationship between oral reading rate and severity of stuttering. *Journal of Speech Disorders, 9,* 161–173.

Bloodstein, O. (1948). *Conditions under which stuttering is reduced or absent.* Unpublished doctoral dissertation, University of Iowa, Iowa City.

Bloodstein, O. (1950). Hypothetical conditions under which stuttering is reduced or absent. *Journal of Speech and Hearing Disorders, 15,* 142–153.

Bloodstein, O. (1958). Stuttering as an anticipatory struggle reaction. In J. Eisenson (Ed.), *Stuttering: A Symposium.* New York: Harper & Row.

Bloodstein, O. (1960a). The development of stuttering: I. Changes in nine basic features. *Journal of Speech and Hearing Disorders, 25,* 219–237.

Bloodstein, O. (1960b). The development of stuttering: II. Developmental phases. *Journal of Speech and Hearing Disorders, 25,* 366–376.

Bloodstein, O. (1961a). The development of stuttering: III. Theoretical and clinical implications. *Journal of Speech and Hearing Disorders, 26,* 67–82.

Bloodstein, O. (1961b). Stuttering in families of adopted stutterers. *Journal of Speech and Hearing Disorders, 26,* 395–396.

Bloodstein, O. (1974). The rules of early stuttering. *Journal of Speech and Hearing Disorders, 39,* 379–394.

Bloodstein, O. (1975). Stuttering as tension and fragmentation. In J. Eisenson (Ed.), *Stuttering: A Second Symposium.* New York: Harper & Row.

Bloodstein, O. (1987). *A handbook on stuttering* (4th ed.). Chicago: National Easter Seal Society.

Bloodstein, O. (1995). *A handbook on stuttering* (5th ed.). San Diego, CA: Singular.

Bloodstein, O. (1997). Stuttering as an anticipatory struggle reaction. In R. F. Curlee, & G. M. Siegel (Eds.), *The Nature and Treatment of Stuttering: New Directions* (2nd ed., pp. 169–181). Boston: Allyn & Bacon.

Bloodstein, O. (2001). Incipient and developed stuttering as two distinct disorders: Resolving a dilemma. *Journal of Fluency Disorders, 26*, 67–73.

Bloodstein, O. (2002). Early stuttering as a type of language difficulty. *Journal of Fluency Disorders, 27*, 163–167.

Bloodstein, O., & Gantwerk, B. F. (1967). Grammatical function in relation to stuttering in young children. *Journal of Speech and Hearing Research, 10*, 786–789.

Bloodstein, O., & Ratner, N. B. (2008). *A handbook on stuttering* (6th ed.). Clifton Park, NY: Thomson Delmar Learning.

Bluemel, C. (1932). Primary and secondary stammering. *Quarterly Journal of Speech, 18*, 187-200.

Bluemel, C. S. (1957). *The riddle of stuttering*. Danville, IL: Interstate Publishing Co.

Boberg, E., & Kully, D. (1985). *Comprehensive stuttering program*. San Diego, CA: College-Hill Press.

Boberg, E. Yeudall, L. T., Schopflocher, D., & Bo-Lassen, P. (1983) The effect of an intensive behavioral program on the distribution of EEG alpha power in stutterers during the processing of verbal and visuospatial information. *Journal of Fluency Disorders, 8*, 245-263.

Boehmler, R. M. (1994). *The treatment of stuttering as a speech-flow disorder*. Unpublished manuscript.

Boemio, A., Fromm, S., Braun, A. R., & Poeppel, D. (2005). Hierarchical and asymmetric temporal sensitivity in human auditory cortex. *Nature Neuroscience, 8*(3), 389–395.

Böhme, G. (1968). Stammering and cerebral lesions in early childhood: Examination of 802 children and adults with cerebral lesions. *Folia Phoniatrica, 20*, 239–249.

Boone, D. R., McFarlane, S. C., Von Berg, S. L., & Zraick, R. I. (2009). *Voice and voice therapy* (8th ed.). Boston: Allyn & Bacon.

Borden, G. J. (1983). Initiation versus execution on time during manual and oral counting by stutterers. *Journal of Speech and Hearing Research, 26*, 389-396.

Boscolo, B., Ratner, N. B., & Rescorla, L. (2002). Fluency characteristics of children with a history of Specific Expressive Language Impairment (SLI-E). *American Journal of Speech-Language Pathology, 11*, 41–49.

Bosshardt, H.-G. (2006). Cognitive processing load as a determinant of stuttering: Summary of a research programme. *Clinical Linguistics and Phonetics, 20*, 371–385.

Boswell, J. (1791). *The life of Samuel Johnson, LL. D., comprehending an account of his studies and numerous works in chronological order ... the whole exhibiting a view of literature and literary men in Great-Britain for near half a century during which he flourished.*. London: C. Dilly.

Bothe, A. (2004). *Evidence-based treatment of stuttering: Empirical bases and clinical applications*. Mahwah, NJ: Erlbaum.

Botterill, W., & Kelman, E. (2010). Palin parent-child interaction. In B. Guitar, & R. J. McCauley (Eds.), *Treatment of stuttering: Established and emerging interventions*. Baltimore: Lippincott Williams & Wilkins.

Boyce, W. T., Chesney, M., Alkon-Leonard, A., Tschann, J., Adams, S., Chesterman, B., et al. (1995). Psychobiologic reactivity to stress and childhood respiratory illnesses: Results of two prospective studies. *Psychosomatic Medicine, 57*, 411–422.

Brady, J. P. (1991). The pharmacology of stuttering: A critical review. *American Journal of Psychiatry, 148*, 1309–1316.

Brady, J. P., & Ali, Z. (2000). Alprazolam, citalopram, and clomipramine for stuttering. *Journal of Clinical Psychopharmacology, 20*, 287.

Brady, J. P., & Berson, J. (1975). Stuttering, dichotic listening, and cerebral dominance. *Archives of General Psychiatry, 32*, 1449-1452.

Branigan, G. (1979). Some reasons why successive single word utterances are not. *Journal of Child Language, 6*, 411–421.

Braun, A. R., Varga, M., Stager, S., Schulz, G., Selbie, S., Maisog, J. M., et al. (1997). Atypical lateralization of hemispherical activity in developmental stuttering: An H2 (15) 0 positron emission tomography study. In W. Hulstijn, H. F. M. Peters, & P. H. H. M. van Lieshout (Eds.), *Speech production: Motor control, brain research and fluency disorders* (pp. 279–292). Amsterdam: Elsevier.

Brayton, E. R., & Conture, E. G. (1978). Effects of noise and rhythmic simulation on the speech of stutterers. *Journal of Speech and Hearing Research, 21*, 285–294.

Brosch, S., Haege, A., Kalehne, P., and Johannsen, S. (1999). Stuttering children and the probability of remission: The role of cerebral dominance and speech production. *International Journal of Pediatric Otorhinolaryngology, 47*:71–76.

Brown, S.F. (1937). The influence of grammatical function on the incidence of stuttering. *Journal of Speech Disorders, 2*:207–215.

Brown, S.F. (1938a). A further study of stuttering in relation to various speech sounds. *Quarterly Journal of Speech, 24*:390–397.

Brown, S.F. (1938b). Stuttering with relation to word accent and word position. *Journal of Abnormal Social Psychology, 33*:112–120.

Brown, S.F. (1938c). The theoretical importance of certain factors influencing the incidence of stuttering. *Journal of Speech Disorders, 3*:223–230.

Brown, S.F. (1943). An analysis of certain data concerning loci of "stutterings" from the viewpoint of general semantics. *Papers from the Second American Congress of General Semantics, 2*:194–199.

Brown, S.F. (1945). The loci of stutterings in the speech sequence. *Journal of Speech Disorders, 10*:181–192.

Brown, S.F., and Moren, A. (1942). The frequency of stuttering in relation to word length during oral reading. *Journal of Speech Disorders, 7*:153–159.

Brown, S., Ingham, R. J., Ingham, J. C., Laird, A. R., & Fox, P. T. (2005). Stuttered and fluent speech production: An ALE meta-analysis of functional neuroimaging studies. *Human Brain Mapping, 25*(1), 105–117.

Brundage, S., & Bernstein Ratner, N. (1989). The measurement of stuttering frequency in children's speech. *Journal of Fluency Disorders, 14*, 351–358.

Brutten, G. J. (1985). *Communication attitude test*. University of Nebraska-Lincoln. Retrieved November 1, 2012 at http://cens.unl.edu/fluency/pdfs/test.pdf.

Brutten, G. J. (1997). *Communication attitude test*. University of Nebraska-Lincoln. Retrieved November 1, 2012 at http://cens.unl.edu/fluency/pdfs/test.pdf.

Brutten, G. J., & Dunham, S. (1989). The communication attitude test: A normative study of grade school children. *Journal of Fluency Disorders, 14*, 371–377.

Brutten, G. J., & Shoemaker, D. (1967). *The modification of stuttering*. Englewood Cliffs, NJ: Prentice-Hall.

Brutten, G., & Vanryckeghem, M. (2007). *The Behavior Assessment Battery for school-aged children who stutter*. San Diego, CA: Plural Publishers.

Byrd, C. T., Wolk, L., & Davis, B. L. (2007). Role of phonology in childhood stuttering and its treatment. In E. Conture, & R. Curlee (Eds.), *Stuttering and related disorders of fluency* (3rd ed., pp. 168–182). New York: Thieme.

Calkins, S. (1994). Origins and outcomes of individual differences in emotion regulation. In N. A. Fox, & J. Campos (Eds.), *The development of emotional regulation: Biological and behavioral considerations*. Chicago: Society for Research in Child Development.

Calkins, S. D., & Fox, N. A. (1994). Individual differences in the biological aspects of temperament. In J. E. Bates, & T. D. Wachs (Eds.), *Temperament: Individual differences at the interface of biology and behavior*. Washington, DC: American Psychological Association.

Callan, D. E., Kent, R. D., Guenther, F. H., & Vorperian, H. K. (2000). An auditory-feedback-based neural model of speech production that is robust to developmental changes in the size and shape of the articulatory system. *Journal of Speech, Language and Hearing Research, 43*(3), 721–736.

Canter, G. (1971). Observations on neurogenic stuttering: A contribution to differential diagnosis. *British Journal of Communication Disorders, 6*, 139–143.

Caplan, D. (1987). *Neurolinguistics and linguistics aphasiology*. Cambridge, UK: Cambridge University Press.

Carey, B., O'Brian, S., Onslow, M., Block, S., Jones, M., & Packman, A. (2010). Randomized controlled non-inferiority trial of a telehealth treatment for chronic stuttering: The Camperdown Program. *International Journal of Language and Communication Disorders, 45*(1), 108–120.

Caruso, A.J., Abbs, J.H., and Gracco, V. (1988). Kinematic analysis of multiple movement coordination during speech in stutterers. *Brain, 111*:439–455.

Caruso, A. J., Chodzko-Zajko, W., & McClowry, M. (1995). Emotional arousal and stuttering: The impact of cognitive stress. In C. W. Starkweather, & H. F. M. Peters (Eds.), *Stuttering: Proceedings of the First World Congress on Fluency Disorders*. Nijmegen, The Netherlands: International Fluency Association.

Caruso, A. J., Chodzko-Zajko, W., Bidinger, D., & Sommers, R. (1994). Adults who stutter: Responses to cognitive stress. *Journal of Speech and Hearing Research, 37*, 746–754.

Chang, S.-E., Erickson, K., Ambrose, N. G., Hasegawa-Johnson, M., & Ludlow, C. L. (2008). Brain anatomy differences in childhood stuttering. *NeuroImage, 39*(3), 1333–1344.

Chase, C. H. (1996). Neurobiology of learning disabilities. *Seminars in Speech, Language and Hearing, 17*(3), 173–181.

Chmela, K., & Reardon, N. (2001). *The school-age child who stutters: Working effectively with attitudes and emotions*. Memphis, TN: Stuttering Foundation of America.

Chuang, C.K., Fromm, D.S., Ewanowski, S.J., and Abbs, J.H. (1980, November). *Nonspeech articulatory sensori-motor control differences between stutterers and nonstutterers*. Paper presented at the Annual Meeting of the American Speech and Hearing Association, Detroit, MI.

Clarke-Stewart, A., & Friedman, S. (1987). *Child development: Infancy through adolescence*. New York: John Wiley & Sons.

Cohen, J. (1960). A coefficient of agreement for nominal scales. *Educational and Psychological Measurement, 20*, 37–46.

Cohen, M.S., and Hanson, M.L. (1975). Intersensory processing efficiency of fluent speakers and stutterers. *British Journal of Disorders of Communication,* 10:111–122.

Colburn, N., & Mysak, E. D. (1982a). Developmental disfluency and emerging grammar. I. Disfluency characteristics in early syntactic utterances. *Journal of Speech and Hearing Research, 25*, 414–420.

Colburn, N., & Mysak, E. D. (1982b). Developmental disfluency and emerging grammar. II. Co-occurrence of disfluency with specified semantic-syntactic structures. *Journal of Speech and Hearing Research, 25*(421–427).

Colcord, R. D., & Adams, M. R. (1979). Voicing duration and vocal SLP changes associated with stuttering reduction during singing. *Journal of Speech and Hearing Research, 22*, 468–479.

Coleman, T. J. (2000). *Clinical management of communication disorders in culturally diverse children*. Boston: Allyn & Bacon.

Conrad, C. (1996). Fluency in multicultural populations. In L. Cole, & V. R. Deal (Eds.), *Communication disorders in multicultural populations*. Rockville, MD: American Speech-Language-Hearing Association.

Conture, E. (2002). *Stuttering and your child: Questions and answers* (3rd ed.). Memphis, TN: Stuttering Foundation of America.

Conture, E. (2010). *Stuttering and your child: Questions and answers*. Memphis, TN: Stuttering Foundation of America.

Conture, E. G. (1982). *Stuttering*. Englewood Cliffs, NJ: Prentice-Hall.

Conture, E. G. (1990). *Stuttering* (2nd ed.). Englewood Cliffs, NJ: Prentice-Hall.

Conture, E. G. (1991). Young stutterers' speech production. In H. F. M. Peters, W. Hulstijn, & C. W. Starkweather (Eds.), *Speech motor control and stuttering* (pp. 365–384). Amsterdam: Excerpta Medica.

Conture, E. G. (2001). *Stuttering: Its nature, diagnosis, and treatment*. Boston: Allyn & Bacon.

Conture, E. G., Louko, L., & Edwards, M. L. (1993). Simultaneously treating stuttering and disordered phonology in children. *American Journal of Speech-Language Pathology, 2*, 72–81.

Conture, E. G., McCall, G. N., & Brewer, D. W. (1977). Laryngeal behavior during stuttering. *Journal of Speech and Hearing Research, 20*, 661–668.

Conture, E., & Melnick, K. (1999). Parent-child group approach to stuttering in preschool and school-age children. In M. Onslow, & A. Packman (Eds.), *Early stuttering: A handbook of intervention strategies* (pp. 17–51). San Diego, CA: Singular.

Cooper, E. B., & Cooper, C. S. (1993). Fluency disorders. In D. E. Battle (Ed.), *Communication disorders in multicultural organizations* (pp. 189–211). Boston: Andover Medical Publishers.

Cordes, A. (1994). The reliability of observational data: I. Theories and methods for speech-language pathology. *Journal of Speech and Hearing Research, 37*, 264–278.

Cox, N., & Yairi, E. (2000). *Genetics of stuttering: Insights and advances*. Paper presented at the Annual Meeting of the American Speech-Language-Hearing Association, Washington, DC.

Craig, A., & Andrews, G. (1985). The prediction and prevention of relapse in stuttering. *Behavior Modification, 9*, 427–442.

Craig, A., Franklin, J., & Andrews, G. (1984). A scale to measure locus of control of behavior. *British Journal of Medical Psychology, 57*, 173–180.

Cross, D. E., & Cooke, P. (1979). Vocal and manual reaction times of adult stutterers and nonstutterers. (Abstract). *American Speech, Language and Hearing Association, 21*, 693.

Cross, D. E., & Luper, H. L. (1979). Voice reaction time of stuttering and nonstuttering children and adults. *Journal of Fluency Disorders, 4*, 59–77.

Cross, D. E., & Luper, H. L. (1983). Relation between finger reaction time and voice reaction time in stuttering and nonstuttering children and adults. *Journal of Speech and Hearing Research, 26*, 356–361.

Cross, D. E., Sweet, J., & Bates, D. (1985). *Mental imagery and stuttering: Electroencephalographic and physiological characteristics.* Paper presented at the American Speech-Language and Hearing Association Convention, Washington, DC.

Crystal, D. (1987). Towards a "bucket" theory of language disability: Taking account of interaction between linguistic levels. *Clinical Linguistics and Phonetics, 1*, 7–22.

Culatta, R., & Goldberg, S. (1995). *Stuttering therapy: An integrated approach to theory and practice.* Boston: Allyn & Bacon.

Cullinan, W. L., & Springer, M. T. (1980). Voice initiation times in stuttering and nonstuttering children. *Journal of Speech and Hearing Research, 23*, 344–360.

Curlee, R. (1984). A case selection strategy for young disfluent children. *Seminars in Speech, Language and Hearing, 1*, 277–287.

Curlee, R. (1993). Identification and case selection guidelines for early childhood stuttering. In R. Curlee (Ed.), *Stuttering and related disorders of fluency.* New York: Thieme Medical Publishers.

Curry, F., and Gregory, H. (1969). The performance of stutterers on dichotic listening tasks thought to reflect cerebral dominance. *Journal of Speech and Hearing Research, 12*:73–82.

Cykowski, M. D., Fox, P. T., Ingham, R. J., Ingham, J. C., & Robin, D. A. (2010). A study of the reproducibility and etiology of diffusion anisotropy differences in developmental stuttering: A potential role for impaired myelination. *Neuroimage, 52*(4), 1495–1504.

Dalton, P., & Hardcastle, W. J. (1977). *Disorders of fluency.* New York: Elsevier.

Daly, D. A. (1986). The clutterer. In K. St. Louis (Ed.), *The atypical stutterer.* New York: Academic Press.

Daly, D. A. (2006). Predictive cluttering inventory. *International Cluttering Association.* Retrieved November, 2012 from http://associations.missouristate.edu/ICA/.

Daly, D. A., & Burnett-Stolnack, M. L. (1995). Identification of and treatment planning for stuttering clients: Two practical tools. *The Clinical Connection, 8*, 15.

Darley, F. L. (1955). The relationship of parental attitudes and adjustments to the development of stuttering. In W. Johnson, & R. R. Leutenegger (Eds.), *Stuttering in children and adults.* Minneapolis, MN: University of Minnesota Press.

Darley, F. L., & Spriestersbach, D. (1978). *Diagnostic methods in speech pathology* (2nd ed.). New York: Harper & Row.

Davenport, R.W. (1977). *Dichotic ear preferences of stuttering adults.* Unpublished doctoral dissertation, Iowa State University, Ames, IA.

Davidson, R. J. (1984). Affect, cognition, and hemispheric specialization. In C. E. Izard, J. Kagan, & R. Zajonc (Eds.), *Emotion, cognition and behavior.* New York: Cambridge University Press.

Davidson, R. J. (1995). Cerebral asymmetry, emotion, and affective style. In R. Davidson, & K. Hugdahl (Eds.). *Brain asymmetry* (pp. 361–387). Cambridge, MA: MIT Press.

Davis, D. M. (1940). The relation of repetitions in the speech of young children to certain measures of language maturity and situational factors: Parts II & III. *Journal of Speech Disorders, 5*, 235–246.

Davis, M., & Guitar, B. (1976). *Speech rate of elementary school children in Vermont.* Graduate student research paper, University of Vermont, Burlington, VT.

De Nil, L. F. (1995). *Linguistic and motor approaches to stuttering: Exploring unification.* A panel presentation at the Annual Convention of the American Speech-Language-Hearing Association, Orlando, FL.

De Nil, L. F. (2004). Recent developments in brain imaging research in stuttering. In B. Maassen, H. F. M. Peters, & R. D. Kent (Eds.), *Speech motor control in normal and disordered speech* (pp. 113–137). Oxford, UK: Oxford University Press.

De Nil, L. F., & Abbs, J. H. (1991). Kinaesthetic acuity of stutterers and nonstutterers for oral and non-oral movements. *Brain, 114*, 2145–2158.

De Nil, L. F., & Brutten, G. J. (1991). Speech-associated attitudes of stuttering and normally fluent children. *Journal of Speech and Hearing Research, 34*, 60–66.

De Nil, L. F., Jokel, R., & Rochon, E. (2007). Etiology, symptomatology, and treatment of neurogenic stuttering. In E. Conture, & R. Curlee (Eds.), *Stuttering and Related Disorders of Fluency* (3rd ed., pp. 326–343). New York: Thieme.

De Nil, L. F., Kroll, R. M., & Houle, S. (2001). Functional neuroimaging of cerebellar activation during single word reading and verb generation in stuttering and nonstuttering adults. *Neuroscience Letters, 302*, 77–80.

De Nil, L.F., Kroll, R.M., Houle, S., Ludlow, C.L., Braun, A., Ingham, R., et al. (1995, November). *Advances in stuttering research using positron emission tomography brain imaging.* Paper presented at the Annual Meeting of the American Speech-Language-Hearing Association, Orlando, FL.

De Nil, L.F., Kroll, R.M., Kapur, S., and Houle, S. (2000). A positron emission tomography study of silent and oral single word reading in stuttering and nonstuttering adults. *Journal of Speech, Language, and Hearing Research, 43*:1038–1053.

De Nil, L. F., Kroll, R. M., Lafaille, S. J., & Houle, S. (2003). A positron emission tomography study of short- and long-term treatment effects on functional brain activation in adults who stutter. *Journal of Fluency Disorders, 28*, 357–381.

DeJoy, D. A., & Gregory, H. H. (1973). The relationship of children's disfluencies to the syntax, length, and vocabulary of their sentences. (Abstract). *American Speech, Language and Hearing Association, 15*, 472.

DeJoy, D. A., & Gregory, H. H. (1985). The relationship between age and frequency of disfluency in preschool children. *Journal of Fluency Disorders, 10*, 107–122.

Dietrich, S., Barry, S. J., & Parker, D. E. (1995). Middle latency auditory responses in males who stutter. *Journal of Speech and Hearing Research, 38*, 5–17.

Dietrich, M. & Verdolini Abbott, K. (2008). Psychobiological framework of stress and voice: A psychobiological framework for studying psychological stress and its relation to voice disorders. In K. Izdebski (Ed.), *Emotions in the Human Voice (Vol. III, Clinical Evidence).* San Diego: Plural Publishing, 159–178.

DiSimoni, F. G. (1974). Preliminary study of certain timing relationships in the speech of stutterers. *Journal of the Acoustical Society of America, 56*, 695–696.

Donnan, G. A. (1979). Stuttering as a manifestation of stroke. *Medical Journal of Australia, 1*, 44–45.

Dorman, M., and Porter, R. (1975). Hemispheric lateralization for speech perceptions in stutterers. *Cortex,* 11:181–185.

Douglass, L. C. (1943). A study of bilaterally recorded electro-encephalograms of adult stutterers. *Journal of Experimental Psychology, 32,* 247–265.

Drayna, D. (1997). Genetic linkage studies of stuttering: Ready for prime time? *Journal of Fluency Disorders, 22*:237–241.

Duffy, J. (2005). *Motor speech disorders* (2nd ed.). St. Louis, MO: Elsevier, Mosby.

Dunn, L. M., & Dunn, D. M. (2007). *Peabody Picture Vocabulary Test—4 (PPVT-4).* San Antonio, TX: Pearson.

Dworzynski, K., Remington, A., Rijsdijk, F., Howell, P., & Plomin, R. (2007). Genetic etiology in cases of recovered and persistent stuttering in an unselected, longitudinal sample of young twins. *American Journal of Speech-Language Pathology, 16*(2), 169–178.

Edelman, G. (1992). *Bright Air, Brilliant Fire: On the Matter of Mind.* New York: Basic Books.

Elliott, R. L., & Thomas, B. J. (1985). A case report of alprazolaam-induced stuttering. *Journal of Clinical Psychopharmacology, 5,* 159–160.

Ellis, B. J., & Boyce, W. T. (2008). Biological sensitivity to context. *Current Directions in Psychological Science, 17*(3), 183–187.

Ellis, J. B., Finan, D., & Ramig, P. R. (2008). The influence of stuttering severity on acoustic startle response. *Journal of Speech, Language and Hearing Research, 51*(4), 836–850.

Embrechts, M., & Ebben, H. (1999). *A comparison between the interactions of stuttering and nonstuttering children and their parents.* Paper presented at the Fifth Oxford Disfluency Conference, Oxford, UK.

Erickson, R. (1969). Assessing communication attitudes among stutterers. *Journal of Speech and Hearing Research, 12,* 711–724.

Ezrati-Vanacour, R., Platzky, R., & Yairi, E. (2001). The young child's awareness of stuttering-like disfluencies. *Journal of Speech, Language and Hearing Research, 44*(2), 368–380.

Faber, A., & Mazlish, E. (1999). *How to talk so kids will listen and how to listen so kids will talk.* New York: Harper Resources.

Fagan, M. K. (2002). *Stuttering, social-cognitive, and emotional development.* Unpublished manuscript. Columbia, MO.

Felsenfeld, S. (1997). Epidemiology and genetics of stuttering. In R. Curlee, and G. Siegel (Eds), *The Nature and Treatment of Stuttering: New Directions* (ed 2). Boston: Allyn & Bacon, pp 3–23.

Felsenfeld, S., Kirk, K.M., Zhu, G., Statham, D.J., Neale, M.C., and Martin, N.G. (2000). A study of the genetic and environmental etiology of stuttering in a selected twin sample. *Behavior Genetics,* 30:359–366.

Fibiger, S. (1971). Stuttering explained as a physiological tremor. *Quarterly Progress and Status Report, 2–3.*

Fibiger, S. (1972). Further discussion on stuttering explained as a physiological tremor. *Quarterly Progress and Status Report: Speech Transmission Laboratory.* Stockholm, Sweden: Royal Institute of Technology.

Finn, P. (2003). Self-regulation and the management of stuttering. *Seminars in Speech and Language, 24,* 27–32.

Finn, P. (2007). Self-control and the treatment of stuttering. In E. Conture, & R. Curlee (Eds.), *Stuttering and related disorders of fluency* (3rd ed., pp. 344–359). New York: Thieme.

Flechsig, P. (1927). *Meine myelogenetische Hirnlehre.* Berlin, Germany: Julius Springer.

Flugel, F. (1979). Erhebungen von Personlichkeitsmerk-malen an Muttern stotternder Kinder und Jugendicher. *DSH Abstracts, 19,* 226.

Fosnot, S. M., & Woodford, L. L. (1992). *The fluency development system for young children.* Buffalo, NY: United Educational Services.

Foundas, A.L., Bollich, A.M., Corey, D.M., Hurley, M., and Heilman, K.M. (2001). Anomalous anatomy of speech-language areas in adults with persistent developmental stuttering. *Neurology,* 57:207–215.

Foundas, A. L., Bollich, A. M., Feldman, J., Corey, D. M., Hurley, M., Lemen, L. C., & Heilman, K. M. (2004). Aberrant auditory processing and atypical planum temporale in developmental stuttering. *Neurology, 63*(9), 1640–1646.

Fowlie, G. M., & Cooper, E. B. (1978). Traits attributed to stuttering and nonstuttering children by their mothers. *Journal of Fluency Disorders, 3,* 233–246.

Fox, N., & Davidson, R. (1984). Hemispheric substrates of affect: Developmental model. In N. Fox, & R. Davidson (Eds.), *The psychobiology of affective development.* Hillsdale, NJ: Lawrence Erlbaum Associates.

Fox, P. T. (2003). Brain imaging in stuttering: Where next? *Journal of Fluency Disorders, 28*(4), 265–272.

Fox, P.T., Ingham, R., Ingham, J.C., Hirsch, T.B., Downs, J.H., Martin, C., et al. (1996). A PET study of the neural systems of stuttering. *Nature,* 382:158–162.

Fox, P., Ingham, R.J., Ingham, J.C., Zamarripa, F., Xiong, J.-H., and Lancaster, J.L. (2000). Brain correlates of stuttering and syllable production: A PET performance-correlation analysis. *Brain,* 123:1985–2004.

Fraisse, P. (1963). *The psychology of time.* New York: Harper & Row.

Franken, M. J., Kielstra-Van der Schalk, C. J., & Boelens, H. (2005). Experimental treatment of early stuttering: A preliminary study. *Journal of Fluency Disorders* 30, 189–199.

Frankenburg, W. K., & Dodds, J. B. (1967). The Denver Developmental Screening Test. *Journal of Pediatrics, 71,* 181–191.

Fraser, J. (2004). Results of survey on electronic devices. *Stuttering Foundation Newsletter, 3*(Winter), 7.

Fraser, J., & Perkins, W. H. (1987). *Do you stutter: A guide for teens.* Memphis, TN: Speech Foundation of America.

Frattali, C. M. (1998). *Measuring outcomes in speech-language pathology.* New York: Thieme.

Freeman, F. J., & Ushijima, T. (1975). Laryngeal activity accompanying the moment of stuttering: A preliminary report of EMG investigations. *Journal of Fluency Disorders, 1,* 36–45.

Freeman, F. J., & Ushijima, T. (1978). Laryngeal muscle activity during stuttering. *Journal of Speech and Hearing Research, 21,* 538–562.

Gaines, N. D., Runyan, C. M., & Meyers, S. C. (1991). A comparison of young stutterers' fluent versus stuttered utterances on measures of length and complexity. *Journal of Speech and Hearing Research, 34,* 37–42.

Garber, S. F., & Martin, R. R. (1977). Effects of noise and increased vocal intensity on stuttering. *Journal of Speech and Hearing Research, 20,* 233–240.

Garfinkel, H. A. (1995). Why did Moses stammer? And was Moses left-handed? *Journal of the Royal Society of Medicine, 88,* 256–257.

Geschwind, N., & Galaburda, A. M. (1985). Cerebral lateralization: Biological mechanisms, associations, and pathology: I. A hypothesis and a program for research. *Archives of Neurology, 42,* 429–459.

Gibson, E. (1972). Reading for some purpose. In J. F. Kavanaugh, & I. Mattingly (Eds.), *Language by ear and by eye.* Cambridge, MA: MIT Press.

Gildston, P. (1967). Stutterers' self-acceptance and perceived parental acceptance. *Journal of Abnormal Psychology, 72:*59–64.

Gillam, R. B., Logan, K. J., & Pearson, N. A. (2009). *TOCS: Test of Childhood Stuttering.* Austin, TX: Pro-Ed.

Goldberg, G. (1985). Supplementary motor area structure and function: Review and hypothesis. *Behavioral and Brain Sciences, 8,* 567–616.

Goldman, R., & Fristoe, M. (2000). *Goldman-Fristoe Test of Articulation—2 (G-FTA-2).* San Antonio, TX: Pearson.

Goldman-Eisler, F. (1968). *Psycholinguistics: Experiments in spontaneous speech.* New York: Academic Press.

Goldstein, B. (2000). *Cultural and linguistic diversity resource guide for speech-language pathologists.* San Diego, CA: Singular Publishing Group.

Goodstein, L. D. (1956). MMPI profiles of stutterers' parents: A follow-up study. *Journal of Speech and Hearing Disorders, 21,* 430–435.

Goodstein, L. D., & Dahlstrom, W. G. (1956). MMPI difference between parents of stuttering children and nonstuttering children. *Journal of Consulting Psychology, 20,* 365–370.

Gordon, P. A., Luper, H. L., & Peterson, H. A. (1986). The effects of syntactic complexity on the occurrence of disfluencies in 5 year old stutterers. *Journal of Fluency Disorders, 11,* 151–164.

Gottwald, S. R. (2010). Stuttering prevention and early intervention: A multidimensional approach. In B. Guitar, & R. J. McCauley (Eds.), *Treatment of stuttering: Established and emerging interventions* (pp. 91–117). Baltimore: Lippincott Williams & Wilkins.

Gottwald, S., & Starkweather, C. W. (1984, November). *Stuttering prevention: Rationale and method.* Paper presented at the short course presented at the Annual Meeting of the American Speech and Hearing Association, San Francisco, CA.

Gottwald, S., & Starkweather, C. W. (1985, November). *The prognosis of stuttering.* Miniseminar presented at the Annual Meeting of the American Speech and Hearing Association, Washington, DC.

Gottwald, S., & Starkweather, C. W. (1999). Stuttering prevention and early intervention: A multiprocess approach. In M. Onslow, & A. Packman (Eds.), *Handbook of Early Stuttering Intervention* (pp. 53–82). San Diego, CA: Singular.

Gray, J. A. (1987). *The psychology of fear and stress* (2nd ed.). Cambridge, UK: Cambridge University Press.

Greenspan, S. I. (1993). Making time for your child. *Parents*(August), 111–114.

Guenther, F. H. (1994). A neural network model of speech acquisition and motor equivalent speech production. *Biological Cybernetics, 72*(1), 43–53.

Guenther, F. H., Ghosh, S. S., & Tourville, J. A. (2006). Neural modeling and imaging of the cortical interactions underlying syllable production. *Brain and Language, 96*(3), 280–301.

Guitar, B. (1976). Pretreatment factors associated with the outcome of stuttering therapy. *Journal of Speech and Hearing Research, 19,* 590–600.

Guitar, B. (1978). Between parent and (stuttering) child. *WMU Journal of Speech, Language and Hearing, 14,* 3–5.

Guitar, B. (1997). Therapy for children's stuttering and emotions. In R.F. Curlee, and G.M. Siegel (Eds), *Nature and Treatment of Stuttering: New Directions* (ed 2). Boston: Allyn & Bacon, pp 280–291.

Guitar, B. (1998). *Stuttering: An integrated approach to its nature and treatment* (2nd ed.). Philadelphia: Lippincott Williams & Wilkins.

Guitar, B. (2000). Emotions, temperament and stuttering: Some possible relationships. Paper presented at the Fifth Oxford Disfluency Conference, Oxford, UK.

Guitar, B. (2003). Acoustic startle responses and temperament in individuals who stutter. *Journal of Speech Language and Hearing Research, 46,* 233–241.

Guitar, B. (2004). Burn your textbooks! Evidence-based practice in stuttering treatment. In A. Packman, A. Meltzer, & H. F. M. Peters (Eds.), *Theory, research and therapy in fluency disorders: Proceedings of the fourth world congress in fluency disorders.* Nijmegen, The Netherlands: Nijmegen University Press.

Guitar, B., & Bass, C. (1978). Stuttering therapy: The relation between attitude change and long-term outcome. *Journal of Speech and Hearing Disorders, 43,* 392–400.

Guitar, C., & Fraser, J. (2007). *Stuttering: Basic clinical skills [DVD].* Memphis, TN: Stuttering Foundation of America.

Guitar, B., & Grims, S. (1977, November). *Developing a scale to assess communication attitudes in children who stutter.* Paper presented at the annual meeting of the American Speech-Language-Hearing Association, Atlanta, GA.

Guitar, B., & Guitar, C. (2003). *Do you stutter: Straight talk for teens [DVD].* Memphis, TN: Stuttering Foundation of America.

Guitar, B., Guitar, C., & Fraser, J. (2006). *Stuttering and your child: Help for parents [DVD].* Memphis, TN: Stuttering Foundation of America.

Guitar, B., Guitar, C., Neilson, P. D., O'Dwyer, N. J., & Andrews, G. (1988). Onset sequencing of selected lip muscles in stutterers and nonstutterers. *Journal of Speech and Hearing Research, 31,* 28–35.

Guitar, B., Kopff-Schaefer, H., Donahue-Kilburg, G., & Bond, L. (1992). Parent verbal interaction and speech rate. *Journal of Speech and Hearing Research, 35,* 742–754.

Guitar, B., & Marchinkowski, L. (2001). Influence of mothers' slower speech on their children's speech rate. *Journal of Speech, Language and Hearing Research, 44,* 853–861.

Guitar, B., & McCauley, R. J. (2010). *Stuttering treatment: Established and emerging approaches.* Baltimore: Lippincott Williams & Wilkins.

Guitar, B., & Reville, J. (1997). *Easy talker: A fluency workbook for school age children.* Austin, TX: Pro-Ed.

Habib, M., Daquin, G., Milandre, L., Royere, M. L., Rey, M., Lanteri, A., et al. (1995). Mutism and auditory agnosia due to bilateral insular damage: Role of the insula in human communication. *Neurpsychologia, 33*(3), 327–333.

Hadders-Algra, M., & Forssberg, H. (2002). Development of motor function in health and disease. In H. Lagercrantz, M. L. Hanson, P. Evrard, & C. H. Rodeck (Eds.), *The newborn brain: Neuroscience and clinical applications.* Cambridge, UK: Cambridge University Press.

Hakim, H. B., & Bernstein Ratner, N. (2004). Nonword repetitions abilities of children who stutter: An exploratory study. *Journal of Fluency Disorders, 29*, 179–199.

Hall, J. W., & Jerger, J. (1978). Central auditory function in stutterers. *Journal of Speech and Hearing Research, 21*, 324–337.

Hall, N. E., Yamashita, T. S., & Aram, D. M. (1993). Relationship between language and fluency in children with developmental language disorders. *Journal of Speech and Hearing Research, 36*, 568–579.

Hampton, A., & Weber-Fox, C. (2008). Non-linguistic auditory processing in stuttering: Evidence from behavior and event-related brain potentials. *Journal of Fluency Disorders, 33*(4), 253–273.

Hannley, M., & Dorman, M. (1982). Some observations on auditory function and stuttering. *Journal of Fluency Disorders, 7*, 93–108.

Harrison, E., Bruce, M., Shenker, R., & Koushik, S. (2010). The Lidcombe Program with school-age children who stutter. In B. Guitar, & R. J. McCauley (Eds.), *Treatment of stuttering: Established and emerging interventions* (pp. 150–166). Baltimore: Lippincott Williams & Wilkins.

Haynes, W. O., & Hood, S. B. (1978). Disfluency changes in children as a function of the systematic modification of linguistic complexity. *Journal of Communication Disorders, 11*, 79–33.

Helliesen, G. (2002). *Forty years after therapy: One man's story.* Newport News, VA: Apollo Press.

Helm, N. A. (1979). Management of palilalia with a pacing board. *Journal of Speech and Hearing Disorders, 44*, 350–353.

Helm, N. A., Butler, R. B., & Canter, G. J. (1980). Neurogenic acquired stuttering. *Journal of Fluency Disorders, 5*, 269–279.

Helm-Estabrooks, N. (1986). Diagnosis and management of neurogenic stuttering in adults. In K. St. Louis (Ed.), *The atypical stutterer.* New York: Academic Press.

Helm-Estabrooks, N. (1992). *Aphasia diagnostic profiles.* Chicago: Applied Symbolix.

Helm-Estabrooks, N. (1999). Stuttering associated with acquired neurological disorders. In R. Curlee (Ed.), *Stuttering and related disorders of fluency* (2nd ed., pp. 255–268). New York: Thieme.

Helm-Estabrooks, N., & Kaplan, E. (1989). *Boston stimulus boards.* Chicago: Applied Symbolix.

Hernandez, L. M. (2001). *A normative investigation of the speech-associated attitude of preschool and kindergarten children.* Masters, University of Central Florida, Orlando.

Herndon, G. Y. (1967). A study of the time discrimination abilities of stutterers and nonstutterers. *Speech Monographs, 34*, 303–304.

Hickok, G. (2001). Functional anatomy of speech perception and speech production. *Journal of Psycholinguistic Research, 30*, 225–234.

Hickok, G., & Poeppel, D. (2001). The cortical organization of speech processing. *Nature Reviews Neuroscience, 8*, 393–402.

Hill, D. (2003). Differential treatment of stuttering in the early stages of development. In H. H. Gregory, J. H. Campbell, C. Gregory, & D. Hill (Eds.), *Stuttering therapy: Rationale and procedures* (pp. 142–185). Boston: Allyn & Bacon.

Hill, H. E. (1954). An experimental study of disorganization of speech and manual responses in normal subjects. *Journal of Speech and Hearing Disorders, 19*, 295–305.

Hillman, R. E., & Gilbert, H. R. (1977). Voice onset time for voiceless stop consonants in the fluent reading of stutterers and nonstutterers. *Journal of the Acoustical Society of America, 61*, 610–611.

Hiscock, M., & Kinsbourne, M. (1977). Selective listening asymmetry in preschool children. *Developmental Psychology, 13*, 217–224.

Hiscock, M., & Kinsbourne, M. (1980). Asymmetry of verbal-manual time sharing in children: A follow-up study. *Neuropsychologia, 18*, 151–162.

Hodge, G., Rescorla, L., & Ratner, N. (1999, November). *Fluency in toddlers with SLI: A preliminary investigation.* Paper presented at the Annual meeting of the American Speech-Language-Hearing Association, San Francisco.

Hodson, B. W. (1986). *The assessment of phonological processes—Revised.* Austin, TX: Pro-Ed.

Hodson, B. W., & Paden, E. (1991). *Targeting intelligible speech: A phonological approach to remediation* (2nd ed.). Austin, TX: ProEd.

Hood, L. (1987, November). *Middle latency responses in stutterers.* Paper presented at the Annual Meeting of the American Speech-Language-Hearing Association, New Orleans, LA.

Howell, P., & Van Borsel, J. (2011). *Multilingual aspects of fluency disorders.* Tonawanda, NY: Multilingual Matters.

Howell, P., El-Yaniv, N., & Powell, D. J. (1987). Factors affecting fluency in stutterers when speaking under altered auditory feedback. In H. F. M. Peters, & W. Hulstijn (Eds.), *Speech motor dynamics in stuttering* (pp. 361–370). New York: Springer.

Howie, P. M. (1981). Concordance for stuttering in monozygotic and dizygotic twin pairs. *Journal of Speech and Hearing Research, 24*, 317–321.

Howie, P. M., & Andrews, G. (1984). Treatment of adult stutterers: Managing fluency. In R. Curlee, & W. Perkins (Eds.), *Nature and treatment of stuttering: New directions* (pp. 425–445). San Diego, CA: College-Hill Press.

Hubbard, C. P., & Yairi, E. (1988). Clustering of disfluencies in the speech of stuttering and nonstuttering preschool children. *Journal of Speech and Hearing Research, 31*(2), 228–233.

Ingham, R. J. (1979). Comment on "Stuttering therapy: The relation between attitude change and long-term outcome". *Journal of Speech and Hearing Disorders, 44*, 397–400.

Ingham, R.J. (2001). Brain imaging studies of developmental stuttering. *Journal of Communication Disorders, 34*:493–516.

Ingham, R. J. (2003). Brain imaging and stuttering: Some reflections on current and future developments. *Journal of Fluency Disorders, 28*, 411–420.

Ingham, R. J., & Andrews, G. (1973). Details of a token economy stuttering therapy programme for adults. *Australian Journal of Human Communication, 1*, 13–20.

Ingham, R. J., Fox, P. T., Ingham, J. C., Zamarripa, F., Martin, C., & Jerabek, P. (1996). Functional-lesion investigation of developmental stuttering with positron emission tomography. *Journal of Speech and Hearing Research, 29*, 1208–1227.

Ingham, R. J., Gow, M., & Costello, J. M. (1985). Stuttering and speech naturalness: Some additional data. *Journal of Speech and Hearing Disorders, 50*(2), 217–219.

Ingham, R. J., Ingham, J. C., Finn, P., & Fox, P. T. (2003). Toward a functional neural systems model of developmental stuttering. *Journal of Fluency Disorders, 28*, 297–302.

Ingham, R., Cordes, A., & Finn, P. (1993). Time-interval measurement of stuttering: Systematic replication of Ingham, Cordes, & Gow (1993). *Journal of Speech and Hearing Research, 36*, 1168–1176.

Ingham, R., Cordes, A., & Gow, M. (1993). Time-interval measurement of stuttering: Modifying interjudge agreement. *Journal of Speech and Hearing Research, 36*, 503–515.

International Classification of Functioning, Disability, and Health: ICF. (2001). Geneva, Switzerland: World Health Organization.

Ito, T. (1986). Speech dysfluency and the acquisition of syntax in children 2–6 years old. (Abstract). *Folia Phoniatrica, 38*, 310.

Jaffe, J., & Anderson, S. W. (1979). Prescript to Chapter 1: Communication rhythms and the evolution of language. In A. W. Siegman, & S. Feldman (Eds.), *Of speech and time: Temporal speech patterns in interpersonal contexts.* Hillsdale, NJ: Lawrence Erlbaum Associates.

James, W. (1890). *The principles of psychology.* New York: Holt & Co.

Jancke, L., Hanggi, J., & Steinmetz, H. (2004). Morphological brain differences between adult stutterers and non-stutterers. *BMC Neurology, 4*, 23.

Janssen, P., Kraaimaat, F., & Brutten, G. (1990). Relationship between stutterers' genetic history and speech associated variables. *Journal of Fluency Disorders, 8*, 39–48.

Jensen, P.J., Sheehan, J.G., Williams, W.M., and LaPointe, L.L. (1975). Oral-sensory-perceptual integrity of stutterers. *Folia Phoniatrica, 27*:106–115.

Johnson, W. (1942). A study of the onset and development of stuttering. *Journal of Speech Disorders, 7*, 251–257.

Johnson, W. (1955). A study of the onset and development of stuttering. In W. Johnson, & R. R. Leutenegger (Eds.), *Stuttering in children and adults.* Minneapolis, MN: University of Minnesota Press.

Johnson, W., & Associates. (1959). *The onset of stuttering.* Minneapolis, MN: University of Minnesota Press.

Johnson, W., & Brown, S. F. (1935). Stuttering in relation to various speech sounds. *Quarterly Journal of Speech, 21*, 481–496.

Johnson, W., Darley, F., & Spriestersbach, D. (1952). *Diagnostic manual in speech correction: A professional training workbook.* New York: Harper & Brothers.

Johnson, W., Darley, F., & Spriestersbach, D. (1963). *Diagnostic methods in speech pathology.* New York: Harper & Row.

Johnson, W., and Inness, M. (1939). Studies in the psychology of stuttering: XIII. A statistical analysis of the adaptation and consistency effects in relation to stuttering. *Journal of Speech Disorders, 4*:79–86.

Johnson, W., and Knott, J.R. (1937). Studies in the psychology of stuttering: I. The distribution of moments of stuttering in successive readings of the same material. *Journal of Speech Disorders, 2*:17–19.

Johnson, W., & Rosen, L. (1937). Studies in the psychology of stuttering: IV. A quantitative study of expectation of stuttering as a process involving a low degree of consciousness. *Journal of Speech Disorders, 2*, 95–97.

Johnson, W., and Solomon, A. (1937). Studies in the psychology of stuttering: IV. A quantitative study of expectation of stuttering as a process involving a low degree of consciousness. *Journal of Speech Disorders, 2*:95–97.

Johnson, K. N., Walden, T. A., Conture, E. G., & Karrass, J. (2010). Spontaneous regulation of emotions in pre-school children who stutter: Preliminary findings. *Journal of Speech Language and Hearing Research, 53*(6), 1478–1495.

Jokel, R., De Nil, L. F., & Sharpe, K. (2007). Speech disfluencies in adults with neurogenic stuttering associated with stroke and traumatic brain injury. *Journal of Medical Speech-Language Pathology, 15*(3), 243–262.

Jones, J. E., & Niven, P. (1993). *Voices and silences.* New York: Charles Scribner's Sons.

Jones, M., Onslow, M., Packman, A., Williams, S., Ormond, T., Schwartz, I., et al. (2005). Randomized controlled trial of the Lidcombe Programme of early stuttering intervention. *British Medical Journal, 331*, 659–661.

Jones, R. K. (1966). Observations on stammering after localized cerebral injury. *Journal of Neurology, Neurosurgery and Psychiatry, 29*, 192–195.

Kagan, J. (1981). *The Second Year: The Emergence of Self-Awareness.* Cambridge, MA: Harvard University Press.

Kagan, J. (1989). Temperamental contributions to social behavior. *American Psychologist, 44*, 668–674.

Kagan, J. (1994a). The realistic view of biology and behavior. *The Chronicle of Higher Education, 5*, A64.

Kagan, J. (1994b). *Galen's prophecy: Temperament in human nature.* New York: Basic Books.

Kagan, J., & Snidman, N. (1991). Temperamental factors in human development. *American Psychologist, 46*(8), 856–862.

Kagan, J., Reznick, J. S., & Snidman, N. (1987). The physiology and psychology of behavioral inhibition in children. *Child Development, 58*, 1459–1473.

Kang, C., Riazuddin, S., Mundorf, J., Krasnewich, D., Friedman, P., Mulliken, et al. (2010). Mutations in the lysosomal enzyme-targeting pathway and persistent stuttering. *New England Journal of Medicine, 362*(8), 677–685.

Karlin, I. W. (1947). A psychosomatic theory of stuttering. *Journal of Speech Disorders, 12*(3), 319–322.

Karniol, R. (1992). Stuttering out of bilingualism. *First Language, 12*(38), 255–283.

Karrass, J., Walden, T. A., Conture, E. G., Graham, C. G., Arnold, H. S., & Hartfield, K. N. (2006). Relation of emotional reactivity and regulation to childhood stuttering. *Journal of Communication Disorders, 32*, 402–423.

Kasprisin-Burrelli, A., Egolf, D. B., & Shames, G. H. (1972). A comparison of parental verbal behavior with stuttering and nonstuttering children. *Journal of Communication Disorders, 5*, 335–346.

Kay, D. (1964). The genetics of stuttering. In G. Andrews and M. Harris (Eds.), *The Syndrome of Stuttering.* London: The Spastics Society Medical Education and Information Unit, 132-143.

Kelly, E. (1994). Speech rates and turn-taking behaviors of children who stutter and their fathers. *Journal of Speech and Hearing Research, 37*, 1284–1267.

Kelly, E., & Conture, E. (1992). Speaking rates, response time latencies, and interrupting behaviors of young stutterers, nonstutterers, and their mothers. *Journal of Speech and Hearing Research, 35*, 1256–1267.

Kelly, E., Smith, A., and Goffman, L. (1995). Orofacial muscle activity of children who stutter. *Journal of Speech and Hearing Research, 38*:1025–1036.

Kelman, E., & Nicholas, A. (2008). *Practical intervention for early childhood stammering.* Milton Keynes, UK: Speechmark.

Kempf, L., & Weinberger, D. R. (2009). Molecular genetics and bioinformatics: An outline for neuropsychological genetics. In L. Kempf, & D. R. Weinberger (Eds.), *The genetics of cognitive neuroscience.* Cambridge, MA: MIT Press.

Kent, R. D. (1981). Sensorimotor aspects of speech development. In R. D. Alberts, & M. R. Peterson (Eds.), *The development of perception: Psycho-biological perspectives.* New York: Academic Press.

Kent, R. D. (1984). Stuttering as a temporal programming disorder. In R. F. Curlee, & W. H. Perkins (Eds.), *Nature and treatment of stuttering: New directions* (pp. 283–301). San Diego, CA: College-Hill Press.

Kent, R. D. (1985). Developing and disordered speech: Strategies for organization. *American Speech, Language and Hearing Association Reports, 15*, 29–37.

Kent, R. D. (1993). Speech intelligibility and communicative competence in children. In A. P. Kiser, & D. B. Gray (Eds.), *Enhancing children's communication: Research foundations for intervention* (Vol. 2, pp. 223–229). Baltimore: Brooks Publishing.

Kent, R. D. (1997). *The speech sciences.* San Diego, CA: Singular Publishing Company.

Kent, R. D. (2000). Research on speech motor control and its disorders: A review and prospective. *Journal of Communication Disorders, 33*, 391–428.

Kent, R. D., & Perkins, W. (1984). *Oral-verbal fluency: Aspects of verbal formulation, speech motor control and underlying neural systems.* Unpublished manuscript.

Kent, R. D., & Vorperian, H. K. (1995). Anatomic development of the craniofacial-oral-laryngeal systems: A review. *Journal of Medical Speech-Language Pathology, 3*, 145–190.

Kent, R. D., & Vorperian, H. K. (2007). In the mouths of babes: Anatomic motor and sensory foundations of speech development. In R. Paul (Ed.), *Language Disorders from a Developmental Perspective: Essays in Honor of Robin Chapman* (pp. 56–80). Mahwah, NJ: Lawrence Erlbaum.

Kenyon, E. L. (1942). The etiology of stammering: Fundamentally a wrong psychophysiologic habit in control of the vocal cords for the production of an individual speech sound. *Journal of Speech Disorders, 7*, 97–104.

Kidd, K. K. (1977). A genetic perspective on stuttering. *Journal of Fluency Disorders, 2*, 259–269.

Kidd, K. K. (1984). Stuttering as a genetic disorder. In R. F. Curlee, & W. H. Perkins (Eds.), *Nature and Treatment of Stuttering: New Directions* (pp. 149–169). San Diego, CA: College-Hill Press.

Kidd, K. K., Heimbuch, R. C., Records, M. A., Oehlert, G., & Webster, R. L. (1980). Familial stuttering patterns are not related to one measure of severity *Journal of Speech and Hearing Research, 23*, 539–545.

Kidd, K. K., Kidd, J. R., & Records, M. A. (1978). The possible causes of the sex ratio in stuttering and its implications. *Journal of Fluency Disorders, 3*, 13–23.

Kidd, K.K., Reich, T., and Kessler, S. (1973). A genetic analysis of stuttering suggesting a single major locus. *Genetics,* 74:(2, Part 2)s137.

Kimura, D. (1961). Cerebral dominance and the perception of verbal stimuli. *Canadian Journal of Psychology,* 15:166–177.

Kinsbourne, M. (1989). A model of adaptive behavior related to cerebral participation in emotional control. In G. Gianotti, & C. Caltagirone (Eds.), *Emotions and the Dual Brain.* New York: Springer-Verlag.

Kinsbourne, M., & Bemporad, E. (1984). Lateralization of emotion: A model and the evidence. In N. Fox, & R. Davidson (Eds.), *The Psychology of Affective Development.* Hillsdale, NJ: Lawrence Erlbaum Associates.

Kinsbourne, M., and Hicks, R. (1978). Functional cerebral space: A model for overflow, transfer and interference effects in human performance: A tutorial review. In M. Kinsbourne (Ed), *Asymmetrical Function of the Brain.* Cambridge, UK: Cambridge University Press, pp 345–362.

Kleinow, J., and Smith, A. (2000). Influences of length and syntactic complexity on the speech motor stability of the fluent speech of adults who stutter. *Journal of Speech, Language, and Hearing Research, 43*:548–559.

Kline, M. L., & Starkweather, C. W. (1979). Receptive and expressive language performance in young stutterers. (Abstract). *American Speech, Language and Hearing Association, 21,* 797.

Kloth, S. A. M., Kraaimaat, F. W., Janssen, P., & Brutten, G. J. (1999). Persistence and remission of incipient stuttering among high-risk children. *Journal of Fluency Disorders, 24*(4), 253–265.

Kloth, S., Janssen, P., Kraaimaat, F., & Brutten, G. (1995). Speech-motor and linguistic skills of young stutterers prior to onset. *Journal of Fluency Disorders, 20,* 157–170.

Kloth, S., Janssen, P., Kraaimaat, F., & Brutten, G. (1998). Child and mother variables in the development of stuttering among high-risk children: A longitudinal study. *Journal of Fluency Disorders, 23,* 217–230.

Knott, J.R., Johnson, W., and Webster, M.J. (1937). Studies in the psychology of stuttering: II. A quantitative evaluation of expectation of stuttering in relation to the occurrence of stuttering. *Journal of Speech Disorders, 2*:20–22.

Kolk, H., & Postma, A. (1997). Stuttering as a covert repair phenomenon. In R. F. Curlee, & G. M. Siegel (Eds.), *Nature and Treatment of Stuttering: New Directions* (2nd ed., pp. 182–203). Boston: Allyn & Bacon.

Kramer, M., Green, D., and Guitar, B. (1987). A comparison of stutterers and nonstutterers on masking level differences and synthetic sentence identification tasks. *Journal of Communication Disorders,* 20:379–390.

Kroll, R.M., De Nil, L.F., Kapur, S., and Houle, S. (1997). A positron emission tomography investigation of post-treatment brain activation in stutterers. In W. Hulstijn, H.F.M. Peters, and P.H.H.M. van Lieshout (Eds), *Speech Production: Motor Control, Brain Research and Fluency Disorders.* Amsterdam: Elsevier, pp 307–319.

Kroll, R. M., & Scott-Sulsky, L. (2010). The Fluency Plus Program: An integration of fluency shaping and cognitive restructuring procedures for adolescents and adults who stutter. In B. Guitar, & R. J. McCauley (Eds.), *Treatment of Stuttering: Established and Emerging Interventions* (pp. 277–311). Baltimore: Lippincott Williams and Wilkins.

Kully, D., & Langevin, M. (1999). Intensive behavioral treatment for stuttering adolescents. In R. Curlee (Ed.), *Stuttering and Related Disorders of Fluency* (2nd ed., pp. 139–159). New York: Thieme.

Langevin, M., Kully, D., Teshima, S., Hagler, P., & Prasad, N. G. N. (2010). Five-year longitudinal treatment outcomes of the ISTAR Comprehensive Treatment Program. *Journal of Fluency Disorders, 35,* 123–140.

Langevin, M., Packman, A., & Onslow, M. (2010). Parent perceptions of the impact of stuttering on their preschoolers and themselves. *Journal of Communication Disorders, 43*(5), 407–423.

Langlois, A., & Long, S. H. (1988). A model for teaching parents to facilitate fluent speech. *Journal of Fluency Disorders, 13,* 163–172.

Langlois, A., Hanrahan, L. L., & Inouye, L. L. (1986). A comparison of interactions between stuttering children, nonstuttering children, and their mothers. *Journal of Fluency Disorders, 11,* 263–273.

LaSalle, L. (1999, November). *Temperament in preschoolers who stutter: A preliminary investigation.* Paper presented at the Annual Meeting of the American Speech-Language-Hearing Association, San Francisco, CA.

LaSalle, L., & Conture, E. (1995). Eye contact between young stutterers and their mothers. *Journal of Fluency Disorders, 16,* 173–199.

Lauter, J.L. (1995). Visions of speech and language: Noninvasive imaging techniques and their applications to the study of human communication. In H. Winitz (Ed), *Current Approaches to the Study of Language Development and Disorders.* Timonium, MD: York Press, pp 277–390.

Lauter, J. L. (1997). Noninvasive brain imaging in speech motor control and stuttering: Choices and challenges. In W. Hulstijn, H. F. M. Peters, & P. H. H. M. van Lieshout (Eds.), *Speech Production: Motor Control, Brain Research, and Fluency Disorders* (pp. 233–258). Amsterdam: Elsevier.

Lazare, A. (1981). Current concepts in psychiatry: Conversion symptoms. *New England Journal of Medicine, 305,* 745.

LeDoux, J. E. (1996). *The emotional brain: The mysterious underpinnings of emotional life.* New York: Simon & Schuster.

LeDoux, J. E. (2002). *Synaptic self: How our brains become who we are.* New York: Viking.

Lee, B. S. (1951). The artificial stutter. *Journal of Speech and Hearing Disorders, 16,* 53–55.

Lefton, L. A. (1997). *Psychology* (6th ed.). Boston: Allyn & Bacon.

Lewis, M. (2000). Self-conscious emotions: Embarrassment, pride, shame and guilt. In M. Lewis, and J.M. Haviland-Jones (Eds), *Handbook of Emotions* (ed 2). New York: Guilford Press.

Lidz, T. (1968). *The person: His development throughout the life cycle.* New York: Basic Books.

Liebetrau, R., and Daly, D. (1981). Auditory processing and perceptual abilities of "organic" and "functional" stutterers. *Journal of Fluency Disorders,* 6:219–231.

Lincoln, M., & Onslow, M. (1997). Long-term outcome of an early intervention for stuttering. *American Journal of Speech-Language Pathology, 6,* 51–58.

Lindsay, J. S. (1989). Relationship of developmental disfluency and episodes of stuttering to the emergence of cognitive stages in children. *Journal of Fluency Disorders, 14*(4), 271–284.

Logan, K., & Conture, E. (1995). Length, grammatical complexity, and rate differences in stuttered and fluent conversational utterances of children who stutter. *Journal of Fluency Disorders, 20,* 35–61.

Luchsinger, R. (1944). Biological studies on monozygotic and dizygotic twins relative to size and form of the larynx. *Archiv Julius Klaus-Stiftung fur Verergungsforchung, 19,* 3–4.

Maassen, B., Kent, R. D., Peters, H. F. M., van Lieshout, P. H. H. M., & Hulstijn, W. (2004). *Speech motor control in normal and disordered speech.* Oxford, UK: Oxford University Press.

MacNeilage, P. (1987). The evolution of hemispheric specialization for manual function and language. In S. P. Wise (Ed.), *Higher Brain Functions* (pp. 285–309). New York: John Wiley and Sons.

Maguire, G., Franklin, D. L., Vatakis, N. G., Morgenshtern, E., Denko, T., Yaruss, J. S., et al. (2010). Exploratory randomized clinical study of pagoclone in persistent developmental stuttering: The Examining Pagaclone for Persistent Developmental Stuttering Study. *Journal of Clinical Psychopharmacology, 30*(1), 48–56.

Maguire, G., Riley, G., Franklin, D. L., & Gumusaneli, E. (2010). The physiological basis and pharmacologic treatment of stuttering. In B. Guitar, & R. J. McCauley (Eds.), *Treatment of stuttering: Established and emerging interventions* (pp. 329–354). Baltimore: Lippincott Williams and Wilkins.

Maguire, G., Yu, B. P., Franklin, D. L., & Riley, G. D. (2004). Alleviating stuttering with pharmacological interventions. *Expert Opinion in Pharmacotherapy, 5,* 1565–1571.

Mahr, G., & Leith, W. (1992). Psychogenic stuttering of adult onset. *Journal of Speech and Hearing Research, 35,* 283–286.

Manning, W. H. (2010). *Clinical decision making in fluency disorders* (3rd ed.). Clifton Park, NJ: Delmar, Cengage Learning.

Mansson, H. (2000). Childhood stuttering: Incidence and development. *Journal of Fluency Disorders, 25*(1), 47–57.

Market, K. E., Montague, J. C., Buffalo, M. D., & Drummond, S. A. (1990). Acquired stuttering: Descriptive data and treatment outcomes. *Journal of Fluency Disorders, 15,* 21–33.

Marshall, R. C., & Starch, S. A. (1984). Behavioral treatment of acquired stuttering. *Australian Journal of Human Communication Disorders, 12,* 87–92.

Martin, R., Haroldson, S. K., & Triden, K. A. (1984). Stuttering and speech naturalness. *Journal of Speech and Hearing Disorders, 49*(1), 53–58.

Maske-Cash, W., & Curlee, R. (1995). Effect of utterance length and meaningfulness on the speech initiation times of children who stutter and children who do not stutter. *Journal of Speech and Hearing Research, 38,* 18–25.

Mattes, L. J., & Omack, D. R. (1991). *Speech and language assessment for the bilingually handicapped.* Oceanside, CA: Academic Communication Associates.

Matthews, S., Williams, R., & Pring, T. (1997). Parent-child interaction therapy and dysfluency: A single-case study. *European Journal of Disorders of Communication, 32,* 346–357.

Max, L., Guenther, F. H., Gracco, V. L., Ghosh, S. S., & Wallace, M. E. (2004). Unstable or insufficiently activated internal models and feedback-biased motor-control as sources of dysfluency: A theoretical model of stuttering. *Contemporary Issues in Communication Science and Disorders, 31,* 105–122.

McCauley, R. J., & Fey, M. E. (2006). *Treatment of language disorders in children.* Baltimore: Paul H. Brookes Publishing Co.

McClean, M. D. (1990). Neuromotor aspects of stuttering: Levels of impairment and disability. In J. Cooper (Ed.), *Research Needs in Stuttering: Roadblocks and Future Directions (ASHA Reports, 18)* (pp. 64–71). Rockville, MD: American Speech-Language-Hearing Association.

McClean, M. D., & McClean, A. (1985). Case report of stuttering acquired in association with phenytoin use for post-head-injury seizures. *Journal of Fluency Disorders, 10,* 241–255.

McClean, M. D., Kroll, R. M., & Loftus, N. S. (1990). Kinematic analysis of lip closure in stutterers' fluent speech. *Journal of Speech and Hearing Research, 33,* 755–760.

McDearmon, J. R. (1968). Primary stuttering at the onset of stuttering: A reexamination of data. *Journal of Speech and Hearing Research, 11,* 631–637.

McDevitt, S. C., & Carey, W. (1978). A measure of temperament in 3–7-year-old children. *Journal of Child Psychology and Psychiatry and Allied Disciplines, 19,* 245–253.

McDevitt, S. C., & Carey, W. (1995). *Behavioral style questionnaire.* West Chester, PA: TempraMetrics.

McFarlane, D. H., & Prins, D. (1978). Neural response time of stutterers and nonstutterers in selected oral motor tasks. *Journal of Speech and Hearing Research, 21,* 768–778.

Merson, R. M. (2003). *Auditory sidetone and the management of stuttering: From Wollensack to SpeechEasy.* Paper presented at the International Stuttering Awareness Day Online Conference.

Meyers, S. C., & Freeman, F. J. (1985a). Interruptions as a variable in stuttering and disfluency. *Journal of Speech and Hearing Research, 28,* 428–425.

Meyers, S. C., & Freeman, F. J. (1985b). Mother and child speech rate as a variable in stuttering and disfluency. *Journal of Speech and Hearing Research, 28,* 436–444.

Miles, S., & Ratner, N. (2001). Parental language input to children at stuttering onset. *Journal of Speech, Language and Hearing Research, 44,* 1116–1130.

Milisen, R. (1938). Frequency of stuttering with anticipation of stuttering controlled. *Journal of Speech Disorders, 3:*207–214.

Milisen, R., & Johnson, W. (1936). A comparative study of stutterers, former stutterers and normal speakers whose handedness has been changed. *Archives of Speech, 1,* 61–86.

Millard, S. K., Edwards, S., & Cook, F. (2009). Parent-child interaction therapy: Adding to the evidence. *International Journal of Speech-Language Pathology, 11*(1), 61–76.

Millard, S. K., Nicholas, A., & Cook, F. (2008). Is parent-child interaction therapy effective in reducing stuttering? *Journal of Speech, Language and Hearing Research, 51*(3), 636–650.

Miller, B., & Guitar, B. (2009). Long-term outcome of the Lidcombe Program for early stuttering intervention. *American Journal of Speech-Language Pathology, 18,* 42–49.

Miller, S. (1993). *Multiple measures of anxiety and psychophysiologic arousal in stutterers and nonstutterers during nonspeech and speech tasks of increasing complexity.* Unpublished doctoral dissertation, University of Texas at Dallas.

Mineka, S. (1985). Animal models of anxiety-based disorders: Their usefulness and limitations. In A. H. Tuma, & J. Mase (Eds.), *Anxiety and the Anxiety Disorders.* Hillsdale, NJ: Lawrence Erlbaum Associates.

Minifie, F. D., & Cooker, H. S. (1964). A disfluency index. *Journal of Speech and Hearing Disorders, 29,* 189–192.

Molt, L.F. (1997). *Event-related cortical potentials and language processing in stutterers.* Paper presented at the 2nd World Congress on Fluency Disorders, San Francisco, CA.

Molt, L.F., and Guilford, A.M. (1979). Auditory processing and anxiety in stutterers. *Journal of Fluency Disorders, 4:*255–267.

Moncur, J. P. (1952). Parental domination in stuttering. *Journal of Speech and Hearing Disorders, 17,* 155–165.

Moore, B. J., & Montgomery, J. K. (2007). *Making a difference for America's children: Speech pathologist in public schools* (2nd ed.). Greenville, SC: Super Duper Publications.

Moore, W. H., Jr., & Haynes, W. O. (1980). Alpha hemispheric asymmetry and stuttering: Some support for a segmentation dysfunction hypothesis. *Journal of Speech and Hearing Research, 23,* 229–247.

Morgenstern, J. J. (1956). Socio-economic factors in stuttering. *Journal of Speech and Hearing Disorders, 21,* 25–33.

Murphy, B. (1999). The school-age child who stutters: Dealing effectively with guilt and shame. *Practical ideas for the school clinician [DVD].* Memphis, TN: Stuttering Foundation of America.

Murray, H. L., & Reed, C. G. (1977). Language abilities of preschool stuttering children. *Journal of Fluency Disorders, 2,* 171–176.

Myers, F. (2002). *Putting cluttering on the map: Looking back/looking ahead.* Paper presented at the annual meeting of the American Speech-Language-Hearing Association, Atlanta, GA.

Myers, F. (2011). Treatment of cluttering: A cognitive-behavioral approach centered on rate control. In D. Ward, & K. S. Scott (Eds.), *Cluttering: A Handbook of Research, Intervention and Education* (pp. 152–174). Hove, UK: Psychology Press.

Myers, F. L. (1978). Relationship between eight physiological variables and severity of stuttering. *Journal of Fluency Disorders, 3,* 181–191.

Myers, F. L., & St. Louis, K. (1986). *Cluttering: A clinical perspective.* San Diego, CA: Singular.

Myers, F., & St. Louis, K. (2007). *Cluttering [DVD].* Memphis, TN: Stuttering Foundation.

National Institute of Neurological Disorders and Stroke (2011). *Mucolipidoses fact sheet.* Retrieved November 2, 2012 from http://www.ninds.nih.gov/disorders/mucolipidoses/detail_mucolipidoses.htm.

Namasivayam, A. K., van Lieshout, P. H. H. M., McIlroy, W., E., & De Nil, L. F. (2009). Sensory feedback dependence hypothesis in persons who stutter. *Human Movement Science, 28*(6), 688–707.

Navon, D. (1984). Resources—A theoretical stone soup. *Psychological Review, 91:*216–234.

Neilson, M.D. (1980). *Stuttering and the control of speech: A systems analysis approach.* Unpublished doctoral dissertation, University of New South Wales, Kensington, Australia.

Neilson, M. D., & Neilson, P. D. (1987). Speech motor control and stuttering: A computational model of adaptive sensory-motor processing. *Speech Communication, 6*(325–333).

Neilson, M. D., & Neilson, P. D. (1988). *Sensory-motor integration capacity of stutterers and nonstutterers.* Paper presented at the Second Australian International Conference on Speech Science and Technology, Sydney, Australia.

Neilson, M. D., Howie, P. M., & Andrews, G. (1987). *Does foetal testosterone play a role in the aetiology of stuttering?* Paper presented at the Fifth International Australasian Winter Conference on Brain Research, Queenstown, New Zealand.

Neilson, P. D., & Neilson, M. D. (2005a). An overview of adaptive model theory: Solving the problems of redundancy, resources, and nonlinear interactions in human movement control. *Journal of Neural Engineering, 2,* S279–312.

Neilson, P. D., & Neilson, M. D. (2005b). Motor maps and synergies. *Human Movement Science, 24,* 774–797.

Neilson, P. D., Neilson, M. D., & O'Dwyer, N. J. (1992). Adaptive model theory: Application to disorders of motor control. In J. J. Summers (Ed.), *Approaches to the Study of Motor Control and Learning.* Amsterdam: Elsevier Science Publishers.

Neilson, P. D., Quinn, P. T., & Neilson, M. D. (1976). Auditory tracking measures of hemispheric asymmetry in normals and stutterers. *Australian Journal of Human Communication, 4,* 121–126.

Nelson, N. W. (1998). *Childhood language disorders in context: Infancy through adolescence.* Boston: Allyn & Bacon.

Netsell, R. (1981). The acquisition of speech motor control: A perspective with direction for research. In R. Stark (Ed.), *Language Behavior in Infancy and Early Childhood.* New York: Elsevier-North Holland.

Neumann, K., & Euler, H. (2010). Neuroimaging and stuttering. In B. Guitar, & R. J. McCauley (Eds.), *Stuttering Treatment: Established and Emerging Interventions* (pp. 355–377). Baltimore: Lippincott Williams & Wilkins.

Neumann, K., Euler, H., Wolff von Gudenberg, A., Giraud, A. -L., Lanfermann, H., Gall, V., & Preibisch C. (2003). The nature and treatment of stuttering as revealed by fMRI: A within- and between-group comparison. *Journal of Fluency Disorders, 28,* 381–411.

Neumann, K., Preibisch, C., Euler, H., Wolff von Gudenberg, A., Giraud, A.-L., Lanfermann, H., et al. (2005). Cortical plasticity associated with stuttering therapy. *Journal of Fluency Disorders, 30,* 23–29.

Nippold, M. A. (1990). Concomitant speech and language disorders in stuttering children: A critique of the literature. *Journal of Speech and Hearing Disorders, 55,* 51–60.

Nippold, M. A. (2007). *Later language development: School-age children, adolescence, and young adults* (3rd ed.). Austin, TX: Pro-Ed.

Nippold, M. A., & Rudzinski, M. (1995). Parents' speech and children's stuttering: A critique of the literature. *Journal of Speech and Hearing Research, 38,* 978–989.

Nittrouer, S., Studdert-Kennedy, M., & McGowan, R. S. (1989). The emergence of phonetic segments: Evidence from the spectral structure of fricative-vowel syllables spoken by children and adults. *Journal of Speech and Hearing Research, 32,* 120–132.

Ntourou, K., Conture, E. G., & Lipsey, M. W. (2011). Language abilities of children who stutter: A meta-analytical review. *American Journal of Speech-Language Pathology, 20*(3), 163–179.

Nudelman, H. B., Herbrich, K. E., Hess, K. R., & Hoyt, B. D. (1992). A model of the phonatory response time of stutterers and fluent speakers to frequency-modulated tones. *Journal of the Acoustical Society of America, 92,* 1882–1888.

Nudelman, H. B., Herbrich, K. E., Hoyt, B. D., & Rosenfield, D. B. (1987). Dynamic characteristics of vocal frequency tracking in stutterers and nonstutterers. In H. F. M. Peters, & W. Hulstijn (Eds.), *Speech Motor Dynamics in Stuttering.* Wien, Austria: Springer-Verlag.

Nudelman, H. B., Herbrich, K. E., Hoyt, B. D., & Rosenfield, D. B. (1989). A neuroscience model of stuttering. *Journal of Fluency Disorders, 14,* 399–427.

Nurnberg, H. G., & Greenwald, B. (1981). Stuttering: An unusual side effect of phenothiasines. *American Journal of Psychiatry, 138,* 386–387.

O'Brian, S., Onslow, M., Cream, A., & Packman, A. (2003). The Camperdown Program: Outcomes of a new prolonged-speech treatment model. *Journal of Speech Language and Hearing Research, 46,* 933–946.

O'Brian, S., Packman, A., & Onslow, M. (2004). Self-rating of stuttering severity as a clinical tool. *American Journal of Speech-Language Pathology, 13,* 219–226.

O'Brian, S., Packman, A., & Onslow, M. (2008). Telehealth delivery of the Camperdown program for adults who stutter: A phase I trial. *Journal of Speech, Language, and Hearing Research, 51,* 184–195.

O'Brian, S., Packman, A., & Onslow, M. (2010). The Camperdown Program. In B. Guitar, & R. J. McCauley (Eds.), *Treatment of Stuttering: Established and Emerging Interventions* (pp. 256–276). Baltimore: Lippincott Williams & Wilkins.

Okasha, A., Bishry, Z., Kamel, M., & Hassan, A. H. (1974). Psychosocial study of stammering in Egyptian children. *British Journal of Psychiatry, 124,* 531–533.

Olander, L., Smith, A., & Zelaznik, H. N. (2010). Evidence that a motor timing deficit is a factor in the development of stuttering. *Journal of Speech Language and Hearing Research, 53,* 876–886.

Onslow, M., Andrews, C., & Costa, L. (1990). Parental severity scaling of early stuttered speech: Four case studies. *Australian Journal of Human Communication, 18,* 47–61.

Onslow, M., Andrews, C., & Lincoln, M. (1994). A control/experimental trial of an operant treatment for early stuttering. *Journal of Speech and Hearing Research, 37,* 1244–1259.

Onslow, M., Costa, L., & Rue, S. (1990). Direct early intervention with stuttering: Some preliminary data. *Journal of Speech and Hearing Disorders, 55,* 405–416.

Onslow, M., Harrison, E., Jones, M., & Packman, A. (2002). Beyond-clinic speech measures during the Lidcombe Program of early stuttering intervention. *Acquiring Knowledge in Speech, Language and Hearing, 4,* 82–85.

Onslow, M., Packman, A., & Harrison, E. (2003). *The Lidcombe Program of early stuttering intervention: A clinician's guide.* Austin, TX: Pro-Ed.

Ooki, S. (2005). Genetic and environmental influences on stuttering and tics in Japanese twins. *Twin Research and Human Genetics, 8,* 529–575.

Orton, S. (1927). Studies in stuttering. *Archives of Neurology and Psychiatry, 18,* 671–672.

Orton, S., & Travis, L. E. (1929). Studies of stuttering: IV. Studies of action currents in stuttering. *Archives of Neurology and Psychiatry 21,* 61–68.

Oyler, M. E. (1992, November). *Self perception and sensitivity in stuttering adults.* Paper presented at the Annual Convention of the American Speech-Language-Hearing Association, San Antonio, TX.

Oyler, M. E., & Ramig, P. R. (1995, December). *Vulnerability in stuttering children.* Paper presented at the Annual Convention of the American Speech-Language-Hearing Association, Orlando, FL.

Paden, E. (2005). Development of phonological ability. In E. Yairi, & N. G. Ambrose (Eds.), *Early Childhood Stuttering: For Clinicians, by Clinicians* (pp. 197–234). Austin, TX: Pro-Ed.

Paden, E. P., Yairi, E., & Ambrose, N. G. (1999). Early childhood stuttering II: Initial status of phonological abilities. *Journal of Speech, Language and Hearing Research, 42*(5), 1113–1124.

Paul, R., & Norbury, C. (2011). *Language disorders from infancy through adolescence: Listening, speaking, reading, writing and communicating* (4th ed.). St. Louis, MO: Mosby.

Paulesu, E., Frith, C. D., & Frackowiak, R. S. (1993). Neural correlates of the verbal component of working memory. *Nature, 362*(6418), 342–345.

Pavuluri, M. N., & Passaroti, A. (2008). Neural bases of emotional processing in pediatric bipolar disorder. *Expert Review of Neurotherapeutics, 8*(9), 1381–1387.

Pearl, S. Z., & Bernthal, J. E. (1980). The effect of grammatical complexity upon disfluency behavior of nonstuttering preschool children. *Journal of Fluency Disorders, 5,* 55–68.

Perino, M., Famularo, G., & Tarroni, P. (2000). Acquired transient stuttering during a migraine attack. *Headache, 40,* 170–172.

Perkins, W. H., Kent, R. D., & Curlee, R. F. (1991). A theory of neuropsycholinguistic function in stuttering. *Journal of Speech and Hearing Research, 34,* 734–752.

Peters, H. F. M., & Hulstijn, W. (1984). Stuttering and anxiety: The difference between stutterers and nonstutterers in verbal apprehension and physiologic arousal during the anticipation of speech and non-speech tasks. *Journal of Fluency Disorders, 9,* 67–84.

Peters, T. J. (1968). Oral language skills of children who stutter. (Abstract). *Speech Monographs, 35,* 325.

Peters, T. J., & Guitar, B. (1991). *Stuttering: An integrated approach to its nature and treatment.* Baltimore: Williams & Wilkins.

Pierson, S. M. (2004). *Evaluating validity and reliability of the Teacher Assessment of Student Communicative Competence (TASCC) by comparing students who do and do not stutter.* M. S., University of Vermont, Burlington, VT.

Piertranton, A. (2003, June). *Evidence based practice.* Paper presented at the Special Interest Division 4 Leadership Conference (ASHA), St. Louis, MO.

Pinsky, S., and McAdams, D. (1980). Electroencephalographic and dichotic indices of cerebral intensity of stutterers. *Brain and Language,* 11:374–397.

Pindzola, R., Jenkins, M., & Lokken, K. (1989). Speaking rates of young children. *Language, Speech, and Hearing Services in Schools, 20,* 133–138.

Platt, J., & Basili, A. (1973). Jaw tremor during stuttering block: An electromyographic study. *Journal of Communication Disorders, 6,* 102–109.

Pollard, R., Ellis, J. B., Finan, D., & Ramig, P. R. (2009). Effects of the SpeechEasy on objective and perceived aspects of stuttering: A 6-month, phase 1 clinical trial in naturalistic environments. *Journal of Speech Language and Hearing Research, 52*(2), 516–533.

Ponsford, R. E., Brown, W. S., Marsh, J. T., & Travis, L. E. (1975). Evoked potential correlates of cerebral dominance for speech perception in stutterers and nonstutterers. *Electroencephalography and Clinical Neurophysiology, 39,* 434.

Pool, K. D., Devous, M. D., Freeman, F. J., Watson, B. C., & Finitzo, T. (1991). Regional cerebral blood flow in developmental stutterers. *Archives of Neurology, 48,* 509–512.

Poulos, M. G., & Webster, W. G. (1991). Family history as a basis for subgrouping people who stutter. *Journal of Speech and Hearing Research, 34,* 5-10.

Preus, A. (1981). *Identifying subgroups of stutterers.* Oslo, Norway: Universitetsforlaget.

Prins, D. (1991). Theories of stuttering as event and disorder: Implications for speech production processes. In H. F. M. Peters, W. Hulstijn, & C. W. Starkweather (Eds.), *Speech motor control and stuttering.* Amsterdam: Elsevier Sciences Publishers.

Prins, D. (1999). Describing the consequences of disorders: Comment on Yaruss (1998). *Journal of Speech, Language and Hearing Research, 42,* 1395–1397.

Prins, D., Mandelkorn, T., & Cerf, F. A. (1980). Principal and differential effects of haloperidol and placebo treatments upon speech disfluencies in stutterers. *Journal of Speech and Hearing Research, 23,* 614–629.

Proceedings of the NINCDS workshop on treatment efficacy research in stuttering. September 21–22, 1992. (1993). *Journal of Fluency Disorders, 18(Special issue).*

Quader, S. E. (1977). Dysarthria: An unusual side effect of tricyclic antidepressants. *British Medical Journal, 9,* 97.

Quinn, P. (1972). Stuttering, cerebral dominance, and the dichotic word test. *Medical Journal of Australia,* 2:639–642.

Rahman, P. (1956). *The self-concept and ideal self-concept of stutterers as compared to nonstutterers.* Unpublished masters thesis, Brooklyn College, Brooklyn, NY.

Ramig, P. R. (1993). The impact of self-help groups on persons who stutter: A call for research. *Journal of Fluency Disorders, 18,* 351–361.

Ramig, P. R., Ellis, J. B., & Polland, R. (2010). Application of the SpeechEasy to stuttering treatment: Introduction, background, and preliminary observations. In B. Guitar, & R. J. McCauley (Eds.), *Treatment of stuttering: Established and emerging interventions* (pp. 312–328). Baltimore: Lippincott Williams and Wilkins.

Rapee, R. M., Wignall, A., Psych, M., Hudson, J. L., & Schniering, C. A. (2000). *Treating anxious children and adolescents: An evidence-based approach.* Oakland, CA: New Harbinger Publications, Inc.

Rentschler, G. I., Driver, L. E., & Callaway, E. A. (1984). The onset of stuttering following drug overdose. *Journal of Fluency Disorders, 9,* 265–284.

Riaz, N., Steinberg, S., Ahmad, J., Pluzhnikov, A., Riazuddin, S., Cox, N., et al (2005). Genomewide significant linkage to stuttering on chromosome 12. *American Journal of Human Genetics, 76,* 647–651.

Richels, C. G., & Conture, E. (2007). An indirect treatment approach for early intervention for childhood stuttering. In E. Conture, & R. Curlee (Eds.), *Stuttering and Related Disorders of Fluency* (pp. 77–99). New York: Thieme.

Richels, C. G., & Conture, E. (2010). Indirect treatment of childhood stuttering: Diagnostic predictors of treatment outcome. In B. Guitar, & R. J. McCauley (Eds.), *Treatment of Stuttering: Established and Emerging Interventions.* Baltimore: Lippincott Williams & Wilkins.

Riley, G. (1972). A stuttering severity instrument for children and adults. *Journal of Speech and Hearing Disorders, 37,* 314–322.

Riley, G. (1994). *Stuttering severity instrument for children and adults* (3rd ed.). Austin, TX: Pro-Ed.

Riley, G., & Riley, J. (1979). A component model for diagnosing and treating children who stutter. *Journal of Fluency Disorders, 4,* 279–292.

Ringo, C. C., & Dietrich, S. (1995). Neurogenic stuttering: An analysis and critique. *Journal of Medical Speech-Language Pathology, 3,* 111–122.

Roberts, P., & Shenker, R. (2007). Assessment and treatment of stuttering in bilingual speakers In E. Conture, & R. Curlee (Eds.), *Stuttering and Related Disorders of Fluency* (3rd. ed., pp. 183–210). New York: Thieme.

Roessler, R., & Bolton, B. (1978). *Psychosocial adjustment to disability.* Baltimore: University Park Press.

Rogers, C. R. (1957). The necessary and sufficient conditions of therapeutic personality change. *Journal of Consulting Psychology, 21,* 95–103.

Rogers, C. R. (1961). *On becoming a person: A therapist's view of psychotherapy.* Boston: Houghton Mifflin.

Rommel, D., Hage, P., Kalehne, P., & Johannsen, H. (2000). Development, maintenance, and recovery of childhood stuttering: Prospective longitudinal data 3 years after first contact. In K. Baker, L., L. Rustin, & F. Cook (Eds.), *Proceedings of the Fifth Oxford Disfluency Conference* (pp. 168–182). Berkshire, U.K.: Kevin L. Baker.

Rosenbek, J. C. (1984). Stuttering secondary to nervous system damage. In R. F. Curlee, & W. H. Perkins (Eds.), *Nature and Treatment of Stuttering: New Directions* (pp. 31–48). San Diego, CA: College-Hill Press.

Rosenberger, P. B. (1980). Dopaminergic systems and speech fluency. *Journal of Fluency Disorders, 5*(3), 255–267.

Rosenfield, D., and Goodglass, H. (1980). Dichotic testing of cerebral dominance in stutterers. *Brain and Language,* 11:170–180.

Roth, C., Aronson, A., & Davis, L. (1989). Clinical studies in psychogenic stuttering of adult onset. *Journal of Speech and Hearing Disorders, 54,* 634–646.

Roth, C., Manning, K., & Duffy, J. (2011). *Acquired stuttering in post-deployed.* Paper presented at the Annual Meeting of the American Speech-Language-Hearing Convention, San Diego, CA.

Roy, N. & Bless, D. M. (2000a). Personality traits and psychological factors in voice pathology: A foundation for future research. *Journal of Speech, Language, and Hearing Research, 43,* 737-748.

Roy, N. & Bless, D. M. (2000b). Toward a theory of the dispositional bases of functional dysphonia and vocal nodules exploring the role of personality and emotional adjustment. In R. D. Kent and M. J. Ball (Eds.) *Voice Quality Measurment*. San Diego: Singular Publishing Group, 461-480.

Rousseau, I., Packman, A., Onslow, M., Harrison, E., & Jones, M. (2007). Language, phonology and treatment time in the Lidcombe Programme: A prospective study in a Phase II trial. *Journal of Communication Disorders, 40*, 382–397.

Rubow, R. T., Rosenbek, J., & Schumaker, J. G. (1986). Stress management in the treatment of neurogenic stuttering. *Biofeedback and Self Regulation, 11*, 77–78.

Rustin, L. (1991). *Parents, families and the stuttering child*. London: Whurr.

Ryan, B. P. (1992). Articulation, language, rate, and fluency characteristics of stuttering and nonstuttering preschool children. *Journal of Speech and Hearing Research, 35*, 333–342.

Sackett, D., Straus, S., Richardson, W., Rosenberg, W., & Haynes, R. (2000). *Evidence-based medicine: How to practice and teach EBM*. New York: Churchill Livingstone.

Salmelin, R., Schnitzler, A., Schmitz, F., and Freund, H.-J. (2000). Single word reading in developmental stutterers and fluent speakers. *Brain,* 123:1184–1202.

Salmelin, R., Schnitzler, A., Schmitz, F., Jancke, L., Witte, O.W., and Freund, H.-J. (1998). Functional organization of the auditory cortex is different in stutterers and fluent speakers. *NeuroReport,* 9:2225–2229.

Schiavetti, N., & Metz, D. E. (1997). Stuttering and the measurement of speech naturalness. In R. F. Curlee, & G. M. Siegel (Eds.), *Nature and treatment of stuttering: New directions* (2nd ed., pp. 398–412). Boston: Allyn & Bacon.

Schmahmann, J. D., & Caplan, D. (2006). Cognition, emotion and the cerebellum. *Brain, 129*(Pt. 2), 290–292.

Schwartz, M. F. (1974). The core of the stuttering block. *Journal of Speech and Hearing Disorders, 39*, 169–177.

Scott, L. A., & Guitar, C. (2004). *Stuttering: For kids, by kids [DVD]*. Memphis, TN: Stuttering Foundation of America.

Sedaris, D. (2000). *Me talk pretty one day*. Boston: Little, Brown.

Seeman, M. (1937). The significance of twin pathology for the investigation of speech disorders. *Archive Gesamte Phonetik 1,* Part II, 88–92.

Segalowitz, S. J., & Brown, D. (1991). Mild head injury as a source of developmental disabilities. *Journal of Learning Disabilities, 24*(9), 551–559.

Seider, R. A., Gladstien, K. L., & Kidd, K. K. (1982). Language-onset and concomitant speech and language problems in subgroups of stutterers and their siblings. *Journal of Speech and Hearing Research, 25*, 482–486.

Semel, E., Wiig, E., & Secord, W. A. (1996). *Clinical evaluation of language fundamentals—3*. San Antonio, TX: Psychological Corporation.

Semel, E., Wiig, E., & Secord, W. A. (2004). *Clinical Evaluation of Language Fundamentals-4—Screening Test (CELF-4)*. San Antonio, TX: Pearson.

Sequin, E. (1999). *Communication competence: "Normal" vs. stuttering children in grades 1–5*. Senior Honors Thesis, University of VT, Burlington, VT.

Shapely, K., & Guyette, T. (2010). Review of "TOCS: Test of childhood stuttering". *Mental Measurements Yearbook, 18*, 138.

Shapiro, A. I. (1980). An electromyographic analysis of the fluent and dysfluent utterances of several types of stutterers. *Journal of Fluency Disorders, 5*, 203–231.

Shapiro, A. I., & DeCicco, B. A. (1982). The relationship between normal dysfluency and stuttering: An old question revisited. *Journal of Fluency Disorders, 7*, 109–121.

Shapiro, D. A. (1999). *Stuttering intervention: A collaborative journey to fluency freedom*. Austin, TX: Pro-Ed.

Shaywitz, B., Shaywitz, S., Pugh, K., Constable, R. T., Skudlarski, P., Fulbright, R. K., et al. (1995). Sex differences in the functional organization of the brain for language. *Nature, 373*, 607–609.

Sheehan, J. G. (1970). *Stuttering: Research and therapy*. New York: Harper & Row.

Sheehan, J. G. (1974). Stuttering behavior: A phonetic analysis. *Journal of Communication Disorders, 7*, 193–212.

Sheehan, J. G. (1975). Conflict theory and avoidance-reduction therapy. In J. Eisenson (Ed.), *Stuttering: A Second Symposium*. New York: Harper & Row.

Sherman, D. (1952). Clinical and experimental use of the Iowa Scale of Severity of Stuttering. *Journal of Speech and Hearing Disorders, 17*, 316–320.

Shields, D. (1989). *Dead languages*. New York: Knopf.

Shors, T. J., Weiss, C., & Thompson, R. F. (1992). Stress-induced facilitation of classical conditioning. *Science 257*(5069), 537–539.

Shugart, Y. Y., Mundorff, J., Kilshaw, J., Doheny, K., Doan, B., Waynee, J. (2004). Results of a genome-wide linkage scan for stuttering. *American Journal of Human Genetics, 124A*, 133–135.

Siegel, G. M. (2007, December). Random observations. *ASHA Leader*.

Silverman, E.-M. (1974). Word position and grammatical function in relation to preschoolers' speech disfluency. *Perceptual and Motor Skills, 39*:267–272.

Silverman, F. H. (1988). The "monster" study. *Journal of Fluency Disorders, 13*, 225–231.

Skinner, E., & McKeehan, A. (1996). Preventing stuttering in the preschool child: A video program for parents. *Videotape*. San Antonio, TX: Communication Skill Builders.

Slorach, N., and Noer, B. (1973). Dichotic listening in stuttering and dyslexic children. *Cortex, 9*:295–300.

Smith, A. (1989). Neural drive to muscles in stuttering. *Journal of Speech and Hearing Research, 32*:252–264.

Smith, A., & Goffman, L. (2004). Interaction of motor and language factors in the development of speech production. In B. Maasen, R. D. Kent, H. F. M. Peters, P. H. H. M. van Lieshout, & W. Hulstijn (Eds.), *Speech Motor Control in Normal and Disordered Speech* (pp. 227–252). Oxford, UK: Oxford University Press.

Smith, A., & Kelly, E. (1997). Stuttering: A dynamic, multifactorial model. In R. F. Curlee, & G. M. Siegel (Eds.), *Nature and Treatment of Stuttering: New Directions* (2nd ed., pp. 204–217). Boston: Allyn & Bacon.

Smith, A., & Zelaznik, H. N. (2004). Development of functional synergies for speech motor coordination in childhood and adolescence. *Developmental Psychobiology, 45*(1), 22–33.

Smith, A., Denny, M., Shaffer, L. A., Kelly, E. M., & Hirano, M. (1996). Activity of intrinsic laryngeal muscles in fluent and disfluent speech. *Journal of Speech and Hearing Research, 39*(2), 329–348.

Smith, A., McCauley, R. J., & Guitar, B. (2000). Development of the Teacher Assessment of Student Communicative Competence (TASCC) in grades 1 through 5. *Communication Disorders Quarterly, 22*, 3–11.

Smith, A., Sadagopan, N., Walsh, B., & Weber-Fox, C. (2010). Increasing phonological complexity reveals heightened instability in inter-articulatory coordination in adults who stutter. *Journal of Fluency Disorders, 35*(1), 1–18.

Snidman, N., & Kagan, J. (1994). The contribution of infant temperamental differences to the acoustic startle response [Abstract]. *Psychophysiology, 31(Supplement 1)*, S92.

Sommer, M., Koch, M.A., Paulus, W., Weiller, C., and Buchel, C. (2002). Disconnection of speech-relevant brain areas in persistent developmental stuttering. *Lancet, 360*:380–383.

Sommers, R., Brady, W.A., and Moore, W.H., Jr. (1975). Dichotic ear preferences of stuttering children and adults. *Perceptual and Motor Skills,* 41:931–938.

St. Louis, K. (1991). The stuttering/articulation disorders connection. In H. F. M. Peters, W. Hulstijn, & C. W. Starkweather (Eds.), *Speech motor control and stuttering.* Amsterdam: Excerpta Medica.

St. Louis, K. (1996). Research and opinion on cluttering. *Journal of Fluency Disorders* (Special issue), *21.*

St. Louis, K. (2001). *Living with stuttering: Stories, basics, resources, and hope.* Morgantown, WV: Populore Publishing Company.

St. Louis, K., Myers, F., Bakker, K., & Raphael, L. J. (2007). Understanding and treating cluttering. In E. Conture, & R. Curlee (Eds.), *Stuttering and related disorders of fluency* (3rd ed., pp. 297–322). New York: Thieme.

St. Louis, K., Raphael, L. J., Myers, F. L., & Bakker, K. (2003). Cluttering updated. *ASHA Leader, 4-5,* 20–22.

St. Onge, K. (1963). The stuttering syndrome. *Journal of Speech and Hearing Research, 6,* 195–197.

Stager, S. V., Jeffries, K. L., & Braun, A. R. (2003). Common features of fluency-evoking conditions studied in stuttering subjects and controls: An H(2)150 PET study. *Journal of Fluency Disorders, 28,* 319–335.

Starkweather, C. W. (1980). A multiprocess behavioral approach to stuttering therapy. *Seminars in Speech, Language and Hearing, 1,* 327–337.

Starkweather, C. W. (1981). Speech fluency and its development in normal children. In N. Lass (Ed.), *Speech and Language: Advances in Basic Research and Practice* (Vol. 4). New York: Academic Press.

Starkweather, C. W. (1985). The development of fluency in normal children. In *Stuttering Therapy: Prevention and Intervention with Children.* Memphis, TN: Speech Foundation of America.

Starkweather, C. W. (1987). *Fluency and stuttering.* Englewood Cliffs, NJ: Prentice-Hall.

Starkweather, C. W. (1991). Stuttering: The motor-language interface. In H. F. M. Peters, W. Hulstijn, & C. W. Starkweather (Eds.), *Speech Motor Control and Fluency.* Amsterdam: Excerpta Medica.

Starkweather, C. W., & Myers, M. (1979). Duration of subsegments within the intervocalic interval in stutterers and nonstutterers. *Journal of Fluency Disorders, 4,* 205–214.

Starkweather, C. W., Gottwald, S., & Halfond, M. H. (1990). *Stuttering prevention: A clinical method.* Englewood Cliffs, NJ: Prentice-Hall.

Starkweather, C. W., Hirschman, P., & Tannenbaum, R. S. (1976). Latency of vocalization onset: Stutterers versus nonstutterers. *Journal of Speech and Hearing Research, 19,* 481–492.

Stephenson-Opsal, D., & Bernstein Ratner, N. (1988). Maternal speech rate modification and childhood stuttering. *Journal of Fluency Disorders, 13,* 49–56.

Sternberger, J. P. (1982). The nature of segments in the lexicon: Evidence from speech errors. *Lingua, 56,* 235–259.

Stewart, S. W. (2012). *The greatest moment of my life: One man's story of beating stuttering and becoming a public speaker:* Self-published. Available for about $25 from stephenstewart497@gmail. com.

Stocker, B., & Usprich, C. (1976). Stuttering in young children and level of demand. *Journal of Childhood Communication Disorders, 1,* 116–131.

Stromsta, C. (1957). A methodology related to the determination of the phase angle of bone-conducted speech sound energy in stutterers and nonstutterers. (Abstract). *Speech Monographs* 24:147–148.

Stromsta, C. (1972). Interaural phase disparity of stutterers and nonstutterers. *Journal of Speech and Hearing Research,* 15:771–780.

Stromsta, C. (1986). *Elements of Stuttering.* Oshtemo, MI: Atsmorts Publishing.

Studdert-Kennedy, M. (1987). The phoneme as a perceptuomotor structure. In A. Allport, D. McKay, D. Prinz, & E. Scheerer (Eds.), *Language perception and production.* London: Academic Press.

Subramanian, A., & Yairi, E. (2006). Identification of traits associated with stuttering. *Journal of Communication Disorders, 39*(3), 200–216.

Suresh, R., Ambrose, N. G., Roe, C., Pluzhnikov, A., Wittke-Thompson, J. K., & Ng, M. C. Y. (2006). New complexities in the genetics of stuttering: Significant sex-specific linkage signals. *American Journal of Human Genetics, 78,* 554–563.

Sussman, H., and MacNeilage, P. (1975). Hemispheric specialization for speech production and perception in stutterers. *Neuropsychologia,* 13:19–26.

Swift, W. J., Swift, E. W., & Arellano, M. (1975). Haloperidol as a treatment for adult stuttering. *Comprehensive Psychiatry, 16,* 61–67.

Taylor, G. (1937). *An observational study of the nature of stuttering at onset.* Iowa City, IA: Master's, State University of Iowa.

Taylor, O. (1986). *Treatment of communication disorders in culturally and linguistically diverse populations.* San Diego, CA: College-Hill Press.

Taylor, O. (1994). *Communication and communication disorders in a multicultural society.* San Diego, CA: Singular Publishing Group.

Taylor, R. M., & Morrison, L. P. (1996). *Taylor-Johnson Temperament Analysis Manual.* Thousand Oaks, CA: Psychological Publications, Inc.

Tellis, G., & Tellis, C. (2003). Multicultural issues in school settings. *Seminars in Speech and Language, 24*(1), 21–26.

Theys, C., van Wieringen, A., & De Nil, L. F. (2008). A clinician survey of speech and non-speech characteristics of neurogenic stuttering. *Journal of Fluency Disorders, 33*(1), 1–23.

Thomson, K. S. (2009). *Young Charles Darwin.* New Haven, CT: Yale University Press.

Throneburg, R., & Yairi, E. (1994). Temporal dynamics of repetitions during the early stage of childhood stuttering: An acoustic study. *Journal of Speech and Hearing Research, 37,* 1067–1075.

Till, J. A., Reich, A., Dickey, S., & Sieber, J. (1983). Phonatory and manual reaction times of stuttering and nonstuttering children. *Journal of Speech and Hearing Research, 26,* 171–180.

Toscher, M. M., & Rupp, R. R. (1978). A study of the central auditory processes in stutterers using the Synthetic Sentence Identification (SSI) test battery. *Journal of Speech and Hearing Research, 21,* 779–792.

Trautman, L. S. (2003). SFA conducts survey on satisfaction with electronic devices. *Stuttering Foundation Newsletter, 2*(Fall), 6.

Trautman, L. S., & Guitar, C. (2005). *Stuttering: Straight talk for teachers [DVD].* Memphis, TN: Stuttering Foundation of America.

Travis, L. (1931). *Speech pathology.* New York: Appleton-Century.

Travis, L. E., & Knott, J. R. (1937). Bilaterally recorded brain potentials from normal speakers and stutterers. *Journal of Psychology, 2,* 137–150.

Tudor, M. (1939). *An experimental study of the effect of evaluative labeling on speech fluency.* Unpublished master's thesis, University of Iowa, Iowa City, IA.

Turgut, N., Utku, U., & Balci, K. (2002). A case of acquired stuttering resulting from left parietal infarction. *Acta Neurologica Scandinavica, 105,* 408–410.

Turnbaugh, K. R., Guitar, B. E., & Hoffman, P. R. (1979). Speech clinicians' attribution of personality traits as a function of stuttering severity. *Journal of Speech and Hearing Research, 22,* 37–45.

van Beijsterveldt, C. E., Felsenfeld, S., & Boomsma, D. I. (2010). Bivariate genetic analyses of stuttering and nonfluency in a large sample of 5-year-old twins. *Journal of Speech, Language and Hearing Research, 53*(3), 609–619.

Van Borsel, J., Maes, E., & Foulon, S. (2001). Stuttering and bilingualism: A review. *Journal of Fluency Disorders, 26,* 179–205.

van Lieshout, P., Hulstijn, W., & Peters, H. F. M. (2004). Searching for the weak link in the speech production chain of people who stutter. In B. Maasen, R. D. Kent, H. F. M. Peters, P. van Lieshout, & W. Hulstijn (Eds.), *Speech Motor Control in Normal and Disordered Speech* (pp. 313–356). Oxford, UK: Oxford University Press.

Van Riper, C. (1936). Study of the thoracic breathing of stutterers during expectancy and occurrence of stuttering spasm. *Journal of Speech Disorders, 1,* 61–72.

Van Riper, C. (1954). *Speech correction: Principles and methods* (3rd ed.). Englewood Cliffs, NJ: Prentice-Hall.

Van Riper, C. (1958). Experiments in stuttering therapy. In J. Eisenson (Ed.), *Stuttering: A Symposium* (pp. 273–290). New York: Harper & Row.

Van Riper, C. (1971). *The nature of stuttering.* Englewood Cliffs, NJ: Prentice-Hall.

Van Riper, C. (1973). *The treatment of stuttering.* Englewood Cliffs, NJ: Prentice-Hall.

Van Riper, C. (1975a). The stutterer's clinician. In J. Eisenson (Ed.), *Stuttering: A second symposium.* New York: Harper & Row.

Van Riper, C. (1975b). *Therapy in action. [3 videotapes].* Memphis, TN: Stuttering Foundation of America.

Van Riper, C. (1982). *The Nature of Stuttering* (ed 2). Englewood Cliffs, NJ: Prentice Hall.

Van Riper, C. (1990). Final thoughts about stuttering. *Journal of Fluency Disorders,* 15:317–318.

Van Riper, C., and Hull, C.J. (1955). The quantative measurement of the effect of certain situations on stuttering. In W. Johnson, and R.R. Leutenegger (Eds), *Stuttering in Children and Adults.* Minneapolis: University of Minnesota Press.

van Zaalen, Y., Wijnen, F., & Dejonckere, P. (2011). The assessment of cluttering: Rationale, tasks, and interpretation. In D. Ward, & K. S. Scott (Eds.), *Cluttering: A Handbook of Research, Intervention and Education* (pp. 137–151). Hove, UK: Psychology Press.

Vanryckeghem, M., & Brutten, G. (1993). The Communication Attitude Test: A test-retest reliability investigation. *Journal of Fluency Disorders, 17,* 177–190.

Vanryckeghem, M., & Brutten, G. (1997). The speech-associated attitude of children who do and do not stutter and the differential effect of age. *American Journal of Speech-Language Pathology, 6,* 67–73.

Vanryckeghem, M., Brutten, G., & Hernandez, L. M. (2005). A comparative investigation of the speech-associated attitude of preschool and kindergarten children who do and do not stutter. *Journal of Fluency Disorders, 30,* 307–318.

Vanryckeghem, M., Hernandez, L. M., & Brutten, G. (2001). *The KiddyCAT: A measure of speech-associated attitude of preschoolers.* Paper presented at the Annual Meeting of the American Speech-Language and Hearing Association, New Orleans.

Vanryckeghem, M., Hylebos, C., Brutten, G., & Peleman, M. (2001). The relationship between communication attitude and emotion of children who stutter. *Journal of Fluency Disorders, 26*(1), 1.

Verdolini, K., & Lee, T. D. (2004). Optimizing motor learning in speech interventions: Theory and practice. In C. Sapienza, & J. Casper (Eds.), *Voice Rehabilitation in Medical Speech-Language Pathology: For Clinicians, by Clinicians.* Austin, TX: Pro-Ed.

Viswanath, N. S., Lee, H. S., & Chakraborty, R. (2004). Evidence for a minor gene influence on persistent developmental stuttering. *Human Biology, 76,* 401–412.

Vrana, S. R., Spence, E. L., & Lang, P. J. (1988). The startle probe: A new measure of emotion? *Journal of Abnormal Psychology, 97,* 487–491.

Wakaba, Y. (1998). *Research on temperament of stuttering children with early onset.* Paper presented at the 2nd World Conference on Fluency Disorders, San Francisco.

Walden, T. A., Frankel, C. B., Buhr, A. P., Johnson, K. N., Conture, E. G., & Karrass JM. (2012). Dual diathesis-stressor model of emotional and linguistic contributions to developmental stuttering. *Journal of Abnormal Child Psychology, 40*(4), 633–644.

Wall, M. J. (1980). A comparison of syntax in young stutterers and nonstutterers. *Journal of Fluency Disorders, 5,* 345–352.

Wall, M. J., & Myers, F. L. (1995). *Clinical management of childhood stuttering* (2nd ed.). Austin, TX: Pro-Ed.

Wallen, V. (1960). A Q-technique study of the self-concepts of adolescent stutterers and nonstutterers. (Abstract). *Speech Monographs* 27:257–258.

Walton, P. (2012). *Fun with fluency for the school-age child.* Austin, TX: Pro-Ed.

Ward, D., & Scott, K. S. (2011). *Cluttering: A handbook of research, intervention and education.* Hove, UK: Psychology Press.

Waters, E. (1995). Appendix A: The Attachment Q-Set (version 3.0). *Monographs of the Society for Research in Child Development, 60,* 234–246.

Watkins, K. E., Smith, S. M., Davis, S., & Howell, P. (2008). Structural and functional abnormalities of the motor system in developmental stuttering. *Brain, 131*(Pt. 1), 50–59.

Watkins, R. V. (2005). Language abilities of young children who stutter. In E. Yairi, & N. G. Ambrose (Eds.), *Early childhood stuttering: For clinicians, by clinicians* (pp. 235–251). Austin, TX: Pro-Ed.

Watkins, R. V., Yairi, E., & Ambrose, N., G. (1999). Early childhood stuttering III: Initial status of expressive language abilities. *Journal of Speech, Language and Hearing Research, 42*(5), 1125–1135.

Watson, B. C., & Alfonso, P. J. (1987). Physiological bases of acoustic LRT in nonstutterers, mild stutterers, and severe stutterers. *Journal of Speech and Hearing Research, 30*, 434–447.

Watson, J. B., & Kayser, H. (1994). Assessment of bilingual/bicultural children and adults who stutter. *Seminars in Speech, Language and Hearing, 15*, 149–163.

Weber, C. M., & Smith, A. (1990). Autonomic correlates of stuttering and speech assessed in a range of experimental tasks. *Journal of Speech and Hearing Research, 33*, 690–706.

Webster, R. L. (1974). A behavioral analysis of stuttering: Treatment and theory. In K. S. Calhoun, H. E. Adams, & K. M. Mitchell (Eds.), *Innovative Treatment Methods in Psychopathology*. New York: John Wiley & Sons.

Webster, W. G. (1993a). Evidence in bimanual finger tapping of an attentional component to stuttering. *Behavioural Brain Research, 37*, 93–100.

Webster, W. G. (1993b). Hurried hands and tangled tongues: Implications of current research for the management of stuttering. In E. Boberg (Ed), *Neuropsychology of Stuttering*. Edmonton, Alberta, Canada: University of Alberta Press, pp 73–111.

Webster, W. G. (1997). Principles of brain organization related to lateralization of language and speech motor functions in normal speakers and stutterers. In W. Hulstijn, H. F. M. Peters, & P. H. H. M. van Lieshout (Eds.), *Speech Production: Motor Control, Brain Research and Fluency Disorders*. Amsterdam: Elsevier.

Weiller, C., Isensee, C., Rijntes, M, Huber, W., Müller, S., Bier, D. et al. (1995). Recovery from Wernicke's aphasia: A positron emission tomographic study. *Annals of Neurology, 37*(6), 723–732.

Weiner, A. E. (1981). A case of adult onset of stuttering. *Journal of Fluency Disorders, 6*, 181–186.

Weiss, A. L., & Zebrowski, P. (1992). Disfluencies in the conversations of young children who stutter: Some answers about questions. *Journal of Speech and Hearing Research, 35*, 1230–1238.

Weiss, D. A. (1964). *Cluttering*. Englewood Cliffs, NJ: Prentice-Hall.

Welch, J., & Byrne, J. A. (2001). *Jack: Straight from the gut*. New York: Warner Books.

West, R. (1931). The phenomenology of stuttering. In R. West (Ed), *A Symposium on Stuttering*. Madison, WI: College Typing Company.

West, R., Nelson, S., & Berry, M. (1939). The heredity of stuttering. *Quarterly Journal of Speech, 25*, 23–30.

Westby, C. E. (1979). Language performance of stuttering and nonstuttering children. *Journal of Communication Disorders, 12*, 133–145.

Wexler, K. B., & Mysack, E. D. (1982). Disfluency characteristics of 2-, 4- and 6-year old males. *Journal of Fluency Disorders, 7*, 37–46.

Wiig, E. (2002). *Putting cluttering on the map: Looking back/looking ahead*. Paper presented at the Annual Meeting of the American Speech-Language-Hearing Association, Atlanta, GA.

Wijnen, F. (1990). The development of sentence planning. *Journal of Child Language, 17*(3), 651–675.

Wilkenfeld, J., & Curlee, R. (1997). The relative effects of questions and comments on children's stuttering. *American Journal of Speech-Language Pathology, 6*, 79–89.

Williams, D. E. (1978). The problem of stuttering. In F. Darley, & D. Spriestersbach (Eds.), *Diagnostic Methods in Speech Pathology* (pp. 284–321). New York: Harper & Row.

Williams, D.E. (2004). *The genius of Dean Williams*. Memphis, TN: Stuttering Foundation of America.

Williams, D. E., Darley, F., and Spriestersbach, D. (1978). Appraisal of rate and fluency. In F. Darley, and D. Spriestersbach (Eds), *Diagnostic Methods in Speech Pathology* (ed 2). New York: Harper & Row, pp 256–283.

Williams, D. E., Melrose, B. M., & Woods, C. L. (1969). The relationship between stuttering and academic achievement in children. *Journal of Communication Disorders, 2*, 87–98.

Williams, D. E., Silverman, F. H., & Kools, J. A. (1968). Disfluency behavior of elementary-school stutterers and nonstutterers: The adaptation effect. *Journal of Speech and Hearing Research, 11*, 622–630.

Williams, D. F. (2006). *Stuttering recovery: Personal and empirical perspectives*. Mahwah, NJ: Lawrence Erlbaum.

Williams, K. T. (2007). *Expressive Vocabulary Test - 2nd edition (EVT-2)*. San Antonio, TX: Pearson.

Wingate, M. E. (1964). Recovery from stuttering. *Journal of Speech and Hearing Disorders, 29*, 312–321.

Wingate, M. E. (1983). Speaking unassisted: Comments on a paper by Andrews et al. *Journal of Speech and Hearing Disorders, 48*, 255–263.

Wingate, M. E. (1988). *The structure of stuttering: A psycholinguistic approach*. New York: Springer-Verlag.

Winnicott, D. W. (1971). *Playing and reality*. New York: Routledge.

Wood, F., Stump, D., McKeehan, A., Sheldon, S., & Proctor, J. (1980). Patterns of regional cerebral blood flow during attempted reading aloud by stutterers both on and off haloperidol medication: Evidence for inadequate left frontal activation during stuttering. *Brain and Language, 9*, 141–144.

Woods, C. L., & Williams, D. E. (1976). Traits attributed to stuttering and normally fluent males. *Journal of Speech and Hearing Research, 19*, 267–278.

Woods, S., Shearsby, J., Onslow, M., & Burnham, D. (2002). Psychological impact of the Lidcombe Programme in early stuttering intervention. *International Journal of Language and Communication Disorders, 37*, 31–40.

Woolf, G. (1967). The assessment of stuttering as struggle, avoidance, and expectancy. *British Journal of Disorders of Communication Disorders, 2*, 158–171.

World Health Organization (1980).*International classification of impairments, disabilities, and handicaps: A manual of classification relating to the consequences of disease*. Geneva: World Health Organization.

Wu, J., Maguire, G., Riley, G., Fallon, J., LaCasse, L., Chin, S., et al. (1995). A positron emission tomography [18F]deoxyglucose study of developmental stuttering. *NeuroReport, 6*:501–505.

Wynne, M. K., & Boehmler, R. M. (1982). Central auditory function in fluent and disfluent normal speakers. *Journal of Speech and Hearing Research, 25*, 54–57.

Yairi, E. (1981). Disfluencies of normally speaking two-year old children. *Journal of Speech and Hearing Research, 24*(490–495).

Yairi, E. (1982). Longitudinal studies of disfluencies in two-year old children. *Journal of Speech and Hearing Research, 25,* 155–160.

Yairi, E. (1983). The onset of stuttering in two- and three-year old children: A preliminary report. *Journal of Speech and Hearing Disorders, 48,* 171–178.

Yairi, E. (1997a). Early stuttering. In R. F. Curlee, & G. M. Siegel (Eds.), *Nature and Treatment of Stuttering: New Directions* (2nd ed.). Boston: Allyn & Bacon.

Yairi, E. (1997b). Home environment and parent-child interaction in childhood stuttering. In R. F. Curlee, & G. M. Siegel (Eds.), *Nature and treatment of stuttering: New directions* (2nd ed., pp. 24–48). Boston: Allyn & Bacon.

Yairi, E., & Ambrose, N. G. (1992a). A longitudinal study of stuttering in children: A preliminary report. *Journal of Speech and Hearing Research, 35,* 755–760.

Yairi, E., and Ambrose, N.G. (1992b). Onset of stuttering in preschool children: Selected factors. *Journal of Speech and Hearing Research, 35*:782–788.

Yairi, E., & Ambrose, N. G. (1996). *Disfluent speech in early childhood stuttering.* Unpublished manuscript. Stuttering Research Project. University of Illinois, IL.

Yairi, E., & Ambrose, N. G. (1999). Early childhood stuttering I: Persistency and recovery rates. *Journal of Speech Language and Hearing Research, 42*(5), 1097–1112.

Yairi, E., & Ambrose, N. G. (2005). *Early childhood stuttering: For clinicians by clinicians.* Austin, TX: Pro-Ed.

Yairi, E., & Lewis, B. (1984). Disfluencies at the onset of stuttering. *Journal of Speech and Hearing Research, 27,* 154–159.

Yairi, E., Ambrose, N. G., & Cox, N. (1996). Genetics of stuttering: A critical review. *Journal of Speech and Hearing Research, 39,* 771–784.

Yairi, E., Ambrose, N. G., Paden, E., & Throneburg, R. (1996). Predictive factors of persistence and recovery: Pathways of childhood stuttering. *Journal of Communication Disorders, 29,* 51–77.

Yaruss, J. S. (1998). Describing the consequences of disorders: Stuttering and the International Classification of Impairments, Disabilities, and Handicaps. *Journal of Speech, Language, and Hearing Research, 41,* 249–257.

Yaruss, J.S. (1999). Utterance length, syntactic complexity, and childhood stuttering. *Journal of Speech, Language and Hearing Research, 42*:329–344.

Yaruss, J. S., & Conture, E. G. (1995). Mother and child speaking rates and utterance lengths in adjacent fluent utterances: Preliminary observations. *Journal of Fluency Disorders, 20*(3), 257–278.

Yaruss, J. S., & Quesal, R. W. (2006). Overall Assessment of the Speaker's Experience of Stuttering (OASES): Documenting multiple outcomes in stuttering treatment. *Journal of Fluency Disorders, 31,* 90–115.

Yaruss, J. S., Coleman, C. E., & Quesal, R. W. (2007a). *Overall Assessment of the Speaker's Experience of Stuttering—School age.* Unpublished assessment instrument.

Yaruss, J. S., Coleman, C. E., & Quesal, R. W. (2007b). *Overall Assessment of the Speaker's Experience of Stuttering—Teenager.* Unpublished assessment instrument.

Yaruss, J. S., Murphy, B., Quesal, R. W., Reardon-Reeves, N., & Flores, T. (2004). *Bullying and teasing: Helping children who stutter.* Pittsburgh: Stuttering Therapy Resources.

Yaruss, J.S., Newman, R.M., and Flora, T. (1999). Language and disfluency in nonstuttering children's conversational speech. *Journal of Fluency Disorders, 24*:185–207.

Yaruss, J. S., Pelczarski, K., & Quesal, R. W. (2010). Comprehensive treatment for school-age children who stutter: Treating the entire disorder. In B. Guitar, & R. J. McCauley (Eds.), *Treatment of Stuttering: Established and Emerging Interventions* (pp. 215–244). Baltimore: Lippincott Williams & Wilkins.

Yaruss, J. S., Quesal, R. W., & Reeves, L. (2007). Self-help and mutual aid groups as an adjunct to stuttering therapy. In E. Conture, & R. Curlee (Eds.), *Stuttering and Related Disorders of Fluency* (3rd ed., pp. 256–276). New York: Thieme.

Young, M. A. (1961). Predicting ratings of severity of stuttering. *Journal of Speech and Hearing Disorders, Monograph Supplement, 7,* 31–54.

Young, M. A. (1981). A reanalysis of "Stuttering therapy: The relation between attitude change and long-term outcome". *Journal of Speech and Hearing Disorders, 46,* 221–222.

Young, M. A. (1984). Identification of stuttering and stutterers. In R. F. Curlee, & W. H. Perkins (Eds.), *The Nature and Treatment of Stuttering: New Directions* (pp. 13–30). San Diego, CA: College-Hill.

Zebrowski, P. (1991). Duration of the speech disfluencies of beginning stutterers. *Journal of Speech and Hearing Research, 34*(3), 483–491.

Zebrowski, P. (1995). Temporal aspects of the conversations between children who stutter and their parents. *Topics in Language Disorders, 15*(3), 1–17.

Zebrowski, P. (2007). Treatment factors that influence therapy outcomes of children who stutter. In E. Conture, & R. Curlee (Eds.), *Stuttering and Related Disorders of Fluency.* New York: Thieme.

Zebrowski, P. M., & Kelly, E. (2002). *Manual of stuttering intervention.* Clifton Park, N.Y.: Singular.

Zebrowski, P. M., Weiss, A. L., Savelkoul, E. M., & Hammer, C. S. (1996). The effect of maternal rate reduction on the stuttering speech rates and linguistic production of children who stutter: Evidence from individual dyads. *Clinical Linguistics and Phonetics, 10,* 189–206.

Zenner, A. A., Ritterman, S. I., Bowen, S. K., & Gronhovd, K. D. (1978). Measurement and comparison of anxiety levels of parents of stuttering, articulatory defective, and normal-speaking children. *Journal of Fluency Disorders, 3,* 273–283.

Zimmerman, I., Steiner, V., & Pond, R. (1979). *Preschool language scale.* San Antonio, TX: Psychological Corp.

Zimmermann, G. N. (1980). Articulatory dynamics of fluent utterances of stutterers and nonstutterers. *Journal of Speech and Hearing Research, 23,* 95–107.

Zimmermann, G. N., & Knott, J. R. (1974). Slow potentials of the brain related to speech processing in normal speakers and stutterers. *Electroencephalography and Clinical Neurophysiology, 37,* 599–607.

Zimmermann, G. N., Smith, A., & Hanley, J. M. (1981). Stuttering: In need of a unifying conceptual framework. *Journal of Speech and Hearing Research, 24,* 25–31.

AUTHOR INDEX

A

Abbs, J.H., 54, 55, 275, 276
Absher, R.G., 52
Achenbach, T.M., 259
Adams, M.R., 54, 55, 100, 190
Ahern, G.L., 38
Ainsworth, S., 248
Alfonso, P.J., 54, 55
Ali, Z., 314
Allen, G.D., 82
Allen, S., 124, 186
Allman, J.M., 38
Alm, P.A., 46, 51, 59, 327
Ambrose, N.G., 15–17, 23, 26, 29, 35, 43–45, 48, 65, 83, 84, 101, 103, 106, 116, 117, 120, 122, 134, 143, 194, 195, 217
Anderson, J., 59, 69, 104, 156, 192
Anderson, S.W., 85
Andre, S., 156
Andrews, C., 151, 196, 238
Andrews, G., 15–17, 19, 23, 42, 44, 47, 55, 62, 63, 78, 81, 83, 85, 91, 94, 96, 99, 116, 121, 124, 147, 151, 153, 158, 159, 164, 167, 196, 211, 213, 221, 235, 238, 273, 294, 295, 311, 312, 314, 315, 321, 326
Andy, O.J., 323
Annenberg, W., 11
Aram, D.M., 83
Arellano, M., 314
Arndt, J., 83
Aronson, A.E., 324, 332
Arthur, G., 84
Augustyn, M., 217
Ayres, J.J.B., 78, 105, 226
Azrin, N.H., 221

B

Bacon, F., 21, 78, 79, 174, 217, 225, 228
Baer, D., 222
Baker, D.J., 54
Bakker, K., 327, 328, 333
Bankson, N., 191
Barasch, C.T., 52, 53, 273
Baratz, R., 323
Barry, S.J., 53, 140
Basili, A., 124
Bass, C., 158, 295
Bates, D., 55
Baumgartner, J.M., 324–326, 332
Beal, D.S., 32, 48
Beck, J.S., 225
Beitchman, J., 15
Bemporad, E., 38, 104, 295, 297
Bennett Lanouette, E., 329
Berk, L.E., 65

Bernstein Ratner, N., 79, 81, 83, 118, 140, 143, 234, 245, 263
Bernthal, J.E., 81, 118, 191
Berry, M.F., 46, 83
Berry, R.C., 151
Berson, J., 53
Bhatnager, S.C., 323
Bidinger, D., 59
Biederman, J., 75
Bijleveld, H., 319
Bishry, Z., 83
Black, J.W., 32, 33
Bloch, E.L., 68
Block, S., 313
Blood, G.W., 10, 53
Blood, I.M., 10, 53
Bloodstein, O., 9, 14–19, 23, 33, 35–37, 45, 49, 55, 63, 65, 66, 68, 79, 83, 85, 94, 98, 101, 103, 106, 113, 115, 116, 118, 120, 123, 124, 134, 253, 261, 322
Bloom, L., 81
Bluemel, C.S., 15, 101, 110
Boberg, E., 49, 294, 311
Boehme, G., 46, 185
Boehmler, R.M., 52, 53, 269, 294, 300, 301
Boelens, H., 239
Boemio, A., 92
Bo-Lassen, P., 49, 294
Bollich, A.M., 32, 33, 47, 323
Bolton, B., 132
Bond, L., 104, 186, 226, 234, 248
Boomsma, D.I., 44
Boone, D.R., 192
Borden, G.J., 55
Boscolo, B., 83
Bosshardt, H.G., 58
Boswell, J., 225
Bothe, A., 220, 228
Botterill, W., 245
Bowen, S.K., 85
Boyce, W.T., 68
Brady, J.P., 53, 314
Brady, W.A., 53
Branigan, G., 82
Braun, A.R., 38, 50–52, 92, 276
Brayton, E.R., 52
Breitenfeldt, D., 313
Brewer, D.W., 9
Brosch, S., 17
Brown, D., 46
Brown, S.F., 18, 32, 51, 52, 56
Brown, W.S., 49
Bruce, M., 254, 285, 288
Brundage, S., 81
Brutten, G.J., 16, 37, 47, 56, 72, 85, 105, 110, 125, 154, 157, 172, 174, 194, 202, 245, 285

Note: Page numbers followed by f indicate figures; those followed by t indicate tables.